THE ILLUSTRATED GUIDE TO PROFESSIONAL

HAIRCARE &

T66999

HUGH BAIRD COLLEGE
BALLIOL ROAD
BOOTLE L20 7EW
TEL: 0151 353 4454

646.
74
POP

4 5

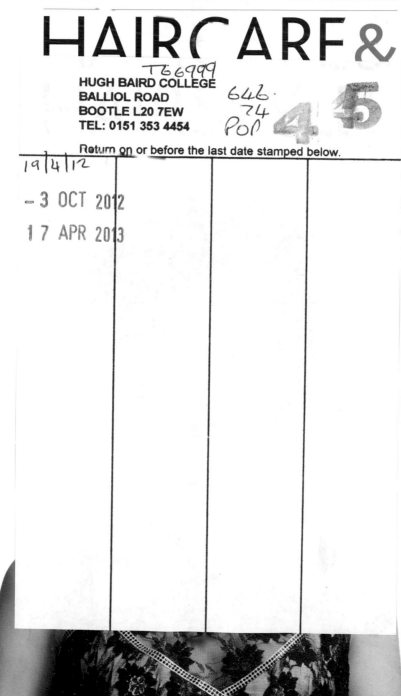

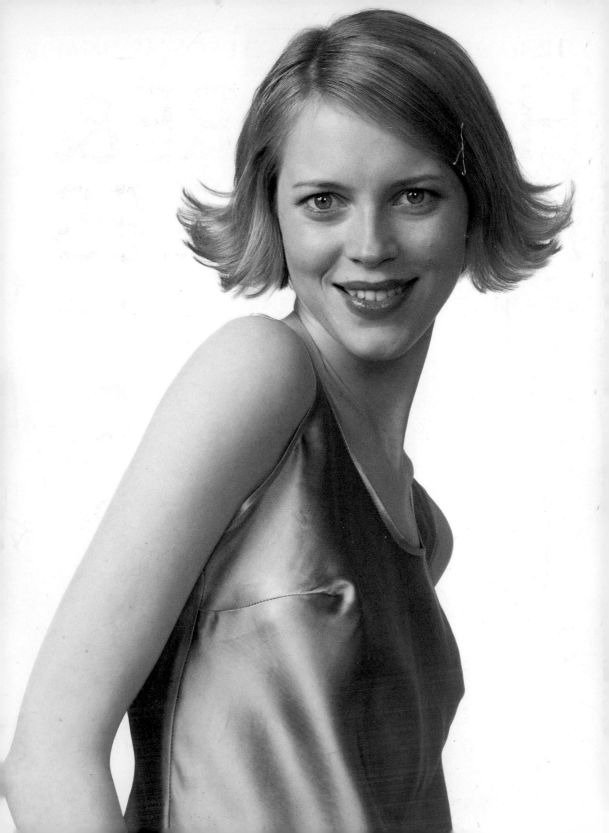

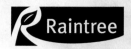

A RIVER JOURNEY

The Amazon

Simon Scoones

A RIVER JOURNEY

The Amazon	The Ganges
The Mississippi	The Nile
The Rhine	The Yangtze

A River Journey: *The Amazon*
Text copyright © 2004 Raintree
Series copyright © 2004 Raintree
Published by Raintree, a division of Reed Elsevier, Inc..

Book design: Jane Hawkins
Picture Research: Shelley Noronha, Glass Onion Pictures
Maps: Tony Fleetwood

The author would like to thank Alex Shankland and Jose Assuncão for their help.

Copyright Permissions
Raintree
100 N. Lasalle, Suite 1200
Chicago, IL 60602

Library of Congress Cataloging-in-Publication Data

Scoones, Simon.
  The Amazon / Simon Scoones.
    p. cm. -- (A river journey)
Includes bibliographical references and index.
  ISBN 0-7398-6069-0 (library binding hardcover)
  1. Amazon River Region--Description and travel--Juvenile literature.
I. Title. II. Series.
  F2546.S45 2003
  918.1'1--dc21

                    2002155377

Printed in Hong Kong.
1234567890
08 07 06 05 04

The maps in this book use a conical projection, and so the indictor for North on the main map is only approximate.

Picture Acknowledgments
Cover Dr Morley Read/Science Photo Library; title page Michel Roggo/Still Pictures; 2 Edward Parker/Still Pictures; 5 Jane Hawkins; 6 Simon Scoones; 7 Simon Scoones; 8 top Simon Scoones, below Panos/A. Bungeroth; 9 South American Pictures/Tony Morrison, inset Art Wolfe/Science Photo Library; 10 Simon Scoones, inset Richard Packwood/Oxford Scientific Films; 11 Tony Morrison/South American Pictures; 12 Tony Morrison/South American Pictures; 13 left Tony Morrison/South American Pictures, right South American Pictures; 14 Tony Morrison/South American Pictures, Simon Scoones; 15 Hart/Reflejo; 16 Dr Morley Read/Science Photo Library; 17 left Sinclair Stammers/Science Photo Library, right Partridge Films Ltd/Oxford Scientific Films; 18 Fred Hoogervorst/Panos; 19 Arabella Cecil/Panos; 20 Julia Waterlow/Eye Ubiquitous; 21 left Edward Parker/Still Pictures, right Sue Cunningham/SCP; 22 Simon Scoones; 23 top Edward Parker/Still Pictures, bottom Gregory Ochocki/Science Photo Library; 24 top Douglas Faulkner/Science Photo Library, bottom Kevin Schafer/Still Pictures; 25 Steve Bowles/ South American Pictures, bottom K. Gillham/Robert Harding; 26 Tony Morrison/South American Pictures; 27 top Edward Parker/Still Pictures, right Simon Scoones; 28 Robert Harding; 29 Mark Edwards/Still Pictures, inset Edward Parker/South American Pictures; 30 Ken Gillham/Robert Harding; 31 Jean Chrisstophe Vie/Still Pictures; 32 K. Gillham/Robert Harding, inset Simon Scoones; 33 Sue Cunningham/SCP, bottom Karen Ward/South American Pictures; 34 Ken Gillham/Robert Harding; 35 Tony Morrison/South American Pictures; 36 Jevan Berrange, inset Hellier Mason/Still Pictures; 38 Nigel Dickinson/Still Pictures; 39 top Geospace/Science Photo Library, inset Herbert Giradet/Still Pictures, bottom Topham Picture Point; 40 Martin Wendler/Still Pictures; 41 Sue Cunningham/ SCP; 42 left Jacques Jangoux/Science Photo Library, right Tony Allen/Oxford Scientific Films; 43 Tony Morrison/ South American Pictures; 44 Ken Gillham/Robert Harding; 45 left Mark Edwards/Still Pictures, right NASA/Still Pictures

Contents

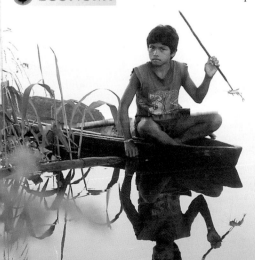

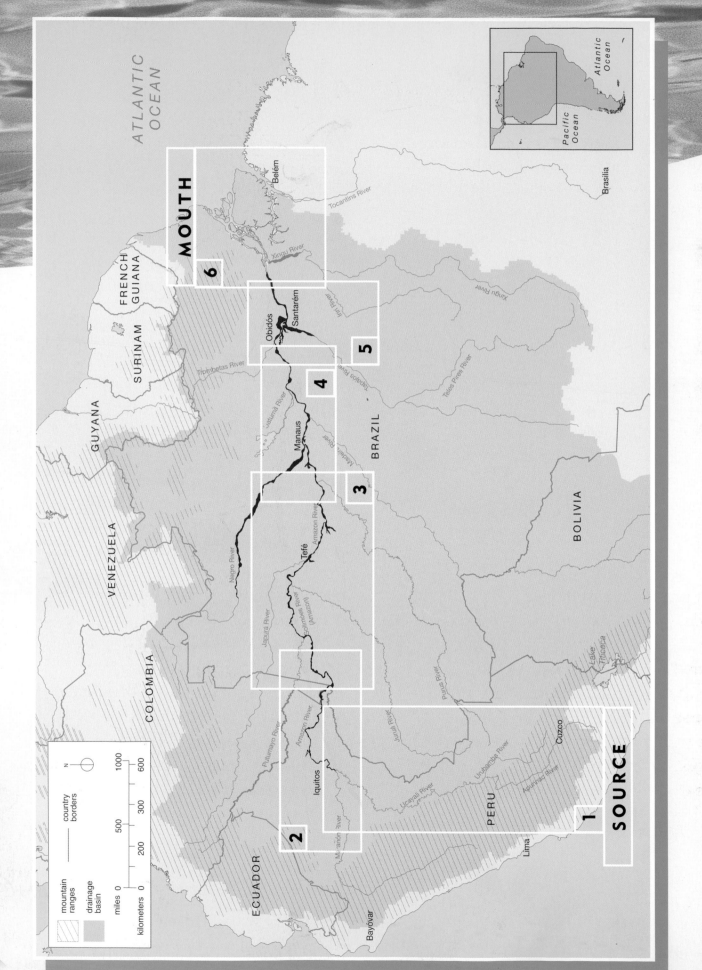

Your Guide to the River

USING THEMED TEXT As you make your journey down the Amazon, you will find topic headings about that area of the river. These symbols show what the text is about.

NATURE   Plants, wildlife, and the environment

HISTORY   Events and people in the past

PEOPLE   The lives and culture of local people

CHANGE   Things that have altered the area

$ ECONOMY   Jobs and industry in the area

USING MAP REFERENCES Each chapter has a map that shows the section of the river we are visiting. The numbered boxes show exactly where a place of interest is located.

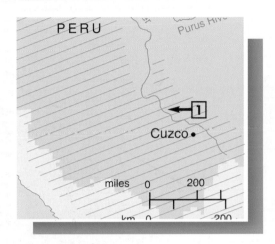

The Journey Ahead

Our journey begins in Peru, high up in the Andes Mountains. Here the Urubamba River, one of the Amazon's tributaries, is born. From here we head north, following the river as it gushes down the mountain slopes into a huge low-lying region. Then the river winds its way through the world's largest area of tropical rain forest. This is one of the few places left on Earth where plants and animals have yet to be discovered. Beyond the city of Iquitos, the Amazon River makes a sharp turn east, following the equator, and enters the country of Brazil. Finally we reach the Atlantic coast, nearly 1,864 miles (3,000 kilometers) away. Here, where the Amazon spills into the ocean, the river is so wide you cannot see across to the other bank.

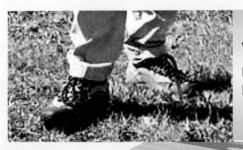

We begin our journey in the snowy peaks of the Andes. Get your hiking boots on and bundle up!

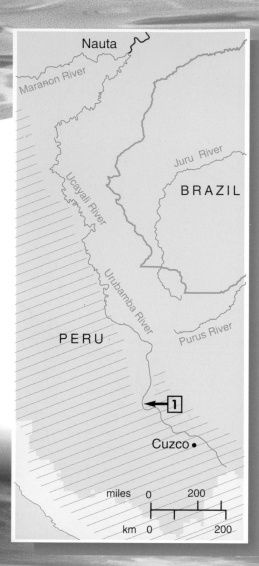

Nauta

Marañon River

Juru River

BRAZIL

Ucayali River

Urubamba River

PERU

Purus River

1

Cuzco •

miles 0   200

km 0   200

1. A River with Many Beginnings

IT IS HARD TO SAY EXACTLY where the Amazon River begins, because it is fed by so many other rivers. It probably begins in the "altiplano" (the high plains) of the Andes Mountains. Here the land collects the melted ice and rainwater that flow off the high peaks. These marshy areas form the Urubamba River, one of the Amazon's tributaries.

Below: The ancient city of Machu Picchu is one of the wonders of the world. It takes four days to walk here along an Inca trail, so many tourists take a train ride instead.

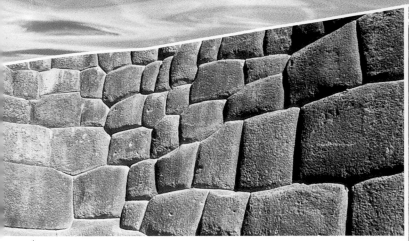

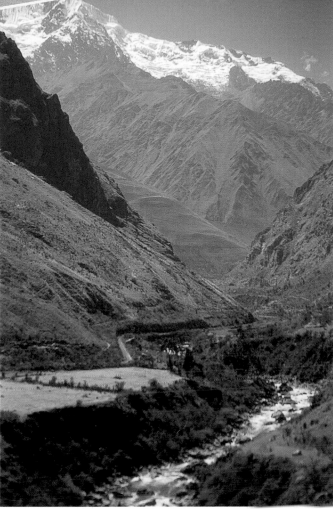

Above: The Incas were skilled architects and engineers. Many of their stone walls still stand.
Right: The Urubamba River is joined by thousands of tiny mountain streams. Its force can cut a path through valleys, such as this one, in the Andes Mountains.

📖 HISTORY A *sacred valley*

The Urubamba River valley is known as the sacred valley of the Incas. The Incas were a people that settled here about 800 years ago. The valley became their storehouse for food.

The Incas developed farming techniques to cope with the steep mountain environment. By cutting into the slopes, they created terraced fields that look like giant steps in the mountains. The Incas watered their fields by draining water from the Urubamba River, through channels carved from the rock. Some channels flowed through their streets and brought water to their homes.

The Incas had one of the world's most sophisticated ancient civilizations. The vast Inca empire was dotted with majestic cities, which were linked by stone-paved roads, steps, and pathways across the mountains and beyond. The Incas could easily travel from place to place, trading food and other goods.

The Inca empire was conquered by the Spanish in the 1500s, and their civilization was destroyed.

💲 ECONOMY *Machu Picchu tourists*

Today thousands of tourists flock to the Urubamba valley each year to marvel at the ancient city of Machu Picchu. MAP REF: 1 Machu Picchu is perched on a narrow ridge, 984 feet (300 meters) above the Urubamba River. The city remained hidden for 500 years, until an American archaeologist named Hiram Bingham visited the area in 1911. After a tip-off from a local farmer, Hiram Bingham crawled up steep slopes and fought his way through thick jungle vines and trees until he found the ruins.

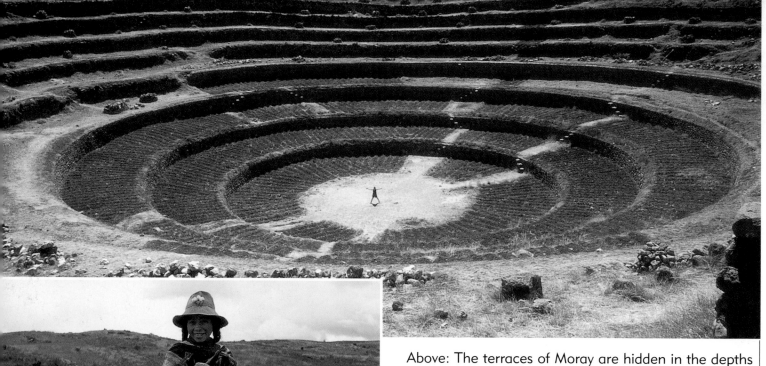

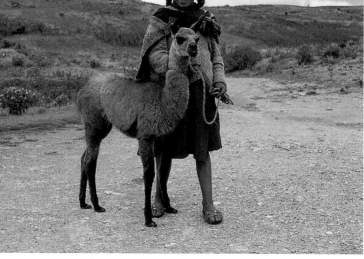

Above: The terraces of Moray are hidden in the depths of the Incas' sacred valley. Here, the Incas tried out new crops. The person in the middle shows you how enormous the terraces are.

Left: A young Quechua girl with an alpaca. Her hat and shawl are made from alpaca wool.

$ ECONOMY *Potatoes, llamas, and alpacas*

The local people in this region are named after the Inca language they speak, called Quechua. Many Quechua people are descendants of the Incas. Like the Incas before them, the Quechua depend on the Urubamba River and the fertile silt it leaves behind. They learned from their ancestors how to farm the land without damaging it. By growing different crops together, or by changing crops from year to year, Quechua farmers keep a balance of nutrients in the soil. Quechua communities also care for each other and help their neighbors, just as the Incas did.

The Quechua grow more than 400 different types of potato and rear herds of llama and alpaca. Llamas are strong, and can transport goods that are too heavy for people to carry. The Quechua also eat llama meat. The llama's woolly cousin, the alpaca, is another very useful animal. The Quechua weave alpaca wool into warm garments and turn alpaca hides into coats, to keep them warm through the worst of the cold Andean winter.

It is very difficult to make a living in this harsh environment. Some Quechua farmers have abandoned their land. They have moved down into towns in the Urubamba valley, where they sell goods to tourists.

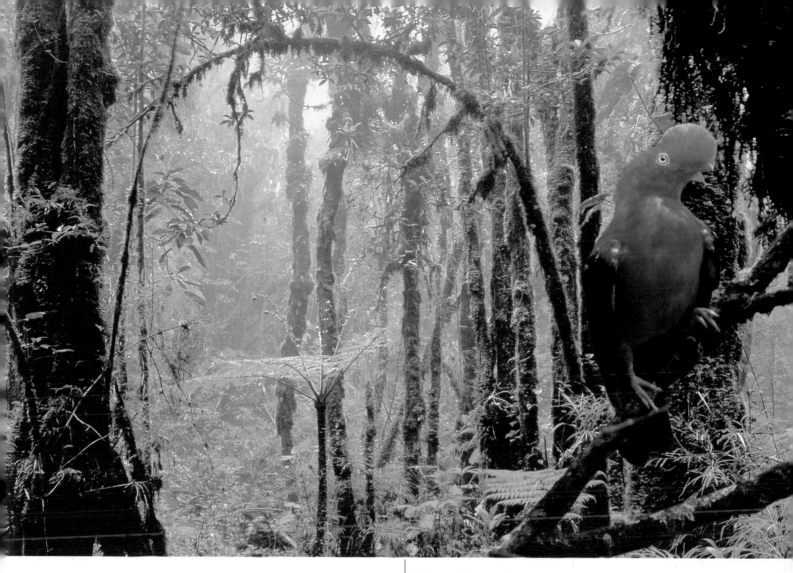

NATURE *A blanket of cloud*

The mountain slopes high above the Urubamba River can receive 20 feet (six meters) of rainfall in a year. These slopes are often covered in a blanket of water vapor. In such a damp, misty environment, a belt of "cloud forest" sucks water from the clouds, acting like a huge sponge. The water is released slowly, dripping off the trees and plants. Because the process is so slow, the valley below does not get too much water at once, so floods and landslides are rare.

Walking into a cloud forest is like entering a magical kingdom in every shade of green. With all the water around, plants cling to

Above: Plants that live on other plants, like ferns, orchids, and bromeliads, are called epiphyte or "guest plants."

every branch and tree trunk and create a hanging garden. In the cloud forest you can find more types of plants in a small area than you can find in all of Europe. Many of these plants are only found here. The cloud forest has its own special animals and birds, too, such as the many kinds of frogs that live in the undergrowth or in pools of water on the ground.

The Urubamba River twists and turns through mountain gorges until it turns north. Then, the river and its tributaries slide down the high mountains into the foothills of the Andes. When it leaves the mountains, the Urubamba changes its name to the Ucayali River. The dramatic fall in elevation gives the river extra energy. It flows fast and furiously, eroding its bed and banks, and carrying rocks, soil, leaves, and branches downstream. Wild, foaming rapids form on the river's surface as it crashes into boulders that block its path. These boulders provide perfect perches for kingfishers and herons. They can hunt for fish in the river's turbulent currents.

The change in altitude brings warmth and more rain. As the water on the ground warms up, it evaporates, rises, and turns into water vapor. Torrential tropical downpours can follow when there is so much moisture in the air. With the change in climate, tropical rain forest replaces the cloud forest in these hot, sticky lowlands.

Right: A kingfisher waits for a fish in the waters of the Ucayali River.
Below: Rapids form on the surface of the river as the water crashes around the rocks.

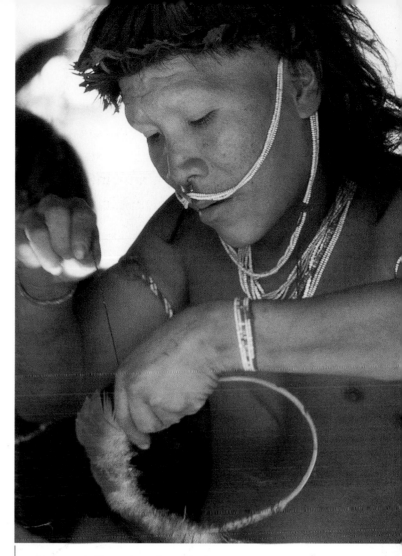

Above: A Peruvian AmerIndian

🖐 PEOPLE *Indians of the Amazon*

American Indians (known as AmerIndians) have lived in these tropical rain forests for 15,000 years. During the last Ice Age, their ancestors moved across to the Americas from central Asia. When the first Europeans explored the Amazon basin in the 1500s, about two million AmerIndians lived in different parts of the forest.

Today, however, there are probably only 250,000 AmerIndians left in the Amazon basin. Some were killed by the European settlers, who took over large areas. Many more were forced into slavery, or died from diseases such as measles, which they caught from the Europeans.

During our journey, we will meet and learn more about the Indians. Each AmerIndian group has developed its own way of life over generations. Some live together in settled villages. Others are nomads, and move every few days in search of food in the forest or the river. Because they are trying to maintain traditional ways of life, dozens of groups either have no, or little, contact with outsiders.

🐇 NATURE *The real Amazon*

Near the town of Nauta, in eastern Peru, an important event happens. The Ucayali River, that we are traveling on is joined by the Marañón River. The Marañón also began its journey in the Andes mountains. It has come 1,118 miles (1,800 kilometers) to this point, one-and-a-half times farther than the entire length of the Rhine, which is the longest river in western Europe. Now the Marañón River joins the Ucayali, and one vast channel of water is formed. From here onward, our river is called the Amazon.

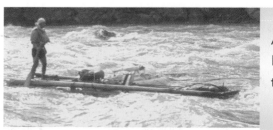

AmerIndians build log rafts, bound up by liana vines. Let's take one of these rafts and head north through the tropical rain forest, don't forget your paddle!

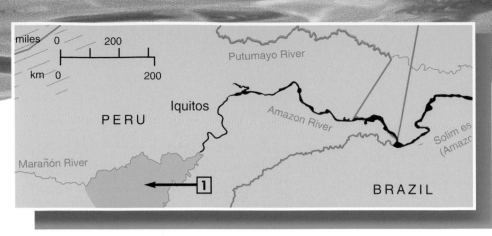

miles 0 200
km 0 200

Putumayo River

Iquitos

PERU

Amazon River

Solim es
(Amazo

Marañón River

1

BRAZIL

2. Toward the Three-Way Frontier

MANY SMALLER RIVERS JOIN THE AMAZON in the lowlands of Peru. Some of these begin in Colombia to the north and in Ecuador to the west. The Amazon River now flows over very flat land, but the flow is still powerful because there is so much water pouring off the mountains. With all that energy, the Amazon wears away its bed and banks. Its channel is deep and wide by the time we reach the city of Iquitos.

Below: The Amazon wears away the outside of its channel, and deposits silt on the inside. That is why the river bends, or meanders, into the snaking shapes you see here.

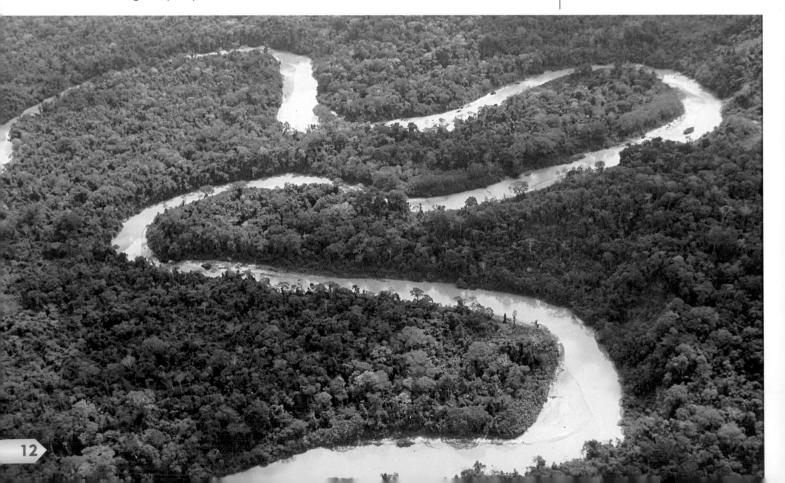

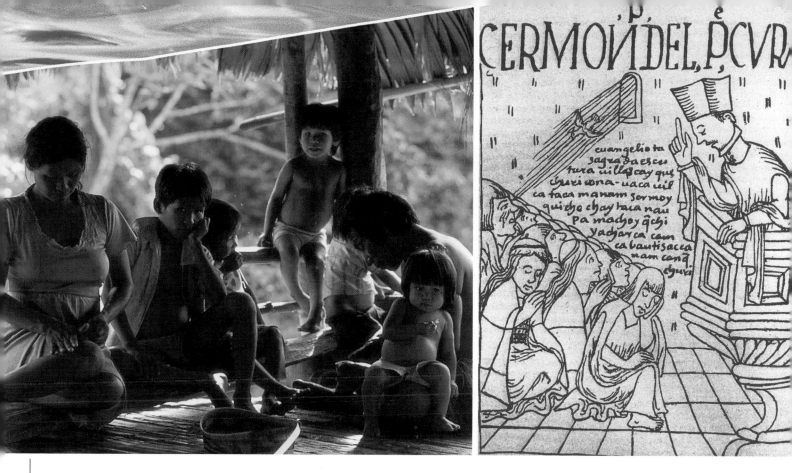

Above left: The Yagua people live near the city of Iquitos. Since the first Europeans arrived, the Yagua have refused to speak Spanish and have kept their own language and system of beliefs. They are one of many AmerIndian groups who still seek advice and help from their own priests, called shamans.

Above right: When the Spanish missionaries came to South America, they tried to make AmerIndians become Christians. This old engraving shows a Spanish priest explaining his religion to AmerIndians in a church.

📖 HISTORY **Explorers and Missionaries**
Francisco de Orellana was the first European to reach this stretch of the Amazon, when he traveled from Ecuador to the Atlantic coast in 1541. He was surprised to see great settlements of Indians living by the river. Like many Europeans of the time, Francisco de Orellana thought AmerIndians were primitive. He believed they needed to be "civilized" by European ideas and traditions. But in fact, the AmerIndians had intelligent and developed cultures.

Although Orellana saw the AmerIndians as inferior, he required their help to find food in the Amazon environment.

Later, Catholic missionaries came from Europe to convert AmerIndians to Christianity. The missionaries tried to learn AmerIndian languages, so they could explain their faith more easily. But AmerIndians had their own belief systems. Their gods were connected to the river, the trees, the earth, the Sun, and the Moon. They resisted Catholic beliefs, and killed many of the missionaries.

$ ECONOMY *No roads to Iquitos*

Iquitos, on the banks of the Amazon, is a city with 400,000 inhabitants. It is also the largest city in the world that cannot be reached by road. The only way to get to Iquitos is by boat along the river, or by air. There are almost no cars in Iquitos, because there are no roads to bring them in. Instead, bicycles and three-seater motor carts fill the streets. Ferries, called *collectivos*, take people and goods across the river. And, because of the Amazon's deep, wide channel, boats can take passengers from Iquitos all the way to the Atlantic coast, 2,299 miles (3,700 kilometers) away.

The center of Iquitos is full of activity. People trade goods among themselves and with people from outlying villages. Markets on the banks of the river sell fruit, fish, vegetables, tobacco, and timber. At the food stalls you can buy a local delicacy, like turtle meat soup, or fried or steamed monkey. Or you could try *palmeta*, a local soup made from river fish.

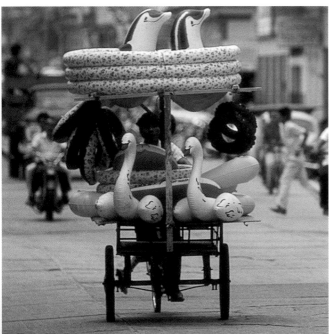

Left: In Iquitos, a town without cars, pedal power is very important.
Below: These cashews on sale in Iquitos's market have several uses. The outer flesh, called the apple, can be squeezed to make delicious juice. The nut in the middle also makes a delicious snack, either raw or roasted.

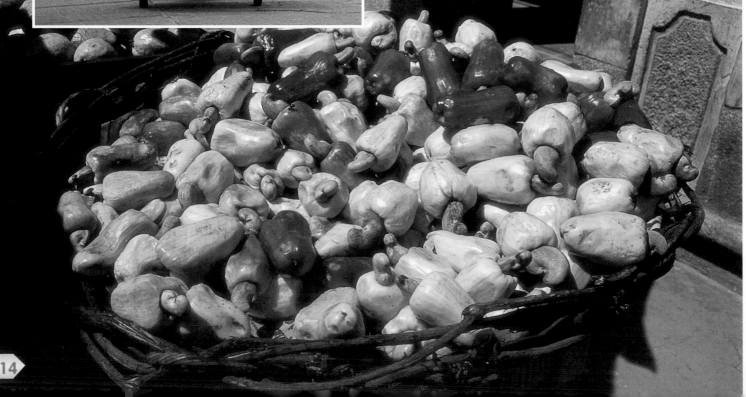

Above: These houses have been built along the river bank in Iquitos. The photograph was taken in the dry season. Imagine how this looks in the rainy season when the river level has risen.

✋ PEOPLE *Living with the river*

Because they live so close to the river, the people of Iquitos have to cope with changing water levels in different seasons. Thousands of people make their homes on the edge of the city, where they build houses from whatever materials they can find, such as bamboo and corrugated iron. But this land floods every year when the river rises. People here must switch from bicycles to canoes to get around.

To keep dry, many people build their houses on stilts. Other houses are built on balsa wood logs. Balsa wood is very light and floats easily, so the houses can float when the river level rises.

$ ECONOMY *The oil business*

Iquitos is the center for exploring the oil and natural gas reserves that lie beneath the rock in this part of the Amazon basin. The Amazon's oil has become big business. Nearly one fourth of all the oil that the United States imports comes from here. Once the oil is pumped from the ground, it is either sent by pipeline, or taken by barge along the river, to the Loreto oil refinery near Iquitos. There, the crude oil is heated and separated into different parts, such as benzine, kerosene, and gasoline.

Refined oil from this part of the Amazon basin is now pumped through the Norperuano Pipeline. This is Peru's longest pipeline and stretches for 497 miles (800 kilometers). It goes right over the Andes, all the way west to the port of Bayóvar on the Pacific Ocean.

➡ CHANGE *The impact of oil*

Oil has improved the lives of many people in the Amazon basin by bringing jobs and wealth to the area. But it has also brought new risks and problems. In October 2000, 5,500 barrels of oil were spilled into the Marañón River. The river water was polluted over a vast area. Some of the leaked oil spread into the nearby Pacaya Samiria Reserve, **MAP REF: 1** Peru's largest protected area, where it caused enormous damage.

For the 20,000 people that depend on the river's water, the effects of the oil spill have been devastating. Fish catches are much smaller than they were before the spill, because so many fish were poisoned or suffocated by the oil. This has deprived local people of their main food source. Many AmerIndians have developed skin diseases and stomach infections from drinking or washing in the polluted water.

✋ PEOPLE *The Urarina people*

The Urarina are a peaceful Indian tribe who have lived around the Marañón River for hundreds of years. Now their livelihood is threatened by outsiders who are moving into their homeland.

Hidden in this swampy area of forest, the Urarina clear small gardens to plant crops such as manioc, corn, and banana. They fish in the river, and are experts at hunting

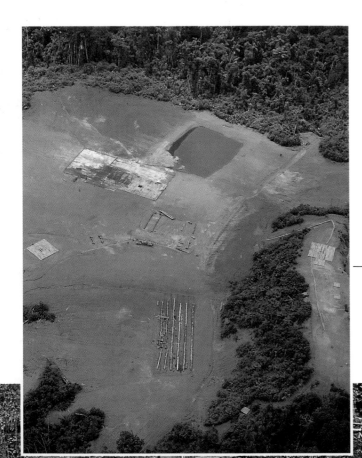

Left and below: The dark square on the left is an abandoned oil well. The forest below has been cleared to make room for a settlement, and an oil pipeline runs across the burned tree stumps.

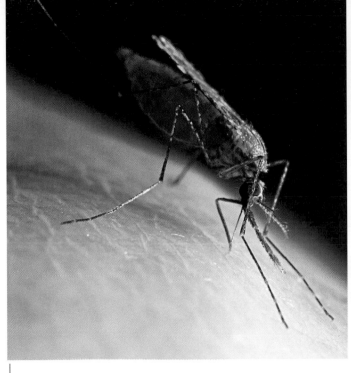

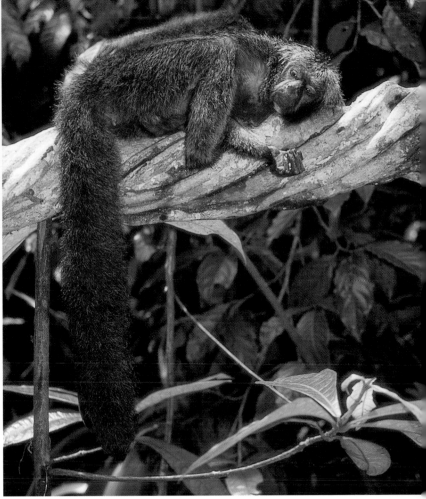

Above: Female anopheles mosquitos spread the malaria parasite in their saliva. The parasite can be transferred to humans if the mosquito bites them.
Right: Poachers in the Urarina lands hunt and kill saki monkeys for their beautiful tails.

animals. But oil companies searching for oil, logging companies cutting down trees, and even tourists in search of a different experience, have all come in contact with the Urarina.

Because they are not used to outside contact, the Urarina do not have any natural protection from outside diseases. This means they are at great risk of getting sick from contact with new people. The results can be devastating. In recent years, many Urarina people have caught deadly diseases, such as malaria and cholera. Diseases like these could threaten their very existence.

Poachers are also a serious problem. They sneak onto Urarina land to catch local saki monkeys. The Urarina have formed their own protection squads, called "river wolves." Divided into teams of four, the river wolves take turns guarding their territory against poachers. They also watch the river and try to stop poachers from using poison to catch fish. Poison can kill the wildlife in whole sections of the river.

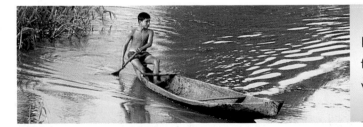

Let's ride in a dugout canoe to the three-way frontier of Peru, Colombia, and Brazil. From there, we will cross the border into Brazil.

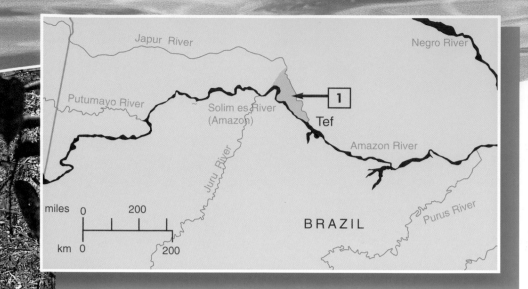

3. An Amazing World

WHEN WE LEAVE PERU AND ENTER BRAZIL, the name of the Amazon River changes again. On this stretch of our journey, the river is called the Solimões. It snakes east for a few hundred miles, surrounded by unbroken rain forest. Here, the river and the rain forest are home to an extraordinary number of living things. A tenth of all the plant, animal, and insect species on Earth live in this area.

Left and below: Rain forest trees form a huge umbrella, called a canopy, over the life below. The tallest trees are supported by gigantic buttress roots, which keep them from falling.

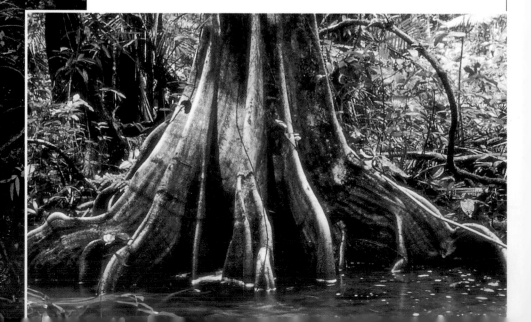

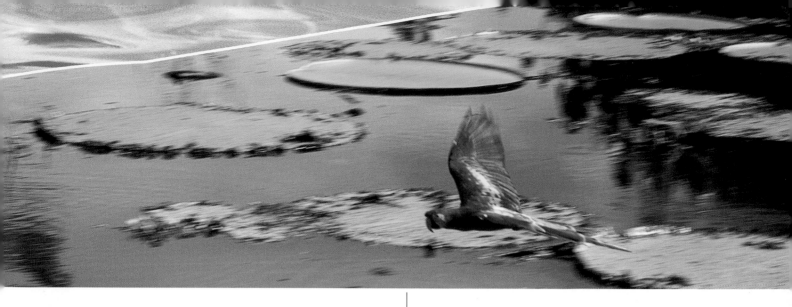

NATURE *The rain forest cycle of life*

All the world's rain forests are close to the Equator. Rain forest trees and plants can grow every day of the year, because of the abundant rain and sunshine. The hot, wet conditions also speed up the rate at which dead leaves and branches decompose on the forest floor. Many types of fungi help to break down this rotting material, and then the nutrients they contain can be used again. A network of tree roots on the forest floor sucks up some of these nutrients before they are washed away by the rain, or seep into the underlying soil.

By recycling the nutrients, rain forest trees grow to amazing heights. The tallest trees, such as the kapok, can be 130 feet (40 meters) high. To keep them from falling, the trees are supported by gigantic buttress roots. Other plants and vines grow along the branches of these forest giants. The trees also provide food and habitats for animals and birds. Some trees have leaves with special drip-tips that shield the land from tropical downpours. In this way, the trees create a vast umbrella that protects

the human, plant, and animal life of the rain forest.

Rainwater drains into the river from the surrounding forest. It carries some of the nutrients in soil particles, or dissolved in the water that was not absorbed by tree roots. These nutrients provide food for an abundance of life in the river itself.

Scientists estimate that there may be 3,000 types of fish in the river. New species are being found all the time. The murky depths of the river are home to many strange life-forms, such as transparent catfish, and electric fish, which hunt without sight.

Where the water is calm, Victoria Regia lilies grow across the surface of the river. Spikes underneath the pads keep fish from nibbling. The lily pads provide a useful platform for nimble-footed birds that search for insects on the water's surface.

PEOPLE *Living in the rain forest*

In order to survive in the rain forest, the AmerIndians have developed a deep understanding of it. They have learned that the soil loses its fertility if they plant crops year after year. To give the soil a chance to recover, they move on to a new patch of forest.

AmerIndians also know that cutting down trees cuts off the supply of nutrients to the soil. So they use the forest resources without cutting down trees. The sap from one tree makes a fire starter, and another tree's bark makes very strong rope. Hitting the hollow trunks of the drum tree is an excellent way to send messages echoing through the forest. The AmerIndians also use some plants to decorate themselves,

making bright dyes from seeds, bark, and leaves. They even use some soft, spongy leaves as toilet paper.

Whether they are visiting a friend or a neighbor, or even going to school, most people on this stretch of the river travel by canoe. AmerIndians can make a canoe from a single tree trunk. At times of conflict in the past, some groups carved canoes big enough for 30 warriors out of just one of the forest giants. To make sure they last for years, the people fill their canoes with water when they are not in use. That stops the wood from drying out and splitting. In their canoes, AmerIndians hunt fish like the

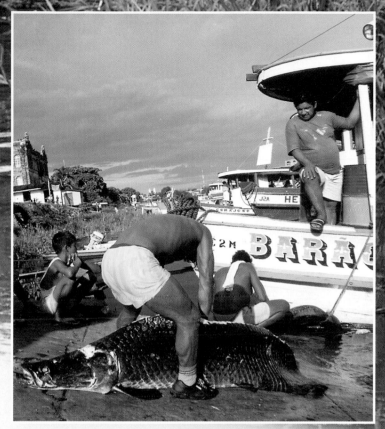

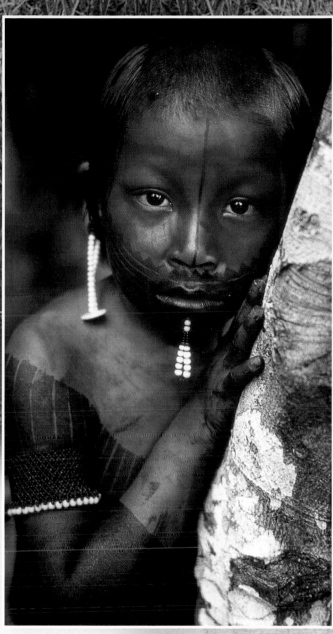

Left: An AmerIndian boy paddles his canoe on the Amazon River

Above: A small *pirarucu* is caught. *Pirarucu* fish can be up to 13 feet (four meters) long, and may weigh as much as a cow!

Right: This AmerIndian child's skin is painted with vegetable dye patterns. The red dye on his face is made from curucum seeds.

pirarucu, the world's largest freshwater fish.

Indians also use the rain forest to make music. They carve a kind of flute from a piece of bamboo, or the hollow leg bone of an animal. Gourds also make good instruments. Gourds are made from the dried and hollowed skin of fruits such as pumpkin and squash. The gourds are filled with seeds or stones from the riverbank to make a percussion instrument known as a maraca. The rattling sound of maracas is heard at parties and festivals all over Brazil.

To protect the land used by different groups of AmerIndians, there are now 29 Indian reserves in the Amazon basin. This helps to protect forest traditions and knowledge, so the people can pass on their expertise to future generations.

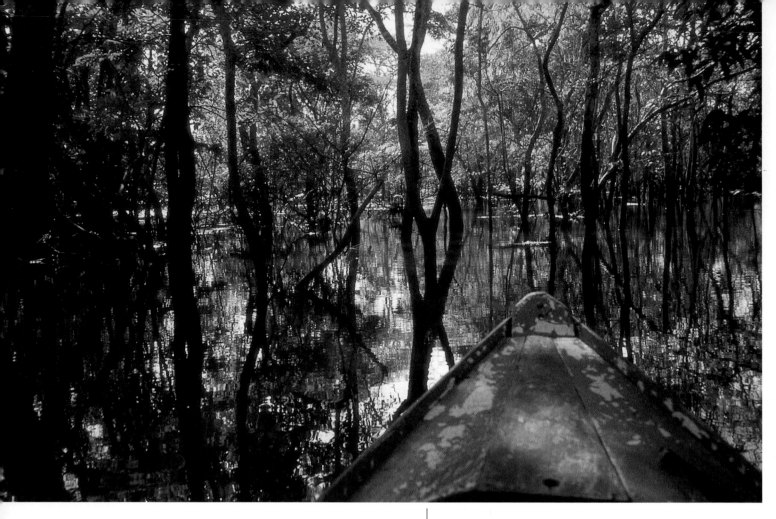

Rising waters

Although rain showers happen all year in the Amazon basin, most rain falls between January and March. During this wet season, rainwater pours off the land and surges down the tributaries into the main river channel. The swollen river rises 66 feet (20 meters), and floods an area larger than the state of Mississippi. In this season the Amazon holds more water than the next eight largest rivers on Earth combined.

The water level spills over the land and rises in the *igapós*, the parts of the forest that are permanently flooded. But the river floods other parts of the forest, too. That creates a maze of seasonal islands and extra water channels. In the flooded forest,

Above: In the wet season, some parts of the river can be reached only by boat. This flooded forest land provides extra fishing grounds.

insects fall from the treetops and provide food for fish. Fish such as the fruit-eating *tambaqui* help to disperse seeds. They eat the fleshy outsides, and the seeds pass straight through the fish, ending up somewhere else in the water. Meanwhile, predators such as *caimans*, members of the alligator family, hunt their prey among the reeds.

In the rain forest canopy, groups of monkeys jump from tree to tree, feeding on leaves and fruits. The white *uacari* monkey lives only in the flooded forest, eating the seeds of unripe fruits. These agile animals can leap up to 98 feet (40 meters) from one tree to another. They have no fur on their heads at all, and their faces are bright red. Sloths are not so athletic. But to move around the flooded forest in search of their next meal, sloths have learned to swim.

By October, the tropical downpours are less frequent and less heavy. During this relatively dry season, the river level drops, and much of the flooded forest is dry land once again. Some channels of water become completely cut off, forming small lakes in the forest.

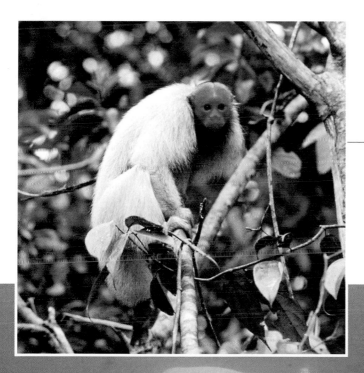

✋ PEOPLE A *handsome young bôto*

A myth surrounds the pink dolphin, another resident of the flooded forest. These beautiful creatures, called *bôto*, feed off small fish in the *igapós*. They are the only dolphins that can bend their necks.

During the Feast of St. John every June, people gather to eat, dance, and have a good time. The *bôto* is said to visit the party disguised as a handsome young man, but he has to wear a hat to hide the nostrils on top of his head.

The *bôto* dances with the first beautiful woman he meets, persuading her to come with him to the bottom of the river. It is traditional to ask any man who is wearing a hat to take it off, to check that there is no *bôto* among the guests!

Left: Local people say that the red faces of the *uacari* monkeys remind them of the sunburned faces of Europeans.
Below: The *bôto* or pink dolphin is almost blind. It uses sonar to find its way through the murky waters of the Amazon River.

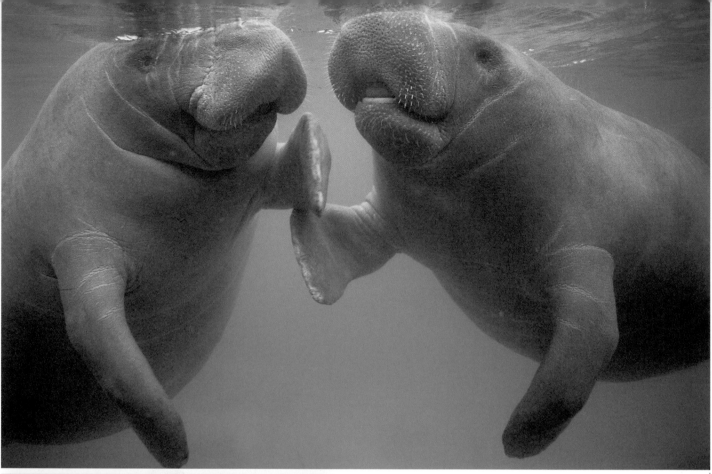

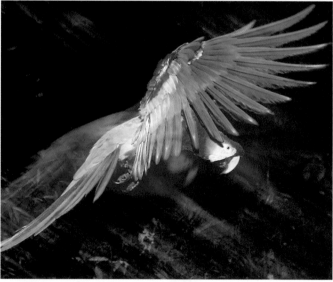

Above: Manatees are gentle and inquisitive animals. Some people think that the myth of mermaids is based on sightings of manatees. Left: Scarlet macaws sometimes eat wet clay from the river bank. No one knows exactly why, but the clay may help settle their stomachs after a meal of sour fruits and berries.

🖐 NATURE The Mamirauá

The Japurá River joins the Solimões River near the town of Tefé. A reserve called Mamirauá [MAP REF: 1] sits in the watery triangle between the two rivers. During the wet season, the water here rises 39 feet (12 meters), making it the largest protected area of flooded forest in Brazil. *Mamirauá* is an AmerIndian word for a baby manatee. The manatee is one of the many unusual animals that lives here. It can grow up to 10 feet (three meters) long, and has a seal-like body with a powerful flat tail.

The Mamirauá Reserve helps to protect some of the world's endangered species. It also gives scientists a chance to learn more about them. Eighty researchers are based here to study the flooded environment.

Mamirauá is different from other reserves in an important way. Instead of banning local people from using the area's resources, the government takes their needs into account. Some parts of the reserve are strictly protected, but the 5,000 people who live here can fish and collect wood in other parts. Local people help manage the reserve. So the lives of both the people and the wildlife of Mamiraua can be maintained.

$ ECONOMY *Medicines and poisons*

Scientists know that some rain forest plants have medicinal qualities. These qualities have helped cure illnesses for centuries. The bark of one tree contains quinine, one of the oldest cures for malaria. The study of rain forest plants continues, in the hope of finding cures for other illnesses.

AmerIndians have always used the forest for different medicines. They collect a nut called *guaraná*, known as the "red gold" of the Amazon. Today, *guaraná* is often ground into a powder and mixed with milk. Drinking one of these *guaraná* milkshakes is said to give you extra energy. AmerIndians have introduced us to different foods, too. *Cacao* are native rain forest trees. They produce large red fruits, the seeds of which are used to make chocolate.

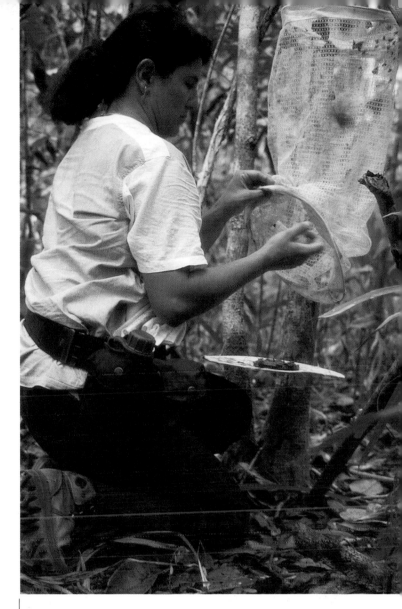

Above: A scientist In the Mamiraua Reserve collects samples of rain forest plants.

Not all Amazonian plants are used to heal or nourish. One plant, called *curare*, is used as a poison. If a monkey high in the rainforest canopy is struck by a dart smeared with *curare*, it quickly loses its grip and falls to the ground.

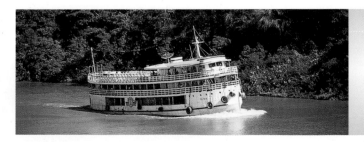

It is a long way to Manaus, our next stop. Let's ride on one of the paddle steamers that have traveled the river for more than a hundred years.

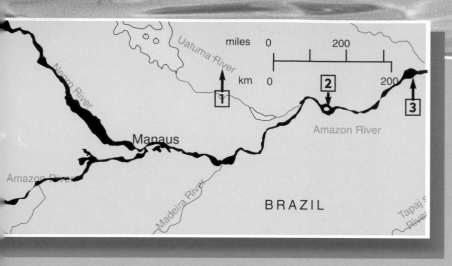

miles 0 200
km 0 200

Uatuma River

Negro River

Amazon River

Manaus

Amazon River

Madeira River

Amazon River

BRAZIL

Tapajós River

1 2 3

4. The Meeting of the Waters

MANAUS CAN BE CALLED the Brazilian capital of the Amazon Basin. Near here, the Solimões River meets another great river — the Rio Negro, or "black river." The milky Solimões River is colored by the silt carried from the slopes of the Peruvian Andes. But the Negro River is the color of black tea. This river began in the lowland forests, and its color comes from the litter of rotting plants. The two rivers flow side by side until the waters finally mix together. Then the river changes its name back to the Amazon for the last time.

Below: The Negro River and the Solimões River flow side by side for a while, after they meet in Brazil.

PEOPLE *Floodplain communities*

People who live along this stretch of the river grow crops on the flat land on either side of the water. This land they use is called the *várzea*, or floodplain. In the wet season, the river spreads over the floodplain, depositing fertile silt. At this time of year, members of the *várzea* communities who live in two-story stilt houses near the river have to move upstairs. Fish is an essential part of every *varzeán* family's diet. Children learn to fish almost before they can walk.

Above: Preparing manioc is a group effort. The process is a long one, and the whole community helps with each stage.
Right: The *Cabaclos* have learned that these palm berries make good wine. The people weave the palm leaves into baskets to carry the berries, and twist a strip of palm trunk into a handle.

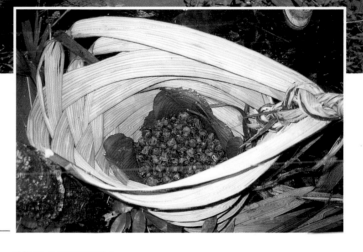

$ ECONOMY *Farming the floodplain*

When the water level recedes, people clear away the undergrowth and grow food on the fertilized land. Many families rely on the crops that they can grow themselves. The most important of these is manioc, a large root crop that grows well here. When the manioc tubers are big enough, farmers dig them up, peel them, and boil them down to a pulp. Then, they squeeze out all the liquid to get rid of poisonous juices. Once it has been dried, the manioc pulp is pounded into flour, which is called *farinha*.

PEOPLE *Survival skills*

Many of the people who live in *várzea* communities have mixed ancestry. Their ancestors were AmerIndian, European, and African. These people are called *Caboclos*, and they have retained many of the forest survival skills used by their AmerIndian ancestors.

Caboclos build temporary shelters in the forest. With strong beams and roofs made of palm fronds carefully woven together, these shelters can keep them dry during the heaviest rainstorm. At night, *Caboclos* sleep in hammocks suspended from hooks attached to the shelters' beams.

HISTORY *The rubber boom*

About 150 years ago, people in Manaus struck gold! They discovered that a sticky liquid called latex, collected from rubber trees by AmerIndians, could make them rich. The invention of tires in Europe meant that rubber became a valuable resource in Manaus. New types of steamboats could transport vast amounts of rubber downriver. Then, it could be exported to Europe. Manaus became a major port, and the population grew from 5,000 in 1865 to 50,000 by 1900.

The boom in rubber brought great wealth to Manaus. Rubber barons displayed their fortunes by building huge mansions and palaces. Manaus became the second city in Brazil to have electricity. The opera house, built in 1896, was a symbol of the city's new wealth and international importance. This building is made of Scottish wrought iron and Italian stone. It is decorated with 36,000 French tiles and has chandeliers made of Italian crystal and French bronze.

But by the early 20th century, British traders had smuggled rubber seeds out of South America and set up rival rubber plantations in southeast Asia. This new competition meant that the glory days of the rubber boom in Manaus were over.

Below: The beautiful colored dome of the opera house in Manaus still stands out as a reminder of the city's past. But now it is surrounded by the new giants, modern skyscrapers.

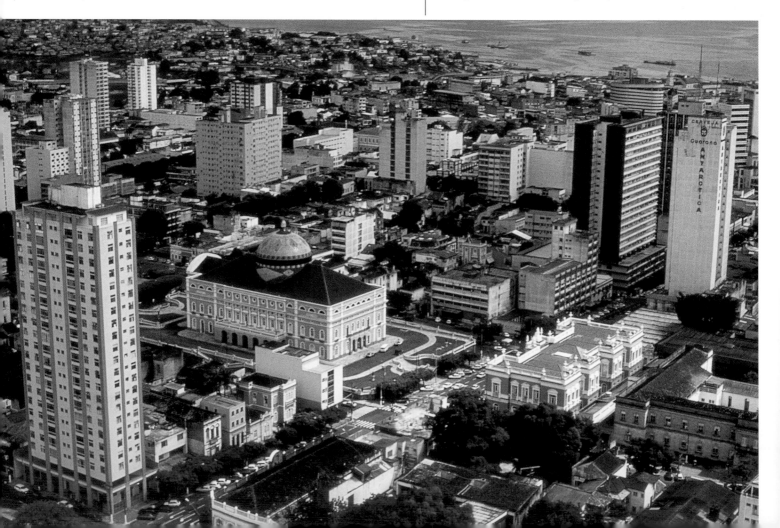

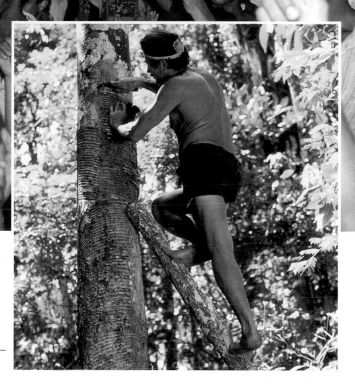

Above: These rubber tappers are members of a union, and work together to protect their livelihood.
Right: This *seringueiro* is making a diagonal cut into the bark of a rubber tree. Then, he will attach a cup to collect the latex that drips from the tree.

$ ECONOMY *Saving a way of life*

Today, the rubber boom is just a distant memory, but rubber tapping remains a way of life for many. Each rubber tapper, called a *seringueiro*, looks after about 200 rubber trees. Every day, he takes a trail through the forest to set up the cups that will collect latex. On the return journey, the *seringueiro* takes a different trail, and picks up the latex from a previous trip. Back home, he heats the latex over a fire, which solidifies it. He then sells this to a rubber trader.

Chico Mendes will always be remembered by the *seringueiros*. Born into a rubber tapping family, Chico was a member of the rubber tappers' union, an organization that protected the rights of the *seringueiros*. He saw that cattle ranchers and other landowners were taking over forests that were used by the *seringueiros*. Chico came up with the idea of setting up "extractive reserves." These are areas set aside for collecting latex and other natural products without cutting down the trees. But the competition for land was fierce and sometimes became violent.

In 1988 Chico was assassinated by one of his enemies. But Chico's "extractive reserves" still safeguard the future of the *seringueiros* and the forest.

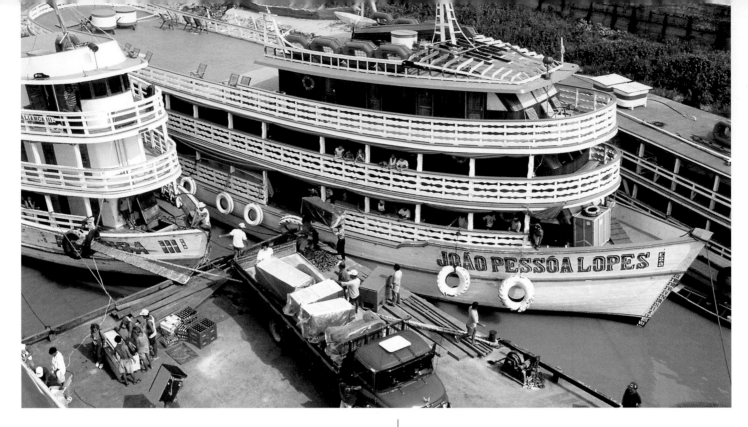

$ ECONOMY *A free-trade zone*

Despite the slump in the rubber trade, Manaus has revived its fortunes. Because it is a "free-trade zone" the city is now an important industrial center for 400 electronics companies. A "free-trade zone" means that companies do not have to pay taxes on goods coming in and out of Manaus, which saves them a lot of money.

Companies can transport their products to and from Manaus's airport, and then fly them all over the world. The port of Manaus can harbor ships, which travel all the way down to the coast. This extra trade brings more money to the area, but it is not all good news. Some local people have lost their jobs because modern electronics factories have replaced them with machines. The machines can produce goods even more cheaply.

Above: The port of Manaus has a special dock to handle changes in the water level. Ships can travel here from the coast, which is 900 miles (1,450 kilometers) away.

➡ CHANGE *River power*

All these companies create a great demand for energy. At this stage, the Amazon River is too slow and wide to be used to produce energy. But there are about 80 tributaries that feed into the Amazon. When these are dammed, hydroelectric power can be produced.

Some of the dams have not succeeded. Nearly 30 years ago, engineers started building the Balbina Dam MAP REF: 1 on the Uatumã River near Manaus. The dam was finally finished in 1987, and the dam wall towered 164 feet (50 meters), rising above the tops of the trees. But because the land is fairly flat, the river water has spread over a vast area behind the dam. It has flooded 583,166 acres (236,000 hectares) of forest.

Many local people think the Balbina Dam is a disaster. The Waimiri Artoari Indians who lived here were forced to leave their homes. They didn't receive compensation, nor have they benefited from the new source of electricity. And the dam's reservoir has become a swamp. Mosquitoes carrying diseases, such as malaria and yellow fever, have multiplied. Plants have grown over the surface of the shallow, stagnant water.

Weeds and dead leaves from the trees rot in the water, releasing millions of tons of methane and carbon dioxide. These gases pollute the atmosphere, and add to the problem of global warming.

The flat landscape creates another problem. There are no steep slopes, so the water does not flow fast enough through the dam's turbines to generate power. In fact, the dam generates only a third of the energy originally estimated. All that water, flooding all that land, only creates enough power to run the air conditioners in downtown Manaus.

Below: Behind the Balbina Dam, the drowned forest trees have been left to rot in the water. The reservoir is so shallow that some pieces of land break the surface of the water.

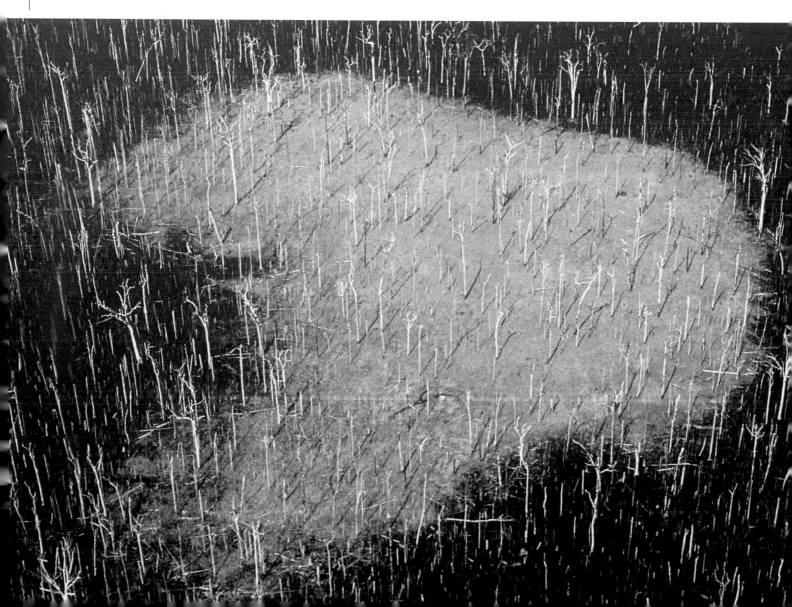

Adventure vacations

The city of Manaus is a growing center for ecotourism. This kind of tourism could help protect the traditional way of life and the natural environment. It also creates new jobs for local people in hotels, lodges, restaurants, and boats. There is an ecotourism lodge on Silves Island, MAP REF: 2 186 miles (300 kilometers) from Manaus. Some of the money made from visitors is used to protect the area's lakes and create health services for local people. But ecotourism has problems. By visiting remote areas, people disturb the environment. Some ecotourist attractions are foreign owned, and local people share only a few of the benefits.

To reach Silves Island we travel to Itacoatiara, where the road ends. The rest of the five-hour journey is by *voadeira* — a canoe with a powerful engine. We may hear the call of a *japim* as we travel upriver. The *japim* bird copies the songs of other birds. It can even sound like a child crying.

We can try to catch piranhas in the flooded forest, using pieces of meat as bait. But piranha fishing is difficult for beginners. These fish can nibble away the meat at lightning speed.

Are you brave enough to go into the flooded forest at night? There are tarantulas, snakes, and caimans everywhere, and eyes glint red by flashlight all around us.

Left: This piranha will make a good lunch for visitors. AmerIndians don't just eat piranhas — they use the razor-sharp teeth as nail files, or to sharpen their weapons!
Below: By visiting hotels built among the trees of the forests, tourists can experience life in the Amazon, but still have luxury and comfort. This tower lookout helps tourists spot forest birds.

Welcome to Ariaú Jungle Tower

Bem vindo ao Ariaú

PEOPLE   *A dance contest*

Tourists can enjoy the rich culture of the Manaus region in other places, too. There is a festival called *Boi Bumbá*, the Ox Dance, that is held on Parantins Island, MAP REF: 3 over a June weekend. This is the region's largest and most famous festival. The music and dance tell an ancient story of Catirina and her husband Francisco. When she was pregnant, Catirina had a craving for ox tongue. Francisco killed his master's best ox to keep her happy. But Francisco was thrown in prison for his crime. He was only freed when a man with magic powers, called Pajé, brought the ox back to life.

Each year, two dance and music troupes from Manaus compete in acting out the story. After three days of singing and dancing, the judges choose the winners. Winning first prize is a cause for great celebration by both the dancers and their supporters.

Below: The Boi Bumbá, or Ox Dance, on Parantins Island

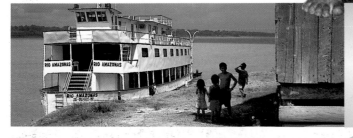

We still have 994 miles (1,600 kilometers) to go before we reach the Atlantic Ocean. Let's buy a hammock in Manaus so we can sleep on the ferry.

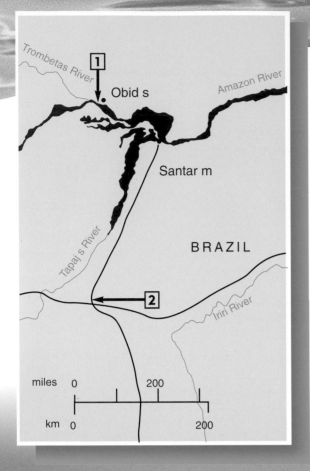

The Amazon Floodplain

FROM MANAUS, WE CONTINUE TO TRAVEL EAST. The Amazon River is now a muddy brown, colored by all the silt it is carrying. After we reach the town of Santarém, we meet another tributary called the Tapajós River. This river flows up from the south. Its water is clear blue because, unlike the Amazon, it doesn't carry much silt with it.

Below: Sandbars like this one at Alter do Chão are made from silt that the river deposits as it slows down. Some sandbars get so high they can cut off parts of the river.

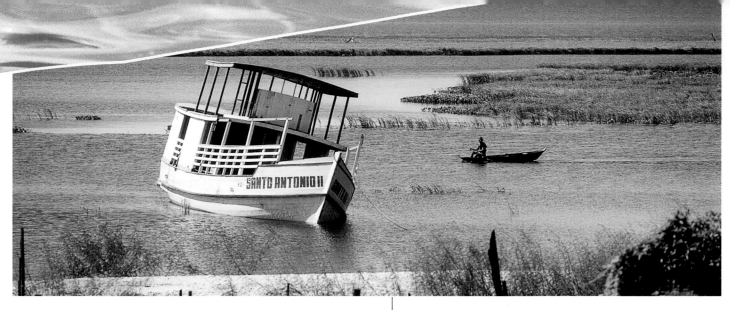

Above: The water of the Tapajós River is a clear blue. It joins the muddy Amazon beyond the town of Santarém.

🐰 NATURE The Óbidos Narrows

Forty million years ago, the movement of the earth's plates pushed up the land to form an enormous inland sea between two mountain ranges called the Guyanan Shield and the Brazilian Shield. The huge sea cut a deep channel between the mountains, as it began its journey to the Atlantic Ocean.

Today, this inland sea is part of the Amazon River. The channel that was cut between the two mountain ranges all those years ago is called the Óbidos Narrows. MAP REF: 1 The river shrinks to a third of its width as it is forced through the Narrows, and that makes the water flow faster. This is the deepest and narrowest point on the Brazilian Amazon. The Óbidos Narrows forms a natural gateway to the final stretch of the Amazon River's journey to the sea.

📖 HISTORY Guarding the fort

When the Portuguese controlled Brazil during the 1600s, they built a fort overlooking the river at Óbidos. Because the channel is so narrow, they could see across the river from the fort. They could keep watch for attacks from their enemies. During the early days of Portuguese rule, Óbidos was the largest town on this stretch of the river. Now the town is less important, but the old fort is a tourist attraction.

🐰 NATURE Tides and sediment

By this stage, the Amazon floodplain is vast. The river has deposited great mounds of sediment. The sediment makes sandy beaches on the inside bends of the river, where the current is weak. Beyond the river's banks, the land is flat as far as you can see. Much of this land is covered in water during the wet season, when the river bursts its banks. Even though we are still about 497 miles (800 kilometers) from the coast, the ocean's tides can push seawater this far up the river.

Over thousands of years, some sea creatures, such as sting rays, have moved upriver with the tides and now live here, far inland. Amazingly, they have been able to adapt successfully to the freshwater environment.

$ ECONOMY *Hidden treasure*

Beneath the rain forest along this stretch of the river, the land is rich in natural resources. There are supplies of important minerals, such as copper, bauxite, and manganese. More than a million people have come to the Amazon basin in search of gold. Large swathes of forest have been turned into mud baths, where people dig, hoping to make their fortunes. Life as an Amazon gold digger is very hard, however, and most people leave empty-handed.

NATURE *Searching for gold*

The Tapajós River valley is the largest gold-mining region in the Amazon basin. Tiny specks of this precious metal can be found in the silt of the Tapajós River. Gold diggers add liquid mercury to separate the gold from the

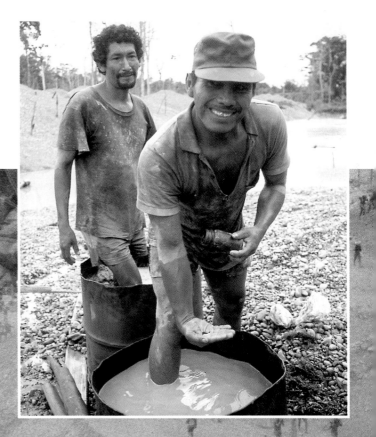

silt. But for every two pounds (one kilo) of gold produced, nine pounds (four kilos) of mercury is released into the environment. Some of the mercury escapes into the atmosphere as a poisonous gas, and more of it is washed into the soil or the river. Once the mercury is in the river, fish absorb it into their systems.

Mercury poisoning is very dangerous to humans. Too much mercury in the bloodstream causes tunnel vision and alarming changes in behavior. Acute poisoning can cause brain damage and even death. People can be poisoned by breathing air polluted by mercury or by eating fish contaminated by mercury.

Because fish is the main item in their diet, thousands of people who live on the banks of the Tapajós River have mercury poisoning. In the gold mining town of Itaituba along the Tapajós River, over one third of the miners have dangerously high levels of mercury in their blood.

➡ CHANGE *Dredging the Tapajós*

Plans are in place to change the shape of the Tapajós River by dredging a 621-mile (1,000-kilometer) section of the water. The dredged section will run upstream from Santarém, making the channel deeper and wider. If this happens, much bigger cargo ships will be able to take goods up the Tapajós River. Then, they will be able to travel along the Amazon itself, all the way to the ocean.

Farmers who live far from the Amazon River are delighted by these plans. The wider channel will let them transport grains to markets in the United States and Europe. There the grains are sold as cattle feed. But many local people are not so happy. Dredging will churn up silt and pollute the water. Waste from big cargo ships could make pollution even worse. Other people are worried about increased flooding in the wet season. The new channel will bring more water surging down the Tapajós River.

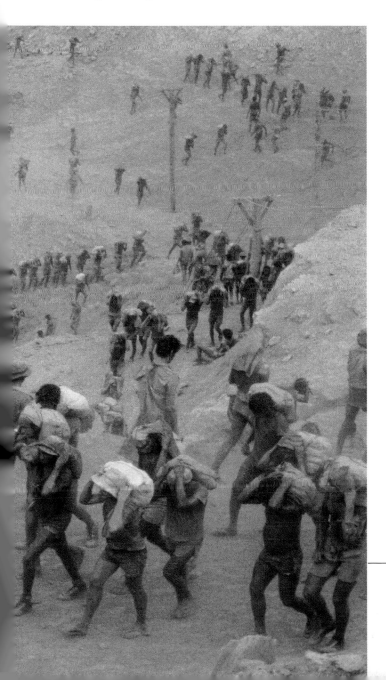

Left: More than one million miners or *garimpeiros*, work in the goldfields of the Amazon River basin. They all hope to make their fortunes, but only a few will ever strike it rich.

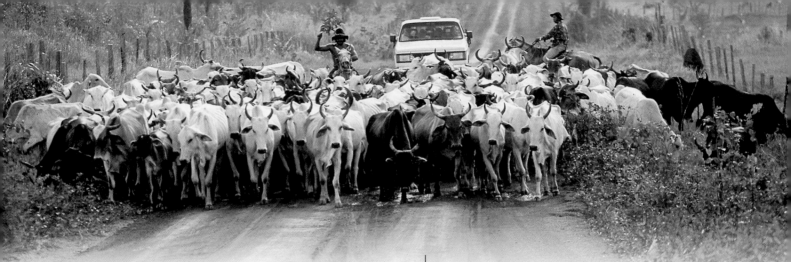

$ ECONOMY *Opening the Amazon*

Since the 1970s the Brazilian government has been encouraging people from overcrowded parts of Brazil to start a new life in the Amazon basin. Road building has opened up areas and linked river settlements to the outside world. The Trans-Amazonian Highway runs for 3,107 miles (5,000 kilometers) across the region, and Santarém is connected to southern Brazil by a 1,081-mile (1,741-kilometer) road. MAP REF: 2 Other roads have been built illegally by logging companies. Tropical hardwoods like mahogany, earn loggers a fortune in Japan, North America, and rich European countries.

These roads act like magnets, attracting new settlers. Families move in and clear patches of forest to grow food. Other large areas are cleared by ranchers to make new pasture for raising cattle, or by companies growing crops in massive plantations.

A satellite image of the Amazon region, such as the one on the opposite page, shows how much forest is being chopped down. Nearly 232,000 square miles (600,000 square kilometers) of rain forest in Brazil has been destroyed since 1970. That area is

Above: Cattle ranching is one of the most destructive uses of land. After only ten years, the land can look like a desert.

the same size as the state of California. Now deforestation is speeding up. In 2000, 2,316 more square miles were destroyed than were destroyed five years earlier.

Once the forest is gone, the soil quickly loses its fertility. Without the network of tree roots, nutrients are no longer recycled. Instead, they are easily washed away in a heavy rain shower, along with the soil. Some of this ends up in the river, adding to the river's already heavy load. With fewer trees, the nutrient supply to the river declines. That leaves less food for the Amazon's fish. AmerIndian communities suffer, because their land is lost forever. The entire ecosystem declines.

➡ CHANGE *Future frontiers*

Up to a fourth of the remaining rain forest in Brazil could be cut down over the next 20 years. More roads, dams, and gas pipelines are all planned as part of a project called "Advance Brazil." With this project the Brazilian government hopes to open up more of the Amazon basin to farming, mining, and logging.

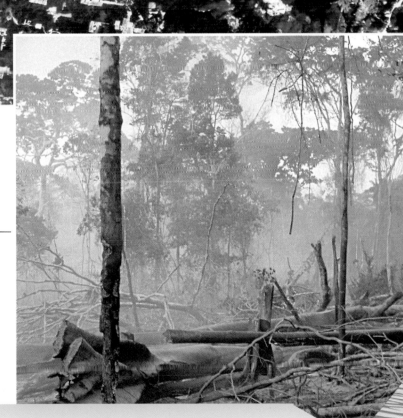

Above: A satellite image of part of the Amazonian rain forest. The lighter areas show where the land has been cleared of trees.
Right: This close-up photograph shows the devastating effects of deforestation.

New jobs will be created, and the new industries can make money for the whole country. But "Advance Brazil" is likely to cost as much as $40 billion. Its effect on the rest of the rain forest may be disastrous.

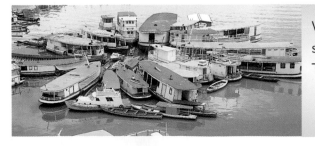

We have nearly finished our journey. The final stage takes us across the delta to the river's mouth. There are hundreds of channels in the vast delta.

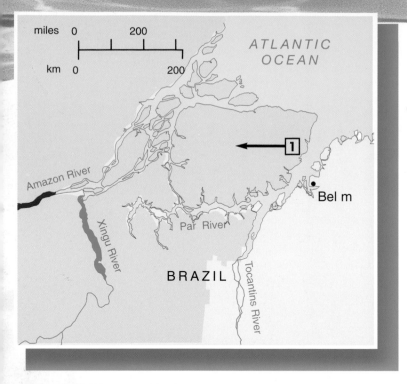

miles 0   200

km 0   200

ATLANTIC OCEAN

1

Amazon River

Xingu River

Par River

Belém

BRAZIL

Tocantins River

Below: When the Amazon River gets close to the Atlantic Ocean, it splits up into a maze of silty channels and islands.

6. Belém and the Delta

ON THE LAST STRETCH OF OUR JOURNEY, the Amazon River is very wide, and very deep. About 66 million gallons (250 million liters) of water drain from it into the Atlantic Ocean every second. Here, the river splits into a maze of channels, and dumps vast quantities of silt to form a delta. The islands of silt, like Marajó, the biggest, are home to many people. From Marajó, we will sail down the Pará River to the port of Belém. This is our final destination, close to the river's mouth.

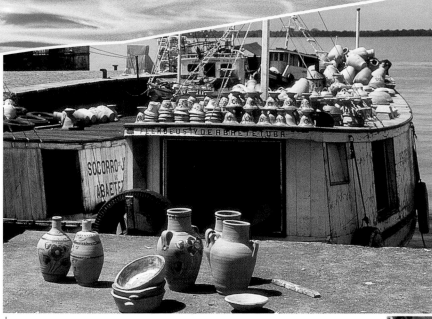

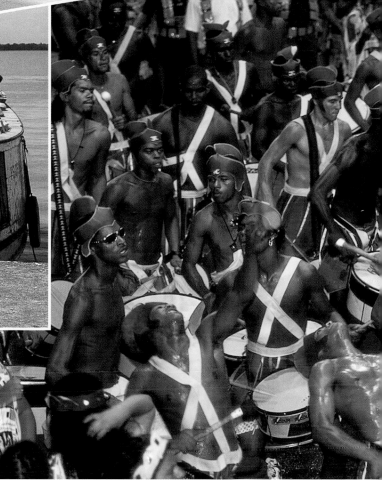

Above: Pots from Marajó Island wait to be shipped to other parts of Brazil for sale.

Right: Drums of different shapes and sizes are an important part of dances and festivals all over Brazil. The prevelance of drums in the beat of the music reflects the African heritage of many Brazilians.

📖 HISTORY *Master potters*

Marajó MAP REF: 1 is one of the largest river islands in the world. It covers an area the size of Maryland. Today, 250,000 people live there, but people have been living on Marajó for about 2,000 years. Archaeologists have found pottery buried in the ground, which gives us clues about life all those years ago.

The Aruã Indians used to live on Marajó Island. The Aruã were one of the bravest AmerIndian groups who fought the Portuguese, but they had disappeared entirely by the 1700s. The Aruã were masters of pottery.

Today, the way people make pots on Marajó is much the same as the Aruã before them. They take clay from the river bank, design and shape it into pots, and bake the pots hard in the sun before decorating them.

✋ PEOPLE *Songs of slavery*

Music and dancing on Marajó Island is also influenced by the past. Runaway African slaves found Marajó a good place to hide from their Portuguese masters. Some of those ex-slaves wrote the songs for a popular dance called the *Carimbó*. This is named after a tall drum, made from tree bark covered with deerskin on one end.

The *Carimbó* dance tells tales of sorrow. It recalls how the slaves missed their African homeland. But the dance is fun, too. Men and women dance to the rhythm of the drum in a big circle. When the women throw their handkerchiefs on the floor, their partners have to pick them up — with their mouths. That takes practice!

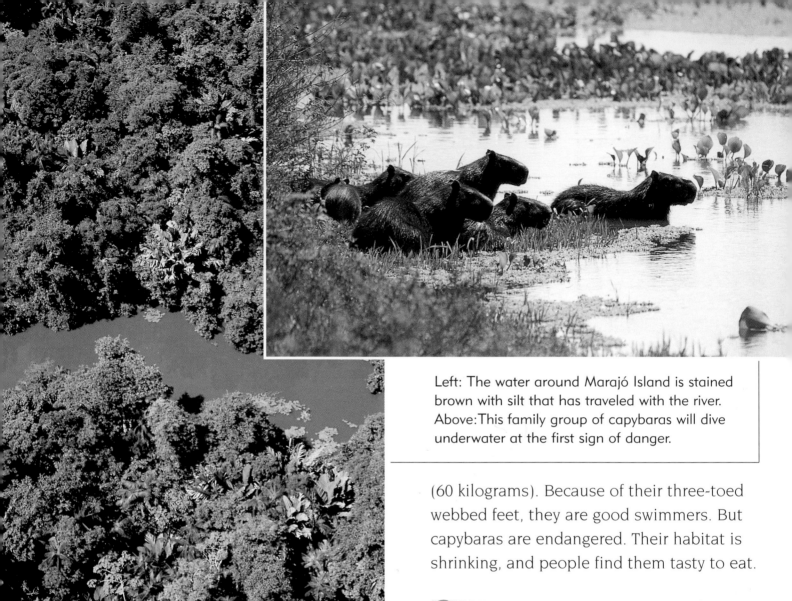

Left: The water around Marajó Island is stained brown with silt that has traveled with the river. Above: This family group of capybaras will dive underwater at the first sign of danger.

NATURE *Giant rodents*

Marajó Island is just above sea level. During the wet season in spring, parts of the island are submerged under water. Families of capybaras live in this soggy environment near the water's edge. Capybaras are the world's largest rodents. They are a little like hamsters, but they can be over three feet (one meter) tall and weigh up to 132 pounds (60 kilograms). Because of their three-toed webbed feet, they are good swimmers. But capybaras are endangered. Their habitat is shrinking, and people find them tasty to eat.

$ ECONOMY *Swimming buffalo*

Farmers have cleared many of the trees in the east of Marajó Island. This has created a large area of grassland, called a savanna. Here, farmers grow a wide range of fruits and vegetables, as well as rice.

Other farmers rear large herds of cattle and water buffalo. According to local legend, water buffalo were introduced to Marajó 100 years ago, when a ship was wrecked off the island's shores. These bulky animals cope well with Marajó's marshy, muddy grassland. They put their heads

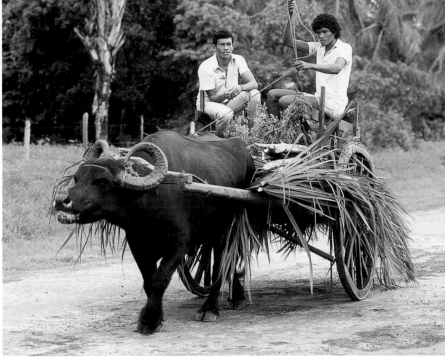

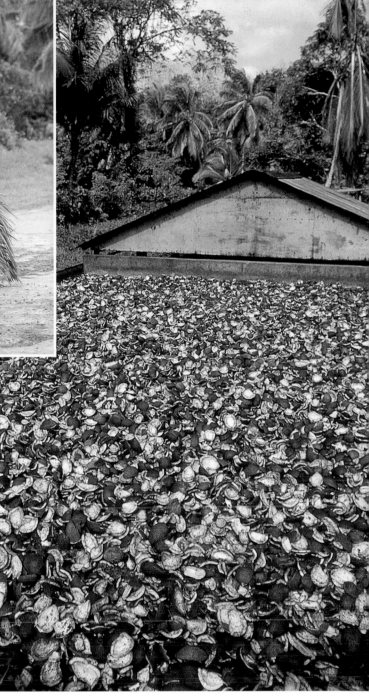

Above: Water buffalo are good work animals. Their meat and hides are the main trade on Marajó Island. Right: Coconut shells must dry in the sun before the outer fiber can be removed.

underwater to graze the flooded pasture, and they don't mind swimming.

➡️ CHANGE *Coconut shell cars*

900 families who live on Marajó Island have found a way to make money from their large supply of coconuts. Farmers sell fibers from coconut shells to a car company. These hairy fibers are used in seats, head rests, and sun visors of new cars that are sold in Brazil.

Through this new use of their coconuts, farmers earn more money than they used to. This new industry is good news for the environment, too. Unlike the synthetic materials that are often used in car parts, coconut fibers can be recycled. And, if extra coconut fibers are burned, they do not pollute the air with synthetic chemicals.

🐰 NATURE *Surfing the wave*

The ocean tides are very strong at the full moon in February and March, when spring tides pull the ocean water up the river channel. When the ocean whips back on the river, it makes a wave 10 feet (3 meters) high. Surfers arrive each year to surf the wave, called the *pororoca*. Some surfers can ride this wave for forty-five minutes!

HISTORY Boom, bust, and boom

In 1616 Belém became the first European base along the Amazon. The Portugese sent cocoa beans and spices from the Amazon basin to the outside world, but they also sent AmerIndian slaves. Fighting between Europeans and AmerIndians left many dead on both sides. The trade in slaves ended in 1888 when slavery was finally abolished in Brazil.

Like Manaus upstream, Belém earned a new lease on life from rubber. It was brought here from all over the Amazon basin in the 1900s. Today, Belém is the gateway to the world for all the treasures of the Amazon. Nearly two million people now live here.

ECONOMY Ver-O-Peso market

From Belém, a great quantity of timber from the Amazon's forest begins its journey to market. Three-quarters of the timber is sold to Brazilians, but a lot more timber is exported each year.

In the city the Ver-O-Peso ("see the weight") market was originally a place for buying and selling slaves. Today, Ver-O-Peso is a market for anything that has been transported down the river. The fish hall displays fish for eating, as well as more exotic kinds that could end up in an aquarium. Here you can buy nuts, fruit and herbs, woven straw sieves, bottled snakes, even amulets to protect you from evil spirits.

ECONOMY An Amazonian smoothie

There is great excitement along Belém's waterfront when big boats loaded with *açaí* arrive. Açaí is a fruit of a palm tree that grows on the delta's river islands. People make a healthy fruit "smoothie" by mixing *açaí* with manioc flour. Açaí ice cream is tasty, too.

To collect *açaí* fruit, children climb the palm trees to reach the bunches of fruit at the top. Açaí growers harvest from the trees, instead of cutting them down. Harvesting in this way is an example of how people can make a living from the the environment while leaving it intact for future generations to use and enjoy.

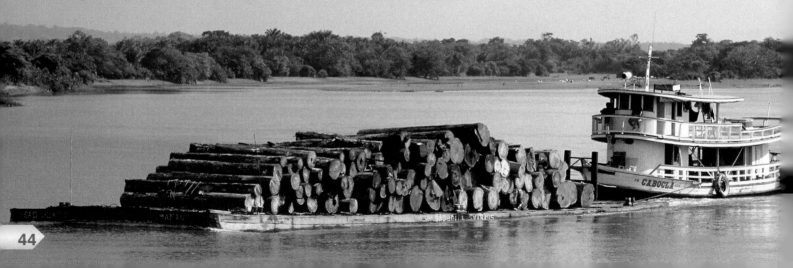

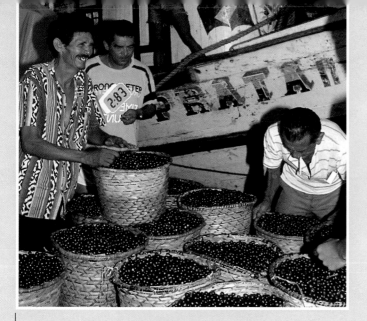

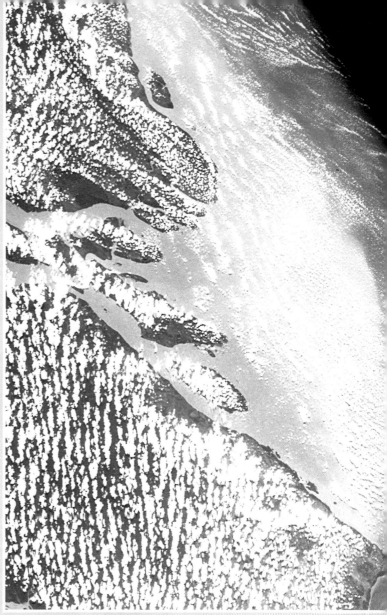

Above: *Açaí* fruit are unloaded at the waterfront in Belém, ready for sale in the market.
Right: This satellite photograph shows the Amazon River meeting the Atlantic Ocean. You can see the plumes of silt spreading into the ocean.
Below: A load of timber is transported to market down the Amazon River.

At the end of our journey, the Amazon River is 150 miles (240 kilometers) wide. If we stand on one bank, it is impossible to see across this vast stretch of water to the other side. Every day the river deposits over a million tons of silt into the ocean. Some of those particles of silt may have come with us on our journey, all the way from the Andes Mountains.

The Amazon falls three miles (5,000 meters) in the first 621 miles (1,000 kilometers) of its journey to the Atlantic Ocean.

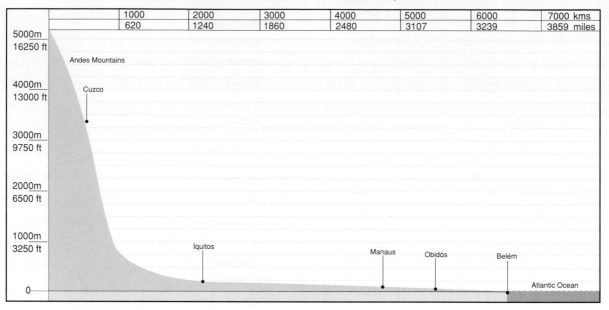

	1000	2000	3000	4000	5000	6000	7000 kms
	620	1240	1860	2480	3107	3239	3859 miles

5000m / 16250 ft
Andes Mountains
4000m / 13000 ft
Cuzco
3000m / 9750 ft
2000m / 6500 ft
1000m / 3250 ft
Iquitos
Manaus
Obidós
Belém
Atlantic Ocean
0

Further Information

Useful websites

www.korubo.com/
An exploration to find an isolated Amazon tribe, the Tsohon-Djapa Indians. This site ncludes a photo gallery.

www.amazonwatch.org/
Amazon Watch works with people in the Amazon basin to protect the environment and the rights of AmerIndians.

//www.pbs.org/journeyintoamazonia/
A well-illustrated website that looks at different issues in the Amazon Basin.

www.pbs.org/wgbh/nova/shaman/
The site explores the Yanomami Indians and their way of life.

www.eduweb.com/amazon.html
Life in the Ecuadorian Amazon and the Quichua people who call it home. Includes games and online activities.

www.ran.org/info_center/index.html
The Rainforest Action Network website with lots of information and learning activities for school.

Photographic sites

www.grid.inpe.br/images.html
Satellite photos of the Amazon and its surrounding forest. The text on this site is in Spanish.

www.amazon-ecotours.com/Photos.htm
Photos of the upper parts of the Amazon river in Peru.

www.amazonthefilm.com
Photos, a quiz, and part of a film about the Amazon river

Books

Kallen, Stuart A. *Life in the Amazon Rain Forest*. Farmington Hills, Mich: Gale Group, 1999.

Montgomery, Sy. *Encantado: Pink Dolphin of the Amazon*. Boston: Houghton Mifflin, 2002

Pirotta, Saviour, and Becky Gryspeerdt (illustrator). Chicago: Raintree, 1999.

Glossary

amulet   something worn as protection against evil

architect   someone who designs new buildings, parks and bridges

archaeologist   someone who studies the remains of ancient civilizations

bank   side of a river

bauxite   mineral produced from rock, used to make aluminum

canal   artificial channel of water, cut for navigation or irrigation

Catholicism   beliefs and practices of the Catholic Church

cereal   farm crops that produce grains such as wheat

channel   passage through which a river flows

cholera   disease of the stomach

confluence   place where two rivers meet

current   flow of water in a certain direction

dam   barrier that holds or diverts water

decompose   rot and break down

deforestation   clearance of trees from land that was once covered by forest

delta   geographical feature at the mouth of a river, formed by the build-up of sediment

descent   downward change in height

diarrhea   bacterial infection of the stomach

downstream   toward the mouth of the river

drainage basin   area of land drained by a river and its tributaries

dredge   clear or deepen a waterway or port, by scooping or sucking up sediment

ecotourism   touring natural habitats in a way that tries to minimize environmental damage

floodplain   flat part of a river valley that is submerged during floods

gradient   steepness of land, or steepness of the fall of water

habitat   natural home of animals and plants

malaria   parasitic disease carried by mosquitos

manganese   hard, greyish white metal used to strengthen steel

mercury   silvery white, poisonous metal

nomads   people who move around to find work or food or water

nutrients   food. Plants use minerals as food

parasite   living thing that feeds off another living thing, without helping its host in any way

plantation   large farm

plate   part of the earth's crust

poacher   someone who hunts or fishes illegally on someone else's land

predator   animal that hunts and eats other animals

rapids   fast-moving stretches of water

sap   watery liquid that flows through a plant, carrying nutrients like sugars, salts, and minerals

shaman   priest who has special abilities to contact the spirit world

silt   a deposit of the matter that settles to the bottom of liquid. Silt is smaller than sand, but larger than clay.

sonar   system using sound waves that can travel underwater and spot any objects that may lie ahead

source   where a river begins

tides   rise and fall of an ocean's water as it is pulled by the Moon and the Sun

tributary   stream or river that flows into a larger stream or river

tuber   fleshy stem or root of a plant

tunnel vision   problem with eyesigh that means you can only see in front of you and not to the side

upstream   toward the source of the river

yellow fever   disease carried by mosquitos

Index

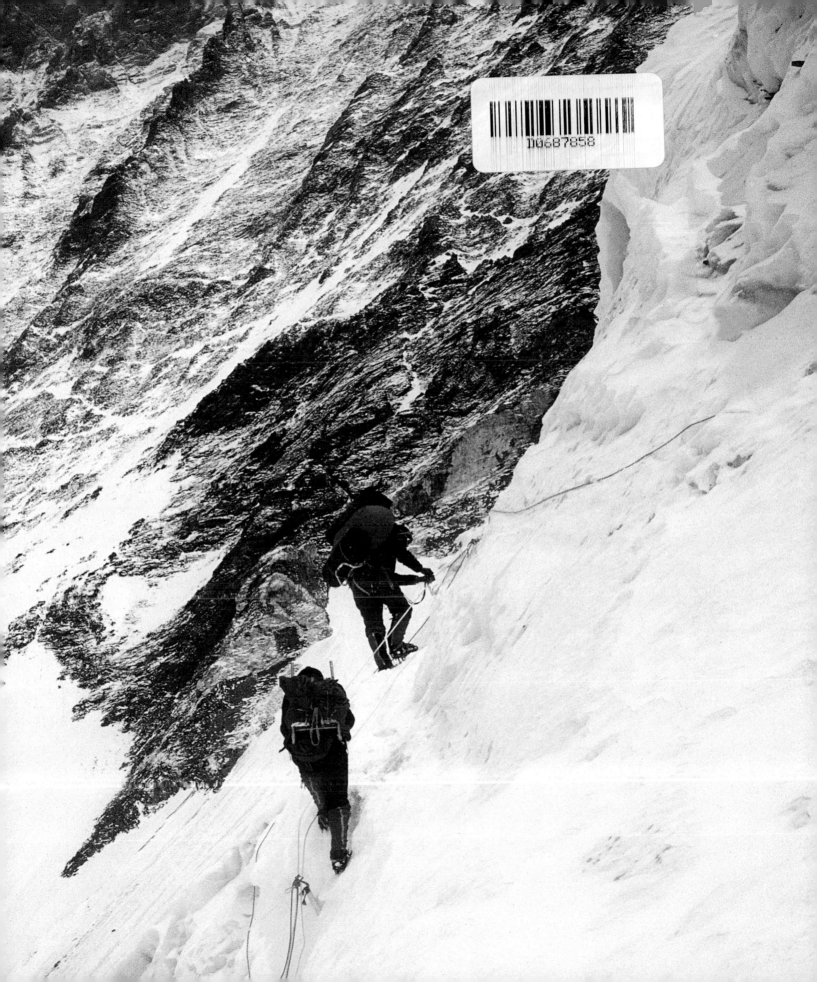

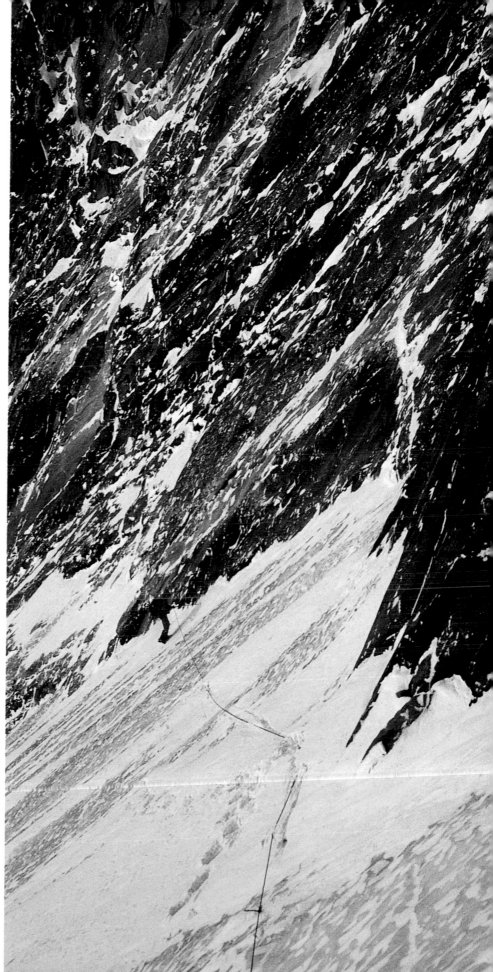

'All history is legend. Every era, indeed almost every generation, aspires to a different ideal and it is this ideal that alters one's view of the individual phases of history.'

EGON FRIEDELL

'One hundred years had elapsed since the beginnings of mountaineering before the Matterhorn could be conquered and a further 100 years of experience were necessary before thoughts turned to the possibility of climbing the most difficult faces on the 8000m peaks. Today, these walls present a similar set of problems for the new generation of mountaineers as the North Face of the Matterhorn once did for those climbers operating after the First World War.'

REINHOLD MESSNER

On the North-West Face of Annapurna I. The traverse at about 6000m into the big gully in the centre of the face.

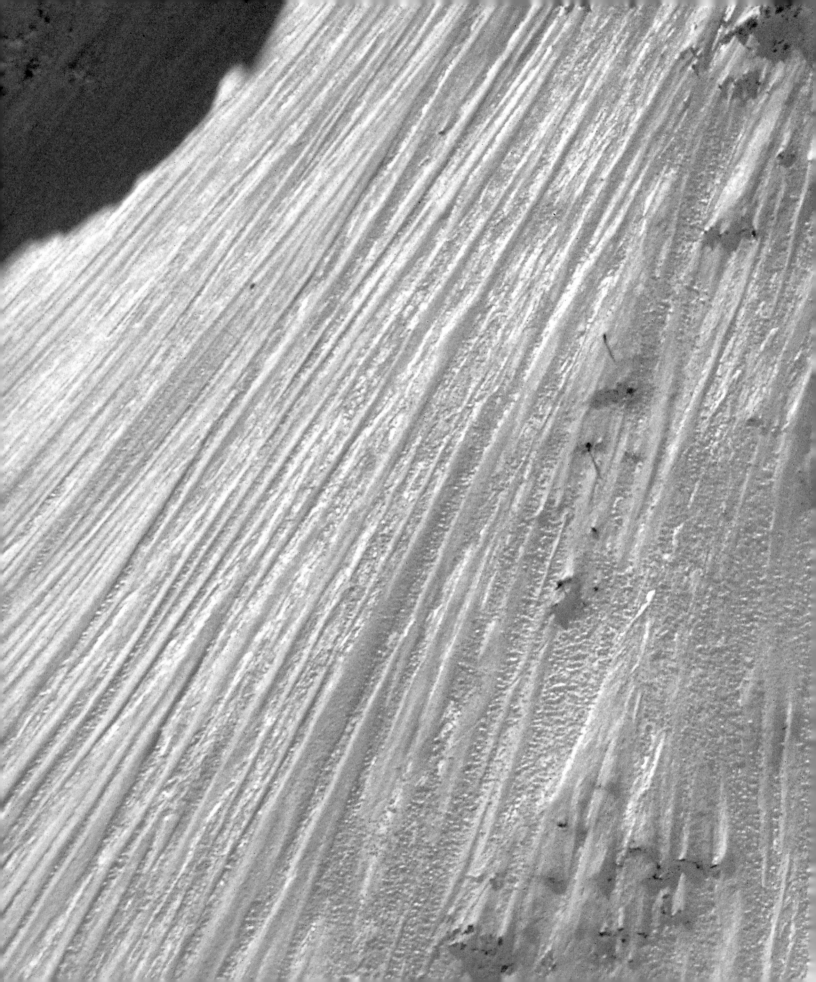

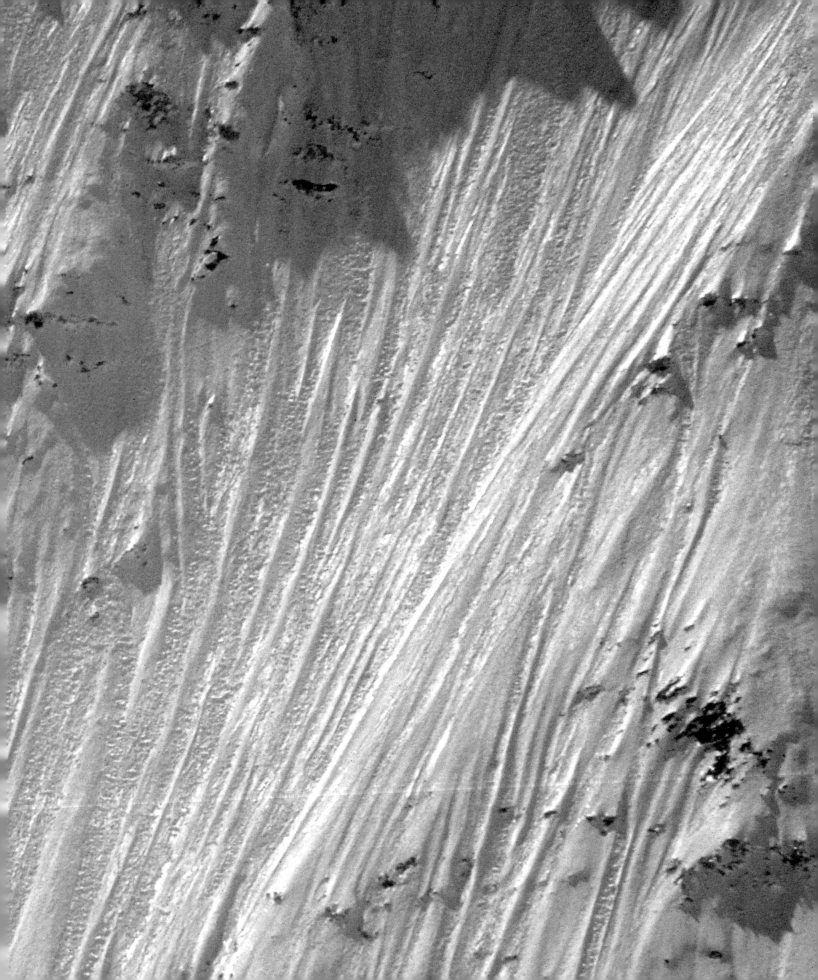

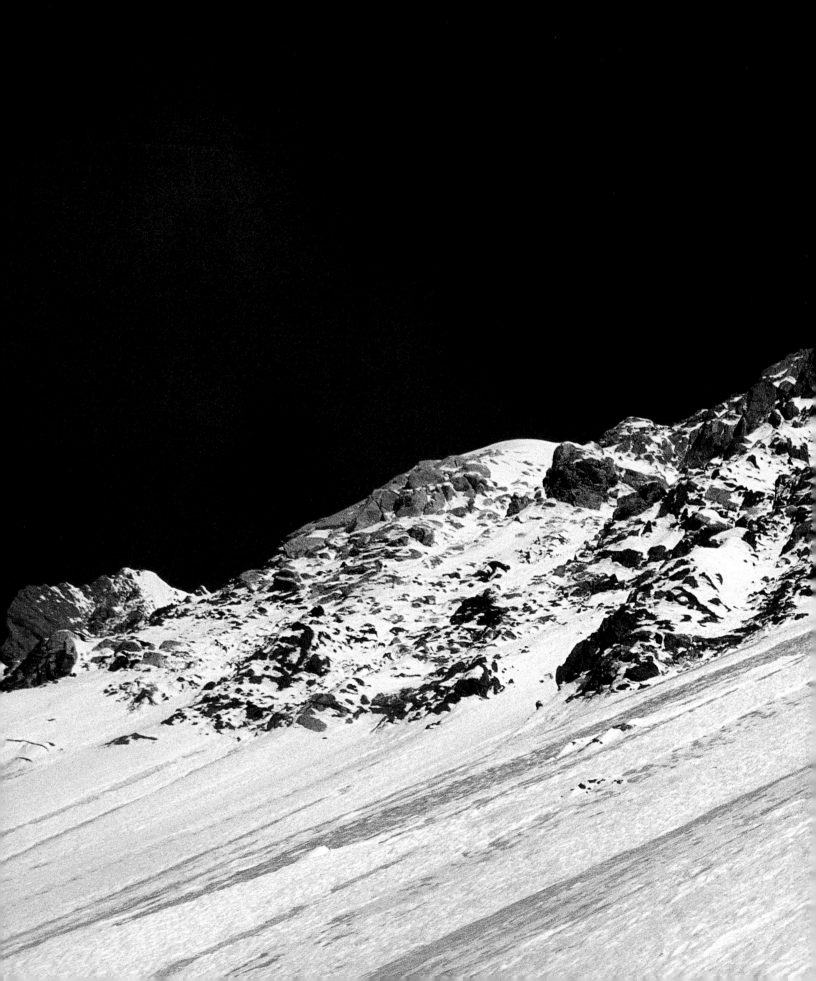

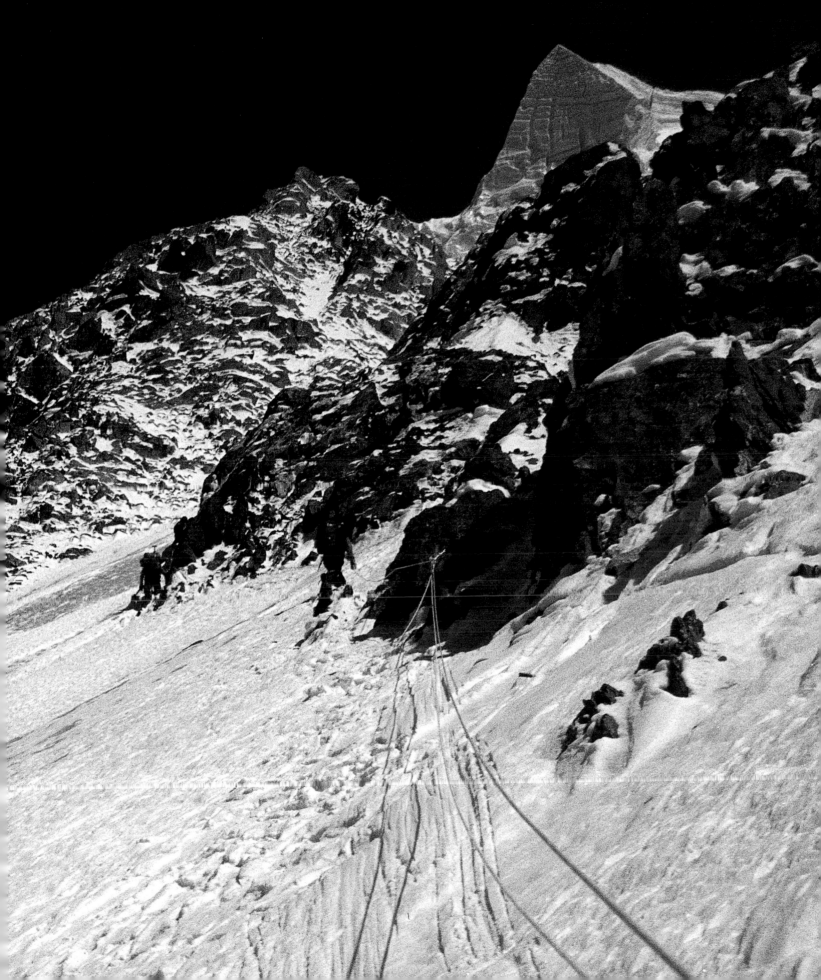

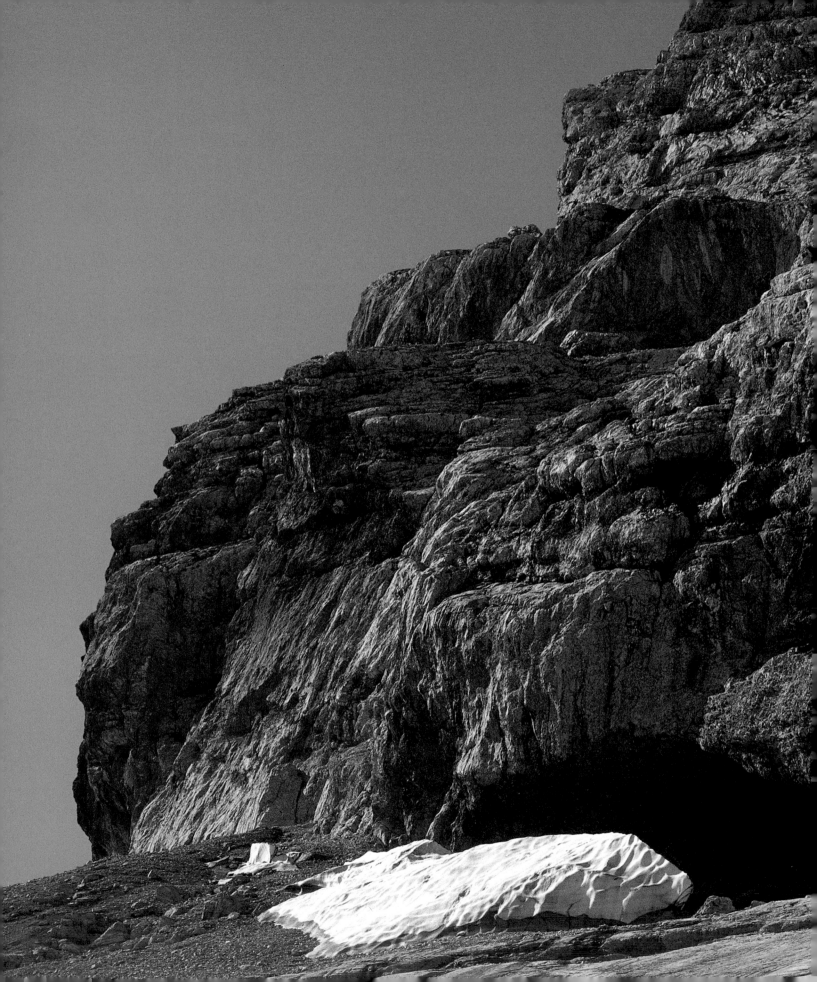

REINHOLD MESSNER

THE BIG WALLS

From the North Face of the Eiger to the South Face of Dhaulagiri

TRANSLATED BY TIM CARRUTHERS

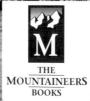

THE
MOUNTAINEERS
BOOKS

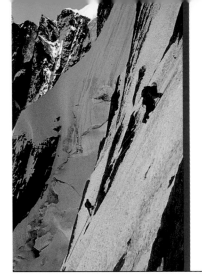

The camp on the big ice field below the summit wall on the South Face of Aconcagua (Andes, 1974).

Climbing the ice-covered Walker Spur on the Grandes Jorasses (Alps, 1966).

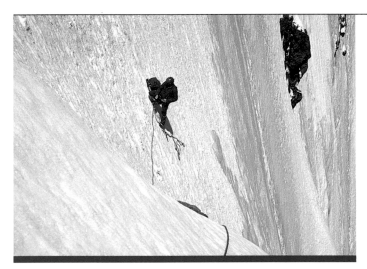

On the Breach Wall of Kilimanjaro (East Africa, 1978).

The Ogre from the summit of Latok II after the first ascent of the West Face (Karakorum, 1997).

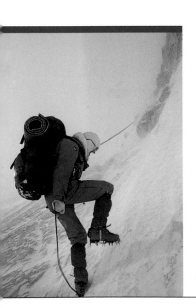

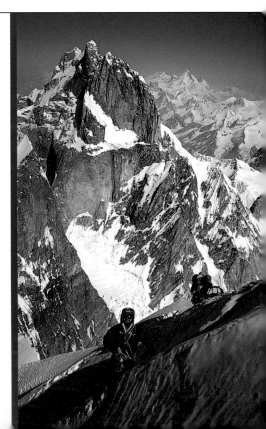

'On all my mountaineering excursions, the most important thing was never the summits, nor the successes or the fame. Ultimately, the most important thing was the discoveries I made about myself, discoveries that are always new and that have taught me again and again to view the relationship between myself and my surroundings, my world, in new ways.'

REINHOLD MESSNER

Descent in a snow storm after the first ascent of the North-West Face of Annapurna (Himalaya, 1985).

Contents

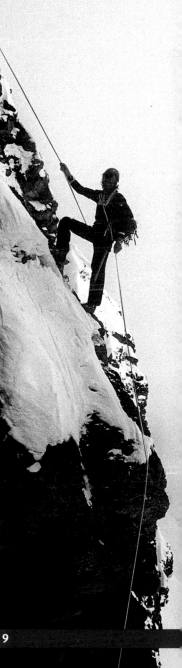

Reinhold Messner retreating from the South Face of Dhaulagiri (Himalaya, 1977).

9

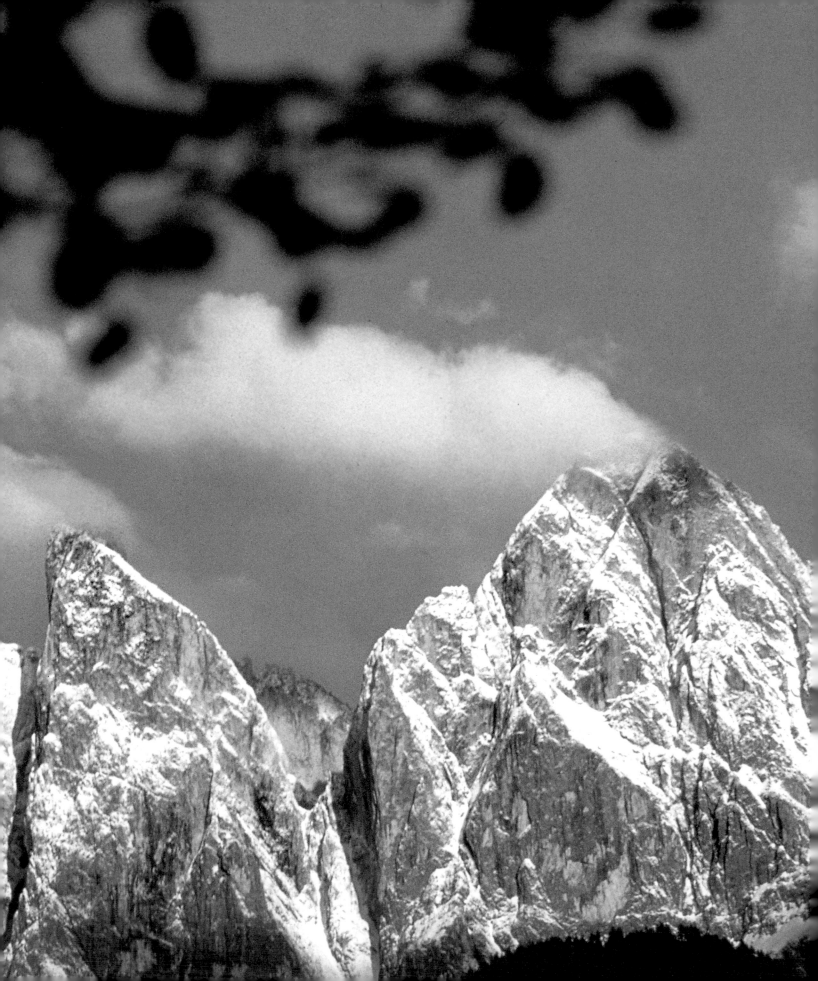

WALLS AND SUMMITS

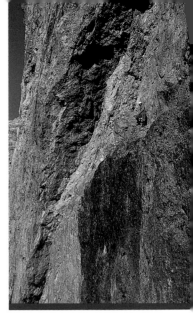

Since childhood I have been fascinated by the Big Walls. When at the age of 16, together with my younger brother Günther, I climbed the North Face of the Sass Rigais in our local Geislerspitzen I had already heard about the Eiger North Face but knew nothing of the Aconcagua South Face or the Rupal Flank. Thus it was the Eigerwand that was the distant goal for which we secretly strove.

That we did not attempt it that same summer was due to the fact that our respect for this great face was as nebulous as its reputation. In those days I also held all other mountaineers in high regard, naturally placing myself at the bottom of the pecking order, and if one of them invited me to join him on a route I invariably seconded. In doing so I learnt a great deal. From Sepp Meyer, a church tower roofer from South Tyrol, I learnt how to set up belays; from Heini Holzer from South Tyrol, a chimney sweep, how to dismiss those worries which I had initially when doing extreme routes on the big faces.

Although to begin with I was mainly concerned with overcoming the difficulties of any particular mountain route, with the more distant mountains the summit suddenly took on a far greater importance. The summit, the point at which all towering lines converge, reached after days, often even weeks of climbing, had something liberating, something releasing, something final about it, even though the descent has to follow an ascent and even though, on

seven and eight thousanders, the descent is often even more dangerous that the climb itself.

Every mountaineer chooses his mountains for different reasons, and today in the age of alpinism as a leisure pursuit, all reasons are legitimate. I found the greatest personal satisfaction – a kind of release – on high summits, reached by climbing hard Big Walls.

It was neither records nor sensation and glory which attracted me, but much more the challenge; those possibilities on the mountain which lie somewhere between the taboo and the 'maybe it is possible after all', a sporting game which in earlier centuries would have been called adventure. It does not consist of the search for danger, still less in playing with death; it is that 'step into the unknown', which occurs between the start of the climb and the summit and shapes the whole range of inner tensions.

You do not have to be a daredevil in order to brave the Big Walls. Experience, tenacity, mental preparation, planning and above all discipline are necessary in order to be capable of mastering those unexpected borderline situations.

Playfulness and seriousness, success and failure, life and death so often keep close company up there, as do heat and cold, sunshine and storm, rock and ice.

Nevertheless, no one who takes their first tentative steps into these borderline areas is a

On the middle section of the North Face of Sass Rigais.

(left): Furchetta (left) and the North Face of Sass Rigais in the Geisler Group, Dolomites.

HISTORY AND LEGENDS

We mountaineers constantly feed our desires with new ideals. Yet throughout it is the 'Big Walls' that have remained a constant, even if what each successive generation of mountaineers describes as a 'problem' has continued to increase in difficulty, height and danger. Every era of mountaineering has found its own challenges and the successes, told in the language of their own time, have given a conclusive picture of the spirit of the age. As if the problems and solutions were not merely invented!

In order to be true to the history of great wall mountaineering and in order not to falsify the stories that go with it, in this book I allow every generation a chance to speak – with their dreams, and in the language of their time – all those who on the mountain were not merely looking for the summit. Thus, the original reports remain at the heart of this account, even if the authors are still idealizing. These original reports, and the unfalsified statements of the protagonists, are the sources of those emotions which mirror the feeling of life of 'Big Wall mountaineering'.

'Lammer did not consider the myth of invincibility a deterrent but a challenge.'

FRITZ SCHMITT

hero. A hero amongst mountaineers does not survive very long. Knowing no fear he would merely perish, never to return.

Only man, man with all his everyday fears and weaknesses, his powers of reason and his instinctive desire to survive, has a chance up there. Only those who maintain respect in the face of these Big Walls, a respect which is absolutely necessary in order to survive on them, can manage this.

Sometimes when I climbed it all went easily and elegantly and when making the decision whether to turn back or to carry on everything was so logical, without problems or danger. It seemed as if nothing was meant to go wrong, everything could be solved quickly or changed and adapted to suit the situation. And then suddenly, perhaps just a little while later, nothing more could be changed. I felt as if there were no way out. And every step I took was determined by the mountain or by the forces of nature and was heavy with Fate.

To escape from such life-threatening situations when they last for longer periods is certainly not easy. If one believes the tales of the heroes, they fought against Death, rebelled against it and thus overcame it. I do not believe them.

For my part, I have never consciously tried to overpower death, never defended myself against it.

On those occasions when there has been a prolonged threat to my life, I have instinctively withdrawn into myself and surrendered myself to what was coming as if in a state of intoxication or shock.

Memories from a few of these borderline situations still live on in my mind and as I sit here writing down the most exciting of them I can see the clear starry sky over Mont Blanc just as it was on the bivouac on the Walker Spur. I can feel the soles of my boots slipping in the exit cracks of the North Face of the Eiger, feel the icy wind on my face on the summit ridge of Aconcagua. Gasping for breath, I cower on the summit rocks of the Matterhorn North Face, while loose snow-slides pour over me. For days I have been descending the Diamir Valley – alone, exhausted, half dead, my brother missing – after the Rupal Face on Nanga Parbat.

The expeditions or routes which ran smoothly and which we mention just in passing are quickly forgotten. But there are others that are not so easy to talk about and that cause upset. These are the ones I will never forget. They lie considerably deeper. Their shadows, fears and experiences will accompany me for a lifetime. They are my 'treasures', brought down from the Big Walls.

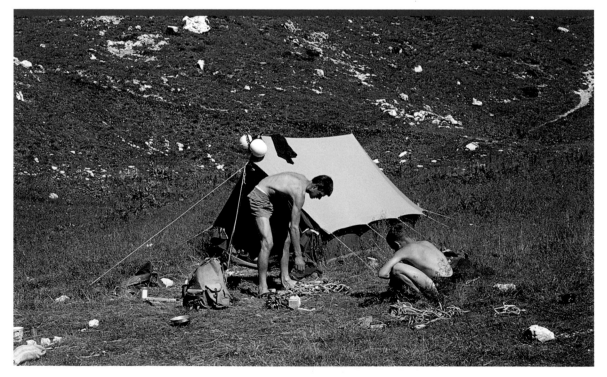

Reinhold Messner with Heini Holzer in 1966 in their camp at the Coldaisee in the Civetta, from where they achieved a dozen big walls in just two weeks.

BIG WALLS – LAST PROBLEMS

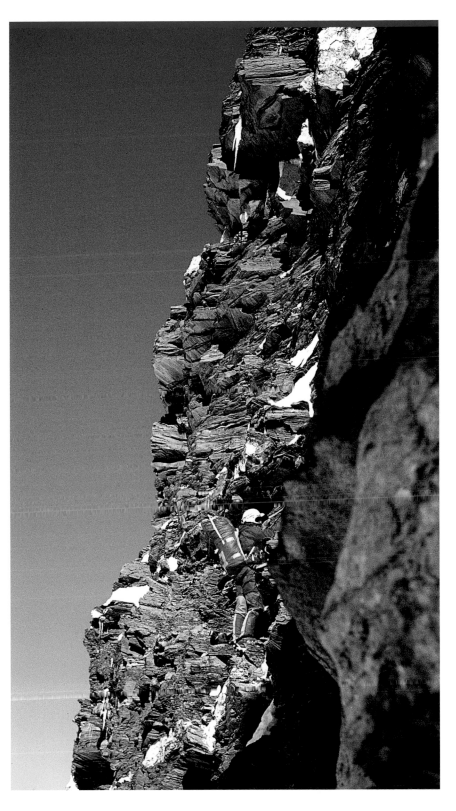

In the years following the First World War the first of the extremely difficult faces of the Alps were climbed. In fact Preuss, Haupt and Dibona had already become amazingly skilled at free climbing but had not yet had the chance to prove this on the biggest faces. It is true that Dibona had been the first to climb the mighty South Face of the Croz dell'Altissimo, but he had failed on the North Face of the Furchetta, as did Hans Dülfer shortly after him. The summit fall line of the Civetta North-West Face had also proved too big, too difficult and too unpredictable an undertaking given the stage of development of alpinism at the time. The East Faces of Monte Rosa and the Watzmann had already been climbed in the second half of the nineteenth century and surpassed the greatest of the Dolomites' faces in terms of length and sheer dimensions, but they lacked that extraordinary technical difficulty, that steepness that distinguishes a flank from a 'Big Wall' and turns it into a 'last problem'. Steepness and level of difficulty were the ingredients that Emil Solleder was looking for on the great Dolomite walls in the mid-twenties and about which he wrote in his essay 'Die letzten grossen Wandprobleme in den Dolomiten' (the Last Big Wall Problems in the Dolomites).

But it was in the Western Alps that these so-called 'last problems' were sought, where, in addition to the pure rock climbing difficulties, there were also ice passages to contend with, and where sudden changes in the weather and bivouacs were also a part of the game.

We know that later on difficult routes were established in all the climbing areas of the world and that there are still countless 'last problems' to be resolved. Although the greatest mixed routes in the world were technically no more difficult than those in the Alps, they were much bigger, covered in ice and much more dangerous. Thus the giant flanks in the Andes, in the Pamirs, in the Himalaya and in the Karakorum are more risky , and it is there that people still look for, and find, what for the last 100 years have been referred to as the 'last problems'.

At 6200m on the South Face of Lhotse. This Yugoslavian attempt in 1981 got as far as the summit ridge.

THE NOTION OF IMPREGNABILITY

The North Face of the Liskamm (left) and the Matterhorn in the Valais Alps.

It is the Big Walls that provide the best canvas for the portrayal of mountaineering development and achievement up to the present day. And the changing motives, echoed in the differing reports of the mountaineers from the various eras, are best documented in relation to these walls.

To the mountaineers of today it may well seem like a fairytale that 100 years ago there were still many great mountain faces in the Alps on which not a single route had been climbed; hidden faces that for decades had attracted the interested glances of the best alpinists.

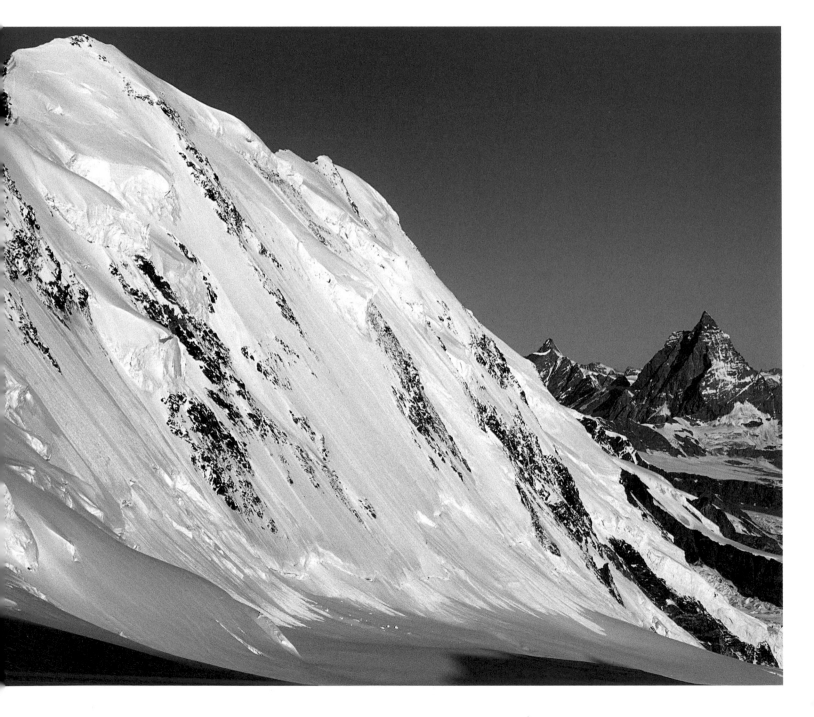

Big Walls cannot be confused. Like human faces, each wall has its own personality, none is like any other. In their form, their structure, their rock type, their height, they are just as diverse as human personalities. Yes, walls have a personality.

All these walls have their own story too. It is not just the story of their conquering, when a route into the uncertain is pieced together like a puzzle from cracks and traverses, overhangs and hidden corners into an overall picture. Successes and tragedies form part of it as well. Only with the repeated attempts at climbing them are these walls graded and evaluated, feared and yet climbed over and over again. How often did walls lose their reputation with the passage of time, only to be rediscovered at a later date? But a word of caution: every great achievement only carries the relative stamp of the ultimate for a couple of decades. Thereafter there are new goals, new dimensions, new benchmarks.

The topic of the 'Big Walls' has not yet been exhausted, even after half a dozen eras – from the 'Walls of the Alps' to the 'Walls of the World' the final chapter of the encounter of man versus mountain has not yet been written. What pessimists have maintained for 100 years is nothing more than obfuscation; like foggy weather, it passes.

Unfortunately, original accounts are not available for all the first ascents of famous walls; during the last decade in particular, routes have been successfully climbed about which we know little far away from the famous peaks.

Beatrice Tomasson left little recorded information about her climb on the South Face of the Marmolada. Otto Schück too wrote little about the Watzmann East Face and Nicolas Jaeger uttered not one syllable about his attempt on the South Face of Lhotse. There are gaps in the Big Wall chronicles.

Initially, it was the high mountains which modern mountaineers were interested in climbing. Financial interests played a part in the conquering of the summits. Horace Bénédict de Saussure, a naturalist from Geneva, offered a large reward for the first person to find the route to the summit of Mont Blanc, or indeed climb it, before finally climbing it himself. The man who initiated the first ascent of the Grossglockner thirteen years later was the Prince-Bishop of Gurk, Franz von Salm-Reifferscheid. Archduke Johann of Austria was the driving force behind the ascent of the Ortler.

Above all, however, it was humankind's innate curiosity that was satisfied by the myth of impregnability. It was this that consistently held them back and challenged them at one and the same time. Between the East Face of Monte Rosa and the South Face of Dhaulagiri, there are almost 130 years and 8000km as the crow flies. But the difference in the spirits of those who climbed them is not great.

The race to climb the Big Walls began after the ascent of the Matterhorn. This mountain had stood as a symbol of impregnability until 1865. In the same year Adolphus Warburton Moore and his friends, accompanied by their guides Jakob and Melchior Anderegg, dared to climb the Brenva Flank of Mont Blanc. Thus the era of 'conquering' the great Alpine summits drew to a close and, in 1872, Taylor and the Pendlebury brothers from England, guided by Ferdinand Imseng and Gabriel Spechtenhauser, forced a route up the highest mountain face in the Alps, the avalanche-prone East Face of Monte Rosa. In spite of the length and the danger of the route – on the ice the guides had always shown their tenacity and skill – initially there were no accidents, until 1881, when Marinelli, Imseng and Pedranzini were swept to their deaths by an ice avalanche. Thereafter, for almost 100 years, the East Face of Monte Rosa East Wall held true to the idealized notion portrayed in mountaineering literature, where it promised only danger, death and fear.

In 1881 the East Face of the Watzmann was climbed. With this ascent, the boundary of achievement in rock climbing had increased by a whole level of difficulty. Suddenly the Eastern Alps found themselves at the centre of Big Wall mountaineering. The level of rock climbing difficulty, the height of the face and its orientation now became the new criteria for the ultimate challenges.

Thus, even 100 years ago, mountaineering was already concerned with Big Walls and the style of the ascent. Otto Herzog had already climbed the crux pitch on the north side of the Laliderer Wall when he and his partner Karl Hannemann were driven back by the onset of bad weather. He had to leave the first ascent to the Dolomite guides Dibona and Rizzi and the Mayer brothers. In 1911 the Laliderer Wall was considered to be the most difficult route in the world. During the same year, the guides Knubel and Brocherel, together with the

'The first of the three great problems had been overcome, the second was showing resistance and brought defeat and disappointment. But the will to win had not been broken.'

ANDERL HECKMAIR

'On the Troll Wall we transported most of the equipment about 80m higher: 800m of rope, 200 pitons, including several of the American type for the very wide cracks of up to 20cm; 200 expansion bolts, sleeping bags and normal winter equipment, provisions and fuel for about fourteen days and a radio transmitter – altogether about 200kg.'

ODD ELIASSEN

British climbers Jones, Young and Todhunter, established an equally difficult route on the granite slabs of the Grépon's East Face.

Then in 1925 the 'last Big Wall problems' of the Dolomites were solved. Emil Solleder showed what he was capable of with his ascents of the North Face of the Furchetta and, above all, the North-West Face of the Civetta. People began to talk of new dimensions.

In the thirties it was the 'three last problems' of the Alps which made the headlines – the North Faces of the Matterhorn, the Grandes Jorasses and the Eiger. In 1931 the brothers Toni and Franz Schmid climbed the dangerous Matterhorn North Face, a climb which had been attempted many times already and one which even Solleder had cast a loving eye over. With only fifteen rock and ice pitons and with simple Tricouni nails on the soles on their boots, they climbed the dark wall of the Matterhorn in two days, 'an irresponsible but wonderful success', according to Colonel Strutt of the English Alpine Club. In 1932 the Olympic Committee awarded a gold medal for the ascent, the first time that such an award had been bestowed for outstanding mountaineering achievement.

The battle for the North Face of the Grandes Jorasses was to prove even more dogged. There were attempts and there were deaths on this 1200m high rock and ice wall. At his second attempt in 1935 Rudolf Peters, together with Martin Meier, climbed the face to the Pointe Croz, which was the greatest achievement in his life. New twelve-point crampons, an ice axe and the experience gained during the previous year had all helped. The mood amongst the 'mountain vagabonds' was buoyant, their motto was 'higher, steeper, harder!'

Thus it was that the 1800m North Face of the Eiger in the Bernese Alps became the 'last great problem of all'. Unfortunately it was soon stamped with the label 'Wall of Death' as Sedlmayr, Mehringer, Angerer, Rainer, Hinterstoisser, Kurz, Sandri and Menti had all died on it. In 1938 Anderl Heckmair and Ludwig Vörg joined forces with Heinrich Harrer and Fritz Kasparek during their ascent. They made it – just. 'Anything is allowed if you are successful!' was the answer the 'victors' gave to those of their peers who pointed a critical finger at them.

But the French too dared to venture onto the Big Walls. Pierre Alain and Raymond Leininger caused a sensation with their success on the North Face of the Dru. Then it was the turn of the Italians.

Riccardo Cassin, who in 1935 together with Vittorio Ratti had won the 'race' for the North Face of the Cima Ovest, survived a storm on the enormous sweep of slabs on the North-East Face of the Badile in 1937 and in 1938 achieved one of the greatest first ascents in the Alps – the Walker Spur on the Grandes Jorasses! He thus became the most successful mountaineer of his time.

After the Second World War it was not only the equipment which was constantly being improved. Vibram soles, multiple-rung etriers, artificial-fibre ropes, climbing harnesses and safety helmets all came into fashion. The options for travelling were also becoming much more varied and with this the sum of experiences became greater. All these changes brought more room for manoeuvre and improvements in safety. Soon, new direct lines on the Big Walls were being found and climbed, for example on the Civetta Wall, the West Face of the Dru, El Capitan in California and Trollryggen in Norway. Thousand-metre Big Walls were becoming the focus of attention.

For the Eiger North Face Direttissima another style was needed, employing alternating teams and fixed ropes. In February/March 1966 there was a successful attempt on the Eiger Direttissima which took thirty-one days; twenty of those were climbing days. Two-hundred and ten pitons, eight of them drilled, were placed and used on the 1800m face. And that was merely the beginning. How many routes had been added to those on the Eigerwand and the North Face of the Grandes Jorasses in the meantime? Dozens! Most of them, however, were established in the classical style. The 'impregnable' no longer existed.

Although 'Big Wall expeditions' in the style of the Eiger Direct did not yet signify a turning point in alpinism, all of a sudden new opportunities began to present themselves, particularly on the Big Walls of the Himalaya, a phase that would start in earnest in 1970.

Shortly before that, during the Matterhorn Jubilee year in 1965, Walter Bonatti set out to establish a new climb on the wintry North Face of the Matterhorn, thus bringing the classical age of Big Wall climbing in the Alps to a temporary end and at the same time leaving a monument to mountaineering achievement. Now, the myth of the impregnable could once more be revived and applied to the Big Walls of the eight thousanders, where it would grow to reach new and dizzy heights.

THE UPS AND DOWNS OF IMPROVED PERFORMANCE

What we call Big Wall climbing nowadays actually began back in 1865 with the ascent of the Brenva Flank on Mont Blanc. From then on, the route became the objective. As the routes became steeper and steeper, the objectives became lower, but only by a matter of metres and only until the Dolomite walls became the focus of attention.

In 1938, about sixteen years after the North Face of Monte Agnér, the greatest of the difficult Dolomite walls, had been climbed, the North Wall of the Eiger was conquered. It was the most spectacular first ascent in the race for the 'three last problems in the Alps'.

Sixteen years later again, in 1954, a French expedition worked its way up the 3000m high South Face of Aconcagua. Their ascent signified the next step in extreme mountaineering, since the level of difficulty on rock and ice was no less than on the great Alpine faces, yet the size was considerably greater. Furthermore, this route was at almost 7000m above sea level and therefore at an altitude at which the low oxygen pressure means a considerable increase in the overall level of difficulty.

After this 'last problem' it seemed as if it would be impossible to find anything more difficult. Yet once again, another sixteen years on in 1970, the Rupal Wall on Nanga Parbat was climbed, the greatest of the giant faces in the Himalaya. The route up this 4500m-high rock and ice flank leads to the summit of one of the fourteen eight thousanders, at an altitude which man can only endure for a very short length of time and then only after weeks of acclimatization.

In 1986, at long last, the Pole Jerzy Kukuczka led a team up the South Face of K2. After their ascent of this wall people once again spoke of the 'last problem' but, of course, an increase in performance is always possible. After the big faces of Lhotse and Dhaulagiri, even a direct route on the West Face of Makalu is now an objective worthy of serious thought.

It took six mountaineering generations from the conquest of the North Face of Monte Agnér until the first ascent of the South Face of Dhaulagiri, eighty years of attempts, effort, sacrifice and, above all, the countless personal experiences that came out of it.

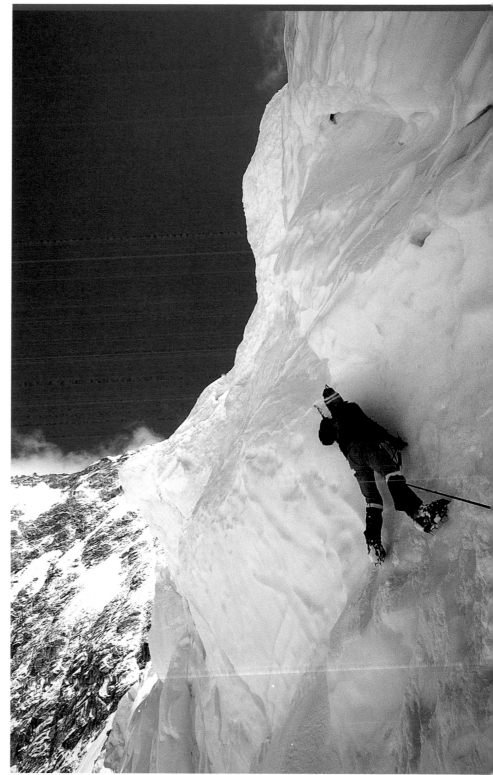

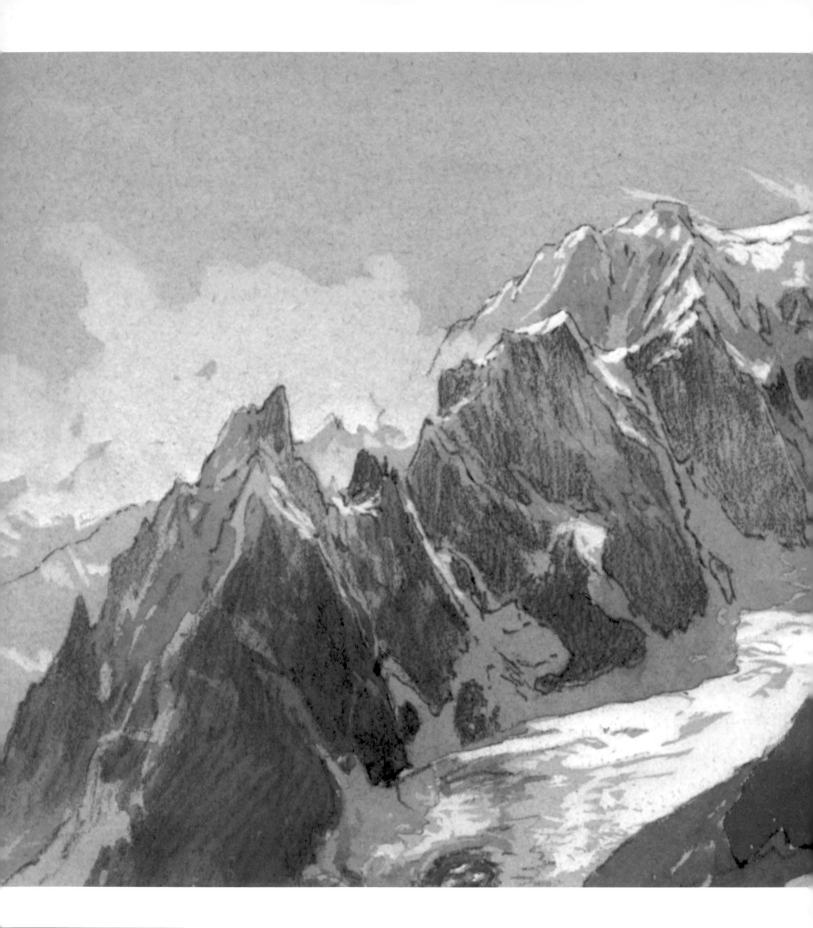

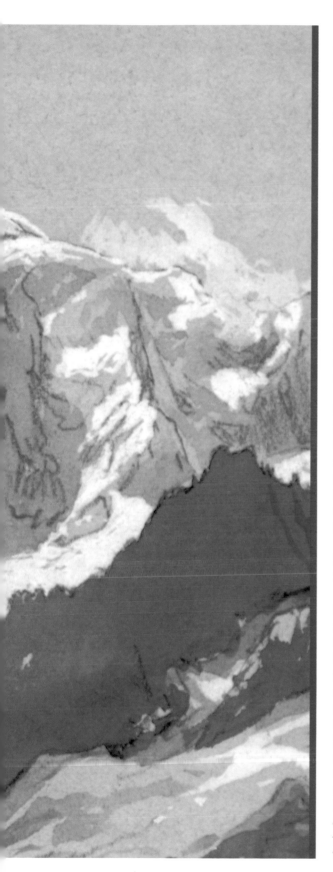

BEGINNINGS

As far as the development of the Western Alps is concerned, the heyday was without doubt the Golden Age of 1855–65. The English stacked up ascent upon ascent. In the Bernese and Valais Alps, their preferred territory, they also achieved great first ascents. But in the Mont Blanc Group too the English and their Swiss guides were celebrating a glittering decade of success on the high mountains of the Alps.

As the sixties became the seventies, increased levels of ability on high mountain routes brought a sea-change in mountaineering, as attention turned to steeper and ever rockier terrain. Once again the Mont Blanc group gained in importance and subsequent developers discovered the Dauphiné. The age of 'alpinism as the pursuit of difficulty' had begun, and it began with the growing curiosity about the unclimbed faces of mountains already climbed and with the race to climb the Big Walls.

For Kennedy, Moore, George, Stephen and Walker, and not least for Whymper, alpinism had become more a matter of conquering and sporting achievement than enjoyment of nature. But eager competition for the highest and most difficult summits, which left hardly any room for the time-consuming, arduous and distracting observations of scientific nature, aroused curiosity, above all a curiosity for even more difficult things.

In 1865 the search for new routes began. Difficulty was sought for difficulty's sake. It became an obsession.

One of the great mountaineering characters during these years was the Briton A.W. Moore, a first class all-round mountaineer, whose great climbs were all undertaken in the period from 1862–65. From Bernina via the Bernese Oberland he roamed the Western Alps until he came to the Dauphiné. His route led him over many summits and across countless passes: Piz Roseg, Gross-Fiescherhorn, Obergabelhorn, Mont Blanc from the Brenva Glacier. Indeed the ascent of Mont Blanc via the Brenva Flank undertaken by Moore, together with G.S. Matthews, both Walkers and the Anderegg guides is not only his most significant achievement, it was a new beginning. For years it was considered to be one of the most important ice routes in the Alps. Today this route still demands experience, stamina and 'careful handling of the ice technology'.

'In the beginnings of alpinism it was only wealthy people who climbed the mountains and even as early as 125 years ago the Viennese Paul Graham used up his entire fortune in order to conquer the most important summits of the Dolomites. Activity, ability and financial means are those things upon which the success of a climber depends, even today. Activity on the one hand may now be the result of enthusiasm and vitality, ability the result of aptitude, training and experience, the financial means are, however, still dependent on possessions and profession.'

REINHOLD MESSNER

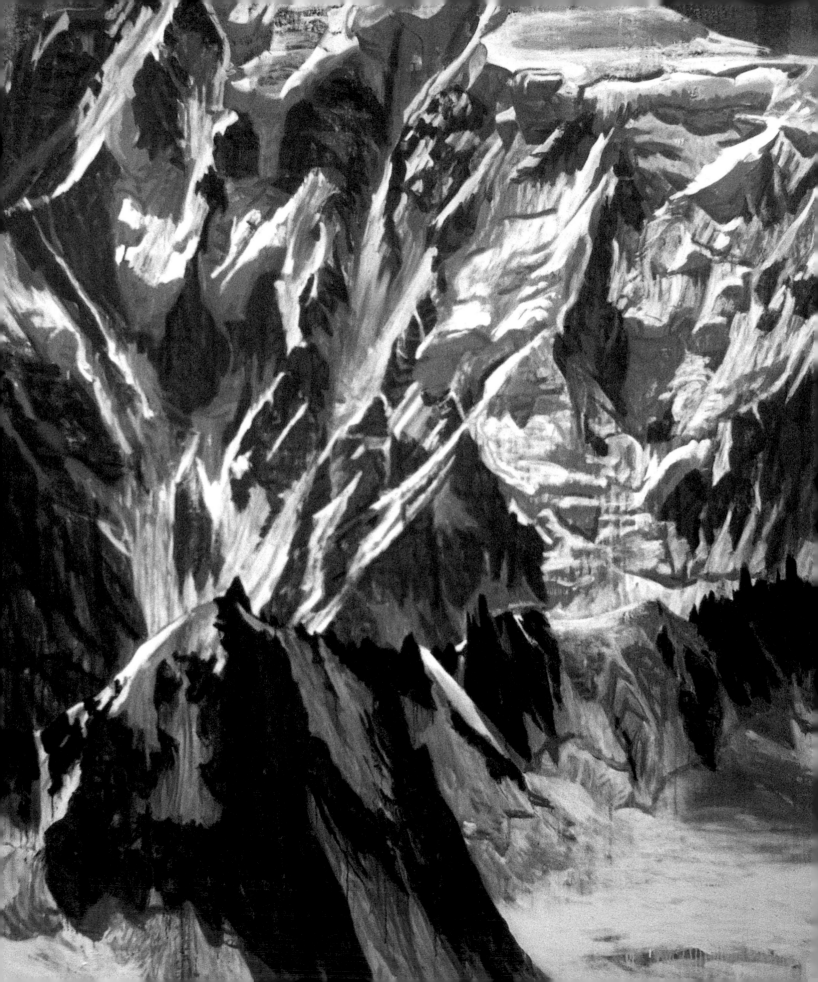

2000 METRES OF ICE AND ROCK

The Brenva Face of Mont Blanc (1300m) is one of the most demanding walls in the Alps, but the East Face of the Monte Rosa is the highest in the entire Alps. Ferdinand Imseng was the first to succeed in climbing it. Whilst hunting for chamois, he had seen the East Wall and persuaded a few Englishmen to venture out with him to attempt his route. Eventually, he also gained the services of their guide, Gabriel Spechtenhauser from Vent in Ötztal, who had thought the wall seemed too risky. Despite being hit by falling ice on 22 July 1872, they still managed to complete their route. Luigi Brioschi achieved a further new climb on the Nordendspitze, also with Imseng. Karl Blodig, together with the guide Christian Ranggetiner, was successful on a third route, reaching the Silbersattel between the Nordend and the Dufourspitze summits.

In the Eastern Alps there is one route that can be compared with the first ascent of the Monte Rosa East Face – the Schück gully on the Ortler. From the Ferner to the Ortler plateau it is said there is no one place on the climb where it would be possible to sit down and rest. In 1879 Otto Schück set off from 'end of the world Ferner' and together with P. Dangl and P. Reinstadler climbed to the left of the Martly Ridge – which A. v. Krafft, L. Freidmann and R.H. Schmitt were to climb in 1889 without a guide – up to the summit of the Ortler. Eleven and three quarter hours after they had set off from Sulden all three were on the top!

(facing page): **Mont Blanc from the South-East with the Brenva Face. The Brenva Spur is on the right of picture. Oil painting by Julian Cooper.**

> 'This tour is the most monumental that a kindly fate in the mountains has ever granted me.'
> — JULIUS KUGY

ON THE EAST FACE OF MONTE ROSA

The Monte Rosa, a massif, which towers high over the Po plain with its shining snow fields and many peaks, is not only one of the most famous four thousanders in the Alps; this mountain is linked with many legends. From the east, the Italian, side it appears in splendour without compare. Its summit tips are like the crenellations atop an enormous fortress wall; it creates a mighty impression, particularly on mountaineers.

This giant East wall can be compared to no other flank in the Alps and has remained a challenge right up to the present day. In the Alps there is no other wall which, in terms of height and savage grandeur, represents such a danger area as the Monte Rosa East Face. There are 3000m difference in altitude between the summit ridge and the valley floor. In the morning the sun takes hours to reach the highest roof terraces of the village of Macugnaga in the valley.

When in 1872, 'in two days work', the Dufourspitze was climbed for the first time from Macugnaga, people knew that that this ice climb was superior to anything which had been climbed up to that point. The news of the success on the East Face of Monte Rosa was of interest above all to the high Alpine circles. Eight years passed before the wall was climbed again and today it is still seldom climbed. There are reasons for this: the East Face is not only a very long and demanding route, in parts it is also extremely difficult. In addition to that comes the danger of imminent avalanche, against which both the most capable and the fastest, the most experienced and the beginner are helpless. Above all, the middle section of the face is threatening, and cost the third party, Damiano Marinelli with guides Imseng and Pedranzini, their lives. Marinelli's party, while traversing the central part of the face on an August afternoon in 1881, was swept to its death in a 50m-wide ice avalanche. Only the porter Corsi, who had not yet set foot in the gully, escaped the fall. Ever since he brought the news of the catastrophe back down to the valley the notorious gully has been called the Canale Marinelli.

Thus the first avalanche victims came early on Monte Rosa. Snow cornices tumbling down from the summit ridge; seracs falling from the hanging glaciers; stones loosened by the sun; masses of new snow which begin to slide; everything falls into this one channel, which has to be crossed by anyone climbing the East Face. The traverse of the gully can only be justified

> 'And anyone who should say that the most difficult route only leads to the same summit as the most gentle, to him I would say no. For individually and subjectively we have certainly reached a different height than that broad-arched snow dome, which year in year out patiently bears the tracks of hundreds on its back.'
> — OTTO SCHÜCK

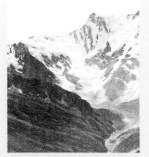

Monte Rosa from the East with the Macugnaga Glacier.

between midnight and the morning. In 1883 Karl Schulz, with the guides Alexander Burgener and Clemens Perren, made a successful attempt at the East Face in record time in favourable snow conditions. In only eight hours they climbed from the Jägerrücken to the summit. Then, in 1884, from 12–14 August, Ludwig Purtscheller, Emil and Otto Zsigmondy became the first to successfully climb Monte Rosa without a guide. Their route – the East Face.

The face certainly had a feeling of unusual greatness and its awe-inspiring grandeur inspired mountaineers to the extent that the crossing of the Monte Rosa massif from Macugnaga to Zermatt became the dream great mountain tour. The significance of this wall 100 years ago is shown clearly in Dr V. Wessely's report of his experiences.

On 7 August 1900, Franz Hörtnagel, a first class mountain guide from Innsbruck, and his guest Wessely come to Macugnaga planning to turn this dream into reality. But 'dazzling white, the new snow shrouded the shimmering blue seracs on the hanging glacier and the rocks of the summit crest, usually so dark, looked as if they had been dusted with icing sugar', Wessely writes in his report about the tour.

On 9 August they leave the Monte Rosa Hotel and walk up to Capanna Marinelli with food for three days and wood for the mountain hut. 'We climbed up to the left of the glacier, soon leaving the mighty glacier from which the young Anza flows away beneath us to the right, and in two hours we reached the Belvedere, the most popular excursion place for summer tourists in Macugnaga. Five minutes above this point, the side moraines on the right of the Macugnaga glacier are reached and the enormous precipice of the East Face is almost upon you. We pause here and, with the help of the map and all the literature we have collected, we broadly outline our continuation route.' It takes in the Jägerrücken with the Capanna Marinelli, south of that the Marinelli Couloir and on the far side of that the Imseng ridge. From the upper end of the firn, because of the increasing steepness and the shattered nature of the ice wall, the continuation of the path cannot be clearly viewed. From there onwards the plan – depending upon conditions – is to go up and left to the bergschrund with little deviation, to overcome this and, keeping right, to reach the steep walls of the boundary summit.

'Climbing continuously, we push forwards into the impressive landscape, climbing higher and higher up onto the mighty wall. Now to our left a second ridge appears. It towers out of the ice to a lesser extent, it is the Imseng Ridge and with a mixture of curiosity and dread we look down into the dark chasm below which rips through the wall between us and the ridge, into the Canale Marinelli. In silent repose it lies before us, almost peaceful to look at, as if it had never taken human life. Today the thunder of its avalanches is silenced, the mists which shroud the heights have silenced it early. Just once, a giant rock boulder comes crashing down the gully to remind us how deceptive this quiet is.'

The guide sees the Capanna, which is similar to the usual huts of the Western Alps in every way, and which they reach at 4pm. The bare essentials are there, there is some basic crockery but they can find no blankets and there is not even enough straw on the sleeping platform. One of the window-panes is broken and because it is not very welcoming the pair set off again into the open before onset of night to reconnoitre the entry to the Canale Marinelli. They are successful. They manage to find a way through the rocks and with anticipation they look into the ice gully lying ahead of them, scoured smooth by avalanches.

Back at the hut they look once again at their surroundings. 'One would search here in vain for charm, for picturesque beauty, a spiteful wildness and resolute energy are the character of this landscape.'

Night falls, the moon comes out, stars appear. Half-asleep, Hörtnagl and Wessely hear strange noises from high on the face, first a distant rolling of thunder which grows quickly in strength to envelop the hut. Without exchanging a word they listen to the darkness. 'An infernal racket shakes the air; every joint of the hut creaks and groans, the very foundations of the mountain quake in immeasurable rage as, foaming and raging, thundering and rattling, the avalanche roars down to the valley.'

Without a word, they listen to the 'terrible voice of the high mountains'. The avalanche has descended precisely in the spot that in a short time they wanted to reach – the Canale Marinelli.

Time to set off. The gigantic East Face lies in the shadow of the moonlight. Due to the clear sky, however, it is light enough to walk without torches. Reaching the Marinelli Couloir, they tie onto the rope and 'begin that walk which was to become the most serious of the whole route and, indeed, one of the most serious' in Wessely's whole life. They have to carve hand and foot holds out of the solid ice. Hörtnagl takes the lead.

'His ice-axe works feverishly and under his mighty blows step after step grows from the ice, step by step he gains ground. I wait meanwhile at the edge of the ice gully, push the ice-axe handle as far into the hard snow as I can and tie the rope around it, thus securing my friend.' They climb on, 'night and ice'. 'It is reasonably light when we reach the wildly shattered icefall which predominates on the firn slope on which we had been climbing up to now and through the middle of which our route leads. … We have to go around clefts, carefully avoid or climb over seracs. Soon we find ourselves in the middle of a chasm, surrounded by ice towers which might fall at any moment, and shortly afterwards we are once again balancing high up on the edge of a serac, the abyss surrounding us on all sides.'

Once more the scenery changes.

'We step out onto the open wall which towers above us far more steeply than the sections we have already overcome. Great channels run down parallel to each other, as if ploughed by an enormous harrow Each of these channels is 2–3m deep and separated from its neighbours by a narrow firn ridge. There is no doubt about it – it is an avalanche chute!

Following first one of the channels, then one of the separating ridges, we progress right into the middle of the greatest avalanche area which I have ever set foot upon. My glance darts up and down the wall and then out again into the open, over to the countless mountain summits rising up as the new day dawns. As we stop for a moment, to take a break from the steep and strenuous work and to let our lungs rest a while, we can watch the snow sloughs, loosened by the ice-axe, as they run their crazy race down the face. Looking along the whole length of this face, ones glance falls 2000m down to the Macugnaga Glacier, the gaping wide cracks of which seem from here like gentle, hardly perceptible veins. The view down is truly nerve wracking, but also nerve strengthening in a way.

Without allowing ourselves a break we immediately start to tackle the slope above us. As soon as we take the first steps we are aware that the composition of the snow here is completely different. Whilst in avalanche territory all the loose snow was swept off into the depths; here it had settled on the slopes as they were less inclined and we soon broke through it up to our calves and then up to our knees. We shared the unpleasant task of breaking trail in the snow fairly and it took almost an hour until we reached the bergschrund. … It is not merely one cleft but a whole system of clefts, a real icefall, through the remains of which we have to channel our

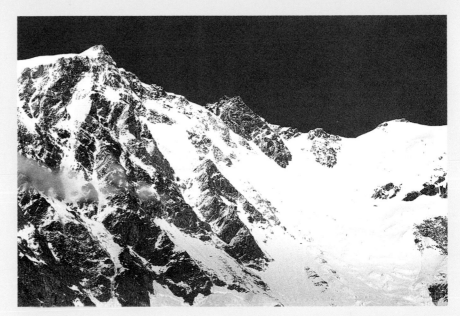

The East Face of Monte Rosa. To the left is the Signalkuppe.

descent. Of course there was hard ice here which hindered our progress no less than the soft snow which we had just overcome. Whereas back there it was our legs that bore the brunt of the hard toil, here it was our arms, weilding the ice-axes, that had to carry out most of the work. It took us half an hour to wind our way through this chaos of cracks and chasms and reach the upper edge. At the same moment we saw, tangibly close it seemed, the rocks of the first false summit. Yet between us and it, dazzlingly smooth in the morning sun, was the glassy ice-wall.'

The extent to which they were exposed as they moved was enormous. All they could see was bottomless, empty space. It was as if the surfaces of the wall had been chopped off and together with the ground on which they were standing, was swaying in the air. At precisely 10 o'clock they set their hands upon the rock wall beneath the summit, and three hours after the start of their climb Hörtnagl and Wessely stood on the summit.

'Once more we glanced down at this enormous wall, which had kept us busy yesterday and today. We could no longer view it in its entire splendour, as a bank of cloud had nestled upon its slopes. Then without stopping we continued. The jagged ridge, the vertiginous bridge upon which deep notches had formed, which stretches between us and the highest summit, is easier under foot than it seems upon first glance. In twenty minutes its solid rocks, which are free from snow, lead us up to the second highest summit in Europe, 4638m above sea level. It is 1.15pm!'

'If I am to tell the truth, the whole truth and nothing but the truth, so let me confess that Monte Rosa seen from Macugnaga is of such grandeur that one simply cannot imagine it. Up to the summit there are 2600m of wall which would make the mouth of any alpinist, or anyone contemplating suicide, water.'

LUIGI VACCARONE

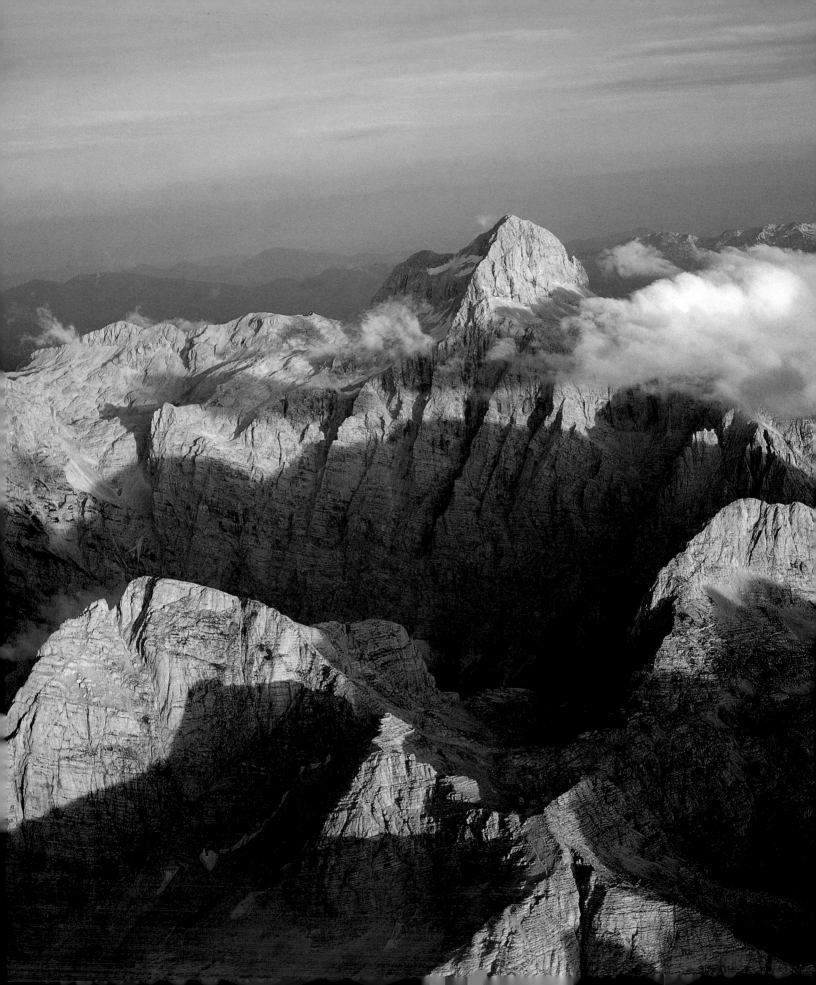

THE BIG ROCK WALLS OF THE EASTERN ALPS

In the 1860s the systematic development of high mountain routes in the Eastern Alps began. In the seventies, interest in the ice climbing areas wanes as big first ascents can no longer be found there. In the Eastern Alps too the initial phase of first ascents has been completed.

Thus attention now turns towards the Big Walls of the Western and Limestone Alps, and in particular the Southern Limestone Alps. The Montasch West Face in the Julian Alps, the Civetta Wall, and the South Face of the Marmolada in the Dolomites are the big objectives.

On 6 June 1881 the Viennese Otto Schück and mountain guide Johan Grill from Ramsau, a man more usually known as 'Kederbacher', climb the almost 1800m-high East Face of the Watzmann and thus establish a route, the like of which is unknown anywhere in the Eastern Alps. Only at the start of the next century are there to be first ascents of a similar scale.

In 1905, the Hochstadel Wall (2678m) in the Lienz Dolomites was first climbed. This rather nondescript mountain – 'the head of the monster' – has a gigantic rock wall, the North Face, which is difficult, exposed and long. K. Doménigg, F. Glatter and F. König manage to climb this tricky route to the summit, starting from the Lavanter Graben, on 9 July 1905. Via ledges, gullies, slabs and three snowfields the route leads up to a giant gorge and then to the West Ridge. The route up to the almost perpendicular steps beneath the summit is clearly marked but frightening nevertheless. In spite of this they make it.

The Triglav (2862m) 'Terglou' or 'Monte Tricorno', is for Julius Kugy 'the King of the Julian Alps'. Already conquered by the Slovenians at a time when the Grossglockner and the Ortler had still not been climbed, it presents a formidable looking prospect when viewed from the North. The North Face of Triglav, almost 1500m high and 3km wide, is one of the highest rock walls in the Eastern Alps, ranking alongside the likes of the North Face of the Hochwanner in the Wetterstein, the North Face of the Schermberg in the Totes Gebirge and the Birnhorn South Face in the Leoganger Steinberge. It is only in 1906 that an ascent of the wall from the Vrata Valley is attempted. The successful climbers are Felix König, Hans Reinl and Karl Doménigg, who in his entire climbing life achieved no fewer than 5000 summits.

In the same year, in August 1906, Gustav Jahn and Franz Zimmer find an easier route. Later still in 1910 Henrik Tuma from Laibach climbs the 'Slovenian Route' together with Joze Komac. The ideal line on the face, however, is the one followed by the Bayerländer Route, climbed in 1926. Today the North Wall offers the climber over thirty routes and variations at almost all levels of difficulty. The most difficult problems were solved by the Slovenian climbers, for whom the Triglav has become a kind of shrine. Great names such as Potocnic, Tominsek, Cop, Jug, Gostisa, Debelakova, Jesih and Fajdiga are intimately connected with it.

In 1910 the first ascent of the South-West Wall of the Croz dell'Altissimo (2339m) in the Brenta is also climbed. This dome to the South of Lasteri, with a sheer face which drops down 1000m into the Val delle Seghe, only then starts to become interesting for climbers. The route on this South-West Wall, which was put up on 16 August 1910 by Guido and Max Meyer with the guide duo Dibona and Rizzi, is one of the most difficult and longest climbs in the Brenta and has remained a fearful tour right up to the present day. The direct line on the North Face of the Kleine Civetta, climbed for the first time in 1910 by the Haupt/Lömpel team, marked the high point of achievement in Big Wall mountaineering pre World War I.

Drawing of the North Face of the Hochstadel by E. Platz.

(facing page): Triglav in the Julian Alps with its famous North Face.

> 'The three highest Walls of the Eastern Alps have left me with values, which sparkle eternally like valuable jewels in the shrine of my mountain memories. Varied is the colour of their moods, like precious stones, and the deeper meaning behind that which we have experienced is only expressed unclearly in the short descriptions we relate.'
>
> LUDWIG SINEK

> 'The route starts at a height of 1200m. The summit of the Hochstadel is 2678m high: 1500m of face climb!'
>
> LUDWIG SINEK

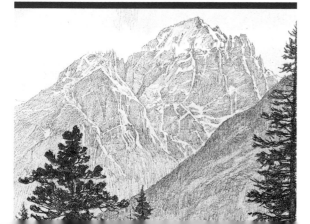

'High above the scree, the cliff hangs in a series of fearful slabs. In between, strangely rotten and pitted, the snow-filled cracks flash brightly, and further up, where the eye would expect to see the open skies, wall upon wall is piled, linked in a wild chaos of interconnecting pillars and ridges, horn-smooth panels set alongside weathered red rocks.'

HANS REINL

'From the very start I was most attracted by those mountains, those walls, those ridges which have something mysterious about them, a quiet, hidden world of the unknown, and the scale of the mountaineering task usually meant more to me than mere difficulty alone.'

LUDWIG SINEK

'When Felix Schickse and Ludwig Sinek arrived one August afternoon at the Slovenian Aljaz Hut intending to climb the Triglav North Wall, the landlady who early in the morning had seen the young Viennese mountaineer Wagner set off with the same intention, due to return that evening, said "It's a sin that you are not afraid of going onto that great wall. The one who set off this morning was young and blond like you," she told us with a motherly concern in her broken German', Sinek writes in his Triglav report. 'The evening was already casting its shadows over this wall, which we had studied for such a long time and observed in reverent amazement. Wagner did not return.'

Let us leave it to Ludwig Sinek to give us his own account of his experiences on the Triglav North Wall.

'Perhaps he left his return too late or changed his plans and wanted to reach the Triglav summit via another route; we thought it certain that he had spent the night up there in the Deschmannhause. It was strange, but why did I keep thinking about the fact that he was young and blond?

Both Felix and I were feeling, as many a mountaineer might feel before such a difficult undertaking, that mixture of emotions, enthusiasm and a certain excitement, when we sought out our mattresses in the hut. We were intending to set off tomorrow at 3am.

We are the only guests in the hut. The silvery light of the moon streams through the window into the sleeping quarters, throwing a great dark cross in shadow onto the brightly lit floor.

Outside, dressed in its night coat, our huge wall towers above. It is all we think of: again and again our thoughts turn to the steep pillars, glide over narrow ledges, floating higher and higher up to the point where the Triglav Glacier shines in the pale light. Will we be successful? I carry this question over into the strangest dream I have had in my life: the last rays of the evening sun light up the Triglav Summit, while the wall is already shrouded in dusk. We are prepared for the ascent. Then the young mountaineer, just returning from his rock climb, appears with a friendly greeting, puts his arm around me like an old friend and shows me the route up the wall, pointing out particularly clearly the starting point. "You should not set off climbing into the middle of the wall, from there it is impossible to get over to the great gorge. Take the gully to the left, you see, the climb goes up this to start with and then slowly moves out to the right, up to the highest section of the wall." He bids us goodbye with a strange, friendly, yet melancholy smile and leaves us again, making his way slowly back along the path from which he had come, from the innermost corner of the valley.

Thus it was that I dreamed that night about our mountain journey on the Triglav North Wall. But Felix stirred quickly from his sleep and woke me. Had I not heard? Outside, it seemed as if Wagner had just returned! We both listened intently, but our ears had deceived us. Only now the wandering moon was no longer casting its light and the shadow from the window onto the floor of the room. Pale and silvery, it shone directly over us, bathing us in our fitful sleep as we thought only of the great wall and the morning. I was not yet fully conscious of the puzzling and mysterious nature of my dream; only later did it really take hold of me. It cannot be self-deception, nor the retrospective transfer in my memory of something that I later experienced.

At 3 o'clock in the morning, by the light of the moon, as Felix and I slowly made our way through the mysteriously quiet Vratatal to the start of the wall, I told him of my dream, describing exactly to him how this unknown climber had looked. Even now I can still remember every last detail, the facial expressions and the clothes, yes even the red symbol of the Austrian Alpine Club in a particular place on his coat, the unique grey pattern of which I had found particularly noticeable. As I was later to experience, it could not have been a trick of the senses.

"This valley feels like a cemetery today", I suddenly say, and my companion looks at me, surprised at my words. Even more silently, we continue our ascent. The cold grey of morning has devoured the silvery magic. We are at the foot of the wall. Felix maintains that this is the start of the route. "No, it is further to the left." We begin to argue loudly about it but I refuse to give way. The sketch of the route I had seen yesterday afternoon had been clear enough – and my dream confirmed it. Our experience on this mighty wall was rich in impressions and well worth all the effort of the day, yet we encountered no great obstacles on the magnificent climb. Gust Jahn's splendid sketch of the route led us up the best line on the huge rock wall and I was more than a little proud to lead my friend, who had complete confidence in me at that time, up the climb without the slightest mistake, even though the route finding on the wall was in parts quite difficult. In spite of this it still took us eight hours to do the climb. Mist surrounded us on the highest part of the cliffs and we were threatened by storms while still on the steep rocks just beneath the Kugy Ledge. We were lucky.

We reached the valley again before dusk. We were the third party to get a glimpse of the secrets of this magnificent wall, something that seemed terribly important to us young, vain fools at the time. And we had not found the slightest trace of our predecessor.'

A week later the body of the dead Wagner was found on a narrow ledge above the foot of the wall. It was no trick of the senses. Down to the very last detail the reality agreed with the picture from Sinek's dream.

Triglav from the North.

'Others will continue to climb the highest walls, as long as the desire and the strength of youth in the mountains continue to woo the Blue Flower of the Romantics.'

LUDWIG SINEK

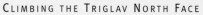

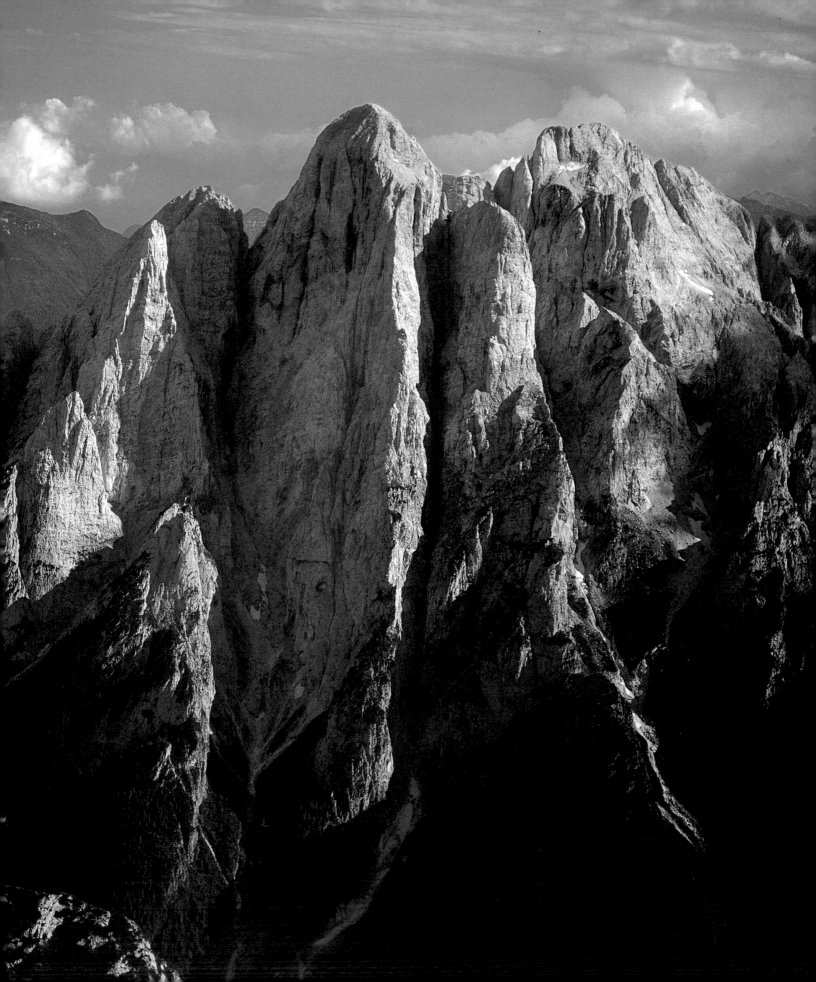

THE BIG WALLS OF THE DOLOMITES

The development of Big Wall climbing has been a story full of strange twists and turns. After the highest faces on the highest mountains of the Alps had been climbed, the young climbing elite turned to the highest limestone faces of the Eastern Alps. After the First World War the objectives were the shorter, but even more difficult, 'last problems' in the Dolomites. After climbing the South Face of the Marmolada, the Agnér North Face and the North Face of the Pelmo, Emil Solleder, the best rock climber of his time, formulated his own list of objectives, 'the Last Big Wall Problems of the Dolomites': Furchetta, North Face; Civetta, North Face and the East Face of Sass Maor. He did the first of these with Fritz Wiessner in summer 1925, the second just two weeks later with Gustav Lettenbauer and the third a year later with Franz Kummer.

Although the actual dimensions of the challenges had shrunk, the difficulties involved had become more and more demanding. And once even the short, perpendicular walls of the Tre Cime had been climbed, attention turned to the 'last big wall problems' of the Alps. Building upon experience thus gained, the post-war period saw the big walls of the Andes come under closer scrutiny and, in the last third of the century, attention shifted to the 'World's Biggest Walls', where the cumulative challenges of size, difficulty and objective danger represent the greatest problem.

Personally, I was lucky enough to have the opportunity of contributing to three of these periods of big wall climbing history with my ascents of the North-East Face of Agnér, the South Face of Burel in the Dolomites – both 1400m high – the North Face and the North Buttress of the Eiger, the South Face of Aconcagua and the Rupal Flank on Nanga Parbat.

After a rich harvest of routes climbed during my 'apprenticeship' at home in the Dolomites, I went to the Western Alps, then to the Andes and finally to the Oooueis, where I was to succeed on the difficult and dangerous North-West Face of Annapurna.

In order to incorporate my own experiences into this book I will include some of my own personal big-wall experiences alongside the respective historical accounts.

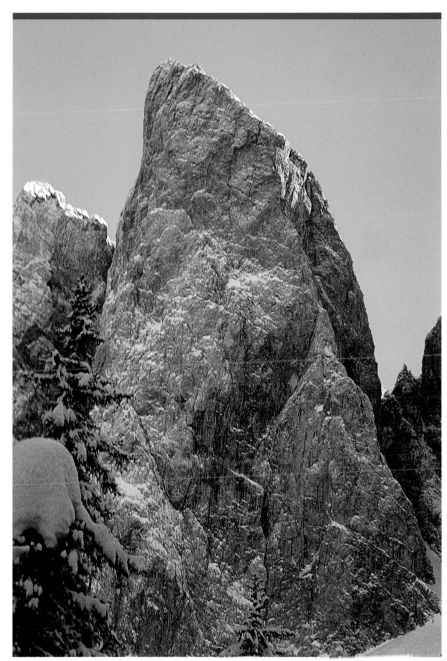

(facing page): The Agnér group in the Pala (Dolomites). Monte Agnér is the peak in the centre, with a 1600m face dropping sheer to the Lucano Valley.

(above): The North Face of the Furchetta is Reinhold Messner's 'local Big Wall'. He has climbed it both in winter and solo.

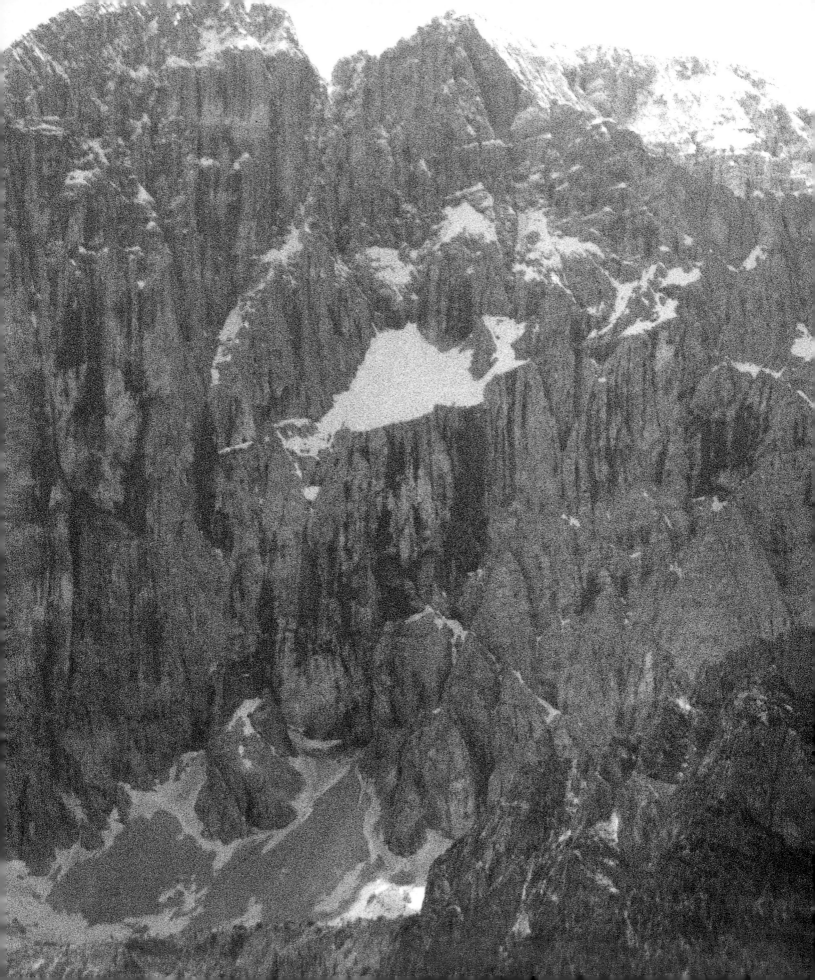

THE CIVETTA WALL

In his essay 'The Last Big Wall Problems of the Dolomites', Emil Solleder turns the spotlight on the North-West Face of the Civetta. For him, this mountain held a magnetic appeal. In August 1925, heavily laden, he hiked up to Alleghe and on to the Coldai Hut after bidding farewell to the departing Wiessner at Caprile, who had injured his hand on the Furchetta and thus felt that it was impossible for him to do any further routes for several days. Solleder arrived at the hut, perched on the eastern spur of the Civetta massif, late in the evening. By the dim light of an oil lamp he could just make out the only two other guests, whose thick accents he recognized as being from Munich. 'Obvious contenders for the North Face,' was his first thought.

'Since my first concern was to keep the purpose of my being there to myself, I thought it better to behave like a humble little mountain finch. However, I did get a little embarrassed when they asked me if I had heard anything about a new route on the Furchetta. Since one display of honesty is deserving of another, when in the course of our conversation they revealed that they intended to attempt the Civetta Wall I told them that I had managed to do the Furchetta with Wiessner. We were soon forging a common plan. The next morning saw us hiking up together to the much-courted objective.

The wall rises in a steep sweep of vertical slabs, and the lower section in particular looks hopeless. We traversed in from the right to a plinth of rock that projects from between two snow ribs that were being raked by stonefall. After chopping our way up an ice field we arrived at a shallow col behind the shattered tower that crowns the col. The left-hand side of the col is formed by a second, black tower that leans against the main wall. It was here that we pulled our kletterschuhe from our rucksacks and here, too, that what we feared might happen did happen; a sudden unearthly howling right above our heads – stonefall! We now stuffed our big boots into a little cave for safety and pulled our rucksacks over our heads, hearts pounding, as the howling came again from above, the stones exploding as they landed on the rock around us.

Moving quickly now, we traversed right from the black tower and headed upwards. Heavy drizzle soaked us through, and the rock became more and more difficult. The tiny holds were glassy with ice from the sprinkling of water, a reminder for us to take the utmost care, since we had left the rope in the rucksack to keep it from getting wet. Wet and shivering, we stood in the earthy notch and scrutinized the possible line of ascent we had spotted from below. It did not look very encouraging. A loose, red crack rises from the notch, leading up to beneath an overhanging bulge and continuing leftwards to join a solid-looking overhanging crack. Since this second crack seems to go a long way up we wanted to attempt it at all costs. Lettenbauer, a most decent climbing companion, did not wish to relinquish the lead and set off along the traverse, belayed by Gaberl and myself. It was a tough piece of work as with slow, calculated movements he carefully edged his way across the exposed wall to the left. At last – it seemed an eternity to me – he was across and called for the second man to follow. The stance was small and poor; we were hard put to get all three of us standing on it. Fully five hours had now passed and strictly speaking we were still only on the entry pitches of the huge face. Yet even this realization could not now induce us to abandon the attempt we had started. I took over the lead and climbed the incipient crack from the stance. A severe overhang right at the start was loose and required extreme caution. Above this, the crack widened slightly and led, still exceptionally difficult, after 50m to a little niche. Here we relieved our rucksacks of the provisions and, deep in thought, watched the stonefall whining and whistling down the face. It still posed no immediate danger to us but how would it be further up, when we stepped onto the easier angled zone of slabs, which were certain to be raked by stonefall from the 900m high wall towering above?

Temporarily at least, the question did not need to be answered; who knew if we would even manage to get that far? In any case, it looked as if it would go above the niche. Directly above the little niche, a

'Away to the south, a proud mountain pushed through the gaps in the mist. Was this real? Never before had I seen a wall like this in the Alps! Soon the huge North-West Face was bathed in the full glow of the evening sun. It stood there, regally, in all its huge width, covered in fresh snow from summit to foot. The time and the energy expended by the very best in their attempts to conquer this virgin beauty had indeed been worthwhile.'

EMIL SOLLEDER

chimney rose, with water running from it. After another rope length we reached the base of the chimney and Lettenbauer immediately set about attacking the wet defile. But there was no way through here, since the chimney petered out, blocked by an 8m basin-like overhang. We still did not admit defeat, though, and while Lettenbauer climbed back down I tried my luck on the vertical wall bounding the chimney on the left. I climbed on small holds up to an arete, traversed around this to the left and moved onto the totally perpendicular and tremendously exposed wall. The severity of the position demanded a running belay, so after 25m I hammered in a piton and looked over to the right to see whether I was already level with the roof of the chimney. I still had to get higher. I managed to climb a further 5m of unusually difficult rock but eventually ground to a halt, standing on tiny footholds below a totally unclimbable section. There was only one way out of this impasse: across rightwards to the chimney! Leaning across to the right, almost out of balance, I forced a piton into the rock to serve as a runner and to give me rope tension for the traverse. I clipped in the last carabiner and stuffed my cap into a little hole in the rock, as the exertions of the last few minutes had made me dreadfully hot. Then I stared across the traverse. Tough luck! Due to the friction caused by the rope running over the rock and zigzagging through the two carabiners, the rope would no longer pull through. It was only with the greatest effort that I managed to tease through the necessary length, centimetre by centimetre. I breathed a deep sigh of relief as I finally wedged myself into the chimney and called down to my companions, who were waiting anxiously 35m below, to follow. Since the rope could not be taken in from my stance, I advised Gaberl to use it to help him climb up to the first piton. My position did not afford me a clear view of the proceedings, but when I estimated that Gaberl must surely have long reached the piton I shouted down to ask him how things were going. Instead of a reply I heard a volley of stones and felt a sudden, sharp tug on the rope. Dismissing my advice to use the rope for aid, Gaberl had fallen and was now hanging free on the exposed wall. It was only due to fact that we were climbing as a rope of three that this ticklish situation turned out to be not too serious, and Lettenbauer soon helped Gaberl back into the safe confines of the chimney. Fortunately he had escaped with nothing worse than a minor injury to his foot. While he was recovering from his fall, Lettenbauer climbed up to join me and after a lengthy struggle we

managed to bring Gaberl, whose movement had indeed been greatly impaired by his injury, up to the stance.

The last few hours had flown by and the day was drawing to its close. It was therefore a matter now of finding a roomy enough spot to bivouac. The very next pitch took us to just such a little ledge. It was too small really for three people but did at least offer us the opportunity of sitting down. I climbed above it for a little way, tackling several difficult sections as I went, and suddenly found myself at the start of the long awaited easier section of the route. With a fresh glimmer of hope that our climb might yet succeed, I abseiled back down to my companions. The lantern was fastened to a rock piton and, by the flickering light of the candle, we ate a cold supper and discussed the prospects for our undertaking. We had gained about 300m today. Above us the wall still reared about 1100m into the dark night and there were still a number of questionable sections to come. Gradually, it grew colder. We tied ourselves to a piton, stuck our feet inside our little bivi tent and pulled it over our heads. It was a long, cramped, hard night but at least we were tolerably warm.

As dawn finally broke at about 4.30am in the morning, thick, grey clouds were moving across towards us from the hidden mass of the Marmolada. Soon after, raindrops began drumming monotonously on the batiste roof of our tent. There was nothing else for it; we had to go down. At 6.00am we began our retreat. The flight down to the base of the chimney was free and airy. The loose traverse back to the notch was again a hard piece of work.

Down at the corrie we were greeted by the midday sun. Remnant tatters of mist were still wafting across the wall as we gazed up at the rocks above the bivouac and the big, as yet unresolved, question mark. We strolled to the hut and decided to descend to the valley that same day, since it would be better to grant both the outer and the inner man some well-deserved rest down there than at the unfriendly and ill-equipped hut, where, furthermore, sleep would be entirely out of the question due to the many little hopping tormentors in residence there. On the first night, even the tried and tested insect repellent, which usually rendered such admirable service in such cases, had failed us.

Two days later, at 1 o'clock in the early morning of 7 August, Lettenbauer and I crawled out of a sweet-smelling hayrick somewhere near Marisons and set off uphill, bound for the Coldai. Gaberl remained behind, since his invalid leg was still troubling him greatly. Gradually, the stars grew pale and a wonderful day dawned. We were soon standing at the now familiar notch and climbed the cracks and chimneys of the sunless face, soaked to the skin by the torrents of water. We came to the last piton, from which I had rigged an abseil back down to the bivouac ledge three days previously, and moved into new and, for us, unknown territory. But how were we to make progress now? A 150m high, steep, yellow wall towered above us. From the corrie it had appeared that a crack or chimney might split this steep step but we now saw that where we had presumed to find a possible way up was, in fact, completely impossible. The only way out of the impasse was to attempt to sidestep the issue. A long, leftwards traverse ended at a splendid waterfall but offered not the slightest possibility of a continuation line. So back it was, and off to the right. Lettenbauer suggested we try a forked crack system but it was so generously supplied with stonefall that we also dismissed this as a possibility. Instead, we traversed further right and now spied a huge corner, whose innermost angle was split by a barely discernible grey crack. The crack seemed to us to be good enough to effect upwards progress, but – oh, the cussedness of inanimate objects! – up above it merged into a belt of yellow, loose overhangs. Nevertheless, I gave it a try. It did not go easily. I was repeatedly forced further and further out to the right until I was finally able make a tension traverse back down and left, turning a dreadfully brittle arete, to get into the crack.

Lettenbauer followed swiftly and safely, retrieving the length of rope used for the tension traverse. If this crack went through the whole of the yellow rock band, by my calculations it should bring us level with the entrance to the gully, which would likely represent the last crux section of the face. Three times I ran out the whole of the 38m rope, belayed to a piton and brought Lettenbauer up. The higher I climbed the more often I was pushed out of the crack and onto the left wall. Slowly, I was approaching a blockage in the crack and it did not bode well, or so I thought. But the section gave in much easier than we had expected and I bridged up past it on good, solid holds. 'A big, fat chimney – and it goes a long way up!' My shout of joy made my companion, sitting it out on the belay, sit up and take notice. The chimney rapidly brought us level with a slabby, triangular pulpit and our confidence grew considerably. If we could just reach the base of the main gully now, the game would surely be won. True, the upper part of the gully was blocked by huge overhangs but the wall to the left did offer various possibilities of effecting upward progress.

Granting ourselves a brief rest, we lightened the load in our small but still heavy rucksack, which my companion had been carrying so courageously all this time. We had actually intended to swap the lead here but since Lettenbauer had no objections I carried on leading. Any worries we might have had about the weather were soon dispelled by a cloudless, deep blue sky. The weather had been unsettled for weeks but this blue sky and a sharp east wind held the promise of good things to come, even if we should be forced to bivouac.

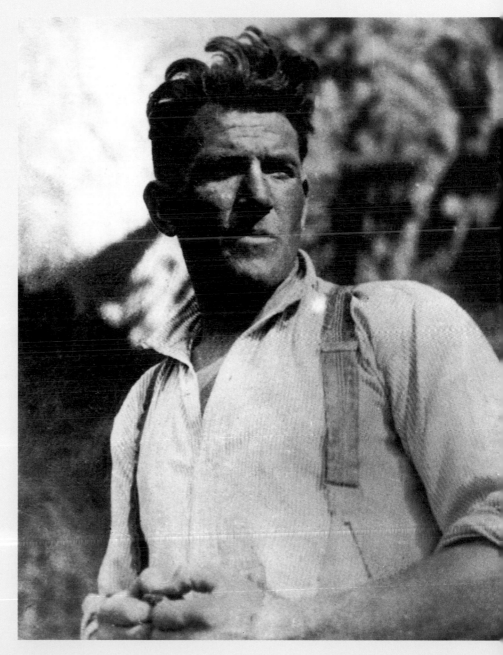

Emil Solleder, mountain guide and prolific Dolomite new-router, was the best rock climber of his time.

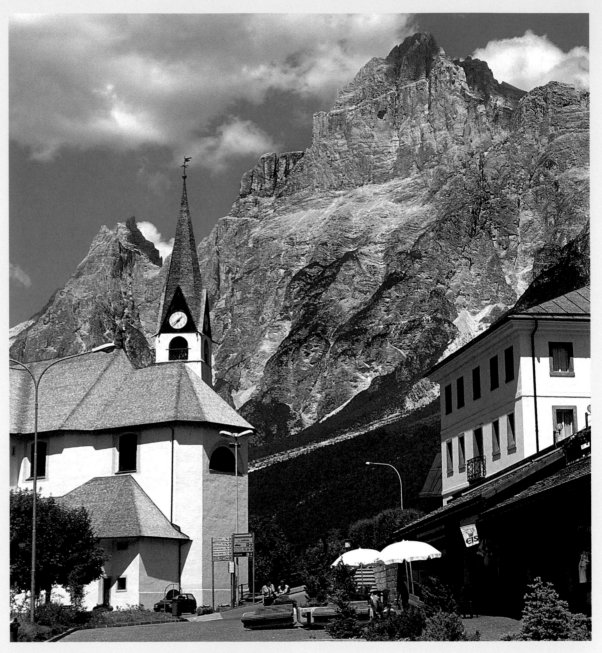

There are bigger walls than the Civetta in the Southern Dolomites. The big faces of the Croda Marcora (pictured), Antelao and Burél are 1500m high.

'No, it is not danger that I look for; for me, climbing is all about other values. When I am hanging up there, when I feel my strength and see the possibilities that unfold and yet decide to renounce my attempt – that, too, makes me happy.'

REINHOLD MESSNER

'In 1929 we heard Walter Stösser from Pforzheim giving a talk on the climbs he had done in the Dolomites. In the course of his lecture he mentioned that, on his fourth ascent of the North-West Face of the Civetta, a big piece of the initial hand traverse had broken off. "The number of ascents may now be limited", he remarked.'

ANDERL HECKMAIR

We were now barely one rope length below the gully and searched for a possible way of getting into it. A little yellow wall, about 8m high, with a crack leading down from its lower edge, seemed to offer the best chance of success. Although the little wall looked more like sandstone, everything else proclaimed a decisive 'impossible'. Contrary to expectations, the crack led up into an area of solid rock and – surprise, surprise – a series of small, favourably sculpted handholds allowed me to climb to within just a few short metres of the base of the gully. Over to the left, still within reach, there was a little hole in the overhang where I attempted to place a piton. Two of my blade pegs proved too weak and bent, but a robust ring piton did the trick. Drooping slightly, but in right up to the ring, it was the only hold on this section. It was the first time that the wall had refused to succumb to pure free-climbing techniques and this at one of the most exposed parts of the climb. My boots scrabbled at the holdless rock. Far up to the left there was a good hold; just one metre higher and I had cracked it! I now knew we had the wall in the bag and as my happy victory call wafted down to my companion it told him much more than any long-winded explanations about our situation could ever have conveyed. Soon we were reunited in the main gully, for so long the object of our desires. The afternoon sun cast its light onto the wall and bathed us in its warming rays. Straightforward climbing up a series of chimney pitches quickly took us higher, until we stood below a vertical precipice, which was, furthermore, running with water. Whereas we had been completely spared from stonefall in the gully, now we were both suddenly, and simultaneously, hit by rocks, reminding us to exercise increased caution. The ascent of the precipice seemed as if it were to become a very damp affair but unfortunately there was no way around it. Paying scant regard to our bodies' requirement for warmth, we plunged right into the icy cold shower bath. To crown it all I then had to place a piton in the capping overhang. Shivering with cold, with wet clothes and dripping boots, I finally landed above the unpleasant section. Yet the ordeal was by no means over. Looming large and imminent, I could see a second, similar, bath ready and waiting for us. Enough was enough. We avoided this section by the exceptionally severe rocks to our left. It led onto rather easier angled terrain and out into the full glare of the afternoon sun. The delicious warmth permeated our bodies and induced us to take a lengthy rest on a rubble-strewn terrace. We dried our clothing as thoroughly as we could and built ourselves a little cairn on the terrace. To the north east, the steep, soaring South Face of the Marmolada, which during the entire ascent had served as a measure for the height of the face still to be climbed, now reminded us not to extend our rest any longer. A 300m wall still separated us from our objective.

We followed the terrace further round to the left to gain a chimney with an unusually hard start. We were finally quitting the gully once and for all. Our rate of progress, swift thus far, gradually became slower, as the increasing difficulty of the climbing and the seemingly endless wall began to drain our mental and physical strength. At one point, I had already put several metres of the hard section behind me when I turned back and swapped my tattered climbing boots for my friend's spare pair, which turned out to be a good size too big for me. The chimney brought us to a terrace-like, independent rock spur left of the big gully, which led to the last steep section of the face. There seemed to be several possible lines hereabouts, although none of them looked particularly promising.

Route finding would present us with few problems now; we simply had to head for a little notch about 200m above us, presently lit up by the setting sun. An overhanging crack brought us to a black and yellow, water-soaked niche, out of which I climbed, on tiny holds, to reach a little crack. A last piton below an overhang went in well, singing as I placed it, until I dropped the hammer, which I had evidently secured insufficiently well during our more rapid climb from the rock spur. As luck would have it, it became lodged just a few metres lower, enabling me to retrieve the errant object. As twilight fell, we climbed higher, moving as quickly as the variable difficulties allowed. I clearly sensed how, after the wearisome passage on the rock and in the race to beat the imminent nightfall, opposing concepts of difficulty gradually merged into a middle line. While the body now perceived any kind of effort as difficult, the nerves were totally blunted even to the unusually difficult sections.

The darkness increased, and our continuation line became lost in a black, ill-defined mass. While we searched with difficulty for a route up to the crest of the ridge and freedom, the mighty outline of the Marmolada had now lost something of its dominant height, which mean that the ridge could no longer be far away. A jackdaw suddenly flitted past close overhead and a cool wind told us the summit was near. We climbed a last loose and overhanging section to stand in the dark, starry night on a snowdrift on the North-East Ridge. The North-West Face of the Civetta was ours!

The rope fell to the ground for the last time as we clasped hands in a firm, wordless handshake. By the eerie, flickering light of the lantern we strolled slowly over loose slabs of rock towards the highest point, barely 40m away from the top of the climb.

Just short of the summit, and with a snowfield within easy reach, we set up the bivouac and squeezed into our little tent. The moon was not yet up, the stars shone faintly and down in the valley grey veils of mist were gathering. Shortly after midnight I looked out of the thin cotton cocoon, as the mist rose from the valley to envelop us in its dark grey embrace. A blood red glow pierced the thick veil – the moon. The glorious atmosphere of this night-time mountain magic completely captivated me. At 2 o'clock in the morning the yellow disc stood victorious above the wreaths of mist and we were able to use its pale light to begin our descent via the unknown South-East flank. Down at the corrie daylight broke around us as we stood and sorted out the rope.'

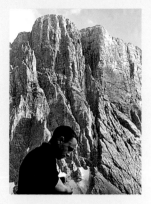

The possibilties that lie to the right of the Civetta Wall (the photo shows the Cima De Gasperi and Cima Su Alto) were only discovered a decade later.

'Three days later, while Gaberl remained behind, still weakened by an injury …, the other two reached the summit to claim both a great victory and the most beautiful route in the Eastern Alps.'

GIUSTO GERVASUTTI

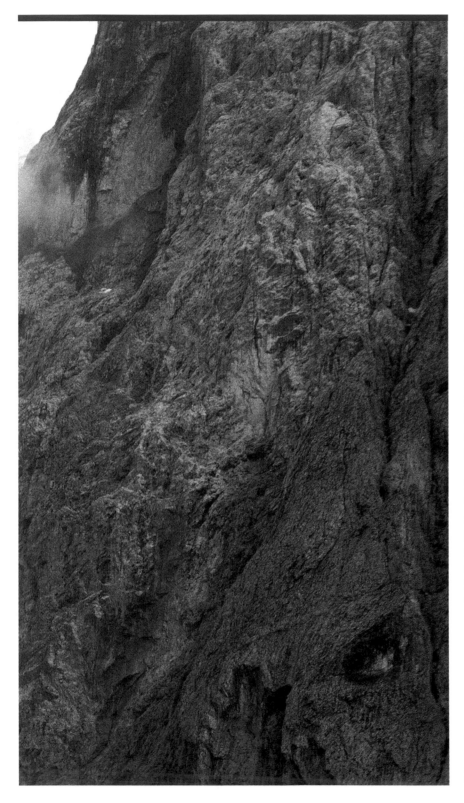

Stylized by Domenico Rudatis as 'the Wall of Walls', the Civetta Wall had fascinated me since childhood. At the age of twenty I climbed half a dozen routes on the North-West Face and in 1967, with Sepp Mayerl, Heini Holzer and Renato Reali, I succeeded on the line to the left of the 'Solleder', which is safer and hardly more difficult than that route. During the climb it became clear to us that although Leo Rittler and Willi Leiner had done a direct variation on the Solleder/Lettenbauer in 1928, they had not actually climbed the middle line on the face as Willi Leiner later seemed to recall.

We are all of us susceptible to memories that deceive us. It is for this reason that I prefer to base this work on contemporary reports rather than on later corrections, since these also often merely represent what we wish was true, or the 'truths' that we repeatedly attempt to convince ourselves of.

Even more than the Civetta Wall, however, it was the big wall of Monte Agnér that captivated me from the beginning; that pillar which – tucked away in an outlying chain of the Pala group – even today leads a Cinderella-like existence, even though it is she, and no other, that may rightly claim to be the greatest and the biggest wall in the Dolomites.

After the first winter ascent of the Solleder on the Civetta by I. Piussi, G. Redaelli and T. Hiebeler in 1963, I ventured – hesitantly at first, it was a very cold winter – onto the North Arete of Monte Agnér and later onto the North Face, beneath a deep covering of snow, finally, together with my brother Günther and Heini Holzer, making the first ascent of the North-East Face, again one of the 'last great big wall problems of the Dolomites'.

The middle section of the North-East Face of Monte Agnér, viewed from the Lucano Valley.

MONTE AGNÉR, NORTH FACE

It took me almost twenty years to climb 'the Big Walls'; twenty years during which I also made numerous other ascents in the mountains and gained more and more experience. I did not of course start with the Big Walls; my first steps were taken on the little objectives, the walking trails and easy rock climbs of my local Dolomites. And I believe that my greatest successes can ultimately be attributed to the fact that for many years – between the ages of five and twenty – I climbed easy and middle grade routes. In this way, I developed the mountaineering instinct that was to help me again and again in later years to cope with those edge-game situations, perhaps even to survive.

Growing up in the Dolomites, I first learned how to rock climb and after I had done many of the big Dolomite faces I did all of the hard ice-face climbs in my home province of South Tyrol. I was thus well practised in both disciplines – rock and ice climbing – before my first trip to the Western Alps.

On top of this, several winter ascents had also given me the opportunity of climbing and gaining experience on mixed ground in the worst conditions imaginable. This gave me an idea of the degree of skill, experience, willpower and self-discipline that are required to make an ascent of a big face on an 8000m peak.

As a prelude to my 'Big Wall' career I climbed the North Face of Monte Agnér, at 1500m the biggest vertical face in the Dolomites. First climbed in 1921 by Francesco Jori, Arturo Andreoletti and Alberto Zanutti, it is still today regarded as one of the greatest routes in the Eastern Alps. I offer it here as one example of many routes in the mountains that can be considered as a kind of preparation for the 'Big Walls'. Jori was a brilliant free climber and, like Angelo Dibona, he knew how to transfer his rock climbing skills to the big mountain faces. Like Paul Preuss he was an advocate of the pure free climbing style and used pitons only in the direst emergency. 'Wherever I might need a piton to succeed, I am better off relinquishing the route', he was often heard to say.

Back then, after my first winter ascent of the Agnér North Face, if anyone had told me that this same Monte Agnér was really just a *klettergarten*, or training ground, I would not only have been disappointed, I would have been furious. Nowadays I know that cliffs like this, compared to the biggest mountain faces in the world, do have something of a crag atmosphere about them and, due to their modest altitude, can never stand serious comparison with the big faces of the Jorasses, Annapurna and Lhotse.

It all depends on the relationship one has with these faces. For a climber used to the Kaisergebirge, the North Face of the Cima Grande would seem huge. Kasparek climbed it in winter as a training route for the North Face of the Eiger.

Training climbs such as this are now found everywhere in the Alps, and in California, South Africa, Norway and the Tatra – everywhere in fact where climbers intent on doing the 'Big Walls' go to prepare themselves. Even if these 'big crags' do play an important role locally for the climbers who live in the vicinity, when viewed in a worldwide context they are still only of secondary importance.

I recently heard of a seventeen-year-old who hitched to Monte Agnér to solo the North Arete. Several days later I met an eighteen-year-old who had ticked off the Walker Spur, the West Face of the Blatiere, the North Face of the Triolet and the North Face of the Courtes, the Cassin Arete on the Torre Trieste, the North Face of the Grosshorn and a few others besides, all in one summer. He had climbed the North Face of the Cima Grande when he was fifteen.

It is not that these young climbers have somehow lost respect for the 'Big Walls'. Nor have they risked anything – the style of their ascents proves this. There has merely been a shift in the dimensions. And if tomorrow they should wish to look for bigger objectives, building on the experiences gained by previous generations of climbers, they will find greater challenges commensurate with their own abilities all over the world – on the 'Big Walls'.

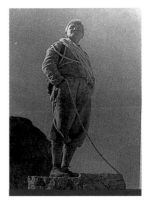

Francesco Jori in the climbing equipment of the 1920s.

'His greatest achievement was undoubtedly the first ascent of the 1500m North Face of Monte Agnér, with Arturo Andreoletti and Alberto Zanutti, one of the most significant climbs in the Dolomites, even today.'

TONI HIEBELER

Reinhold Messner on the first winter ascent of the Jori Route on the North Face of Monte Agnér.

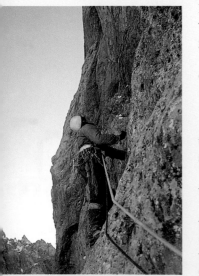

The farmer at Col di Pra merely shook his head, sensing what it was that we had come to do. He sat on his doorstep, killing time. He had brought in the hay and the cows would not need to be milked again until evening. So he crouched where he was and looked up at Monte Agnér. It was keeping the sun off him.

When we returned three days later, the man was still sitting in the doorway; or rather, he was again sitting there.

Our tent still stood on a little patch of meadow at Col di Pra, directly beneath the huge mass of the Agnér Wall. Günther and Heini wanted to stay longer; Erich, one of my seven other brothers, and I wanted to set off homewards.

Down on the road, we cast a glance back at our friends and the North-East Face. A car stopped next to us.

'Are the climbers back from the North Face?' someone asked through the car window.

'Yes, just back.'

'How long did the three of them take?'

'They bivvied the second time on the descent, in the bivvi box below the summit.'

'Where did they start up?'

'Same place Aste tried a few years ago.'

'How do you know Aste tried it?'

'They told us in Taibon.'

'How far did Aste get?'

'Not far; about 400m.'

'What's the route like?'

'Long, free, a bit dangerous. Similar to the "Via Ideale" on the Marmolada d'Ombretta…slabs, waterfalls. No, not as difficult! But it's still a great route.'

'You've done the "Via Ideale" on the Marmolada d'Ombretta?'

'Second ascent', I said proudly.

'What's it like?'

'Without doubt, it's one of the greatest routes in the Dolomites, if not the whole of the Alps. That was some route Aste did! Respect is due!'

'*Aste sono io* – I am Aste', said the man with the week-old stubble.

Powerful handshakes all round! Suddenly there was a friendly atmosphere. He would have been setting off up the North-East Face himself tomorrow if…and we had snatched the new North Face Route on the Civetta from under his nose as well. '*Ci dispiace* –

sorry about that', I said, thinking, 'It was about time.'

He asked if we knew that he was in Taibon when we went for the winter ascent of the North Arete. He had also wanted to do the first winter ascent.

'And now you've climbed the North-East Face?'

'Yes.'

'*Complimenti*.'

'Thank you.'

'The early bird catches the worm, eh?' he said, a little wistfully. 'You've got a good eye for a line and you had better luck than us. How come you went for this new route?'

'I spotted a possible line left of the Jori Route when I set off up the North Arete in winter. There was snow lying in all the features and it gave me a clear picture of the difficulties. I forgot about the face when I was on the North Arete. I studied it again in detail this summer.'

'And how was it?'

'I got down off it three days ago. With Heini Holzer from Meran and my brothers Günther and Erich. That's our tent over there.'

We set off on 17 August with our oversized rucksacks. Erich, our support man, carried the heaviest of them up to the start of the route. The first 400m went quickly. Grade IV at the most. Then, just to the right of the black water streak, we found a bunch of bivi gear, a stove and some food. During the entire climb we were puzzling over who might have been there before us. It was only on the descent that Erich gave us the news, 'They reckon Aste was on it before you.' The old man smiled, a little wryly. 'Yes, Aste tried it too, your wall', he said. Then I understood. It was his wall.

The bearded Aste was not exactly happy, but nor was he angry with us. 'What was it like up there?' he wanted to know.

'We went straight up the buttress above your bivouac. About 400m of nice climbing, but the rucksacks made it hard going.

In the late afternoon we climbed a chimney to reach a little pulpit beneath the steep, grey sweep of slabs of the North-East Face. We set up a nice bivouac there. We had time.'

Then, however, a dark bank of cloud shifted in from the west. As a precaution, we stretched the bivi sack over our sleeping bags. Better to wait for the morning cold than wet through, we thought – gallows humour. We were frightened of storms. We thought about Buscaini, trapped for five days with Silvia Metzeltin on the Jori Route to our right when continuous rain made any further progress impossible. Retreat through the waterfalls and avalanches of stones was out of the question. Cold, hungry and wet…it was a miracle that they had survived at all.

'*Attenti allí acqua* – be careful if it rains', the publican at the 'Locanda al Sasso' in Taibon had warned us.

It's not going to rain, we thought. But it did rain. And how it rained. No, it didn't rain, it poured, it hailed.

Again and again, lightning flashed and thunder rolled. A raging storm had broken and it would not stop.

As the first fragments of rock began to crash onto our bivi bag we dismantled the makeshift roof and fled the little ledge that we had taken such pains to prepare. In darkness, we felt our way back down the chimney to a chockstone, where we spent half of the night huddled together, shivering, frightened. We were scared. Very scared!

Behind everything that we know as adventure, experience, the joy of climbing, behind all this there is always fear.

It is Fear writ large, and danger and hope too. Our place was so small, so full of doubts. We did not want to be afraid, afraid of the waterfalls and the slabs above, afraid of a fall. Down in the valley, before we set off, we had wanted to be brave.

Nevertheless, we were afraid. Initially only of the rain, of the lightning, of the stonefall. The overhangs came later, much later, while far away – somewhere on the Civetta or the Pelmo or somewhere else – the thunder rolled.

Towards midnight the storm abated. There were still no stars to be seen as we felt our way back up the chimney to our little nest; this night was a long one. Nothing had happened – not here nor there – yet we were full of uncertainty. The weather had not improved. So we waited it out. At 9 o'clock in the

morning we continued, climbing up, as retreat seemed too long and dangerous. The slabs were easier than we had thought they would be the day before. With only six peg runners, I climbed more than 200m up the armour of slabs, moving right, then back left of the water streak, always following the freest route.

Heini led the overhanging crack leading up into the exit gully. Up above, a little stream trickled out of the gully, showering us as we climbed. It actually felt like being under the shower. The summit gully was not particularly difficult; just a few wet bits and loose chimneys.

Over on the other side, in the bivi box below the summit, we arranged ourselves for the night. As we were drying our clothes in the morning sun, Erich arrived. He was surprised to see us at the bivi box. Sitting down there in his tent he had no longer thought that our adventure would turn out so well.

We wanted to be going now.

'Maybe I'll find myself another big wall problem for this holiday', the great Aste said. We hoped he would.

'*Arrivederci* – see you again, Aste.'

See you again, Agnér.

The farmer was still sitting outside his hut, staring at us in astonishment.

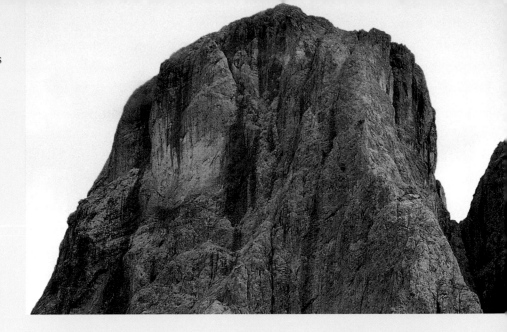

The summit wall of Monte Agnér. The Messner Route takes the black water streak on the left; the chimney system on the right is followed by the Jori Route.

'Compared to his famous brother-in-law Tita Piaz, Checco Jori had a decidedly more even temperament and was possessed of the kind of indescribable modesty that has no truck with flashy self-aggrandise-ment, which made him an even nicer person to be with. As a climber – and this is the unanimous verdict of his partners – Checco Jori was at least the equal of Tita Piaz, if not superior to him.'

BEPI PELLEGRINON

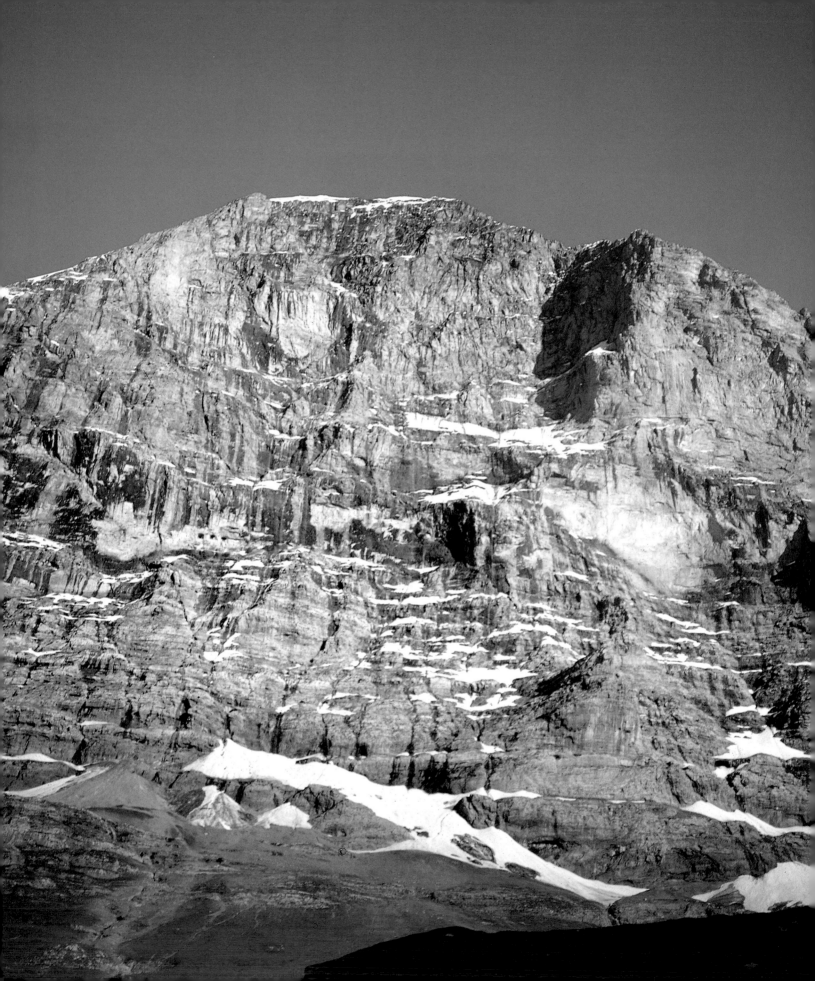

THE LAST GREAT PROBLEMS
OF THE ALPS

The solution to the 'three last problems of the Alps' must be viewed in the context of the young generation of Munich climbers who, in the 1930s, set out to surpass their role models Hans Dülfer, Otto Herzog and Emil Solleder. Little time was spent deliberating the sense of mountaineering; actions spoke louder than words. What else was there to test their youthful energies? In addition to the nascent fascism then prevalent, widespread unemployment meant that climbers of every political persuasion were now more independent.

Hermann Kobel and Emil Solleder had already spoken about the problem of the North Face of the Matterhorn back in 1925, but not a single attempt was then made. Solleder, a master on rock, lacked experience on ice, in common with practically all of the contenders for these 'last great big wall problems in the Alps'! To succeed on the North Face of the Matterhorn it was not enough to be a good rock climber. Fitness, toughness, ice-climbing technique and not least route-finding ability all played an important part.

Then, in 1931, the news suddenly went round the world (there was, of course, no Internet then!) – 'the North Face of the Matterhorn has been conquered!'

Contrary to many people's expectations, It was not Leo Rittler and Hans Brehm who were the conquerors, but the Schmid brothers, and they had kept their plans a complete secret.

There were dozens who knew of this problem and who would have loved to have been the one to solve it. But in the end success fell to just two men – Franz and Toni Schmid. They had travelled by bicycle from Munich and after their successful ascent they cycled back home again.

After dispensing with the steep initial ice field, the two men had attacked the oblique gully system in the middle of the face and bivouacked at the end of it. The frozen rocks of the North Face slanted awkwardly and were loose in parts, and, in addition, the second day brought mist and windblown snow. It was not until the late afternoon that the two brothers reached the summit. Since they could not be seen from below – either on the summit wall or on the descent to the Solvay Hut, where they were trapped by the storm – they were presumed missing.

Although Walter Bonatti's 1965 first ascent of the Direct North Face in winter – and solo – set new standards of classic Alpine mountaineering, his route, although it has been repeated several times, is of secondary importance. The classic route was, and remains, the Schmid Route, as it is more logical.

The next objective was the North Face of the Grandes Jorasses. In the thirties, a trip to the Western Alps was as difficult and awkward an undertaking as an expedition is today. When Gustl Kröner and Anderl Heckmair cycled to Chamonix in July 1931 to attempt the northern precipices of the Grandes Jorasses, they had previously sent their equipment ahead as freight and had to wait around at the foot of Mont Blanc for almost two weeks for it to arrive, a period of time sufficient nowadays to mount a modern, lightweight expedition to an 8000m peak.

If we ignore for a moment several failed attempts by French climbers under the leadership of Armand Charlet, nothing of note was done on the Jorasses Wall in 1932 and 1933. Gustl Kröner, however, was still 'hot for it' and teamed up with Walter Stösser. They turned their attentions first to the North Face of the Matterhorn, hoping to bag the second ascent, but Kröner was killed by stonefall during the attempt.

In 1934 Anderl Heckmair joined forces with Martin Meier, one of the best of the Munich climbers, and Ludwig Steinauer from the Bayerland section of the Alpine Club, for an attempt on the Jorasses Wall. Rudolf Peters and Rudolf Haringer were on the route at the same time. The weather, however, was inclement and the atmosphere between the two parties antagonistic. The Leschaux Hut was then in the process of being renovated and the two teams had to bivouac in a cave and pitch a tent, respectively. One night, during a fearful storm, the Heckmair party

'Black ribs of slanting, verglassed rock requiring the utmost caution. Our objective was the big, tremendously steep, rightwards trending depression that leads up through the middle section of the face and ends high up below the 500m slabby summit headwall.'

— FRANZ SCHMID

'Grandes Jorasses! Like a demon, this face dominated my every thought, my life. I knew about many smaller problems but they did not interest me; I concentrated totally on the big objective.'

— ANDERL HECKMAIR

(facing page): worm's-eye view of the North Face of the Eiger.

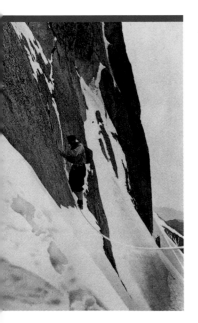

Armand Charlet on the North Face of the Grandes Jorasses.

abandoned their cave for the safety of the half-finished hut. In spite of Heckmair's invitation to move into the hut with them, Peters and Haringer stayed in their tent. When Peters' petrol stove exploded, engulfing the tent in flames, they were all sympathetic of Rudl's plight but only Haringer accepted the renewed offer to come into the hut. Despite the incessant rain, Peters stayed where he was, lying amidst the remains of his equipment. Such a display of stubbornness and obstinacy certainly demanded respect from Heckmair but it did not bring success on the climb. Heckmair departed.

Meier and Steinauer also abandoned their attempt after a bivouac on the face, whereupon Peters and Haringer set off on the face. Armand Charlet, who had already made many attempts on the Jorasses, followed.

When the Charlet team gave up, Peters and Haringer continued undeterred. On the third day on the face, however – the two men were only about 200m below the summit ridge – the weather suddenly took a turn for the worse. As the wind rose and the hail and snow set in, retreat became imperative. The climbers were caught by nightfall while still on the abseils and forced into an emergency bivouac. It was their third night on the face. Ignoring Peters' warnings, Haringer untied from the rope in order to look for a halfway acceptable spot to bivouac. In the process, he suddenly slipped and disappeared into the void. Peters, numb with shock, heard a series of dull thuds, growing fainter ... Then silence.

Rudolf Peters, wet, hungry and desperate, waited and dozed fitfully through the long, cold night. In the morning, he attempted to rescue himself! A portion of the equipment had disappeared down the face with Haringer; even Peters' snow goggles had gone missing. In spite of this, Peters slowly made his way down, half climbing, half abseiling. Snow-blind, at the absolute limit of his endurance, he felt his way back down to the foot of the face. In the afternoon he reached a point a few metres above the bergschrund where, half-blind by now, he drove in his last ice piton as an abseil anchor. 'The sheer effort of dredging up my very last reserves of strength and willpower is something I find inconceivable, even now' (Peters). He reached the tent in the crevasse where they had spent the night before setting out on the North Face and fell into an exhausted sleep. Meanwhile, climbers who had rushed to help found the body of Haringer.

Peters, too, was presumed dead, before he had made his descent. Haringer was buried in Chamonix and Martin Meier occupied the now vacant pillion seat on Peters' motorbike for the long ride back to Munich.

A year later, Peters succeeded on the unbelievable, the impossible – the North Face of the Grandes Jorasses, climbing the Croz Spur with Meier. But by now a second race had already begun, the race for the Walker Spur, the 'last great problem of the Alps'.

With typical determination, Richard Cassin, who had arrived too late for the North Face of the Eiger, hurried to the Grandes Jorasses where, over three days in 1938, together with Ugo Tizzoni and Gino Esposito, he made the first ascent of the climb described as one of the 'most beautiful routes in the Alps'. With this route Cassin, without doubt the best climber in the world at the time, established a line next to the one climbed by Peters and Meier which surpassed the latter in terms of steepness, length and difficulty.

Nowadays, with the Walker Spur having seen several thousand ascents, often in winter (the first being done by Walter Bonatti and Cosimo Zappelli, 1963) and solo (first solo ascent by Alessandro Gogna, 1968), the Croz is once more gaining in significance. The other routes on the North Face of the Grandes Jorasses, climbed later, often in expedition style and in winter, remain second rate by comparison.

'Smooth and absolutely unclimbable' – that was how the Englishman, A.W. Moore described the North Face of the Eiger when he looked down on it from the North-West Ridge after the third ascent of the mountain in 1864. The Eiger had first been climbed in 1858 by Charles Barrington and his guides Christian Almer and Peter Bohren, and all the ridges were done before a small circle of elite climbers began to turn their thoughts to the North Face itself. Willo Welzenbach was one of the first to give serious consideration to the possibility of climbing it, but in the years when attempts were being made he was no longer able to participate, having lost his life on Nanga Parbat in 1934. Although he was not an outstanding rock climber, Welzenbach combined all those other attributes and skills needed to succeed on a face such as the Eigerwand – a mastery of the new rock and ice techniques, calm, strength, stamina, experience gained on big walls and the ability to work well in a

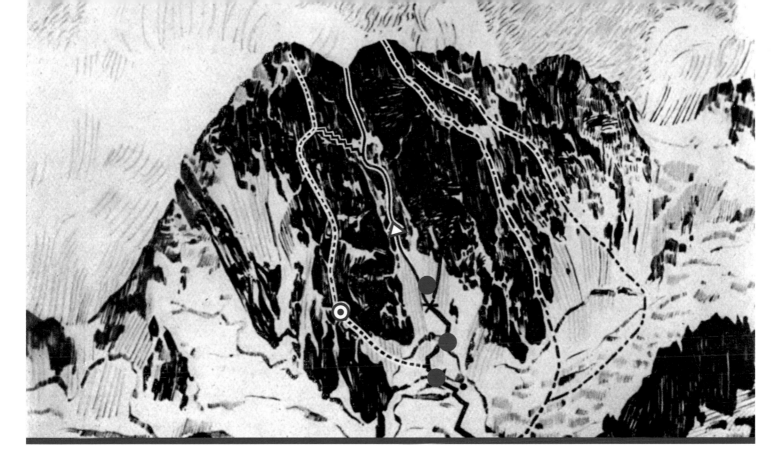

partnership. 'In our Munich climbing club "Hoch-empor" we had a master blacksmith who made pitons for the whole of the Munich climbing frater-nity', Anderl Heckmair recalls. Perhaps Welzenbach had also been shopping?

The first serious attempt – a kind of assault on the North Face of the Eiger – was made by Munich men Max Sedelmayr and Karl Mehringer. Both were excellent climbers – Sedelmayr had made the third ascent of the East Face of Sass Maor. But neither had the necessary experience on ice. And they must surely have deceived themselves about the enormity of their undertaking.

The North Face of the Eiger has a relative height of 1800m! Sedelmayr and Mehringer attacked the first band of cliffs above the initial rocks, following the direct fall line from the summit. Their second, dreadfully cold, bivouac was on the First Ice Field. On the third day, they made only very slow upward progress. The two climbers were being observed from Kleine Scheidegg when mist enveloped the face. Presumably they had their third bivouac on the upper rim of the Second Ice Field. On the fourth day the weather was terrible. When it finally cleared towards midday on day five the two men could be seen. They were still climbing, moving

towards the feature that was later to become known as the Flatiron. Then, mist, storm, stonefall, avalanches – nothing more was seen of Sedelmayr and Mehringer.

The Munich Mountain Rescue Service organized a rescue attempt. But all efforts to help were in vain. When the sun broke through again, the face was plastered with ice and fresh snow. There was not the slightest sign of the missing climbers. Only three weeks later, when the famous Alpine pilot Ernst Udet flew his plane to within 20m of the presumed last bivouac, was one of the climbers spotted – frozen stiff, like a pillar of ice, leaning against the wall; dead.

In 1936, three teams planned to attempt the face: the Munich pair Herbst and Teufel, Berch-tesgaden men Hinterstoisser and Kurz, and Rainer and Angerer from Salzburg. Hinterstoisser and Kurz were two of the best rock climbers in the Eastern Alps. Herbst and Teufel, who had arrived at Kleine Scheidegg at the end of May and had seen that it was still too early for the Eigerwand, suffered a fatal accident while descending from the Schreck-horn at the beginning of July. A few days later Angerer and Rainer made an attempt but turned back due to the bad conditions on the lower part of

Gustl Kröner's drawing of the North Face of the Grandes Jorasses with the lines then considered possible marked.

⬤ = lower bergschrund

⬤ = upper bergschrund

⬤ = high point of attempt Heckmair/Kröner 1931,

△ = presumed site of Brehm/Ritter fall

◉ = high point reached by Heron et al. in 1928

'I feared some kind of competitive free-for-all and made Peters, who had done as little on ice as Haringer, aware of the peculiar dangers of this face.'

ANDERL HECKMAIR

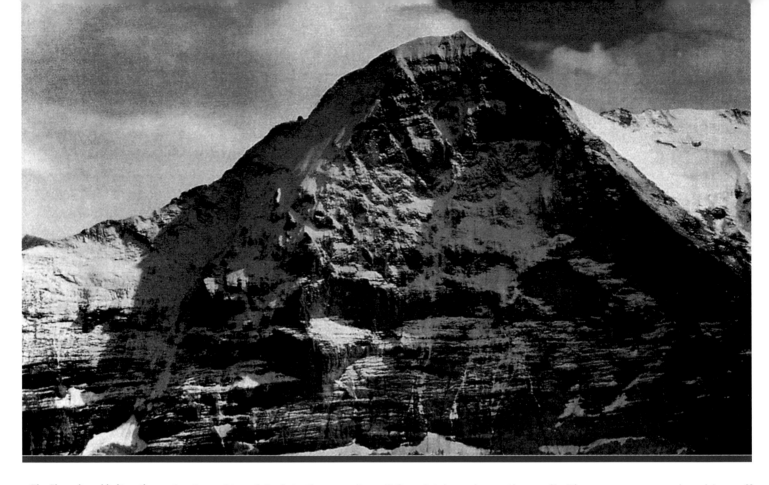

The Eiger viewed in its entire width from the North. To the left is the North-East Face, with the notorious North Face in the middle.

'The North Face of the Eiger is, after all, not some kind of climbing wall, or any old amusement park challenge built for climbers. This cracked and shattered precipice has a history rich in victims and, above all, it reaches deep into the adventurous hearts of whole generations of mountaineers.'

DER SPIEGEL

the face. At 2 o'clock in the morning of the 18 July they set off again, at the same time as Kurz and Hinterstoisser. A short while later the two parties joined forces.

In contrast to Sedelmayr and Mehringer, they took a rightwards detour around the first barrier of cliffs and Hinterstoisser made a crucial tension traverse to gain the First Ice Field, thus solving one of the crux sections of the face. But it was exactly this traverse that was to prove to be the four climbers' undoing, for after retrieving the rope used a handrail they had effectively cut off their only means of retreat. Angerer was injured by stonefall higher up the climb, yet the four men still managed to get as far as the upper rim of the Second Ice Field, where they established their first bivouac. On the second day, mist enshrouded the face. Visibility was nil and they managed only another 200m. Finally, on the third day, they began their retreat. The mist closed in again. They could hardly see a thing.

Three hundred metres lower, completely soaked through, exhausted and frozen stiff, the climbers spent their third night on the face. The weather had deteriorated still further. Torrents of water roared

down the wall. There was snow sloughing off everywhere. On the fourth day they stood, motionless, for hours at the impossible slabs below the Rother Fluh, where they had pulled in the rope after the tension traverse. How to get down now? It was a desperate situation; the rising traverse rightwards would not go. Valuable time elapsed, with 200m of nothing yawning below the climbers. A last attempt ended with Hinterstoisser taking a fall onto the rope. In desperation, they made the fateful decision to abseil directly down the partly overhanging rock step.

Later on, calls for help were heard. But only one person was shouting! The sector linesman of the Jungfrau railway alerted the rescue team, who climbed out of the Gallery Window onto the face that same afternoon. They managed to get to within 100m of the climbers. They could not get any closer.

Was Toni Kurz the sole survivor? Yes, Hinterstoisser had come off and fallen the whole way down, Rainer had frozen to death and Angerer was dead too, strangled by the rope when he fell. Kurz had run out of gear and could not abseil any further. He sat on a tiny rock ledge and the rescuers were unable to reach him. There was nothing they could do. The stonefall continued, the weather was foul, it grew dark ...

When morning came, Toni Kurz was still alive. He shouted for help. Was a miracle about to happen? The guides on the rescue team managed to climb to within about 40m of Kurz. Using one hand – the other had frozen stiff during the horrific bivouac – and his teeth, he unravelled a piece of the rope into several strands and tied them together to form a thread long enough to lower down to his rescuers. They tied on two ropes, some pitons, carabiners and food. Kurz hauled it all up and was finally able to start abseiling, using a carabiner brake and sit sling. But he became stuck at the knot joining the two ropes, 3m above the rescuers. Was it all to be in vain? Yes, it was – Toni Kurz died of exhaustion.

After these attempts, and their fatal consequences, it fell to Hias Rebitsch and Ludwig Vörg to prove that escape from the face in bad weather was indeed possible when, in 1937, they managed successfully to retreat from 'Death Bivouac'.

Then, in the midsummer of 1938, Anderl Heckmair, Ludwig Vörg, Fritz Kasparek and Heinrich Harrer finally completed the first ascent, in four days. High up on the summit wall, the weather turned mean and Heckmair had to gamble everything to lead the party of four – the German and Austrian teams had by then joined forces – safely off the face.

The aura surrounding the North Face, which had arisen as a result of the dramatic first ascent attempts and the adventurous events on the first ascent itself, increased after the Second World War as the route received its first repeats. Numerous tragedies followed.

Even after the first winter ascent (Toni Kinshofer, Walter Almberger, Anderl Mannhardt, Toni Hiebeler, 1961) and the first solo ascent (Michel Darbellay, 1963) the wall remained for a further decade the most feared climb in the Alps.

Now however, after so many ascents that it is impossible to record them all, after helicopter rescues and the cellphone culture, the wall has lost much of its sinister atmosphere. Above all, the successful helicopter rescues have contributed to the fact that – in informed circles at least – the Eigerwand is no longer considered to be the 'Mordwand', or Wall of Death, it once was. Since the 1970s it has lost much of its magic, the spell has been broken.

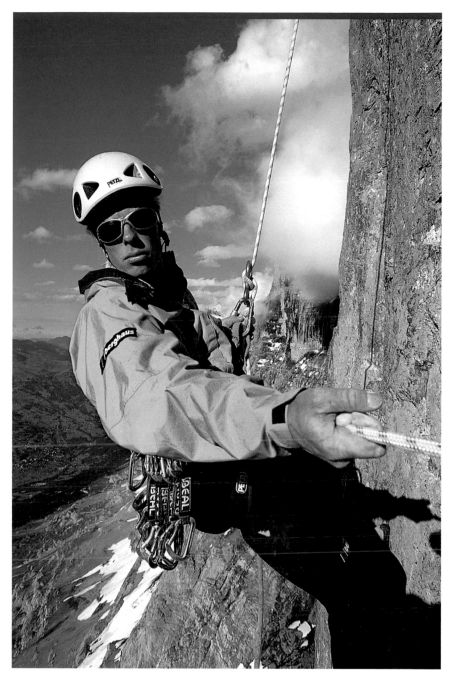

Viewed in this context, with every successful ascent and above all as a result of modern helicopter rescue techniques, the North Face of the Eiger has grown 'smaller'. Although, after the Harlin-Direttissima (winter 1966) and the not-so-logical line of the Japanese Route (summer 1969), many further routes have been added to the face, the Heckmair Route will always be the classic, the ideal line on the North Face of the Eiger.

Robert Jasper, one of the best ice climbers of our times, on one of the modern Eiger routes. Jasper is an excellent all-round mountaineer and has climbed more than a dozen routes on the Eigerwand.

MATTERHORN NORTH FACE

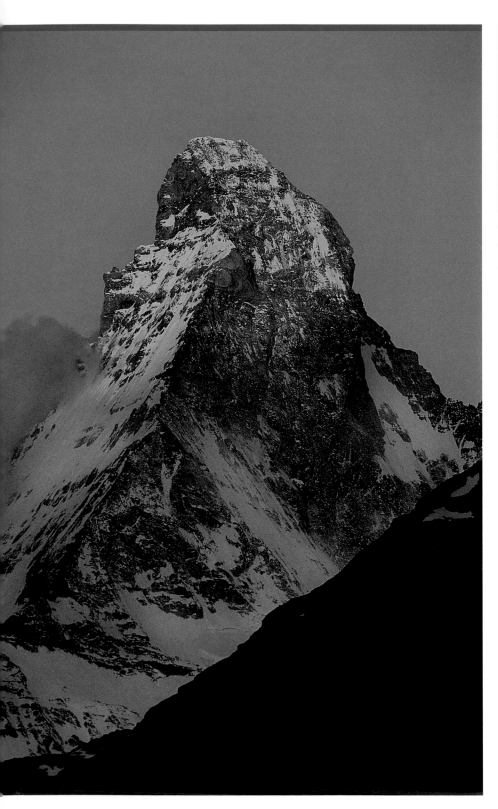

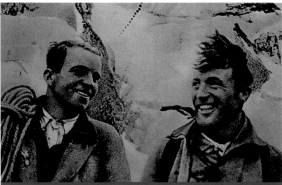

The 'Battle for the Matterhorn' signalled the end of the Golden Age of Mountaineering when all the great Alpine peaks were conquered. The desire to be the first to stand on its summit had eclipsed much of the romantic idealism that had characterized early Alpinism, and had also done much to dispel the superstitious fear of mountain spirits. Rivalry was widespread amongst the leading mountaineers of the day. It was probably for this reason that, in 1865, this 'most beautiful Alpine peak' was climbed by two completely different routes in quick succession – by Whymper and his group via the Swiss Ridge, and by Carel and his friend from the Italian side. The idea that the Matterhorn's North Face might also be climbable did not occur to people for more than another sixty years, at a time when exploration of the difficult faces and ridges in the Alps was approaching its zenith.

And just as the summit of the Matterhorn had exerted a special attraction for mountaineers in the conquest, or peak-bagging, phase of Alpinism, so too the North Face of this elegantly sculpted four-thousander exercised a similar magnetic pull on many of the pioneers in the classical era of hard Alpinism. It was not just the steepness that was challenging, it was also the line.

Today the sight of the North Face of the Matterhorn still provokes enthusiastic reaction in every top climber, even if they know it is loose and really not as difficult as it appears. Its logical line, superlative free climbing and, above all, the fact that the climb leads directly onto the summit of the Matterhorn, are what give the North Face route its reputation.

The North Face of the Matterhorn and the first successful climbers, Toni and Franz Schmid (above).

BORDERLINE SITUATION ON THE MATTERHORN

At the end of July 1974 towards 7 o'clock in the morning, Peter Habeler and I stood indecisively below the Difficult Crack on the North Face of the Eiger. It was warm and therefore everything was so wet that we could not really make up our minds whether to go on climbing or not. On the ledges under the first buttress of smooth rock it was so unpleasant that our rapid progress came to a sudden stuttering halt. To move even ten paces to our left would mean serious danger, as lumps of ice came crashing down. Waterfalls gushed down the Rote Fluh and even above the Hinterstoisser Traverse, the morning air was full of spray. We gave up and climbed back down the face.

That same evening we sat in the Hörnli Hut under the Matterhorn, trying to engage the guides present in conversation. We wanted to learn from them what sort of condition the North Face was in. Our abortive attempt on the Eigerwand was already long forgotten. We had descended to the valley and driven to Zermatt the very same day. On the walk up to the hut, Peter had set a cracking pace.

The guides were all of the opinion that although the face was not exhibiting any signs of being in good condition it must still be possible. We should, however, allow two days and a storm in the afternoon, they said, should not be ruled out. This counsel left us a little uneasy and we passed the evening in the cheerless room leafing through the hut book hoping to find a recent entry for the North Face. We did not find any. Just before we went to bed – Peter was already discussing with some Americans their plans to climb the Normal Route – I met up with a Japanese climber in the outer room who was all equipped in North Wall gear. He was so exhausted that he looked stoned. At first I did not know if what I had here was a 'pothead' or an extreme climber and asked, a little hesitantly, 'Matterhorn North Face?' He nodded and gave me to understand that it had been very hard. 'The face is all iced-up. We bivouacked at the very end of the slanting couloir – spent the whole night on a tiny ledge. It was very cold. We have just come down from the summit.' His friend, also Japanese, had joined us in the meantime and a broad grin crossed his face when he noticed my interest.

This chance night-time meeting strengthened our resolve to have a crack at the North Face the next morning. We checked our equipment that night, put the bare essential bivouac gear into the rucksack and set the alarm clock for 2 o'clock.

When we left the hut shortly after two, there were already numerous parties on the Hörnli Ridge, as the many little glimmering lights betrayed. A Swiss guide heading for the Zmutt Ridge had started the traverse under the North Face ahead of us. Peter and I – still moving together – overtook him while he was carefully belaying his client on a steep ice pitch. The ice was blank in places and we were glad when, as we reached the plateau beneath the North Face, the first grey light dawned.

We stamped our way a few hundred metres further through slushy snow until we were at a place where, from below at least, it looked possible to cross the bergschrund. Directly above us stood a steep ice shield, smooth and unremitting; it led up to the slanting couloir and was mostly as hard as iron. We made straight for the edge of the crevasse, roped up and crossed it without difficulty. The ice in the Great Ice Field was glassy and the climbing not without danger, so we had to keep placing intermediate pitons for protection.

In the meantime the grey mists that had masked the summit of the Matterhorn since the early morning had now covered the surrounding mountain ranges. Above us, they clung around the mountain down to around the 4000m level. Peter and I had made very fast progress to the start of the big traverse and we hoped to be on the summit in a few hours.

The certainty that by late afternoon we would have the North Face behind us mounted as we traversed the last, infamous pitches of verglassed rock in the slanting couloir. Neither of us had hesitated once on the climbing we had done so far.

Everything had gone smoothly and as trouble-free as if we were on a classic Dolomite route. We even managed the steep loose groove without difficulty. We reached the spot, marked by a few items of rubbish, where the Japanese climbers had bivouacked. All this time I had not for a moment felt as if we were on one of the great faces of the Alps. Although the first snowflakes had been whirling around for an hour or so, we were cheerfully confident, perhaps over-confident.

Not until we reached the steeply sloping slabs which led out to the right and onto the easier-angled

> 'The right choice of partner for a particular climbing objective is a basic prerequisite for success. The reciprocal trust must be there, especially in critical situations when it can be a life-saving factor. In all my climbing career to date I have not known a better climbing partner than Peter Habeler, and although we have done relatively few routes together we have always got on brilliantly well together. This is not only due to the fact that Peter is a climber of great ability, is always superbly fit and has a manner which I find appealing, but also a result of his essential character.'
>
> REINHOLD MESSNER

Peter Habeler and Reinhold Messner on the North Face of the Matterhorn during their attempt on the Bonatti Route in the winter of 1966.

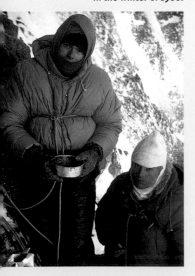

headwall did I suddenly feel that we had begun to lose our command of the situation. Enough snow had fallen by this time to cover all the little ledges and cracks that were to serve as our foot- and handholds. I was in the lead and called back to warn Peter how difficult it was becoming – friction climbing, placing of belay pegs, to say nothing of down-climbing. Moreover, I was no longer sure which was the best way to proceed. I looked left then right – everywhere the same uniformly steep angled slabs. Under the loose layer of new snow the rocks were coated with a thin glaze of ice, which was particularly unpleasant when there were no horizontal footholds to be unearthed anywhere.

Worse still – in the middle of a holdless, smooth slope the rope ran out. I was forced to hammer half a dozen knife-blade pitons into two hairline cracks. It was the only way I could construct a reliable belay.

Once he had climbed up to join me, Peter led through, tension traversing out to the right and then, in the thickening snow, attempting to move back left above me to the edge of a pillar of rock. The original route seemed to take a line out to the right but was swept by perpetual new snow avalanches, leaving him no other choice than this projecting spur. Although it was certainly the steepest piece of rock in the vicinity, at least he did not run the danger of being swept off into the void by the periodic avalanches that came sloughing down. From the stance at the end of his pitch I tried climbing some cracks which rose to the left up to the shoulder of the mountain. Useless. The cracks were channels for snowslides and out of the question. We had to concentrate on the rock spur which, steep and forbidding, rose above us.

Centimetre by centimetre I dragged myself upwards, cleaning off each hold as I went. When a snowslide flowed over me like a waterfall, I would duck, bent almost double, and wait until the icy shower had passed. Then instinctively I would begin again, scrabbling with the tips of my fingers to uncover the holds for the next move. I had been able to place a few pegs and so the slim hope grew in me that I might not plunge unchecked if I suddenly slipped on the icy terrain. I thought I perceived a narrow ledge under the layers of snow and, holding my breath, I gingerly balanced my way up to the left.

The few lulls in the storm permitted snatches of conversation, and while I kept saying that I was on the brink of falling, Peter encouraged me not to give up, to climb just a few more metres up to the shelter of an overhang. Once there I tried to place some pegs for the belay but during my seemingly everlasting search for cracks I soon realized that the standing about was even worse than the climbing. I was chilled and wet. The fine spindrift, which the storm – now graduated into a hurricane – blew inside my clothes, was now melting against my skin.

Another avalanche rattled down on top of me. The overhang, under which we had hoped to find some shelter, was too small to prevent the cascades of snow from sweeping down upon us. When Peter had climbed up on the fixed rope to join me on my stance, he had warmed up slightly. But the pitch that awaited him and the continual bombardment of avalanches would demand all of his skill, despite his best efforts. 'I am glad it's you', I said as he climbed on past me to take over the lead, 'I wouldn't have let anyone else lead this bit.'

The face was plastered with a layer of ice and snow and every time a flash of lightning struck the summit rocks, we would wait for the stones to whir past that we knew must follow. We were both chilled to the bone. A retreat was now out of the question. We laboured up to a spur between the main summit and the shoulder. 'Don't come off now', I heard Peter murmur to himself. He was climbing in a steep groove. Again powder snow avalanches were engulfing him so that for a few minutes at a time I couldn't see him at all. 'Watch me!' he shouted down again. Peter climbed without gloves, hold by hold, in constant danger of slipping off; anyone else would surely have fallen, but not Peter. He inched steadily onwards.

It was not just the rope that bound us together on this storm-battered summit wall; we were linked, too, in a critical situation by the constant fear of lightning – wherever it struck it invariably unleashed a hail of stones. Above us, to the side of us, the stone avalanches hurtled down into the abyss. It was only mutual trust that helped us preserve a measure of calm and climb the next two pitches without a fall.

Suddenly the angle eased, and the rock became more favourably structured and thus easier to climb. It was still snowing and the thunder continued to crash all around us, but we could now make out the summit ridge above us through the cloud and the spindrift. Up there, all the objective dangers that we had been mercilessly exposed to for many hours now would stop; up there lay temporary respite.

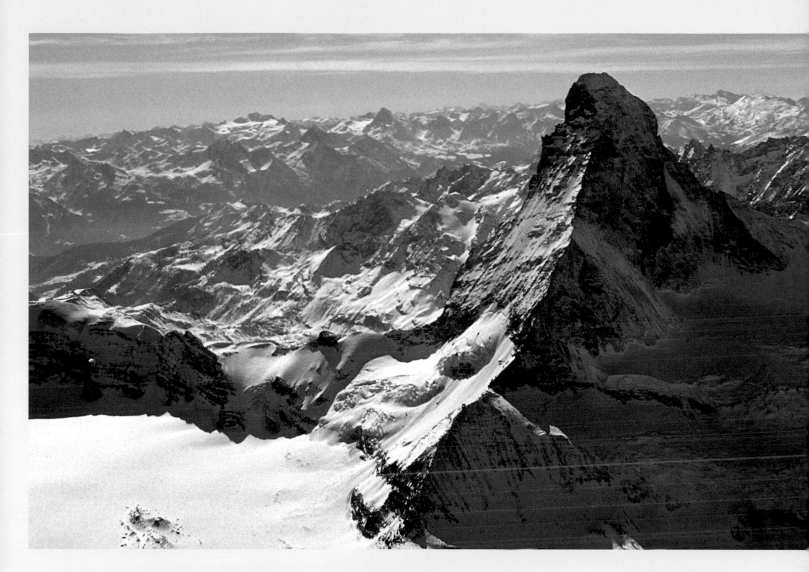

It was already past midday when we shook hands on the ridge. Because of the lightning risk we made haste to get off the exposed summit as soon as possible.

We unroped and climbed down to the Shoulder; from there we could see the whole of the descent route, which neither of us knew from experience, but which was easily distinguished from the number of parties making their way down. In their bright clothing, they were easy to pick out against the grubby snow-covered rocks.

We enjoyed the descent as much as we had enjoyed climbing the central section of the face a few hours before. The guides assisting their clients down step by step were somewhat surprised when we greeted them from above and assumed that we had given up and retreated when the storm broke. Back at the hut they congratulated us warmly, which was doubly pleasing in view of the normally reticent nature of the Swiss Guides.

The Matterhorn, seen from an aeroplane window. The North Face is on the right.

'The knowledge that we are not divided by the Alps but are joined by them in a common bond of unity is the cornerstone that binds us European climbers.'

GUIDO TONELLA

GRANDES JORASSES – THE WALKER SPUR

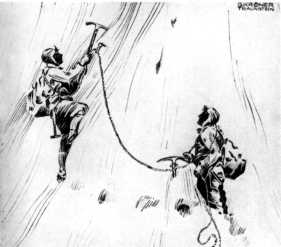

The North Face of the Grandes Jorasses consists of a series of rock buttresses, diminishing in height towards the right of the mountain. They stand hidden away in the great Mont Blanc massif but were nevertheless discovered by mountaineers quite early on. At first, however, this granite face was sketched, then photographed and in 1935 climbed for the first time. But the ideal route, the Walker Spur, was only climbed a few years later. Since then it has ranked as the 'most beautiful extreme route in the Alps'.

Although there are now more than a dozen routes on the North Face of the Grandes Jorasses, the Walker Spur remains the classic and whenever talk turns to the 'Three Great Alpine Faces' one thinks of the huge granite pillar that leads up to the Pointe Walker. Its steepness and compactness give it a special kind of fascination. If the irresistible thing about the Matterhorn is the shape of the mountain, mirrored in its North Face, and the lure of the Eiger is in its sheer size and the logic of the route, with the Walker Spur it is the elegance and directness of the line that challenges the climber.

Profile view of the North Face of the Grandes Jorasses and (above) the climbers during an attempt on the face, first climbed by Rudolf Peters and Martin Meier in 1935.

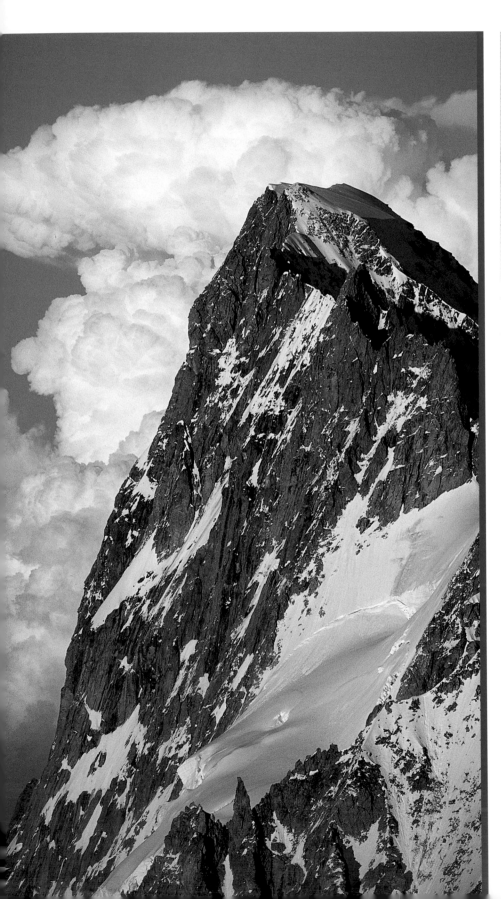

BIVOUAC ON THE WALKER SPUR

We had high hopes for that summer. We had been to the Dolomites to prepare ourselves for the Western Alps and had often discussed the Walker Spur, having seen it described in books as 'the most beautiful route in the Alps'. When Günther, my brother, and I were waiting at Milan station for a connection, several people enquired whether we were returning from Mount Everest – so big were our rucksacks, our faces so sunburnt. For this, our first trip to the Western Alps, we had saved for a year and had run many thousands of metres in training. Now we were waiting for the train that would carry us and our many plans, our dreams and our hopes, to Courmayeur.

We arrived in torrential rain and the next morning we still did not get to see Mont Blanc through the clouds. Nevertheless, we hitch-hiked that day over to Chamonix and from there climbed up to the Argentiere Hut.

The next morning, bright and early, we plodded off towards the foot of the North Face of the Courtes. Snow fell gently on the icy slopes and all the other climbers were heading off down the mountain in groups. Günther and I kept on going and reached the summit in four hours, searching through the mist for the highest point, where we waited in vain for the breath of wind that would cause the clouds to disperse.

The weather remained unsettled and from the summit were we only able to get a brief glimpse the North Face of the Grandes Jorasses. We knew all about the difficult routes on this 1000m-plus face, we carried the image deep within us and only began our descent when the wind had again drawn a thick veil of mist across the gigantic face.

My second trip to the Western Alps coincided with the fine weather period in the autumn of 1966. The fresh snow that had settled on all the mountain faces would not, we thought, present too much of an obstacle to climbing big routes. But the Chamonix guides spoke of too much new snow in the Argentiere Basin and on the Brenva Face and the Grandes Jorasses. 'The Walker Spur is coated with a thin layer of ice right to its base and is practically impossible', one of the locals informed us. But since we had come to Chamonix with the secret desire of doing the Walker, we were at first rather disinclined to believe these rumours.

We consulted the weather reports posted in Chamonix three times a day. They were so promising that even our own discussions seemed over-enthusiastic by comparison. Intoxicated by the prospect of so many fine days, at first we did not really know what decision to make. Encouraged by the continuing fine weather, yet with our feeling of security at the same time undermined by the advice of the locals, we took the rack railway up to Montenvers so that we could get a first-hand impression of the condition of the face.

We spent half an afternoon up there, gawping at the West Face of the Dru, the Bonatti Pillar and the North Face of the Charmoz but training the binoculars again and again on the Jorasses Wall. Although I secretly hankered after doing the Walker Spur I was impressed by the amount of ice on the upper half of the face and I discussed with Sepp Mayerl and Fritz Zambra, the two climbers from East Tyrol in our team of four, which also included Peter Habeler, all the various possibilities for alternative, equally worthwhile routes in the region.

We were gathered around a big telescope and every time Peter looked through it he would adjust it so that when I peered into it after him it would always be focussed on the notorious Red Chimney pitch of the Walker Spur. To be sure, it all looked very wintry but the weather was good and, as Peter was at pains to point out, there was nothing else in the whole Mont Blanc area that could remotely compare with the Walker. So it was that an hour later, against the better judgement of our two elder members, but full of expectancy, we marched across the Mer de Glace to the Leschaux Hut. We would at least make an attempt on the Spur the following day.

Bent under the load of our rucksacks and doggedly determined to adhere to our plan, we plodded along for a time one behind the other in silence. It was only when we were well up the dead glacier that all four of us halted and took a look at the Cassin Route that seemed to be getting whiter and whiter the nearer we came to it.

At that time, Peter's skill as a climber was unsurpassed. He had acquired his Guide's Diploma with Distinction. Even more than his competence on rock, the trainers had admired his all-round ability and his tough self-discipline. His slim, almost frail physique seemed completely unsuited for extreme routes, yet once on a face he was like a cat. His movements radiated power and skill. He could climb

'I knew now who the competition was and in 1935 I wanted at all costs to be the first on the North Face of the Grandes Jorasses.'

ANDERL HECKMAIR

'The pitons that had been hammered into the vertical cliffs of the world famous North Faces of the Grandes Jorasses and the Eiger Frendo and Lachenal, by Terray and Rèbuffat now bore a glorious layer of rust that obscured any clues there might once have been to their origins. They stand as monuments to the perfect protection for an ideal European climbing team.'

GUIDO TONELLA

(facing page): Below the North
Face of the Grandes Jorasses.

(below): Reinhold Messner on
the last section of the Cassin
Route (Walker Spur) on the
Grandes Jorasses.

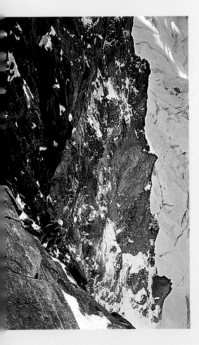

on any type of terrain, be it rock, ice or mixed ground, solo and in winter. Besides talent, he also had that kind of endurance which can only be achieved by unyielding self-discipline and rigorous year-round training. In those days, I would have believed him capable of any of those routes described in extreme climbing circles as 'desperate'.

The Mer de Glace runs like an enormous S from Montenvers right up to the foot of the Grandes Jorasses. To the right of the glacier is the Aiguille du Charmoz, its North Face prey to continual stonefall; to the left stands the Aiguille du Dru, rising against the backdrop of the Aiguille Verte like a mighty, gothic tower carved from granite. The crevasses of the dead glacier were mostly filled with stones, so that to start with we made rapid progress. Further up, isolated blocks of ice were strewn across the glacier, and here and there impressive glacier tables had formed. The sun had melted away the ice around the stones, so that the rocks – some as big as the room of a house – were left perched on slender cones of ice, like monster mushrooms of rock and ice.

During the late afternoon we reached the bivouac shelter on the right bank of the glacier, directly opposite the Walker Spur. It was still dark when we left it the next morning. An icy wind caught us in the face as we opened the door and the rocks in front of the hut were coated with a layer of hoar frost. In the cone of light from our pocket torch, we looked for a way up to the start of the climb. We had to jump over crevasses and negotiate our way around several serac zones. Day was already breaking as we approached the bergschrund and the firn snow was so good that for a brief moment we seriously debated whether we needed to rope up at all. But the thought that we were embarking upon one of the greatest Alpine routes meant that common sense prevailed and we climbed roped – Fritz and I as the lead team, Peter and Sepp following on behind. Everything went well as long as we were able to bypass the isolated patches of rock on the icefield or make use of them purely for belays.

However, further up the ice slope merged into a rock barrier with just a few isolated patches of very steep ice clinging between the rocks. The ice was glassy and hard, often only a thin layer lying on top of smooth granite slabs, and it sounded hollow when I struck it with my ice axe. Two possibilities now remained if we were to make further progress: climb the rocks or the thin ice that coated them. We first tried hacking off the armour of ice and climbing the rock; with a loud splintering noise the plates of ice

came away and went rattling down the mountain, and once we had climbed a section the work of peeling away the huge plaques of ice began anew. Next we tried front-pointing again, a not undangerous dance on a thin veneer of ice.

With each metre of height we gained, the steepness of the face increased. Soon the only ice remaining lay deep inside the cracks and grooves and once, at the end of one of these grooves, I had to make six attempts before I could climb out onto the platform above, each time sinking back onto my last hold.

Completely drained now, I set off up the Rèbuffat Crack. In the meantime, Peter and Sepp had taken over the lead. In these wintry conditions we would only achieve anything by dividing the work in a comradely fashion. The so-called 75m diedre at the end of the first third of the face was so choked with ice that none of the *in situ* pegs were visible. Sepp bridged up the outside of it and then handed over the lead to Peter, each giving of his best.

It was night before the last of us reached the first Cassin bivouac at the end of the pendulum traverse. It was a very clear, starry night and the temperature was correspondingly low. On two sloping ledges we sat close together, two and two, and waited for the morning. Astonished that we had come through it so well after the hazards and extertions of the past day, the whirl of tension and anxiety, doubt and desperation, we began to doze in our bivouac sacks. But the wind, with curious persistency, found its way through our cocoon and kept tearing us out of our half-sleep.

My gaze ranged over mountain ridges, glaciers, savage pinnacles of rock down into the valley beyond … it was all strange, out of reach and somehow inconsequential, silhouettes which memory told me I had seen before. This then was the Walker Spur, and this was me sitting here, freezing and with my toes gone to sleep. There was no way back down, not now. We would have enough pegs and ice screws to get us to the top.

The feeling spread in me that we were now safe, that for the time being there was nothing we could do here in the bivouac and at night. It was a pleasant thought, but nevertheless a little disturbing. Throughout this night, my whole body craved warmth and rest but the night was like a blanket on which I sat. I did not sleep, I no longer shut my eyes even, and tiredness weighed like lead in my arms and legs. I had the strange feeling, and it struck me again in the early hours of the morning, that I could no longer think what I wanted to think. I had no power over my

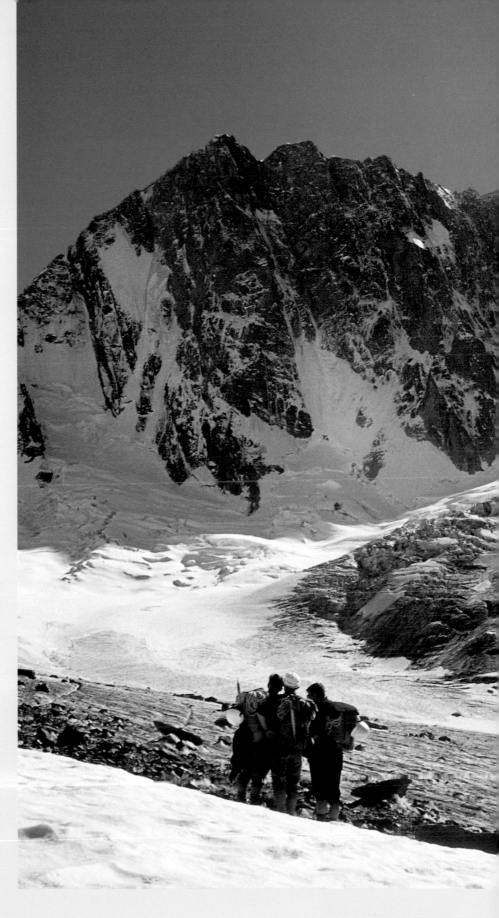

thoughts; they wandered at will and despite my best efforts they always harked back to images that I found disturbing: steep, ice-glazed slabs, chimneys choked with hard-packed snow, vertical buttresses. Maybe it was just the lack of sleep and the cold – it was already getting light now – or perhaps it was the long period of inactivity that crippled my will like sleep a dreaming body.

This state of waking sleep left me as soon as I had put the first rope's length behind me. We climbed the slabs of the Tour Grise and the subsequent arête faster than we had expected that morning. The wind had done some good work here, the arête was dry and it was only when we reached the icefield above that all our efforts were again required. We lost so much time putting on and taking off our crampons that when we reached the Red Chimney we scarcely dared hope that we would reach the summit the same day.

Wearily we looked for the route upwards. We gave up trying to find the pegs buried beneath their armour of ice and hammered in our own instead. How tiring that was! If we had really known from the start just how incredibly tiring it is to climb the Walker Spur when it is completely iced-up we would have happily waited for good conditions, maybe even for several years!

So our pleasure was all the greater when, in the late hours of the afternoon of the same day, we shook hands on the top of the Pointe Walker.

We were happy enough to bivouac on the other side of the mountain during our descent, since we knew that we would reach the hut the following day. During the night it snowed, however, and at regular intervals the snow would slide off our bivouac bags; whenever I moved, the wind blew fine spindrift under the nylon shell of the bag.

Again we froze, the moisture creeping under our clothes. We could not be bothered lighting the stove and set off again before the grey light of morning. We wanted to avoid the avalanche danger after the heavy snowfall and get down to valley early.

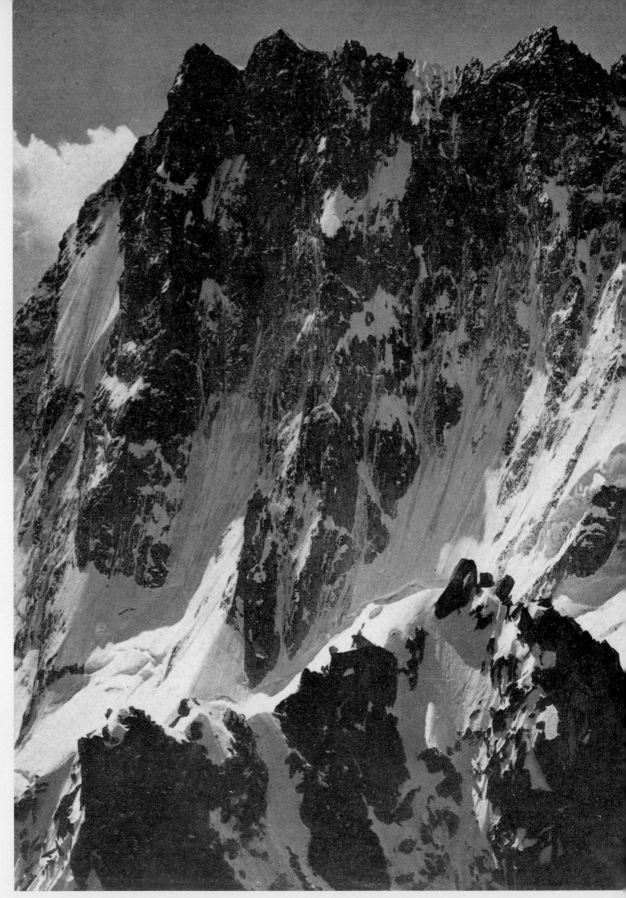

Like the Eigerwand, the 'conquest' of the Jorasses Wall was a story of jealousy, competition and resentment amongst the main protagonists.

'It would be interesting to trace whether jealousy among the many success-oriented climbers might lessen if one were to follow the example of climbers in Russia or Lombardy and introduce an annual competition for mountaineering activities. One such competition is the "Grignetta d'oro", which makes an award each year to honour the climber with the best tally of routes. What counts is a certain number of routes and their difficulty, and anyone who takes even one fall is excluded. The routes are allocated a points score and as far as the Alps are concerned it is the Walker Spur that tops the list.'

REINHOLD MESSNER

THE NORTH FACE OF THE EIGER

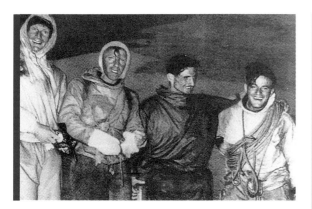

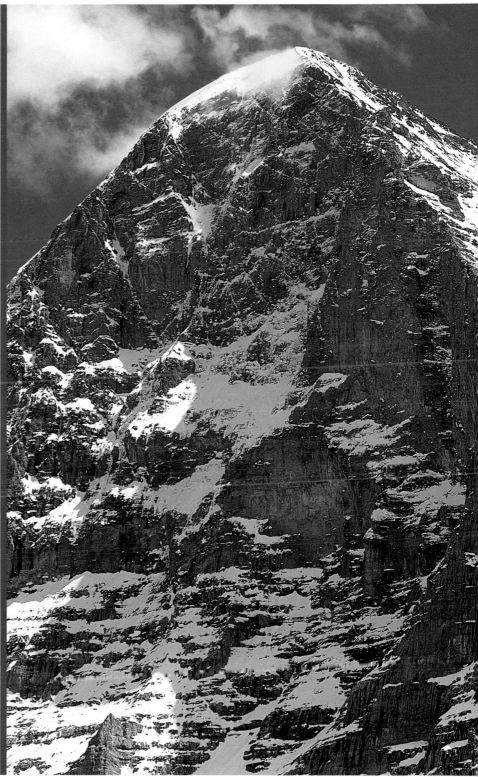

All the fuss and commotion that has surrounded the North Face of the Eiger as a result of the dramatic story of the first ascent and the many tragedies of the fifties and sixties has fortunately now passed. For a quarter of a century, this was the most infamous big face in the world; now, amongst climbers at least, it is considered to be just one of the great West Alpine faces, even if in layman's terms it remains the epitome of 'suicidal alpinism'.

The first successes on the huge faces of the eight-thousanders – more than double the height of the Eigerwand, and in part more difficult – have contributed in no small way to this redefining of the dimensions. Nevertheless, it should not be underestimated, even today.

Viewed from Kleine Scheidegg, the Eiger North Face – according to Professor Brückner the highest precipice in the Alps – exercises a strong fascination. The awesomely steep cliff, with its serried ranks of icefields, certainly appears impregnable, but the structure of the face dictates the line of the classic route so clearly that many extreme alpinists aspire to repeat it. With the exception of the shattered rocks before the Difficult Crack and the easy-angled summit icefield, the face demands the full concentration of the aspirant climber. The frequent alternation between rock and ice climbing, the fact that the route is always wet and at risk from stonefall and the sudden, violent storms give the face a certain merciless character. No other face in the Western Alps so justly deserves the title of a 'big, mixed climb' as the Eigerwand.

The Eigerwand and the first ascent team: Heinrich Harrer, Fritz Kasparek, Anderl Heckmair and Ludwig Vörg (above).

THE EIGERWAND IS CONQUERED

Anderl Heckmair's report, published in the *Völkisher Beobachter* in July 1938 was the first account to appear of the first ascent of the North Face of the Eiger and it is for this reason that I quote at length from it here. The story is told in a realistic way and in the style of the times, and gives the reader a clear insight into the thoughts of the climbers in those bygone days.

'The song you sing of these dramatic events is truly a song of heroes. It is an epic song, full of the names of all those who have fallen during the struggle and of those who were crowned with fame and glory on the shining summits, a song that speaks to us in the eternal language of battle and victory.'

GUIDO TONELLA AND
ANDERL HECKMAIR

The ascent up to the second shattered pillar only seemed difficult because of the great weight of our rucksacks. We had completed this section many times and knew every step of the way and soon – it may have been about two o'clock – we had made it to the spot where we wanted to set up the first bivouac.

It was surprising what kinds of things we had found during this ascent: several pieces of rope still hanging from their pitons, a ripped sleeping bag, a broken off ice axe and then the storm cap of our comrade Kurz who had fallen from the wall. Traces of the many earlier expeditions that had passed this way.

We almost believed we might find the body of Mehringer or one of the Italians, which the wall had not yet released. But at the top of the pillar we found a full rucksack with a note attached to it that read: 'Please do not take anything, this belongs to Kasparek and Harrer!' The Viennese had very cleverly brought their heavy load a considerable way up the face and then climbed down again in order to be able quickly and without unnecessary waste of energy to cover the greatest distance possible on the first day. Thus we knew that they were ready to go.

The night spent bivouacking was really pleasant. We slept well and long and the next morning, after we had got up, cooked and eaten, there was a lovely rosy dawn rising in the sky. Moreover, our barometer had fallen several notches, bad forecast for the next few days. As we were thinking about what was still to be done, the mist that had enshrouded us during the night slowly disappeared. We were standing 600m above the screes and we had a clear view down to Alpiglen and Grindelwald and out into the narrow Lötschen Valley. A blond figure appeared beneath us, a climber forced his way over the edge and Harrer stood before us. A rope-length behind him was Kasparek and then a little further behind Brankowski and Fraissl. At this first meeting we all pulled rather silly faces. We told the Viennese that the barometer had fallen, pointed out the rosy dawn and the approaching cirrus clouds to them and told them that we would probably be climbing back down. In addition, we said, there was no point in three ropes climbing at the same time on such a difficult face. But they wanted to continue. We wished them all luck, chatted a little with them, promised them our help if they should get into danger and then after a 'Sieg-Heil', the first rope, with Kasparek in the lead, disappeared to the left on a traverse which adjoins a fairly difficult crack leading upwards. The others followed. We began our descent.

At 10am we are standing at the foot of the wall once more. The weather has not worsened. We run to the telescope in Alpiglen and follow our comrades' progress up the wall. Kasparek is leading again; he cuts step after step out of the hard ice. Slowly they make the traverse over to the first icefield. The difficulties appear to be great. Carefully and slowly the four work their way up.

Then – all of a sudden – the second rope remains behind. They are hanging in a narrow crack. Fifteen minutes have already passed and now, now they turn back. Fraissl has, he tells us later, suffered an injury in a rock-fall and in addition he is mildly concussed. He grows slightly dizzy from time to time and it was right for him to turn back from the wall with his comrades.

But we hurry up to our camp. One party is still on the wall. We are not in too great a danger from rock-fall. If only the weather stays good. At 6 o'clock the cooker is whistling away. We take time to eat plenty and soon we are asleep on our rubber mattresses in order to draw strength for the exertion of the days ahead.

It is 2 in the morning. The stars are clear in the sky. We have slept really well and are fresh. Quickly we eat just one more hearty meal. As morning dawns

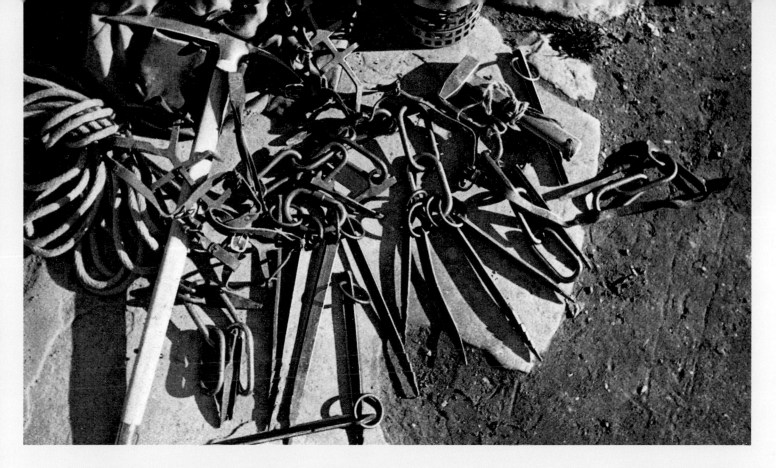

we set off onto the wall. For the last time now. The rivulets of the day, which stream down the thousand crevices of the face, are all iced up. But soon we are up on the pillar once more. We pack our rucksacks, take off the crampons and at 7am we are already tackling the first difficulty, a familiar one, the Hinterstoisser Traverse. It goes surprisingly well. There is still a stout length of rope hanging there, a leftover from the recovery operations of the German Mountain Rescue in 1936. It is a valuable help to us. We carry on quickly. We have to be quick. We have soon overcome the icy section, where a waterfall runs down over the traverse, then we are standing, it may be about 10am, at the foot of the first icefield. And we are already seeing signs of the other team coming down to us: pieces of ice crash down from the second icefield, broken off by Kasparek as he cuts out the steps. The Viennese man's steps have iced over in the night. We cannot use them. Quickly, very quickly, we climb up the steep incline of the mirror-like ice surface in order to get out of the area of ice hail. And we are immediately faced by another difficulty. The traverse to the second icefield is surprisingly hard.

The gully we have to get up is a frozen waterfall. We have to press the teeth of our Grivel crampons sharply into the ice in order to gain any purchase and

then, then we have overcome that obstacle too. Now we continue up the second icefield. To the left, up there on the western edge, is where the two Viennese spent their first night. During the night, probably at about quarter to two I saw the flash of a flame. So they must have brewed hot tea or coffee there. Now we find fresh tracks from today and then, at 11.30, we catch up with our comrades. We stand next to each other, the Viennese and us. And there is only one thing left for it: to continue together, to stick it out, and to fight our way through to victory!

We relieve Kasparek, who has blisters on his hands because of the many steps he has cut, take the lead and off we go up to the third icefield. We have to overcome difficult chimneys. We climb up channels of ice. At 2 o'clock we are up. We are unable to eat, only drink. And so we cut ourselves a stance and make Ovaltine and eat dry toast. The four of us have become a unit.

By three o'clock we have reached the edge of the third icefield. There we find an old piton that Mehringer had hammered in.

Steep walls tower up above us, which no man has ever set foot upon before. The four of us agree unanimously that we must forge ahead as quickly as possible. We agree that the best line to take can only

A selection of the equipment used by the Heckmair/Vörg team ('ironmongery', rope, stove and ice axe).

'The North face of the Eiger – everyone has heard of it. It is only one of many big faces that were conquered in the inter-war period but it is, perhaps, the longest and the most dangerous.'

REINHOLD MESSNER

ANDERL HECKMAIR

be over to the left up a steep gully. The ramp that we find is relatively easy. I take the lead, bring Vörg up and Kasparek and Harrer follow. The difficulties are similar to those on the Kopftörl ridge in the Wilder Kaiser. The ramp leads up for 150m, becoming increasingly narrow and ending at an overhanging ice chimney. On the one side black water ice, on the other side incredibly friable rock. Meanwhile the mist has come down and now shrouds the silent walls. Somewhere down in the depths we sense the valley. The strands of mist creep around the summits and the towers, enveloping everything. We have to find a bivouac site. We reach a small overhang above a precipitous ice ledge and decide to stay. As we stand there next to each other, with no belay, the mist suddenly clears and we look down in horror into the abyss: beneath our feet there is a 1500m vertical drop. We quickly hammer in a few belay pegs, tie ourselves on and, in the most difficult circumstances imaginable, cook a meal and then try to sleep. Our first night on the face. The effort has been incredible. We have climbed 1500m of this terrible wall in one day. Our comrades are tired too. The night grows cold and we sit next to each other on this narrow ledge, shivering, wrapped in the Zdarsky bag waiting for sleep to come.

We sit on our narrow ledge, still roped up. The hours creep past. It grows colder and colder. From time to time one of us sleeps for a short time. Whilst cooking, I ate a tin of sardines in oil. They do not agree with me. I feel sick! Not that as well! But Comrade Kasparek is already up and once again setting up the Primus stove to brew me a hot cup of tea. It must be about 12 o'clock. How touching! Then we doze off again into the new day's dawn.

How many times have we done this, keeping watch through the night? How often have we crouched on decimetre-wide rock ledges with the gaping abyss black and eerie beneath and up above us the light of an occasional star? If only it had not been so cold! We are soaked through from the water channels and the ice walls and now the cold is creeping its way through our clothes. Freezing cold, we shudder the night away.

It gradually grows lighter, thank God. At 5am we rub our numb limbs warm again. All our bones are aching from the uncomfortable position. At 7am we drink hot chocolate; it tastes wonderful. And then we carry on climbing; we want to get as far as possible today. We follow the crack further up to the left. It becomes more and more difficult. We reach a short

section which reminds us of the Dülfer Crack. Just 10m of vertical crack. Ten metres which have to be overcome, which use up all our strength, which are more difficult than anything else before. Once, a hold breaks on me but luckily I have decent protection in. The rock here is incredibly friable. Then we take a detour around the unconquerable overhang that I was unable to climb.

The chimney grows narrower and narrower! And then – an overhang of ice, a roof, caps the chimney, preventing further upward progress. Outside on its edge long icicles hang down. I push myself further into the chimney and further up until I am just beneath the jutting roof. The walls are smooth, black ice. It is impossible to leave the chimney, impossible to climb the overhang.

Impossible? We are already too far up the face. There can be no going back. We have to get up, we have to! It is hopeless to attempt this section, yet we have to overcome it. With my ice axe I smash away at the icicles hanging down behind me. At the back of the crack I bang a piton into the ice, hang a rope through the eye, brace myself against the hard ice of the chimney and now – I have to attempt it – I slowly lean outwards, holding the rope in one hand, further and further out – if only the piton holds! My whole weight is now hanging on it. Now, with my free hand, I reach upwards and outwards, grab hold of a boss of ice. How on earth am I supposed to get up there? It is ridiculous!

Then, the clump of ice breaks; I fall and land heavily back into the chimney. Damn it! I immediately try to get back up to the top. This has to work. Again I bend out backwards, further, further out. I manage to get hold of another lump of ice – it holds. The other hand lets go of the rope, reaches over the overhang. I can get some purchase up there with the ice axe, two or three seconds of inhuman use of strength – it has to work – I manage it, I force myself up over the overhang, I force my way up onto the steep ice-field. Quickly, just a few more metres. The overhang has been conquered. I fashion a stance for both feet on the ice wall and belay my comrades. The crux of the North Face has been cracked!

We have to rest for a few minutes. Then climb blue ice to the right to regain the rock. Meanwhile a plane has appeared. Droning loudly, it flies nearer and nearer to us in steep, banked curves, close in to the wall. We wave to it. Down there in the sunshine lies Grindelwald, with its many scattered houses. We are already very high up. How many metres are there left until we reach the summit? How many difficulties have still to be overcome before we finally have our victory?

We continue. We have get over to the 'Spider'. A very demanding, strength-sapping rope length and other difficult sections are overcome, and then we reach the rock ledge that leads over to the icefield of the 'Spider'. It is about six rope lengths before we reach that point. It is 3 o'clock. We look anxiously to the west. There is a storm approaching – great speed is called for. We leave our Austrian comrades behind and climb into the 'Spider' icefield. I cut steps as quickly as I can so that we will be protected by the rocks up there when the storm breaks. We are in such a hurry that we no longer put in any pitons. We climb unprotected up the steep icefield. Then we hammer in a belay peg. A few metres lower down we can see a small platform, the only place on which we can stand in some sort of comfort. Somehow or other Vörg even manages to sit down.

Meanwhile the clouds have arrived. It grows black as night now, although it is only quarter to four. We are glad to be out of the main avalanche chute. Our comrades traverse beneath us and climb up through the 'Spider'; we can no longer see them in the darkness. Then it begins to hail and now – I look up carefully – there is an avalanche coming down through the ice wall, growing and growing, shooting towards us with incredible speed. We stand open and unbelayed on the icy surface right in the line of firing. I hammer in my ice axe, grab hold of Vörg by the collar and then – now it has reached us – the masses of snow rage down upon us. We only just manage to hold on.

There is more and more of it, the pressure grows immeasurable. We can no longer see anything, it is terrible. How long can I continue to stand here? The avalanche hit me and my axe and splits, spreading itself out, for minutes we stand in the terrible flood, which surges against us threatening to sweep us away.

After many a long minute the force decreases. It becomes somewhat lighter again. We hardly dare to look down to the area where our comrades were standing, out in the open surface, and then – it is a miracle! – they are still there! The avalanche has not dragged them with it down to the depths – it is really a miracle! We are quickly up the few metres to the piton. We call to the Austrians to see if they are all

right. And then we tie two ropes together and go to the aid of Kasparek and Harrer. Kasparek has injured his hand grabbing hold of a piton in the storm of the avalanche. We bandage it for him; we have to get a move on now.

The weather has turned. There will be more avalanches and we are in the funnel into which all the channels of this system run together; we had been exposed to the cumulative force of the avalanches. We must attempt to get up as far we can during what is left of today and then tomorrow, even in these extremely bad weather conditions, to reach the summit. In spite of our enormous tiredness we make good progress. We climb up again now to the left to the exit ramp. Clouds enshroud the mountain. It is snowing slowly and crashing avalanches rage down over the smooth icefields to our right.

At 9 o'clock we are still climbing. Then we find a narrow ledge hardly a metre wide beneath a narrow overhang. We will bivouac here. In the darkness we knock away a few stones and some ice, hammer some belay pitons into the wall above us, hang the Zdarsky bags off the pitons and sit next to each other, huddled beneath the dubious protection of these little tents on this narrow sill in the middle of the Eigerwand.

It is difficult to cook here. We have hardly any room to put the stove. Our second night begins, the third for Kasparek and Harrer. Again it becomes bitterly cold. Small avalanches crash down over us or rustle past us to the side. Vörg lets me rest my head on his back. We are all terribly tired. I soon fall sound asleep. It is 12 o'clock at night. At 6 o'clock we cook ourselves something warm to eat again. Vörg rubs his limbs; he has sacrificed all sleep, sitting uncomfortably the whole night through, in order to let me sleep. And I was not even aware of it. And so, somewhat rested and refreshed, I once again take the lead for the final obstacle of the 300m up to the summit. We traverse from our bivouac site over to the main gully, which should lead us to the top.

The weather has finally taken a turn for the worse. It is snowing. At approximately hourly intervals the avalanches rage down through the gully. When enough snow has settled on the steep flanks for adhesion to be lost, it simply avalanches off. We are always left with about half an hour to get on with the job of climbing, then we search for the most secure place to stop and let the next avalanche pass. The gully is very difficult. It demands our last reserves. At the top it narrows into a chimney which can only be overcome

'The hysteria was so widespread that the Swiss Government called for and finally implemented a legal ban on climbing the North Face of the Eiger. However, several noteworthy Swiss alpinists opposed the ban and worked hard to ensure the subsequent repeal of this senseless law. The stipulation remained that henceforth the Swiss Mountain Rescue should be under no obligation to assist in the event of an accident. This proviso had always existed, however, yet in an emergency the Swiss Mountain Guides had always been on the scene to assist their fellow climbers.'

ANDERL HECKMAIR

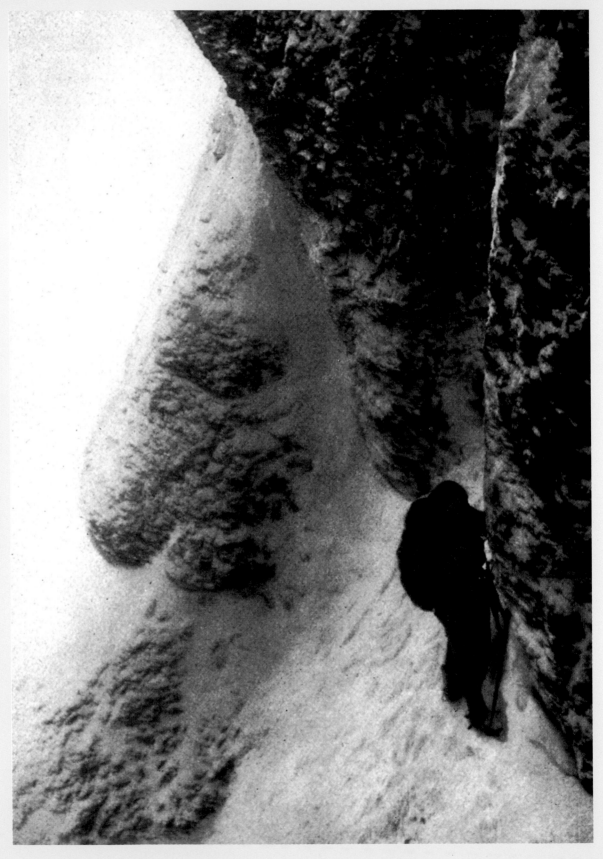

'They revived the miracle of again making the Alps the true stadium of Europe. This was the moment when the great feats of the mountaineer achieved in the public's mind a similar status to the greatest news events of the day, and through which our sport was lent a never before imagined propagandist resonance. All the climbers who experienced that unforgettable period of great failed attempts and great conquests between 1931 and 1938, all the climbers from north and south, will concur with me when I claim that, back then, we had the best experiences ever granted by the myth of mountaineering.'

GUIDO TONELLA

In the Exit Cracks. Anderl Heckmair leading in poor conditions – high wind, new snow, wet and cold.

by summoning all our strength and skill. I snake my way up the most difficult section and bring Vörg up before the next avalanche comes raging down the gully. We find somewhere to stand out of the firing line, but the others are still in the middle of the chimney. And the next avalanche is already on its way. Now we see how it breaks away and as it rushes past us we are able to call down to those below to warn them when it is coming and when the greatest pressure will be. Then, in the middle of the iced up section, the two of them put their rucksacks on their heads and brace themselves against the force. It is a hard thing to do.

Then we are up this section too, but we still have not overcome the last dangers. We have to climb an overhanging ice section and we almost fail in our attempts. I am standing 8m above Vörg in a narrow crack with no footholds. And then, suddenly, I lose my balance, slip and fall; an ice screw comes out and I fly down, only to be caught by Vörg.

The force of the impact throws him off his stance. I come to a standstill with my crampons scraping on the ice and grab tight hold. There, right next to me, is Vörg. He too has only just managed to keep standing. The whole thing has taken a minute perhaps. How lucky we have been. Vörg's hand is bleeding badly. When he caught me one of the teeth of my crampons went into his hand. Quickly we bandage it up.

Suddenly we hear shouts from the summit. In spite of the crazy weather, a Swiss mountain guide has climbed up to the summit via the West Ridge in order to look for us. We hear him clearly but do not answer him. Snow is falling, more and more snow. It would be too easy for him up there, upon hearing our shouts, to venture further down and thus to trigger an avalanche, which could be the death of us all. We climb the final difficult section as if in a dream.

Avalanches continue to rage down the wall. But now we can at least belay each other.

And then – finally, after five hours of battle we have managed to overcome the 140m. One more overhang to go, then we swing up onto the Eastern

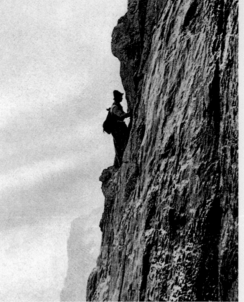

Hias Rebitsch, an exceptional climber of the 1930s, on the Hinterstoisser Traverse in 1937.

ridge, we have cracked it! The Eigerwand has been conquered.

Just the last 150m to the summit to do now. There is a wild snowstorm raging. At the top almost half a metre of new snow has settled.

We stand on the summit of the Eiger. Our joy is unimaginable. Laughing, we look into each other's eyes and shake our injured hands. Harrer, the SS man from Graz, takes a flag out of his rucksack with a Swastika on it and plants it in the snow. The victory is ours! The last big face of the Alps has been conquered. It is 3.30 on a Sunday afternoon. And then, as we climb down the Western ridge, fighting against the snow and the storm, with the ice sticking our eyes together, tiredness again overcomes us. We have been hanging on the face for 61 hours, the others for 86. Very, very difficult hours.

Then we see climbers coming up from the Eiger-Glacier station and we experience the joy of seeing our friends from Germany, who had come to help us if we should be unable to get up the face on our own. We are so tired. We stumble more than walk down along the path and soon everyone knows: German mountaineers, who came together in inseparable camaraderie, have conquered the most difficult wall in the Alps, the North Face of the Eiger.

'In the age of economic ruin and unemployment, a new generation of mountaineers grew up in the impoverished countries of Germany and Austria. They travelled by bicycle, spending their nights in tents and hayricks to save money. For many young climbers, climbing seemed to be a comforting alternative, a solace even. The concept of the 'mountain vagabond' began to achieve common currency.'

FRITZ SCHMITT

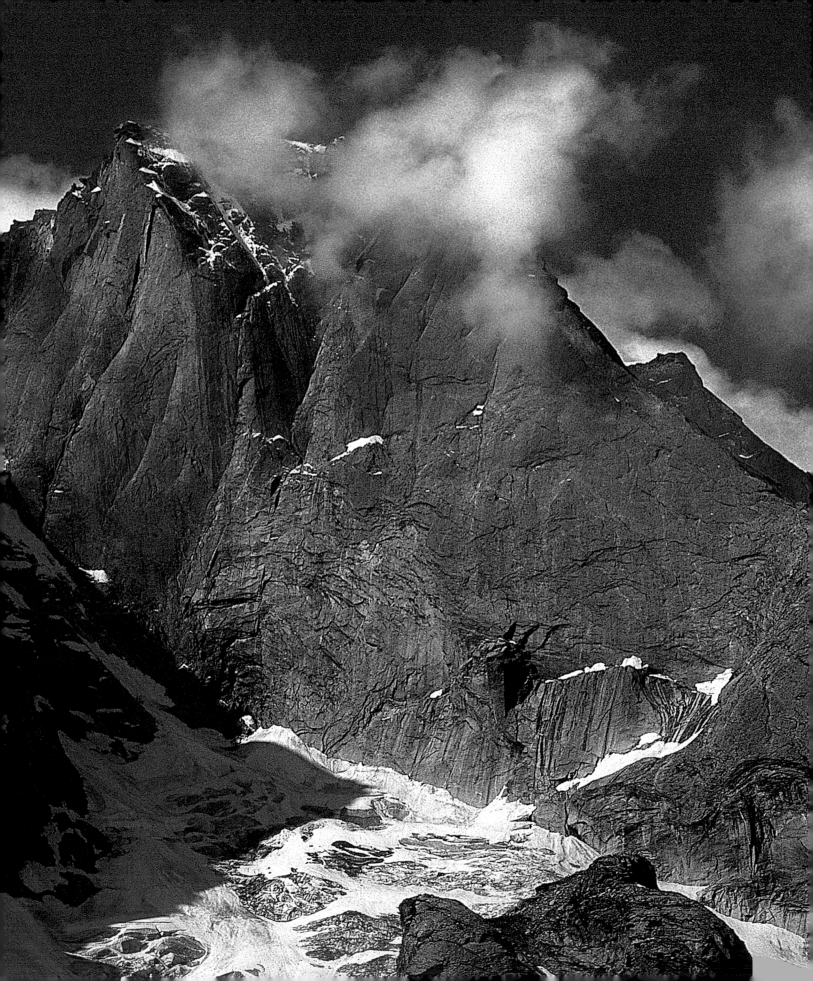

THE CLASSICS

The 'three Great Alpine North Faces' soon became an established concept and the routes to which the appellation referred are now regarded as classics. Later, the Badile Wall, the Zinnen Wall, the North and West Faces of the Dru, the North Face of the Charmoz and many more were added to the list. Each clique then provided its own 'big faces'. Finally, it once more became a private thing.

The French climber Gaston Rèbuffat identified six great mountain faces as the focal point of his life as a mountaineer, while Radovan Kuchař's 'second home' consisted of ten. The North Face of the Eiger was on every list.

With the internationalization of mountaineering, big faces in the Caucasus, on Mount Cook in New Zealand, on Fitz Roy in Patagonia and in Alaska were added, then the Troll Wall in Norway and later still the big walls of the Trango Towers in the Karakorum, Yerupaja and Huandoy in the Andes. Meanwhile, an élite circle of high-altitude mountaineers became devoted to the 'big walls of the world', and when Christophe Profit climbed the three big Alpine faces within 24 hours – solo, first in summer and then, rather more slowly, in winter – a new age had begun.

What an increase in performance this was but, above all, it was the attitude of the protagonists with regard to these big faces that had become different. It was a change in approach so remarkable that I intend to pursue this matter further.

The pioneers of bygone days – those laconic men who went about their business with equal measures of modesty and decisiveness – by 1980 existed only as a memory. The itinerant mountain vagabonds who shunned the comforts of civilized society to spend months on end tentbound beneath some mountain face or other waiting for their 'death or glory' moment had been replaced by young professional mountaineers, who acted swifty and objectively and analysed their successes or failures as one might a sporting event. Although names like 'First Pillar', 'Shattered Pillar', 'Difficult Crack', 'Rote Flüh', 'Swallow's Nest', 'Flatiron', 'Traverse of the Gods' and 'Exit Cracks' still refer to the same features, the corresponding emotions they once aroused have been lost, at least in the mind of those climbers who are still active. Values like 'life or death', 'the rope as

the epitome of splendid cameraderie' or 'battle' no longer find many adherents amongst the present generation of mountaineers – luckily!

The presence of the media, whether TV, Internet or satellite telephone, does not bother these modern-day climbers. What they do find disturbing, even ridiculous, is the 'death wish' mentality exhibited by previous generations of climbers. Nor do the new heroes wish to be associated with any kind of elitist contempt for the public at large; after all, they produce and direct their adventures with a wide circle of interested parties in mind.

Dramatic televised 'rescue shows' or media events like the Dhaulagiri Wall live webcast are now in fashion. However, it is no longer the thrill of death that interest people but the presentation of mountaineering as another normal, routine sporting fixture. Concepts like the 'Myth of the Eiger' might well

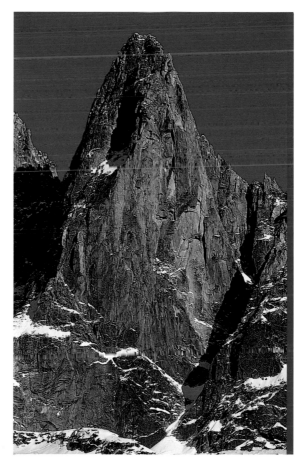

'To defy the most precipitous faces, those that are untouched by anyone, means to search for the mystery.'

GUIDO MAGNONE

'Was the West Face of the Dru really one of the 'last great problems', one that could no longer be surpassed? Those who know the history of alpinism ... will experience strong feelings of misgiving at the use of such superlatives. And yet it is hard to imagine how this 'vertical expedition', this 'superclimb' might ever be surpassed.'

GÜNTHER OSKAR DHYRENFURTH

The North-East Face of the Badile-Nordostwand (facing page) and (near left) the North and West Faces of the Dru are amongst the classic routes of the Alps.

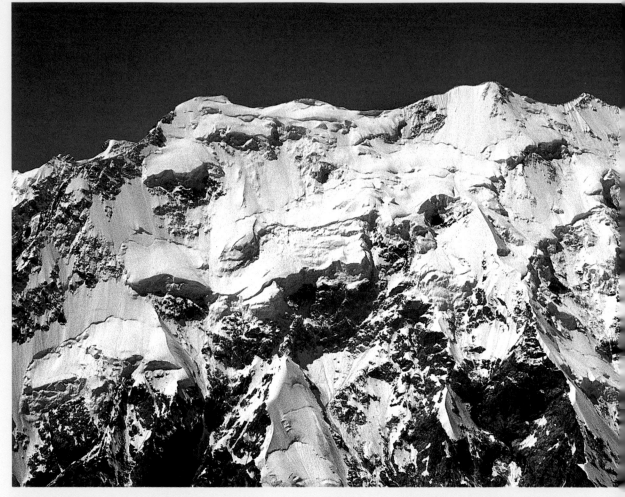

'The highest of the
mountains in the
Caucasus with the
exception of Elbrus
and Kasbek, which
are of volcanic
origin, are
concentrated into a
relatively small
area, the Besingi
Cirque. It could be
said, therefore, that
a climber only gets
a true impression of
the Caucasus when
he has visited the
Besingi Cirque.'

RADOVAN KUCHAŘ

Meanwhile, 'the sun is already high in the sky.
From the snowfields above, one avalanche after
another thunders down to the valley. They boom down
left of us, roar down the gully and disappear into the
abyss. The air current carries the swirling snow dust
up to us. But here on the edge of the buttress we are
safe. I can not imagine that anybody could ever climb
straight up an avalanche chute.'

Kuchař is climbing in rope of three and although
the zones of rock rear up very steeply, calling for
exposed climbing on sound rock, they are very fast.
From time to time jutting overhangs look as if they
might block the way forward but again and again a
horizontal ledge will appear that leads back onto
climbable territory. The three men function well as a
team; nothing can hold them up.

'A climbing team roped together forms an
indivisible whole, joined by the rope in life or death.
The characteristics of its members are skill, prudence
and mutual respect', Kuchař writes. 'An individual

mistake is a mistake made by all. A highly developed
feeling of responsibility for his companions is the
most important character trait of the mountaineer.
Even the most accomplished leader is nothing without
the others. Victory goes to the whole team.'

Yes, if they get up the climb.

'The buttress suddenly becomes more broken, as
the rock walls merge into an easier-angled ridge. After
three pitches the three of us find ourselves standing
on the top of the pillar.' Two-thirds of the face, the
most difficult portion, now lie behind them. Soon the
climbers are directly beneath the seracs, menacing
towers of ice that hang above them like the sword of
Damocles. They are now climbing at the altitude of
Mont Blanc. Tatters of mist appear again on the face,
which now has a cold and eerie feel to it. The wind
whips up tiny ice crystals that penetrate their clothing.

'The mountains are shrouded in a white gloom.
The horizon no longer exists. The world has shrunk to
that one section of ice slope up which we are moving.

We do not register the 1.5km of face below us, nor do we think of the summit – at this moment it seems so far removed from reality. Perhaps the face has no summit. There is nothing to remind us that we are in the Caucasus.'

They finally reach a gully, where they find an excellent spot for a bivouac. But no, they cannot stay in the gully; avalanches might shoot down here during the night. So they carry on. Past and future have become meaningless, the only thing that counts now is 'up'. Their route goes upwards, towards the next band of seracs.

They are now moving at an altitude of 5000m. 'Our damp boots have frozen stone-hard, the cold penetrates through our clothing. The tiniest careless action brings the threat of frostbite. We try to stimulate our circulation by stamping our feet on the ice for a few minutes when belaying.'

Soon it is dark and they still do not have a place to bivouac. Suddenly the gully becomes wider, they traverse right across a broad icefield but have to come back again when they sink up to their knees in loose, unconsolidated snow. Uncertain now, they hope to find a place to spend the night in the serac belt. But the slope is still too steep. Ducking around an arête they at last find a crevasse full of powder snow – an ideal place to bivouac!

'We think things over for a while. With the weather being so uncertain it would probably be best to establish the camp as thoroughly as possible. Although we have got down jackets and "pieds d'elephants", as the section of the down sleeping bag that can be attached to the jacket is known, it is questionable whether we'll be able to continue tomorrow. We therefore decide to dig a snow hole. This is the warmest and safest way of spending the night on a hard route. Digging out the snow and shovelling it away with only an ice axe is a horribly arduous chore. Only one of us can work at a time. Tiredness and the 5000m altitude now start to make themselves felt. After an hour's hard labour the hole is finished. Now we are safe from any bad weather, and from avalanches too.'

The next morning the sun is shining from a dark blue, cloudless sky. They wade through loose snow to the summit. Fear they leave behind, along with the many 4000m peaks and the steep slopes of the North-East Face of Dych Tau now below them. The ascent now belongs to the past, they can finally breathe easily again. They have climbed the greatest big face in the Caucasus and lived through it – until the next big face.

'After a difficult climb is all over the sun seems warmer, the ice whiter and the joy is boundless. After overcoming danger, life seems somehow more valuable.'

Radovan Kuchař died in the Andes below Huascarán, a victim of natural catastrophe. A section of the huge face of Huascarán Norte broke off and the ensuing avalanche destroyed everything in its path as it thundered down to the valley, wiping out the village of Yungay and causing a massive flood.

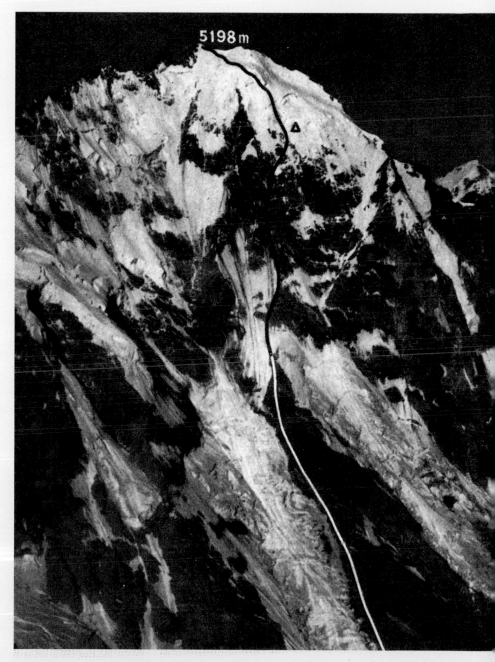

The North-East Face of Dych Tau, situated close to the Besingi cirque.

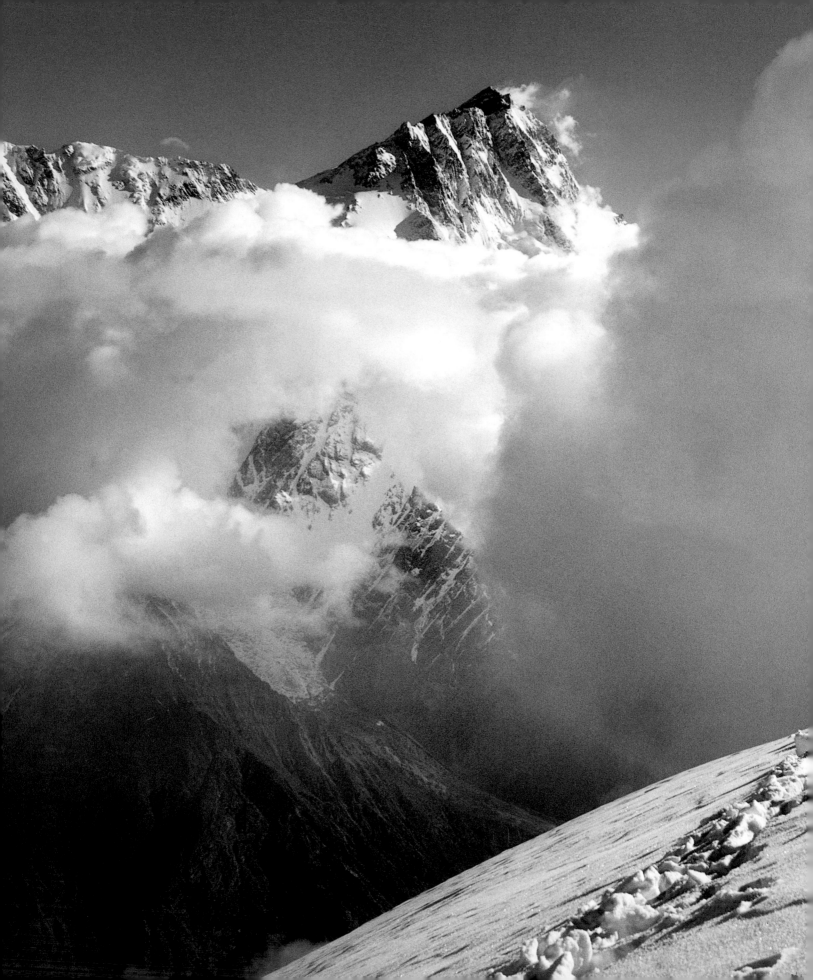

THE WORLD'S BIG WALLS

The concept of the 'Three Great Alpine Faces', which evolved from the 'three last problems' and was expounded by Anderl Heckmair in book form, became an integral part of classic mountaineering. The North Face of the Matterhorn, the North Face of the Grandes Jorasses and the North Face of the Eiger characterize classic extreme alpinism so exactly that until 1970 they represented the holy trinity of pure Alpine climbing. These three faces had repeatedly caused sensation and new combinations of the three were found again and again. Even today, anyone who 'bags' all three is rated as a good mountaineer, even if he need not necessarily be an outstanding climber.

There is no disputing the fact that there are more difficult faces in the Alps, perhaps even more beautiful ones, but there has never been any doubt that these three are 'the three greatest'. The North-West Face of the Civetta, the Laliderer Walls, the Freney Pillar on Mont Blanc, the North Face of the Droites, the North-East Face of the Piz Badile, the West Face of the Dru and many others – all these are big and extremely difficult, but they lack certain specific criteria that would allow them to rank alongside the Big Three.

Apart from the historical context, the almost mythical status enjoyed by these three faces lies in my view in the combination of summit height, relatively high technical difficulties, absolute height of the face, the mixture of ice and rock climbing and not least in the fact that on all three faces there is no easy escape. For many years, these faces were considered to be 'impregnable'. The concept of the 'Big Walls' thus has much to do with the 'myth of impregnability'; something deemed impossible that, despite everything, eventually does become possible.

If we are now to set the indisputable concept of the 'three Great Alpine Faces' next to the new idea of the 'three greatest Big Walls of the World', we must also agree new terms of reference since, if we were to remain true to the aforementioned criteria, all the Big Walls of the Himalayas and the Karakorum would qualify. The South Face of Annapurna and the West Buttress of Makalu would make the shortlist, along with the Rupal Flank of Nanga Parbat, the South Faces of Lhotse and Dhaulagiri,

the South-West Face of Everest and the South Buttress of K2.

Just as for the Alps the final selection included faces from three completely different regions involving different types of climbing – each was of a different type of rock – the concept of the 'greatest Big Walls of the World' should also consider both the geographically most important and highest mountain ranges and the composition of the face, its history and local climate. If we stay with the criteria of summit height, technical difficulty and remoteness and select the highest faces of the various continents or mountain ranges, there can be no doubt about the Big Walls that qualify.

The Rupal Flank of Nanga Parbat is the highest Big Wall in the world and as such obviously the biggest face in the Himalaya region and in Asia. In addition, it leads to the summit of one of the fourteen eight-thousanders. The biggest face in the Americas, the South Face of Aconcagua, leads to the top of the highest peak in the Andes and is also extremely difficult. If we also include the North Face of the Eiger in our selection – as the highest face in the Alps and also one of the original 'three Great Alpine Faces' – we have both a cut-off point and a basis for comparison.

At the current stage of development in mountaineering – the general trend for extreme climbers to break out beyond their local regions like the Pyrenees or the Alps and look to other mountain regions of the world – the 'Big Walls of the World' naturally represent an attractive prospect. Although these do offer numerous three-star objectives, such as the Dych Tau North Face in the Caucasus, the Trollryggen Wall in Norway, the granite monolith of El Capitan in California and the huge ice face of Mount Cook in New Zealand – to name just a few – the Rupal Flank of Nanga Parbat, the South Face of Aconcagua and the North Face of the Eiger still remain the three classic objectives that define the sport of modern mountaineering.

It is interesting to note that during the first ascents of all five of these Big Walls, the climbers found themselves in each case facing borderline situations – near tragedies and actual tragedies – of the kind that were to occur only rarely in the

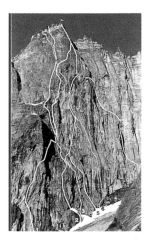

The Trollryggen Wall with a series of routes marked.

'A failed attempt on a "virgin" face of an eight-thousander gives me much more than the successful ascent of a known route.'

REINHOLD MESSNER

(facing page): The summit area of Nanga Parbat from the South (Rupal Flank).

history of mountaineering. And this despite the fact that the protagonists were the leading climbers of their generation.

Today there must be several hundred climbers a year who do the three big north faces of the Alps and since any new terrain in this region is now merely of second-rate importance, to climb all three continues to be the predominant goal of any climber of rank and reputation.

On a world scale, however, things are rather different. Some of the Big Walls in the Himalayas have yet to be conquered and the question arises whether it might not be more interesting to attempt one of the numerous 'virgin' faces than to repeat a 'classic'. Nevertheless, the time will come when a mountaineer's lifetime ambition might be to climb not just the three great faces of the Alps but also the Big Walls of the World, an objective which goes far beyond simply collecting the 8000m peaks, since on the world's Big Walls it is the remoteness and the commitment that count for so much.

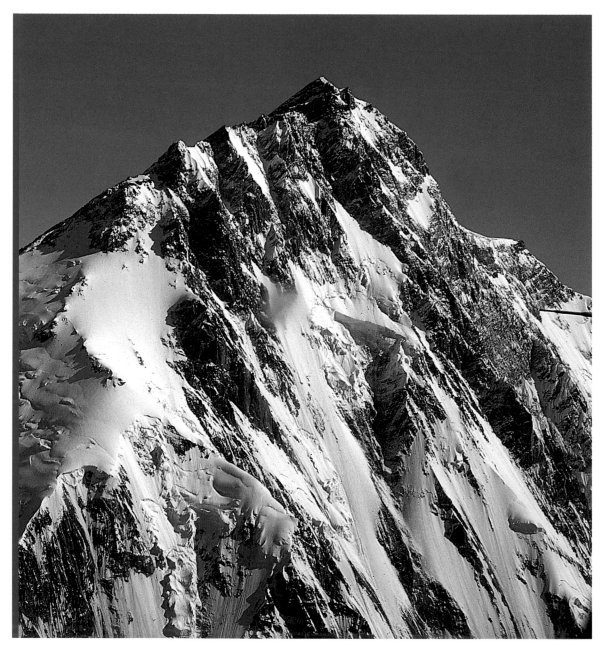

The ascent of the Rupal Face of Nanga Parbat ushered in a new dimension in big wall mountaineering.

ACONCAGUA SOUTH FACE

For many years the South Face of Aconcagua remained unknown amongst climbers, although it was one of the first of the world's Big Walls to be climbed. Even today it is known only to insiders.

Several kilometres wide and 3km high, it towers over the Horcones Glacier. The bleak and barren landscape below the face – dead glaciers, huge piles of rubble and scree and snowfields – is constantly swept by avalanches and has a wild and threatening feel.

The complete isolation and the constant wind in this remote corner of the Horcones Valley accentuate the unpleasant appearance; it is only when viewed from the top, looking down onto the twisted stream of the dead glacier, that the true magnitude and magnificence of the face becomes clear.

In terms of steepness and difficulty, this is a very unevenly balanced face, embracing every level of climbing, from easy loose scrambling to grade VI overhangs, from level snowfields to huge, vertical icefalls. The steep, loose bands of cliffs are particularly unpleasant, as are the sudden and violent storms that rake the face, but the belt of sandstone in the central section of the face and the steep summit icefield on the Direct Route offer really enjoyable climbing.

The highest peak in the Andes is easily reached by its easy-angled Normal Route, a route which, for many extreme climbers, holds no great appeal despite its height above sea level. But to climb the mountain by the South Face represents a different challenge for the modern mountaineer – an adventure that requires skill, experience and stamina.

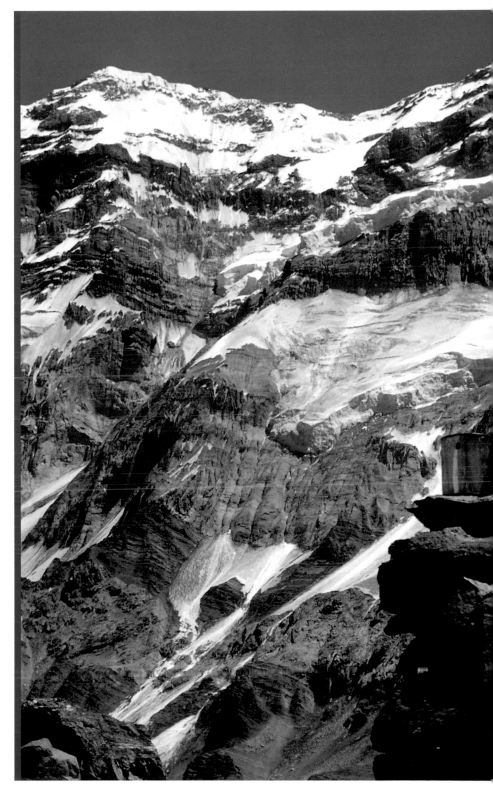

The southern precipices of Aconcagua fall 3000m sheer to the valley. Several difficult routes lead to the South Summit (left) and Main Summit.

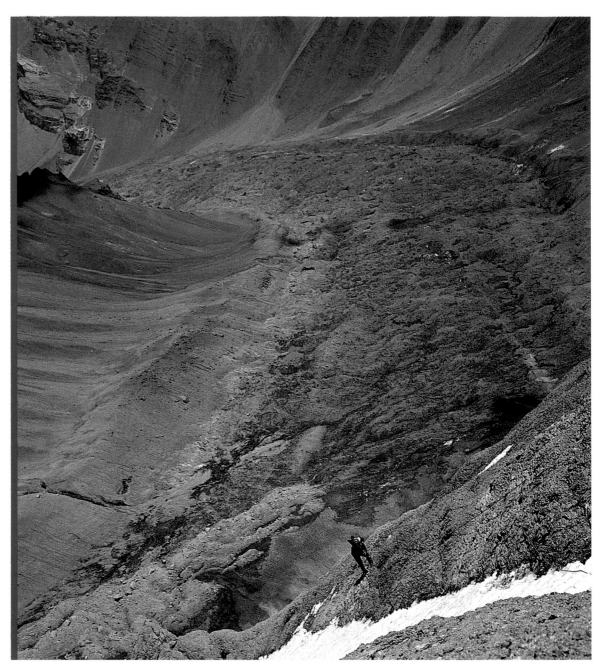

'Nowadays, mountaineering is available to a broad spectrum of the population and is more a question of time than money. Anyone wanting to participate in an expedition, for example, has to be able to take maybe several months off, a period of time well outside most people's annual holiday entitlement. For myself, I chose the uncertain path of the freelance mountaineer in order to maintain the greatest possible independence and to create the prerequisites necessary to pursue great mountaineering objectives, often in series, the world over, for thirty years.'

REINHOLD MESSNER

line across the right-hand section of the face, but although it joined the exit ramp of the French Route it remained a South Face ascent of only secondary importance, since it avoided the central section of the face. Also in 1966, during the International Naturfreunde Andean Expedition under Fritz Moravec, Hans Schönberger and José Luis Fonrouge made a lightning-fast ascent of the face, climbing a new variation on the lower section that joined the French Route below the sandstone belt. Although easier than the French Route, the danger from falling ice is so acute that I would advise against it.

The Direct Finish from the big snowfield to the summit, first climbed by the 1974 South Tyrol Andean Expedition, is an ideal complement to the French Route and the resultant combination now provides the classic line on the face. While the first repeat ascents of the face, by expeditions from Japan and Spain, had all used the French Route, nowadays many parties and solo climbers are increasingly electing to follow the South Tyrol Route to the main summit of Aconcagua.

THE SOUTH FACE OF PEAK COMMUNISM

Not quite as big as the South Face of Aconcagua, but much harder and more dangerous, is the South Face of Peak Communism in the Pamir range. At 2900m high, this was the 'wall of walls' for climbers from the former Soviet Union; it was first climbed in 1968 by E. Myslovsky, A. Ovchinnikov, V. Gluhov and V. Ivanov, who followed a line up its right-hand, or south-west, side, topping out at 7495m above sea level. In later years, a series of even harder climbs were added and although this face was for two decades the most coveted objective for every top-flight mountaineer from the former Eastern Block, it was largely ignored by climbers from the West. Meanwhile, it is the Eastern European mountaineers who have set the pace of modern mountaineering in the Himalaya and Karakorum, too, yet hardly any Westerners have yet dared to rise to the challenges of the Big Walls in the Pamirs.

Perhaps this is due in part to the limited opportunities we once had for travel to the former Soviet Union. We did not attempt to seek out those masterpieces of Eastern climbing art, since problems of a similar dimension also existed in the Karakorum and the Himalayas. These days, however, when almost all of the world's great mountain ranges are readily accessible and big new routes are becoming increasingly rare, it is high time that mountaineers from the Alpine lands and the USA repeated the big faces in Tien Shan and the Pamirs that are the pride and joy of the local climbers there. The South Face of Peak Communism compares very favourably with other big mountain faces; any climber wishing to do the 'big walls of the world' can no longer ignore it.

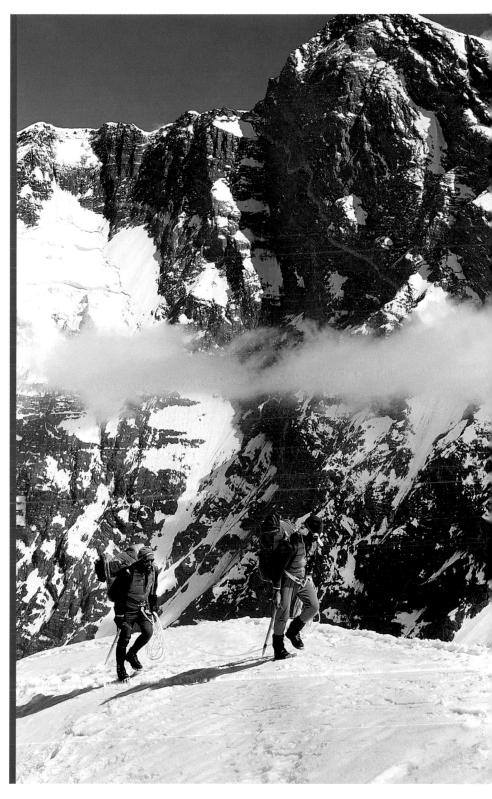

Soviet mountaineers with their typical clothing and equipment. In the background, the South Face of Peak Communism.

NANGA PARBAT SOUTH FACE

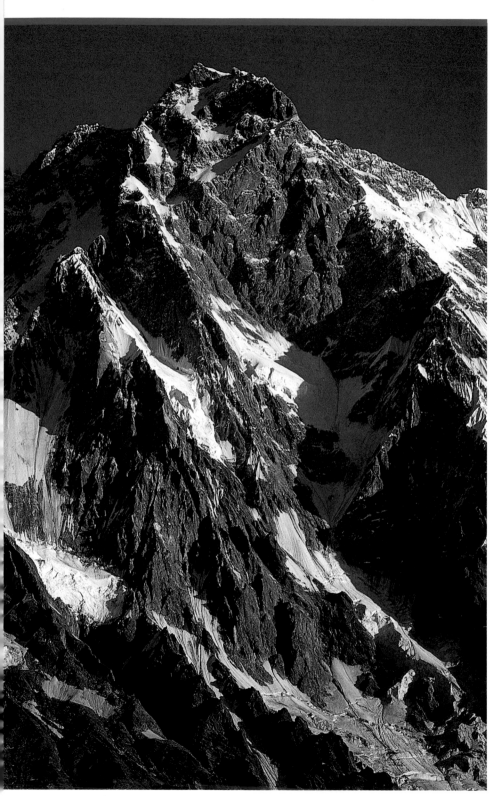

The South Face of Nanga Parbat, also known as the Rupal Flank, rises 4500m above the Tap Alpe and ranks amongst the greatest big mountain faces in the world. It is not as seemingly unapproachable in character as the faces of some of the other eight-thousanders but it is the very contrast with the gentle Alpine meadows that lie immediately below that gives it its special fascination.

When A.F. Mummery, and later Willo Welzenbach and Willy Merkl, saw the Rupal Face, none of them thought it would ever be possible to climb it. Even Hermann Buhl, who had climbed both the Walker Spur and the North Face of the Eiger and is said to have toyed for a while with the idea of attempting the South Face of Aconcagua, considered the South Face of Nanga Parbat to be impossible, after seeing the South-East Flank a few times from above.

Everyone who has ever stood beneath this face, studied it or flown past it has been entranced by this, the 'highest rock and ice wall in the world'. Relatively easy-angled and not too difficult for the first 2000m, the face steepens as it gains height. The route winds its way up through the buttressed middle section of the face and is logical and relatively safe. A series of icefields, rock spurs and gullys lead from the base to the summit of the ninth highest mountain in the world – a challenging prospect for the modern alpinist.

'A period of fine weather is setting in. We will use the days for the first, and maybe the last, summit push. In the evening of 18 June the Messner brothers, accompanied by Werner Haim, Elmar Raab and twelve high altitude porters, go up to Camp 1. ... The next day ... in the early hours of morning they reach Camp 2, which has been totally buried by snow, and immediately start the job of digging it out.' This is how Dr Karl M. Herrligkoffer begins his account of the last summit push in his official expedition report published in *Nanga Parbat – the Killer Mountain*.

HISTORY

In 1963, a reconnaissance expedition under Dr Karl M. Herrligkoffer discovered two possible routes on the Rupal Face, the Toni Kinshofer Route taking a line up to the left to the West Saddle and a Direttissima in the fall-line of the South Shoulder, the elegance and steepness of which is without rival in the Himalaya. A third possibility, the South-East Buttress, was also discussed.

The Central Pillar was first attempted in the winter of 1964. In 1968 a very strong team, the majority of whom had been on the Eiger Direct expedition and had set off from Europe amid much premature praise, reached the Merkl Icefield, the start of the main difficulties. This expedition, like the earlier Rupal Flank expeditions, was under the leadership of Herrligkoffer, and it was to form the basis for the success of the 1970 expedition.

In the summer of 1970, drawing on 75 years of experience on Nanga Parbat, and after one reconnaissance expedition and two failed attempts, the Sigi Löw Memorial Expedition, under the leadership of Dr Herrligkoffer, and with both my brother Günther and I in the team, finally achieved the long-awaited success on the Rupal Flank. Other members of the expedition were: Michl Anderl, Gerhard Baur, Wolf Bitterling, Werner Haim, Alice von Hobe, Max von Kienlin, Günter Kroh, Dr Hermann Kühn, Felix Kuen, Gert Mändl, Elmar Raab, Hans Saler, Peter Scholz, Peter Vogler, and Jürgen Winkler. With the support of such an outstanding team, the five-man summit party pushed the route as far as the Merkl Couloir, the crux of the face.

Thereafter, events moved very quickly. When, on account of the weather, I set off alone to make a lightning attempt on the summit, Günther followed me of his own free will, and together we reached the top. Felix Kuen and Peter Scholz followed a day later. On 28 June the second team summitted and, after a bivouac near the South Shoulder, returned via the route of ascent to Base Camp. On the same day, one day after our successful summit bid, since my brother was suffering from altitude sickness, I felt compelled to descend down the easier Diamir Face. It was for us a descent into despair and from that moment on the expedition took a tragic turn.

Of the eight climbers who had reached the summit of Nanga Parbat by 1970, only two are still alive today. Hermann Buhl fell to his death on 27 June 1957 on Chogolisa in the Karakorum; Günther Messner, my brother, who had stood with me on the summit on 27 June 1970, died two days later at the foot of the Diamir Face, buried under an avalanche; Sigi Löw had been killed eight years before while descending the mountain; Toni Kinshofer, perhaps the best German climber of the post-war era, died in a fall at the Battert just a few years after his Nanga Parbat ascent; Peter Scholz lost his life on the Aiguille Noire; Felix Kuen took his own life on 23 January 1974.

Despite these coincidences, it is nonsense to talk of 'the curse of Nanga Parbat' and if Nanga has become the 'Destiny Mountain of the Germans'. It is not because of any demon reigning there, but because it is so immeasurably bigger than we mortals.

'The fantastic South Face of Nanga Parbat, the Rupal Flank, is the biggest vertical precipice on Earth.'

RICHARD COWPER

'In a fairly big expedition with experienced German and Austrian climbers, Günther and I climbed for some forty days, with breaks, in May and June 1970, on the south face of Nanga Parbat. Most of the time we were at the front of the group.'

REINHOLD MESSNER

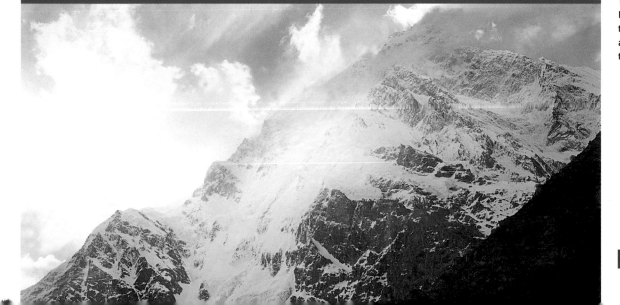

The problems of climbing the Rupal Flank are all to do with the constant bad weather and avalanche danger, in addition to the size and height of the face.

It is thirty years since that first ascent of the Rupal Face, years during which I have climbed other mountains and gained many new experiences. It is said that a man is rejuvenated every seven years, that all his cells are replaced. I wonder, does that also apply to his spirit?

So much has been written in the intervening years of that first ascent of the Rupal Face of Nanga Parbat, of the 'Red Rocket Affair', that the events back then are now sufficiently well known and it is easy to arrive at one's own verdict by studying all of the accounts.

I will not go into detail here of those forty days my brother and I spent on the Rupal Face, days into which we put every last effort in order to conquer this, the world's biggest rock and ice face. The subsequent descent down the Diamir Flank, which offered us our only chance of getting back to the valley alive, remains my hardest mountaineering experience. But it doesn't belong here. It was a descent into despair, not a climb on a Big Wall. Although it is enough for me today just to remember the hours that Günther and I spent on the summit together to arouse those past emotions, now it all appears in a dim light.

During the course of this expedition, I died. Not 'died' in the true sense of the word – I do not believe in resurrection – it wasn't my body that died, but my spirit, my will, my hopes. At the Merkl Gap, I had the feeling that I 'was like a bundle, rolling along behind myself' and later, in the Diamir Valley, my last vestige of hope disappeared. And when I found myself once more, it was a new spirit, a new will, new hopes that carried me along.

When I set off for Nanga Parbat, and above all in all those years before when I had been occupying myself more and more intensively with the attempts on the Rupal Face, I was more concerned with the 'struggle and conquest on Nanga Parbat', and with climbing the highest face in the world. Today, with hindsight, none of this is important. One of the first to climb the Rupal Face – so what?

Yet at the time our every will was directed towards this face. Günther and I wanted to reach the summit if at all possible and behind this wish there was also a generous portion of egoism. This comes over clearly in a letter that Günther wrote home to our parents and

brothers and sisters a few days before the summit bid. Even if at the time our chances seemed slight, we did not relinquish our ambitious hopes.

Rupal Valley, Tap Alpe, 15 June 1970

Dear parents, dear brothers and sisters,
Today we have been on the mountain exactly a month. On 15 May we set up our main camp here on the Tap Alpe. Since then much has happened and changed. The snow has melted for quite a long way up the mountain and the Tap Alpe has become green. It is full of flowers, resembling an English country garden in places. Half-wild yak herds romp around this romantic, wild, basin-shaped, high valley. Scrawny horses come to recover here from the harsh winter.

I am sitting almost exactly above Base Camp and can look across the whole corrie. The Alpe itself is an area of meadow, almost as flat as a table top. In the middle there is a wood. Storms and avalanches have left their mark. Every second tree is withered and leafless. In the evenings our porters often bring us five or six of these withered trees to make a huge campfire.

To the north, directly above us, stands the Rupal Flank, rising 4500m to the summit of the mountain, unbelievably impressive. Two huge moraines border the Alpe to the west and east. To the south the Rupal Peak dominates the valley. It is the much sought-after objective of our 'amateur mountaineers', but so far they have not reached the summit.

In the north-west corner lies our Base Camp, close to two natural springs. They are five minutes away. Our tent village comprises fifteen tents, including porters' tents, kitchen and mess tent and expedition leader's tent. Everything is nicely contained and in the centre of the circle stands a pole with the German and Pakistani flags. Everyone has his own tent where (if it rains or snows) he can write, read, sleep, where he can stow his personal belongings – and find them again. Reinhold and I are sharing a three-man tent. We are nice and comfortable. We also have inflatable mattresses and sleeping bags, of course, and

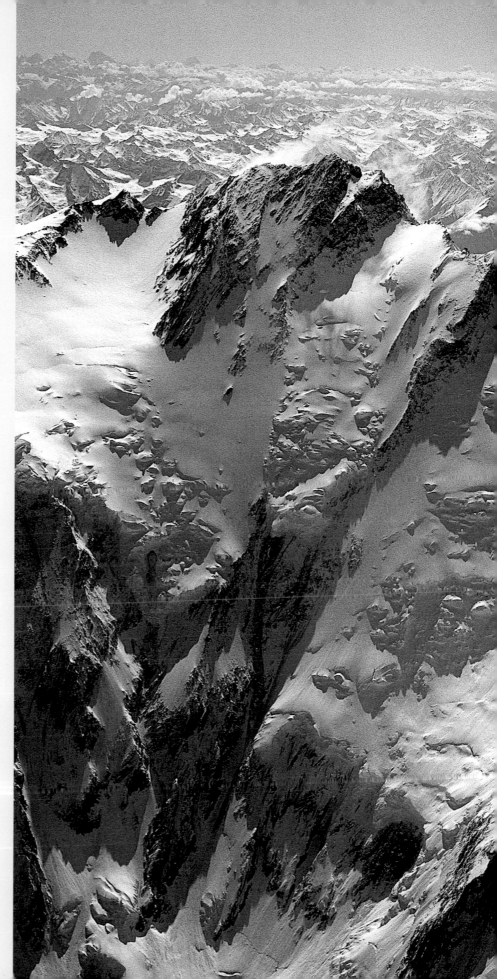

nobody tells us how our own tent should be organized. That was just a brief glimpse of our Base Camp, the mother camp to all our exposed advanced high camps.

Why am I writing a letter, a situation report, today from Base Camp when the letter I wrote in Camp III has not gone off yet? Well, for a good ten days now, all hell has been let loose here; not amongst the team, who have worked together in exemplary fashion, no – it's the weather that's being so shitty. Since 3 June we have had storms practically without a break. Up in the high camps there have been large quantities of new snow every day (a metre and more!). Avalanches thunder down the endless steep flanks. It is very good to know that Reinhold and I have selected the sites for all the camps so far and have been careful to check for avalanche and stonefall danger. Only then did we pitch the tents. Camp I is under a big protruding rock; Camp II below a vertical serac some 20m high with a ridge above that splits the avalanches and sends them thundering down to the left and right of the camp; Camp III is our famous Ice Dome, similarly protected from avalanches. We haven't yet moved into Camp IV (reached it on 3 June; retreated due to snowdrifts).

With the new snow, the face is extraordinarily treacherous. Whenever there is avalanche danger, there is no climbing or load carrying done, even in fine weather. Over the past twelve days all the high camps have had to be evacuated and the whole team has now returned to Base Camp. As you can read in my other letter, Reinhold and I initially spent ten full days at Camp III in a snowstorm waiting for better weather. We stayed on up there as the descent would have been too risky.

Then, on 10 June, we again got a reasonably sunny, calm day and a lot of the snow had either avalanched off or settled. During the course of the day the rest of the team, who had been in Base Camp since 5 June, climbed back up to the high camps. New hope and high spirits seemed to be ushering in a new phase in the expedition's fortunes.

On 11 June Reinhold and I wanted to go up to Camp IV, finally locate a good place for it on the lower edge of the Merkl Icefield, pitch a tent and stock it with food and gear. The food that we had hauled up there on 3 June would have been sufficient for two to three days, by which time the others should have come up with fresh supplies. But in the morning we were greeted by a sleet shower and a black cloud encircling Nanga. Quickly we crawled back into the tent. At 6 o'clock all hell broke loose again. We were really fed up by now. Firstly, we would soon have spent a full two weeks at Camp III at 6000m and secondly we felt it was now absolutely crucial that we got moving again soon. So we decided that on the 12th, or the 13th at the latest, we would go down if the weather really was no better. On 13 June we went back down to Base Camp; thanks to good acclimatization we only took a few hours for the descent.

The weather report from Peschawar was still bad, so the rest of the team (nine men) cleared the high camps again on 14 June (the food supplies had also been running low, since the high-altitude porters had been practically unable to do any carries since 3 June). Today, 15 June, everyone has assembled back at Base Camp (eighteen sahibs, fifteen high-altitude porters and our twenty-five-year-old liason officer). The mist hangs right down to the Tap Alpe and there are frequent light showers. Up on the Rupal Flank, the avalanches are thundering away. As you can imagine, the mood is rather subdued, even if not everyone shows it. As a result of this foul weather, our hopes of getting to the top are getting much slimmer and some people are saying there's not really much sense in it any more.

A few of us don't want to give up on any account; they're saying it's cheaper to stay out here longer than to come out again. At a push we'd like to stay on until 15 June, as experience has shown that the start of the monsoon often brings a period of fine weather.

Unfortunately, food supplies will be a bit short by then and we are already discussing the possibility of some kind of rationing here at Base Camp. Today, for instance, we have bought a young yak for 200 rupees (about 156 deutschmarks), which we will eat over the next few bad weather days. We are also hoping to buy eggs, flour, potatoes and rice from the farmers and eat 'à la Rupal' here at Base Camp, saving our own precious food for the high camps. This way we can avoid suddenly running out of food. We still have a surfeit of tinned vegetables and rhubarb grows wild here in profusion.

As I write, our porters and some local farmers are busy trying to catch the young ox that we'll be spit roasting in the next few days, chasing after the half-wild beast like Stone Age men!

Everyone is fit and healthy, except our youngest, Peter Vogler, who is very poorly. Suffering badly, he managed to drag himself back down from the Winch Camp to Base. The diagnosis is pleurisy. Reinhold and I are fine, despite – or maybe because of – the fact that we have both lost weight. Our noses are peeling again.

Every four or five days the mail runner comes up, an agile little farmer from Tarshing; he brings our post and eggs. He stays overnight and then either rides or drives by jeep back to Gilgit the next day. The road should be OK again now; on the approach march it was a mess and that is why we had to come in on foot. Tomorrow he will ride back to Gilgit with about twenty letters from us, most of which we wote at Camp III during the storms, and the rest of the mail.

School must have broken up by now and we are curious to know where you will all be when we get home. Have Helmuth, Erich and Waltraud received our letters? The post is very slow and I believe that many letters go astray.

The ox has now been slaughtered and we are looking forward to liver, lung and barbecued meat with plenty of vegetables.

You can still write to us until the end of June as we will receive our post in Gilgit, and Rawalpindi too if necessary. How long the return journey will take depends on the weather. In any event it will be at least six days from Base Camp.

Looking forward to seeing you all again soon,

Günther and Reinhold

But there was to be no 'Wiedersehen'. Günther was lost after the traverse of Nanga Parbat. I came back alone – and as a different person.

For years I have had to defend myself against all the persecution and accusations that this Nanga Parbat traverse brought in its wake. I know now that I will not get very far by constantly going over the whys and wherefores of the accident. And I am no longer disappointed about the outcome of the expedition, just sad that Günther is no longer there.

I came to terms with the big disappointment by more or less immersing myself in it completely; I started to listen more to how I felt inside rather than to other people's accusations or to what other people believed they ought to persuade me. For the decision to climb down the Diamir Face I alone bear

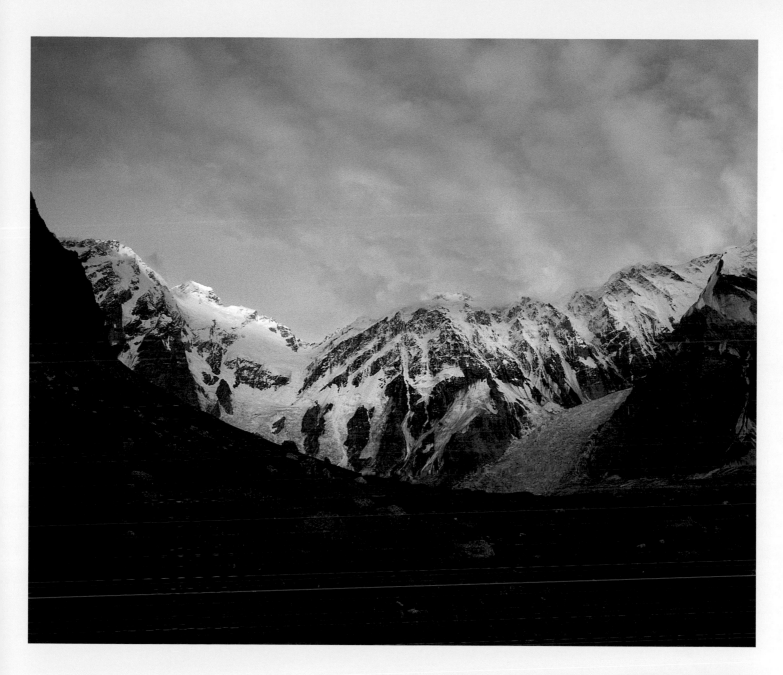

the responsibility. Whether it was the right decision or not, nobody can know. Although many have passed judgement, the truth is we had no other choice.

At the time, bizarre events like these are really desperate affairs but in a way they are good for a young person to experience, for it is such experiences that deepen our sensitivity.

I had the good fortune to 'die' young; it created the prerequisites for me to occupy myself with the fundamental questions of existence.

The Nanga Parbat Odyssey gave me the strength to accept or avoid any future risks and I now view every single hazardous enterprise I undertake, whether it is 'successful' or not, as a necessary part of my life.

For a long time I believed that, after accomplishing the traverse of Nanga Parbat and surviving the many disputes that followed, there was nothing more that could harm me. Yet this belief is also an illusion and to yield to it could be dangerous. So I am prepared for the next disappointment – it is part of the drama of life.

The summit of Nanga Parbat in the last light of evening and the gloomy Diamir Valley, which Reinhold Messner had to descend alone in 1970.

View to the East from the summit of Nanga Parbat, showing the false summit (left) and the col of the Silbersattel.

Experience shows that of the most successful mountaineers of any generation, only half die from 'natural causes'. The others fall to their deaths, freeze to death or otherwise perish in the mountains. Alpine history confirms this situation as a brutal reality; early on, it caused me to think critically about big wall mountaineering. Is it, then, pure chance who 'stays up on the mountain' and who 'survives' or is there some connection between survival and a climber's experience and circumspection? Today I am convinced that one of the most decisive factors for enduring in a borderline situation is the will to survive. I believe that this can even have some influence over objective dangers. I am not saying that one can stop rocks breaking away or hinder the passage of avalanches, only that the mentally well-balanced climber is unlikely to get hit by them. I would even dare to suggest that the climber who is in tune with himself and the world will not normally perish on a mountain. Does this then mean that every mountain accident has a spiritual cause?

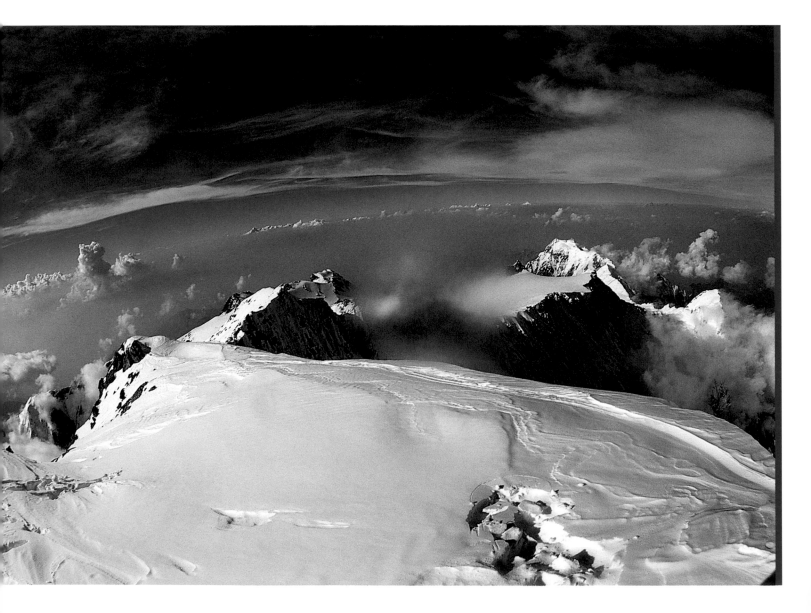

If I survived on Nanga Parbat back in 1970, then it was only because at the time I was posessed by an overwhelming will to survive. For all that, I nevertheless did 'die' and today I feel that I would not survive in such a critical situation. The will to survive that I am talking about here is probably dependent on a person's age, enthusiasm and on his mental balance and peace of mind.

The Nanga Parbat expedition, with all its consequences – the loss of my brother who was at the same time my closest climbing partner, the frostbitten feet, the many arguments and disputes – threw me mentally off balance, at least for a short time. Soon, however, with the help of new activities and new friendships, inner calm, self-knowledge and strength were restored in me.

In recent years, I have become more and more preoccupied with the great mountaineers and their spiritual and psychological constitution – with Mummery, Lammer, Preufl, Shackleton, Mallory, Buhl, Terray, Karl and Lowe.

Let us take Hermann Buhl as an example. The first person to climb Nanga Parbat in 1953, he was sharply criticized after this, his greatest success, and suffered far more from these personal attacks than he himself would ever admit. And yet Buhl did not give up climbing. On the contrary, he went on to climb the most difficult faces of his day in the Western Alps and pursued new expedition objectives. In 1957 he set off for Broad Peak, his second eight-thousander. At the time, Buhl was without dispute the most successful mountaineer in the world, yet he remained a controversial figure. Even former climbing partners were hostile towards him. Was it fame that was responsible for his exclusion from the mountaineering community or was it the man himself who was at fault? Buhl quite obviously suffered as a result and climbed like a man posessed, in a vain attempt to counter these prejudices. Slowly, little by little, he became a different person – he lost his inner balance.

More and more frequently now, I find myself asking what it was that caused Buhl's fabled will to survive to suffer, whether the Buhl who walked over the cornice in thick mist in the Karakorum in 1957 was indeed the same Hermann Buhl who fought his way back alone from the summit of Nanga Parbat in 1953, totally exhausted yet determined to live. Certainly, Buhl did react to the frequent attacks, most of which came from his 'closest circle of friends', and thus squandered some of his vital energy. Each new success brought him more recognition, but also caused more envy. He could not distance himself from it all. Once imprisoned within this vicious circle, did he perhaps even toy with the idea of self-surrender? We will never know.

When Günther and I stood on the summit of Nanga Parbat on 27 June 1970, our will to survive was so great that we were able to find our way down the unknown Diamir Flank. This was only possible because during the descent I retraced at least 1000m of height, step by step, looking for a way out. I climbed back up once because a serac blocked the way, again when a rock step seemed too risky for Günther and a third time when crevasses barred all further progress. I doubt whether today I would still have the psychological strength to get myself out of a similarly life-threatening situation.

These days I see inner harmony as the prerequisite for any climber who seeks to push the frontiers. Without it, he should give up extreme mountaineering, otherwise he would be a potential suicide on a big mountain face. I remain convinced that the psychological erosion caused by years of sustained personal attacks, disappointment and disillusionment and, above all, by a damaged emotional life presents a serious threat on such extreme undertakings. Without noticing it, the protagonist loses, drop by drop, that very will to survive that is so crucial in those borderline situations. Without it, he can no longer instinctively do the correct thing when the situation becomes critical.

Why was it that, in 1965, Walter Bonatti withdrew from extreme mountaineering? Because too many jealous people had begun to gnaw away at his psyche? Or was this step the unconscious reaction of an experienced climber against those extraneous forces that made him unhappy? Was he trying to save his 'eroded' will to survive? I do not know.

In my case, I felt very early that I had to be very careful on this point. Since I have been climbing big mountains for three decades now and recognized this 'Alpine danger' early enough, I am still alive. I am searching for a balance within myself, one that does not crave applause, and am training myself in the art of patient acceptance. It can serve no purpose to try to make sense of the many jealous and critical people, or to punish their triviality with arrogance. Better not to let them anywhere near me. They must not be allowed to affect me, just as the Buddhist remains unaffected by the burdens of the world. Maybe then I can avoid becoming tired of it all and ensure that I, too, do not one day walk off the cornice to my death.

'What is it that causes this ill-will and jealousy amongst climbers? This unimportant question gains in importance when one views the climber as an individualist who spends his free time in the mountains. One might assume that everyone ought to be happy that others have also discovered this fascinating activity, since every fairly executed climbing act enriches the sport of mountaineering. It is interesting to observe that amongst top mountaineers this jealousy does not exist. It only occurs between climbers of differing abilities. I conclude, therefore, that it is the lack of direct competiton in climbing that is the root cause.'

REINHOLD MESSNER

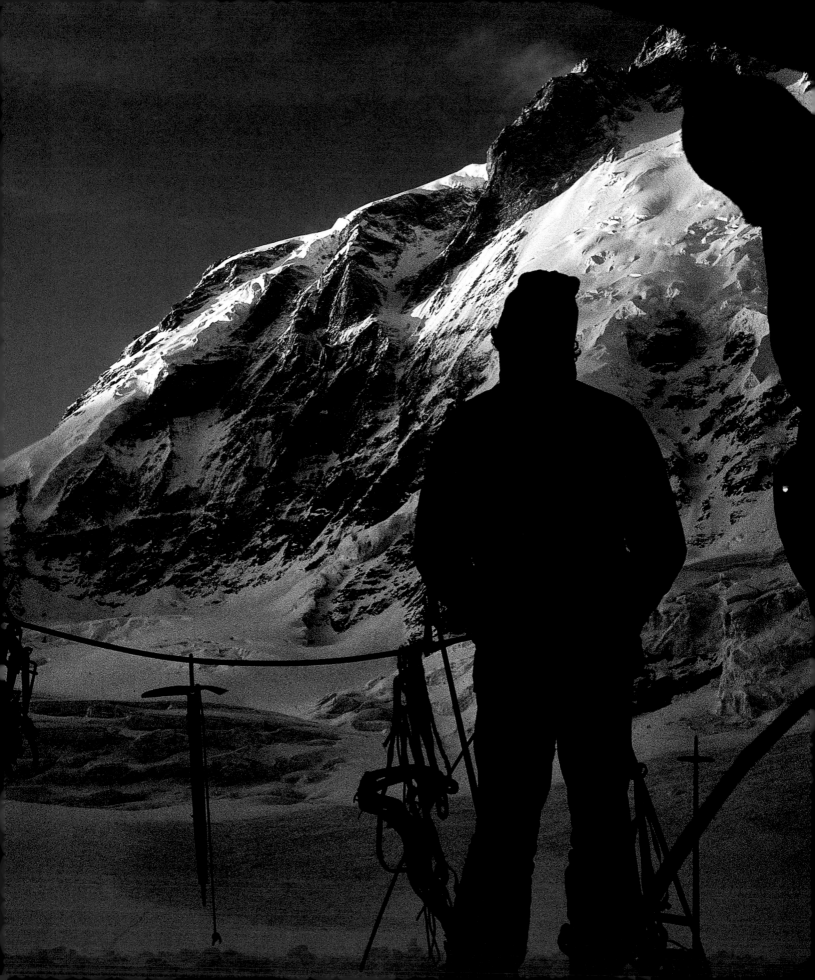

VERTICAL WILDERNESS

To be sure, modern mountaineering is a British, and also a Central European, invention. Further developments were made in the USA, in Japan and, above all, in the countries on the other side of the former Iron Curtain. Finally, it was Slovenian climbers who then took the whole thing one step further. The new routes that have been climbed in the last decade on the South Face of Lhotse, the West Face of Makalu, Gasherbrum IV and Dhaulagiri would have been unthinkable in the 1980s. For me, they demand more respect than the Big Walls of Yosemite or Patagonia, even if many of these have meanwhile been climbed free.

The vertical wilderness of the highest faces of the Andes, the Pamirs and Tien Shan, the Himalayas and Karakorum is beyond compare, since the 'exposure' and commitment there is absolute. In other words, there is no one there to help you in an emergency.

In these places, Big Wall mountaineering is the same as it was in the early days. Only the very best dare to attempt the 'big problems', and drama, failure and tragedy too, unfortunately, are an integral part of the game, just as they were in bygone days on the East Face of Monte Rosa, the Eigerwand and the South Face of Aconcagua.

(facing page): 'Butterfly Valley' beneath the summit wall of the South Face of Manaslu, first climbed in 1972.

THE SOUTH FACE OF MAKALU

Aleš Kunaver, the great expedition leader from Ljubljana in Slovenia, wrote a report on the first ascent of the South Face of Makalu in 1975. His piece clearly describes the beginnings of Big Wall mountaineering on the eight-thousanders.

'This time we returned to Makalu Base Camp to settle an account still outstanding from 1972,' he writes. 'In that year we had not reached the summit, but had come close to climbing the face. We had also learned some useful lessons.'

Kunaver had realized that the organization of the flow of loads being carried up the face needed to be improved and that the periods of 'dead time' in the high camps had to be reduced. This meant further rationalization of the circulation of climbers up on the face. 'We were assisted in both these matters by having a larger team of climbers and a smaller group of Sherpas. We intended to use the Sherpas mainly below Camp II, where the ground suited their experience and abilities.'

Five teams of climbers were to move up the face to a strict timetable, by virtue of careful planning they hoped to keep the lead teams active and the loads moving without bottlenecks. 'The plan was logical in theory, but we did not take it too seriously,' Kunaver says. 'As it turned out, though, only the poor weather

on September 25, 26 and 27 prevented us from implementing our cleverly formulated theories.' The larger number of climbers meant that the work on the face was safer and more reliable. 'Even our "sick battalion" got to 7500m as a support group with their loads. Of the twenty-one members, including the doctor and photographer, nineteen reached Camp IV at 7500m.' They therefore had no problem in finding enough 'candidates' for the summit bid. 'But there were serious risks and dangers inherent in the final stages of the climb, so that not all were considered suitable.'

The sixth Yugoslavian Himalaya Expedition, 'Makalu South Face 1975', began on 17 August when all the members and their equipment were finally assembled in Dharan. Ten Sherpas and 320 porters made up the rest of the cast.

On 19 August the expedition set off for Base Camp, via Dhankuta, Hills, Tumlingtar, Kaandbari, Sedua and Kiki La. The weather was really good. Base Camp was established on 6 September, at a height of 4,950m. 'The first loads went up to the Camp I site on 6 September. On 7 September Camp I was established at 5,850m. On the following two days, Camp I was fully stocked and Camp II prepared. At first we equipped it with two tents but then, because of serious avalanche

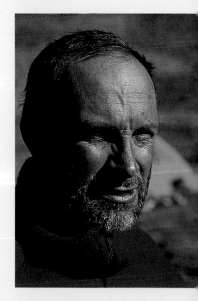

Stane Belak from Slovenia was one of the most successful climbers of his generation.

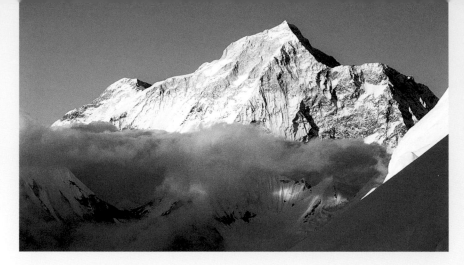

Makalu. On the left, the West Face; on the right, the South Face.

> 'I could not climb the South Face of Makalu. Such an elegant face! Such a clean line! A fascinating route. An ideal climb!'

REINHOLD MESSNER

Retreat from the South Face of Makalu.

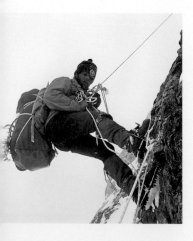

danger, we relocated it in snow holes, where it was safer and where there was more room and better insulation. Eventually, the capacity of this camp was such that it could hold fourteen climbers and, at 6300m, it became the advanced base camp for the face. By 12 September all the load carries for Camps I and II had been completed and ropes had been fixed up to the middle of the face.' Bad weather on the 13th interrupted the work but on 14 September the team pushed the route to 6600m. They later dug a snow hole there with 'room for eight beds'.

'Camp III was established at 7000m on 16 September with two tents capable of accommodating six climbers. We used the next few days to transport loads up to Camp III. Once this job was completed we started fixing ropes to Camp IV. This was accomplished in two stages. On 23 September Camp IV was established at 7500m. The camp was fully equipped over the next few days and the fixed ropes advanced to the difficult traverse.'

Then the heavy snowfalls struck, marooning all the teams in their camps.

All the climbers were pulled back to Base to recover on 27 and 28 September. On 29 September the final push began. The teams set off from Base Camp at one-day intervals to rebuild the camps and push the route higher up the face. 'Camp III was reoccupied on 1 October, Camp IV on 2 October. On 3 October the fixed ropes were pushed out again. The following day, Camp V was established. The summit team now had sufficient back-up. Five climbers carried in support to Camp V at 8050m.'

The following day they completed the route-finding and fixing of the rock sections above Camp V and on 6

October the first summit team set off. 'When the two climbers noticed that their Belak's oxygen apparatus wasn't working properly, Marjan decided to give his set to his friend so he could get to the summit. Stane Belak was the one who had worked hardest on both Makalu expeditions and had done his utmost to force a successful outcome.'

They continued climbing, in good weather, reaching the summit ridge a little after 11 o'clock and heading up this to the top. It was 6 October 1975.

'Belak reached the summit at 4.00pm and Manfreda Marjan, climbing without oxygen, joined him forty minutes later. The climbers maintained radio contact with Base at all times. They regained Camp V safely at 9.00pm.'

The next team set out for the top on 8 October. 'Two of the four climbers ran into difficulties; Cedilnik Danilo was hit on the knee by a falling chunk of ice and Robas Roman had trouble breathng. Both therefore turned back. Nejc Zaplotnik and Ažman Janko continued and reached the summit with no further problems.'

During the preparations for the third summit bid, Boris Erjavec was hit on the head by a falling rock. He was knocked unconscious and left hanging on his jumar clamp. Only his helmet had prevented him from sustaining more serious injuries. 'Boris was helped back down to Base Camp. His companions, Ivč Kotnik and Viki Grošelj pushed on, topping out on 10 October despite strong winds and snowfall, before returning safely to Camp V.

The last team set off just one day later. The pair had two Sherpas in support, who were prepared to carry oxygen bottles up to Camp V for an additional bonus payment but who unfortunately failed to arrive. In spite of this Janez Dovžan and Zoran Bešlin set off for the summit on 11 October. Dovžan summited and returned safely, but Bešlin did not fare so well and failed just 100m below the top. It was also too late for him to make it back to camp that night, and he was forced to bivouac at 8300m on the descent. He returned to Camp V next day. Lower down the face, the men were escorted all the way back to Base Camp.

The expedition was a resounding success, attributable to comradely cooperation. The Slovenians had not only theorized about it, they had lived it too.

THE SOUTH FACE OF DHAULAGIRI

For a long time Dhaulagiri (8167m), a peak that rises high above the subtropical jungle of Nepal, was considered to be the highest mountain in the world. Now, this elegant summit – visible in clear weather from Pokhara – takes its rightful place as the sixth highest of the fourteen eight-thousanders. The local people call it the White Mountain (dawala – white, giri – mountain).

Even its 'Normal Route', the North-East Ridge – first climbed in 1960 by an international expedition led by the Swiss climber Max Eiselin – is rated as being difficult. Its South Flank, described by Professor G.O. Dyhrenfurth as 'one of the most terrifying walls in the Himalayas', is the highest unclimbed mountain face in the world.

Incredibly steep, this giant face is a good 4000m high and was the objective of a small expedition that I organized and led in the pre-monsoon season in 1977. Again I joined forces with Peter Habeler, my tried and trusted partner on Hidden Peak in 1975, and for the extremely difficult and hard enterprise we invited two further top climbers of international repute: Michael Covington, one of the top American rock climbers, and Otto Wiedemann, one of the best young German mountaineers.

But the South Face of Dhaulagiri is more than just a Big Wall. It was secretive and it kept its secrets. Like an oracle I read today the words of an old Ghurka soldier from Bega:

'Dhaulagiri is like five fingers on a hand. The first and last fingers are deadly; the two others too dangerous. Only the forefinger points the way to the summit.'

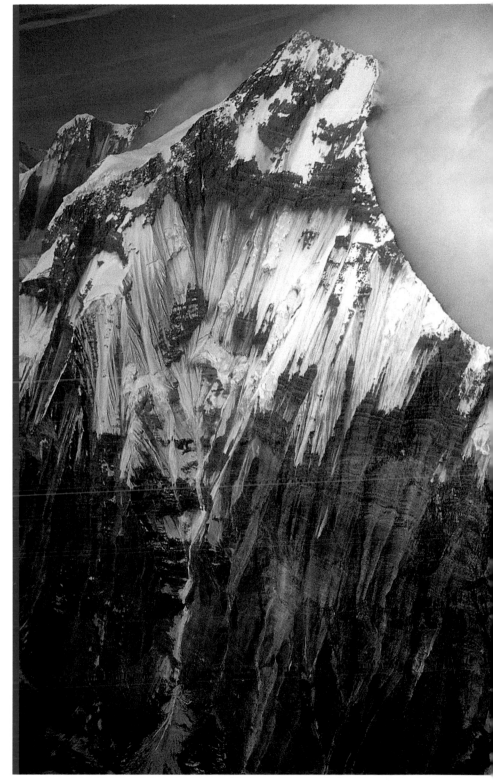

There are three lines up the South Face of Dhaulagiri, although none of them leads directly to the summit: the Buttress on the left (Polish Route), the Buttress to the right of the Central Couloir (Humar Route) and a route up the slabs to the right (Belak/Slovenian Route).

Without taking my left hand from the hold, with my axe I could smash off the icicles that hung like a thick, tattered curtain from the overhang. The sun had come up early and now, at 7.30am on a clear morning, it was already hot and dry. I wondered what it would be like about midday if it was so sultry, so unpleasantly warm now. The light morning breeze from the south-west carried fine crystals of snow that seemed to float in the air, sparkling constantly.

We were in that section of the initial gully on the South Buttress of Dhaulagiri where it narrows into a vertical chasm – mixed ground leading up to an overhanging rock pillar.

Keeping to the right, we climbed up towards a ramp that led upwards for several hundred metres to meet another vertical rock buttress. Above that an incredibly steep icefield clung improbably to the face. We had spotted it in the morning as we approached the foot of the wall – set at an angle of at least 60 degrees. Seen from here, it looked like a church roof rising into the heavens above us.

There was not much snow lying on the loose, dark rocks, so that at first we could climb without crampons. Whenever I was stuck on a stance for a while, belaying Peter, I would crane my neck right back, trying to spot a possible route and make myself feel a little braver. Would it go at all or would our expedition come to an end right here? It had to go; so far, we had always found another possibility.

We had only just put the short traverse into the ramp behind us when I again began to have my doubts; might it not be better to turn back now? The cliffs above us to the left were nothing like the crags you find on an Alpine face; they were huge shattered fragments of rocks stuck randomly to the mountain with seemingly nothing to bind them. It seemed a miracle to me that the whole lot did not come crashing down on top of us.

Despite this ever-present threat I was still happy to be climbing the face. The vertical wilderness I was now entering was the promised land, mysterious, described by no one and therein, somehow, lay its appeal.

The tension eased as we advanced, hold by hold, metre by metre, into this unknown territory. Then, as the face began to lean out above us, obscuring the route ahead, new tensions were created. The fear of

avalanches and stonefall was always there, yet we climbed on. We wanted to know, once and for all, whether this wall was possible or impossible for us, whether it was too risky or whether there was indeed a safe route to the summit.

Step by little step, we traversed up and diagonally right towards the ramp. Far away to our right stood the Annapurna group, wrapped in a thin veil of haze and seemingly belonging to a different world to ours, while down below in the valley the green-black hills of the Nepalese jungle rolled away in close formation to the horizon, with a finely-sketched snow ridge and the summit of Manapati rising in the foreground. Here and there, a white cloud floated above these hills and if one looked closely enough one could just make out trees on the edge of the spurs and, occasionally, birds flying.

Suddenly there was an eagle in the sky. I kicked a bigger step in the soft snow, slammed in the adze of my ice axe and held on tightly, pointing in the direction of the circling bird of prey.

'There's an eagle', cried Peter, who had only just seen it, and he paused, gasping for breath, 'an eagle – over the glacier!' And with that, he turned again to look in the direction of the Annapurnas.

'It's climbing, it's coming nearer!' I called to him excitely.

'Where?' Peter shouted back.

'Almost at the same height as us, between us and the South-East Ridge.'

Peter held on tightly to the belay peg, leant right back and bellowed up to me 'It won't find much up here – it's too steep even for geckos!'

'Or too dangerous', I called down. Then I carried on climbing.

The ice here was at an angle similar to the lower part of the Droites North Face. We came to a rock band barring the way ahead. Above it rose another ice shield, even steeper and more threatening than the last.

We had just reached the lower edge of the rocks when suddenly a snowslide poured over us, giving us such a fright that we considered heading back down to the safety of the valley; we actually thought seriously about giving up once and for all. Our desire to carry on and the decision to give up on this face were at that moment as close together as lightning and thunder.

However, once the spectre had gone, the snow dust had settled and the avalanche had run out down below – it had crashed down onto a kind of prow above us and sprayed out over our heads – we grew a little braver again. More than that, we were curious to see how the route might continue, so we climbed the next rock step in order to study the line ahead.

Meanwhile, we had reached an altitude of 6,150m above sea level. Over to the left we could see the western outliers of the Dhaulagiri group; on the other side, we could make out the whole of the Annapurna Massif.

We ventured out over the rocks for a good half ropelength more, before moving onto the ice shield – the steepest piece of ice climbing I had ever done. Suddenly there was a sharp crack – an avalanche! At that moment we knew that climbing further was out of the question. Not in this weather. There was simply too much new snow; it had been falling day after day. We were still every bit as enthusiastic but good sense prevailed, the good sense that given the prevailing conditions this face was impossible without taking unacceptable risks.

The decision to give up was not too hard to make.

So we determined to give up and, having made our decision to retreat, we didn't hang around too long at our highpoint, since to wait would mean further exposure to danger and any delay would mean that recrossing the glacier would be more strenuous as the snow would certainly have become slushy by now. We abseiled off, experiencing a second avalanche on the way down that merely served to confirm the wisdom of our decision. We congratulated ourselves on having made the only logical choice given the situation.

I now saw the expanses of ice and the loose rocks with fresh eyes, like a relief model of the face rather than a possible route to the summit as they had been just a few hours previously. Everything seemed to have changed now in some mysterious way; even I had changed. And the feeling began to grow that I was immersed in some great lake, not in order to sink to the bottom, but to climb out again. The sun, shining through the mist, soothed my overwrought mind and body and a liberating tiredness washed over me. Placing a rock peg in a crack made me think of flowers blooming on a sun warmed country wall.

The mists came and then went; the crevasses on the glacier below us yawned darkly. Stones rolled and bounced past, rebounding out until they disappeared into the abyss. Judging by the noises in the air, everything was now in motion: the snow under the soles of our boots, the stones, the mist in the valley. For a long time I watched a strip of cloud in the shape of a fish hanging over Annapurna, seeing it change shape and then suddenly dissolve into the blue of the sky.

I would often linger for longer than was strictly necessary on the belay stances and gaze at the jungle far out on the horizon, or at a patch of sky between the clouds. It was as if there was nothing else beyond, only a few secret sensations.

I recalled idly the press contracts we had entered into in connection with this Dhaulagiri adventure and the fact that the provisions cached at our first high camp would soon be exhausted, but neither thought really bothered me in any way.

As we came back into camp, Gyaltsen, one of our Sherpas, was standing in front of the tents. He wore his down jacket over a thick pullover and his boots were unlaced.

It was hot and stuffy in the tents in the midday heat so we went outside to sit in the fresh air. The bright snow slopes stretched out below us now in a blueish light, shimmering, soothing surfaces of snow. The face, with its serac zones and rocky outcrops, formed such a unified image with the glacier and the sky that the mists appeared to boil up everywhere and just as suddenly disappear again from whence they came.

How easy it was to live with this final defeat. Perhaps this was only because I had considered this as a possibility from the very start and had come to terms with it. Not only had I not discounted the possibility of failure, I had also made friends with the idea during our preparations and planning for the climb. From the beginning, as often as I thought about the summit, I was also occupied with the possible early retreat.

The sun had disappeared behind an outcrop of rock and it became cooler. We shivered and lay down on the insulating mattresses inside our tent, snuggling in between clothing, sleeping bags, stoves and provisions. Without saying much, we just rested and relaxed.

After a while Peter began writing in his diary. He glanced at me thoughtfully over the open pages of the book. I returned his gaze and each of us relived the day in the eyes of the other, seeing in them not just Dhaulagiri, but the whole expedition.

We had failed and so there would be no reason to write even a single line about these dramatic hours or about the undertaking as a whole, had the objective

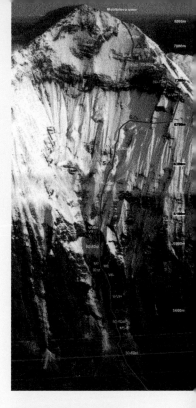

The Humar Route was first climbed in autumn 1999.

'I felt that this retreat was absolutely final, unalterable, like a law. There wasn't the slightest chance of another attempt in the future.'

REINHOLD MESSNER

'We had failed, and yet to fail after all we had been through had still been worth it It was worth it just to have been up there, cut off from the rest of the world.'

REINHOLD MESSNER

been any other summit or the attempted climb on any other mountain face. For, let's face it, who ever speaks of failure?

Yet it is still a powerful feeling just to survive on this 4000m wall of rock and ice, in the drumfire of stonefall and the thundering rage of avalanches. To carry on climbing would have been suicidal. Right up to the point at which we turned back, we had been totally committed to the climb.

We had begun to study the South Face after we had established Base Camp, in a very pleasant spot with little lakes and patches of green moss, at an altitude of 4000m. In terms of steepness, danger and savage grandeur this face really did outdo anything I had ever seen before. Huge icefalls hung poised to fall; now and then a piece broke off and thundered down the face. It would often go on for minutes at a time, the earth shaking, the pressure waves from the avalanche blasting off our feet in a cloud of powder snow when we were still 2km away from the foot of the face.

As a result, we planned to avoid the central section of the face and to attempt instead the left-hand rock buttress, the only justifiable route. Since at that point we had not yet put hand to rock on the face proper, we were confident still, if a little sceptical since it snowed day after day. By 10 o'clock in the morning at the latest it would grow gloomy and avalanches of new snow would join the ice avalanches. In the four weeks we spent at Base Camp, there were only two relatively fine days on which it did not snow.

While we spent our time in a futile search for a possible route, a drama was playing itself out in Base Camp. Bruno Moravetz (Mora), who was in charge of the ZDF camera team, which was supposed to be making a documentary record of the ascent of the face, contracted altitude sickness. The bad weather meant there was no possibility of helicopter evacuation, so I had to send him down to the valley with the expedition doctor, Dr Berghold, and my brother Hansi. It was a life and death matter for him.

As they set off through the snowdrifts for the valley, Mora with the oxygen cylinder strapped to his back, staggering rather than walking, I thought to myself it must have been like this when Scott came staggering back from the South Pole with his last two comrades. The whole of the approach march was now laid out before me like a scene of horror: the rivers and the bridges of ice barely a hand's breadth thick, the narrow gorges and mossy rainforests, the knee-

deep avalanche snow and table-size boulders that we had to scramble over.

It had taken us almost two weeks to get from Pokhara to Base Camp; no one had ever been through the last gorge before us.

From the start, we were in no hurry. It is not my style either to risk everything out of fear of failure or to chase tirelessly after successes. In any case, that would have been dangerous. We had come here to attempt the face and all four of us were equally preoccupied with our own individual ideas of success and failure.

Finally, on 9 April, the four of us – Peter Habeler, Otto Wiedemann, Michael Covington and I – established our first high camp at 5,350m, safely positioned under some rocks.

We were very pleased.

1,350m of height gain from Base Camp was a big deal. Expeditions that operate with tons of gear and lots of Sherpas and oxygen apparatus would have certainly placed one or more intermediate camps. But we had to be economical and were therefore pleased to have accomplished so much height between camps.

The next day we reconnoitred further, but realized that the rock sections on the middle part of the face were incredibly loose. We would have to move on to the literally vertical wall, where the layers of rocks were perched loosely on top of one another like the stones in a dry-stone wall. Slowly the feeling grew that our chances were almost – if not totally – nil. And this although we simply could not believe that with all our experience, knowledge and skill we were unable to find a line up this gigantic wall of rock and ice that gave us any chance of summitting without getting ourselves killed in the process.

On an early morning in April, Peter Habeler and I suddenly decided to attack the middle section of the face. Without fixed ropes, we climbed Alpine-style in order to get as high as possible, as I explained at the beginning. On the initial section there were several gullies and rock steps to overcome, their difficulties far exceeding anything we had met on the North Face of the Eiger. We had passed the 6000m mark and had pushed the route out onto a huge, steep shield of ice when the big avalanche struck. It was a loose new-snow avalanche, no ice, lucky for us. We had the feeling that it was all over for us, that we would be blasted away. It did not blow us away, but our last hope of mastering this face disappeared with it.

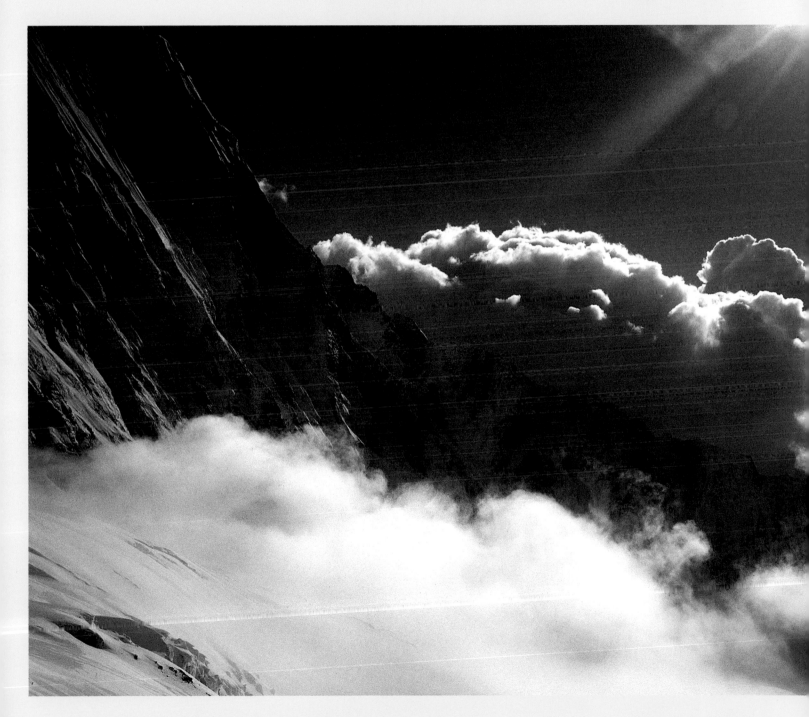

In the hours before midday, the corrie below the South Face of Dhaulagiri is usually shrouded in mist.

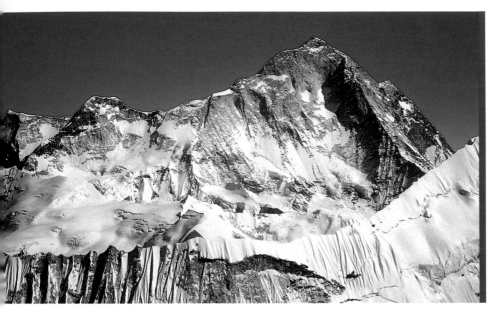

Makalu from the south-west. Two climbers perished on the first ascent of the West Face (right of centre).

'In 1974, with Wolfgang Nairz and other Austrian climbers, I attempted the South Face of Makalu. We got to about 7500m, then we had to give up.'

Reinhold Messner

'This time we returned to Makalu Base Camp to settle an account still outstanding from 1972,' wrote Yugoslavian expedition leader Aleš Kunaver at the beginning of his report on the successful Makalu South Face Expedition of Autumn 1975.

Is it not dangerous for a Big Wall climber to take this attitude? It is the start of the vicious circle of 'victory at all costs'.

I have never returned to any of the eight-thousander walls to attempt for a second time a route I previously failed on. This is not to say that I considered these walls to be impossible – after all, the South Face of Makalu, from which we retreated in 1974, was climbed a year later – it is just that they do not capture my imagination to the same extent as those lines I have not yet attempted.

I never place limits on my dreams just because other people assume that something is impossible; I will only acknowledge it to be so when the mountain itself clearly tells me 'No' at the time. My climbing, therefore, has always been governed by my own set of rules and by the actual conditions prevailing on my routes and expeditions.

To submit to other people's guidelines has never been my thing; I would rather live for a few short decades in a way that I find enjoyable than

live my whole life within the accepted norms, confined by rules and mediocrity. My life requires from me a willingness to accept risk and to recognize the impossible, but only what is impossible for me.

This attitude helps me not to become too presumptious and not to despair when faced with defeat. In contrast, someone who, after every success, always has to chase after another, becomes driven by an anxiety that forces him on to ever greater levels of achievement, until eventually that unavoidable defeat that he has been running away from causes either injury or death or simply knocks him off course. Very few retire on a winning streak.

Ever since I was a young man, my climbing has been a continual up and down affair and it is precisely this process of trial and error that has brought experience, a feeling for the details, a blossoming of my imagination and a deepening of my knowledge. The sensation on that return march from Dhaulagiri – the feeling of wanting it all to go on like that for the rest of my life – gave rise to the same kind of inner calm and harmony as those minutes of liberating nothingness on the summit of Hidden Peak. Anything that can lead to such a release of tension on returning after a harrowing attempt on a climb is more important than the summit or the Big Wall itself.

'The dragon must not die', I wrote as a twenty-year-old, in the recognition that it was only 'the impossible' that kept climbing so fascinating. Today I would phrase it differently: 'Only the secrets can be conquered' – most of all, the secrets that lie within ourselves.

For me, then, the impossible exists only as a concrete fact, never as an inconceivable thing. With this attitude I have not only survived, but survived such 'nightmares of extreme isolation as are encountered by space travellers in science fiction novels and which, on earth, exist almost solely in the Death Zone of the Himalayas beyond the 7500m frontier, where no radio and no signal can summon a rescue helicopter'. With this attitude I have achieved things that others considered impossible – I have survived again and again in the hostile world of the Big Walls.

SUCCESS WITHOUT SUMMIT

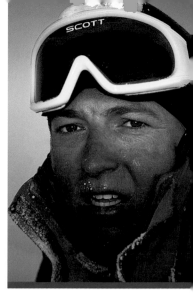

Was it by luck, coincidence or instinct that the Slovenian climber Tomaž Humar reached the summit ridge of Dhaulagiri directly above this 'forefinger' (*see* page 89: 'Dhaulagiri is like five fingers on a hand. ... Only the forefinger points the way to the summit.'), the forefinger that pointed the way for him to achieve his objective?

With new routes on Ama Dablam, Api and Nuptse to his credit, Tomaž Humar has achieved a whole series of 'crazy things'; he is the absolute, undisputed star amongst today's Big Wall mountaineers.

On 2 November 1999 he completed his new route on the 4000m-high South Face of Dhaulagiri I – solo and Alpine style – a climb with difficulties up to VII, ice to 90 degrees, M7+ (the 'M' rating is a mixed climbing rating system applicable to extreme rock/ice climbs). It marked a new watershed in contemporary extreme mountaineering.

Although after his fifth bivouac Humar was no longer able to follow his ideal line, there was no way back either. Nor did the terrain allow him to camp safely. So he traversed diagonally right for 1000m across a couloir and mixed ground to find himself on the Japanese Ridge, where he bivouacked at an altitude of about 7300m – his seventh night on the face. The following day was to be his summit day. Leaving his tent and a large portion of his gear behind, he traversed back into the centre of the face. Unfortunately, things did not go as he had expected, with extremely hard sections of climbing – water ice and dry-tooling – slowing his progress considerably. Imagine it, if you will: M5/M6 climbing in the Death Zone! Humar was forced to bivouac again, at 7800m, without a tent, just a sleeping bag. On day nine he was able to finish his climb, and descended via the Normal Route without summitting first.

Tomaž Humar, the strongest all-round mountaineer of our time, after his ascent of the South Face of Dhaulagiri.

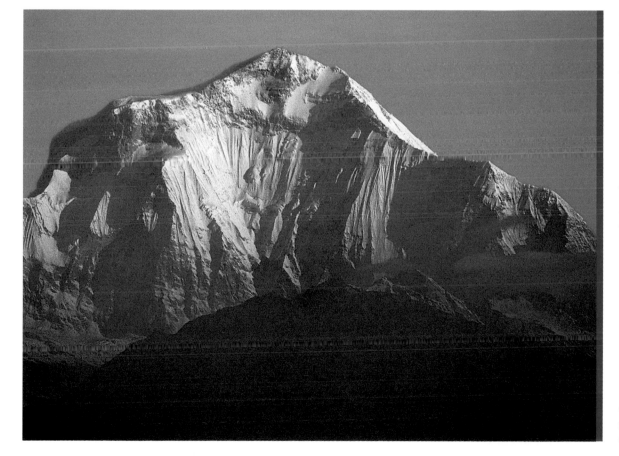

'I know only that at the end I bivouacked at 7800m. I was so exhausted that I was frightened of getting an oedema. It was dreadfully cold. I didn't have a tent, only my sleeping bag.'

TOMAŽ HUMAR

The beautiful concave form of the Dhaula Wall – beautiful but dangerous.

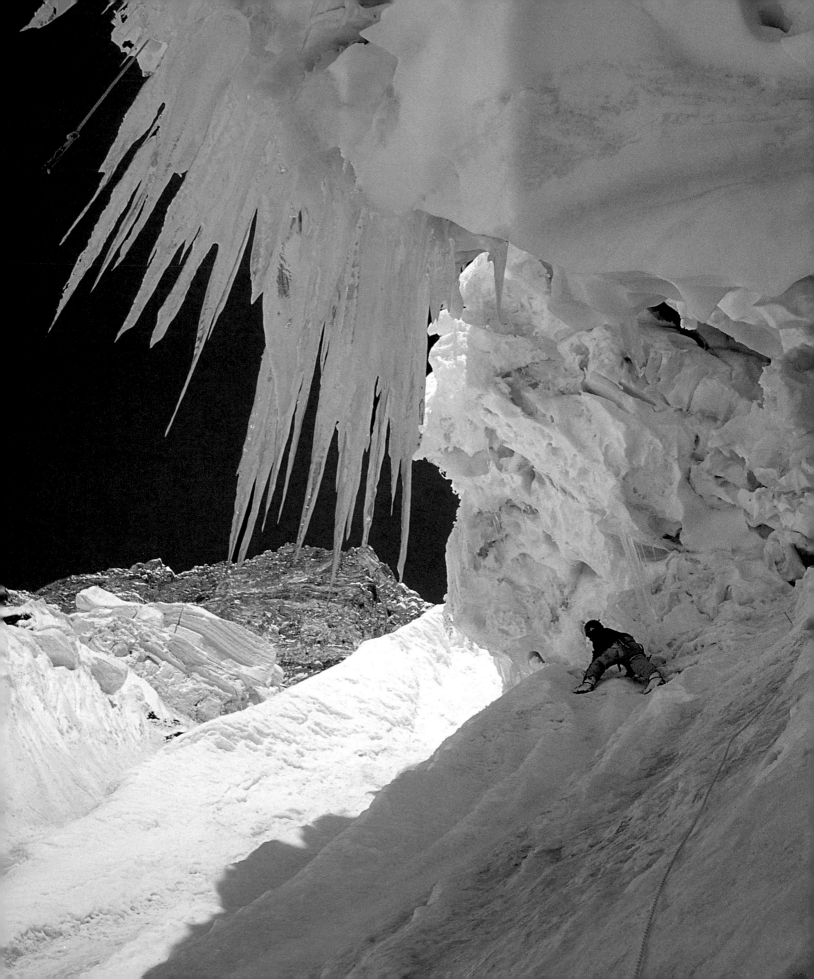

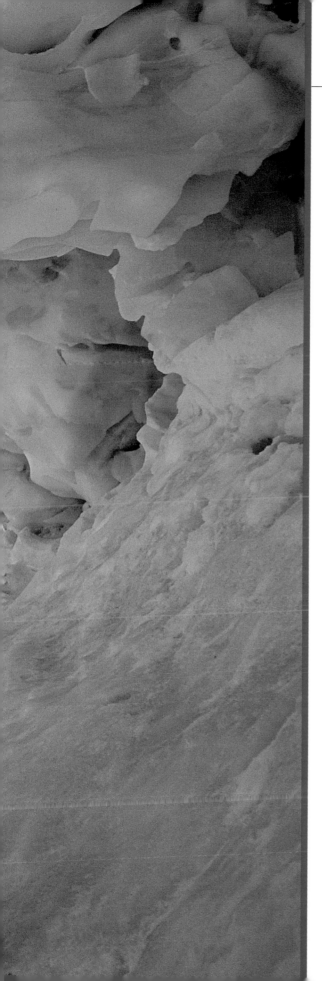

THE BIGGEST WALLS

In this central chapter it is not my intention to present a detailed description of the fifty biggest big walls, or a piece of guidebook literature. Nor do I set out to create a blueprint for repeat ascents. But whoever takes up the challenge of climbing one, a few or even a dozen of these walls will find enough information to prevent the climb becoming a trap.

What I am concerned with here is the feeling common to these big faces, with a few legends and a little additional data, with ideals and ideas – but above all, with the general picture. It is only by viewing things from a distance that the interested observer can gain any kind of perspective on the Big Wall mountaineering scene – a scene that was once mine – and thus rate both the walls and the protagonists in accordance with their true worth.

I had the great good fortune to climb, or at least to take a close look at, Big Walls all over the world. I have also met many climbers who have accomplished much more difficult things than I. And it is only in this way that I have been able to create my own picture of what Big Wall mountaineering really means.

The Big Walls have been the focal point for a good 100 years – on Fitz Roy and on Mount McKinley, from Nanga Parbat to Namcha Barwa, but also in New Guinea, New Zealand, the Antarctic and the Alps. You might ask why it is that I include all the great mountain ranges of the world and all the epochs of mountaineering. It is because 'Big Wall mountaineering' has everywhere been elevated to the position it now enjoys, and will continue to occupy – the royal discipline in mountaineering!

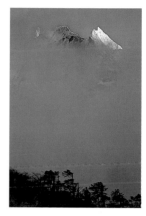

Tamserku in the Solo Khumbu. The Big Walls are both mysterious and dangerous places to be.

'"The Big Walls" are so impressive and at the same time so terrifying that it would be enough for me just to look at them.'

HORST HÖFLER

On the Bonington Route on the South Face of Annapurna, often climbed nowadays.

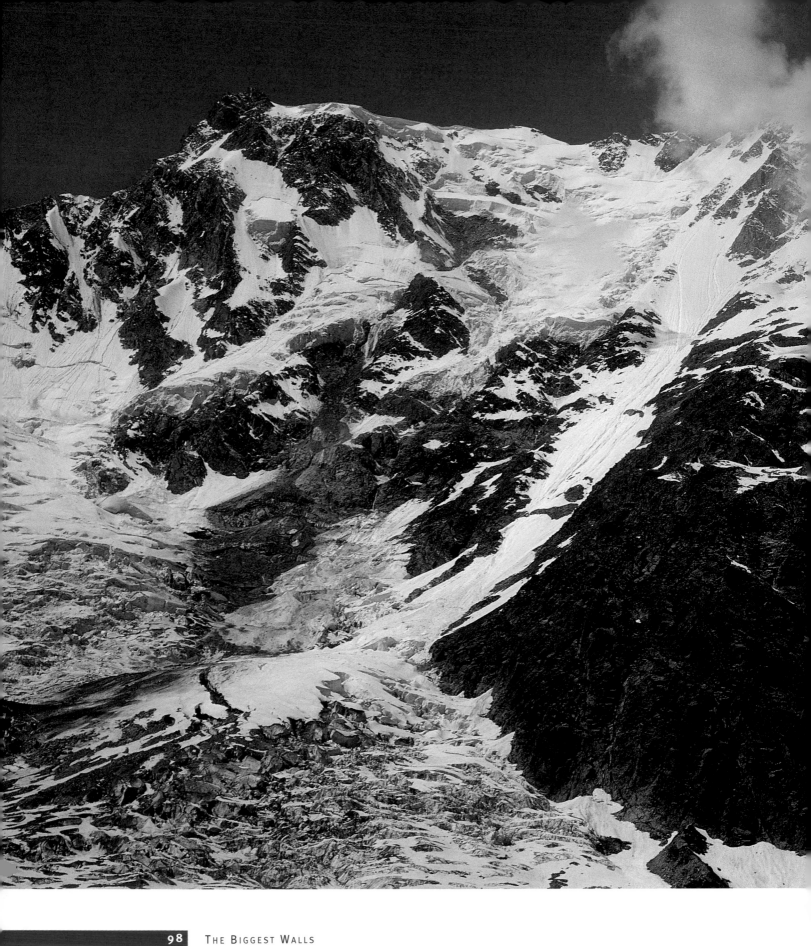

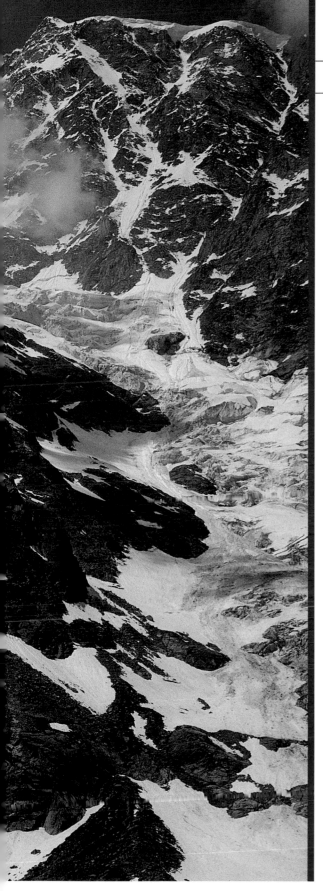

MONTE ROSA, EAST FACE, TAYLOR-PENDLEBURY ROUTE

1872 – VALAIS ALPS

SUMMIT HEIGHT

4634m

HEIGHT OF FACE

Approx. 2400m (between 2250 and 4634m)

DIFFICULTIES

Rock: medium; ice: 55 degrees

TIME

10–15 hours in normal conditions

STARTING POINT

Rodolfo Zamboni Hut (2065m); the best situated hut for the actual ascent of the face is the Damiano Marinelli Hut (3036m); from Macugnaga-Pecetto take the chairlift to Belvedere, continue on foot to the Zamboni Hut, cross the Belvedere Glacier and go over a rock spur (Crestone Marinelli) to the Marinelli Hut.

OVERVIEW

The central section of the face between the Dufourspitze and Nordend is split by the Marinelli Couloir. Cross this at its narrowest point and continue up the southern bounding cliffs (Imseng Spur) to the seracs and rock bands of the final wall.

TIPS

Since the East Face of Monte Rosa is also subject to the process of snow melt due to climate change the best conditions are likely to be found in the early summer. The route should only be started when the temperature is clearly below 0°C and the greater part of the route from the Marinelli Hut should be climbed at night. This is the only way to reduce the avalanche danger to a reasonably acceptable level.

'The Marinelli Couloir was scored by several deep secondary couloirs. Moving out onto this very steep section of hard ice and cutting steps was a gripping affair. The section from the Imseng Spur to the glacier was easy. At 7 o'clock we heard the first thunder of avalanches from the Couloir. That is the serious moment when it becomes clear to you that there can be no going back.'

JULIUS KUGY

The East Face of Monte Rosa – with the Marinelli Couloir in the centre of the picture – is the highest face in the Alps. It was first climbed on 22 July 1872, just a few years after the end of the 'Golden Age' of Western Alpine climbing.

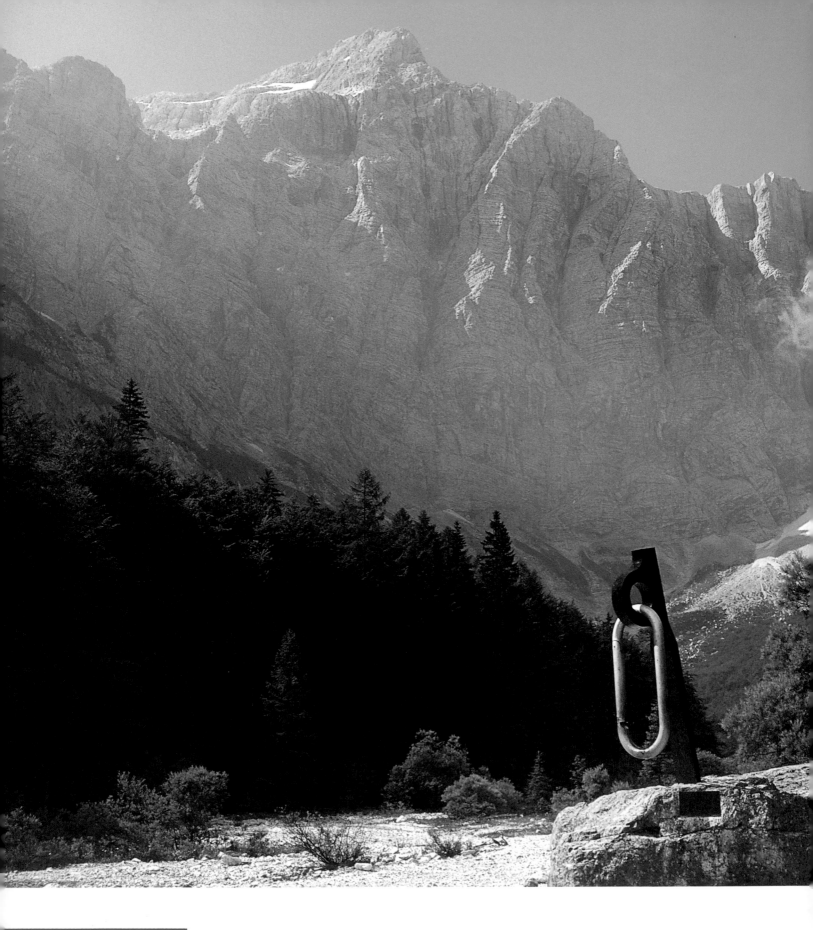

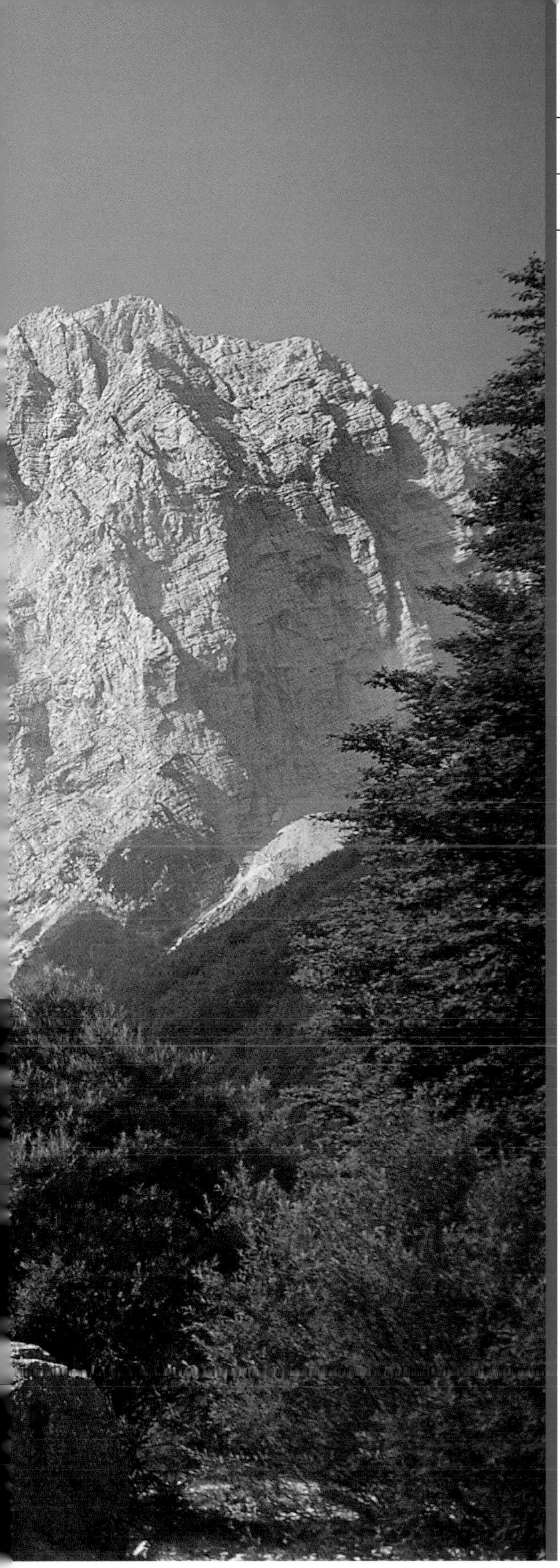

TRIGLAV, NORTH FACE, GERMAN ROUTE/ LONG GERMAN ROUTE

1906 – JULIAN ALPS

SUMMIT HEIGHT

2863m

HEIGHT OF FACE

c. 1400m (between 1460 and 2863m)

DIFFICULTIES

to IV+

TIME

7–9 hours

STARTING POINT

Aljaž-Haus (1015m) in the Vrata Valley, accessible by car from Mojstrana.

OVERVIEW

The central part of the North Face of Triglav Nordwand is defined by three huge buttresses. The 'Deutscher Weg' (German Route) takes a line up the face between the eastern and middle buttresses; its continuation, the 'Langer Deutscher Weg' takes in the upper half of the middle buttress. The summit structure is climbed on its west side via a wide chimney, ledges and gulleys to join the West Ridge, up which the route finishes.

TIPS

Confident climbers should consider the possibility of soloing the lower third of the face ('Deutscher Weg', II–III) in order to save time. A small rack of pegs and nuts is recommended for the 'Langer Deutscher Weg'. In the event of bad weather, escape is possible along the Kugy Terrace below the summit rocks.

'Few climbs have left such a lasting impression on me as this one. Of the three biggest faces in the Eastern Alps, the Triglav Wall seems to me to be the most difficult.'

LUDWIG SINEK

It is on the North Face of Triglav, and in particular on winter ascents of the gullies and couloirs, that the Slovenian alpinists hone their skills for the Big Walls of the world's mountains.

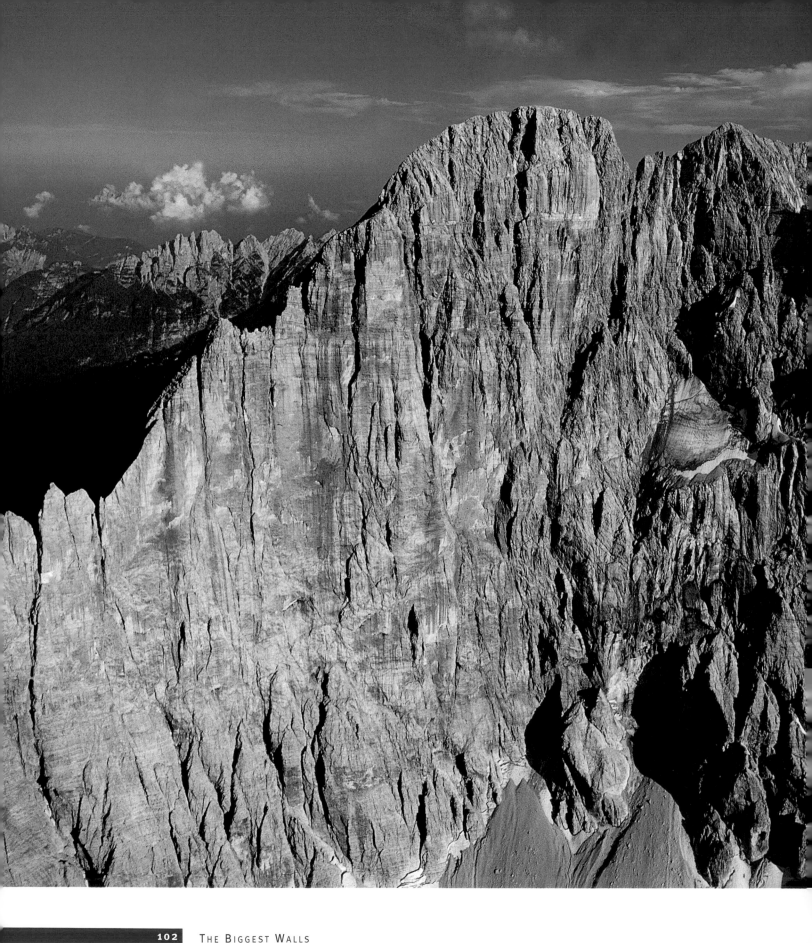

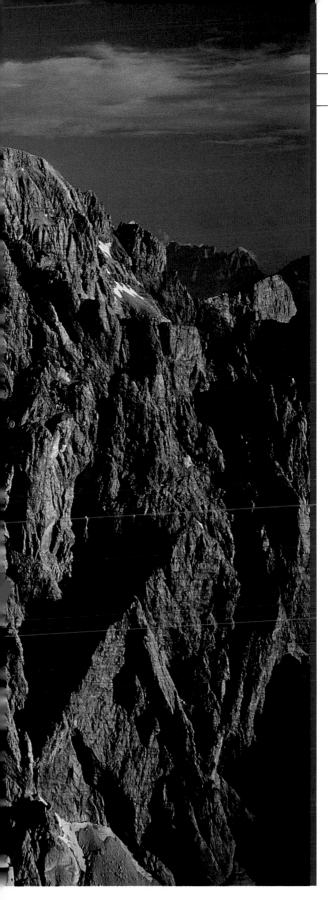

CIVETTA, NORTH-WEST FACE, SOLLEDER ROUTE

1925 – DOLOMITES

SUMMIT HEIGHT

3218m

HEIGHT OF FACE

c. 1000m (between 2200 and 3218m)

DIFFICULTIES

V+/VI, not always the best of rock

TIME

10–12 hours

STARTING POINT

Tissi Hut (2262m), reached on foot from Alleghe.

OVERVIEW

The route starts up the pedestal of rock directly below the summit fall line and follows a series of cracks and chimneys before heading for the firn field situated between the main Civetta summit and the Kleine Civetta (Piccolo Civetta) and then climbing a diagonal groove and a gully to exit left of the summit.

TIPS

Many pitons *in situ* but take a selection of pegs and nuts. Heavy rain increases the danger of stonefall and would make retreat difficult.

'Italian speakers refer unequivocally to the face as "the wall of walls", a reputation that it fully deserves. The face is around 1000m in height, which makes it bigger even than the Marmolada, and several of the routes occupy the status of milestones in the history of Dolomite climbing.'

REINHOLD MESSNER

On 4 August 1925, Emil Solleder and Gustav Lettenbauer succeeded in climbing the Civetta Wall direct to the summit without recourse to a bivouac. For a long time, this was the route against which the best climbers of the day measured themselves.

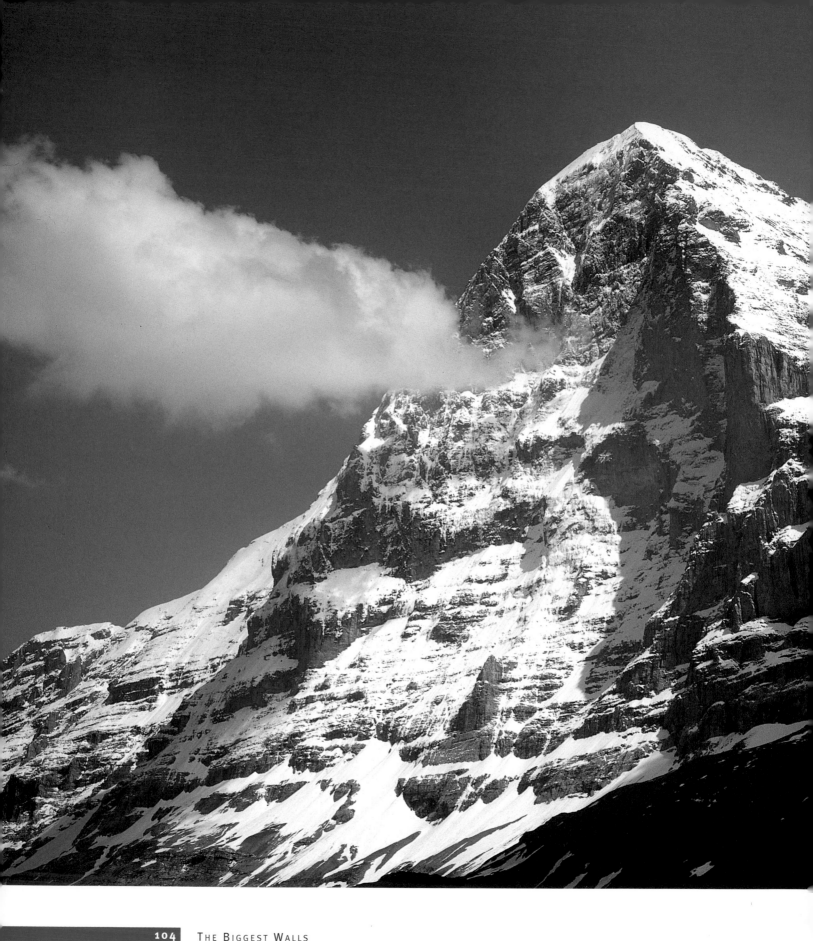

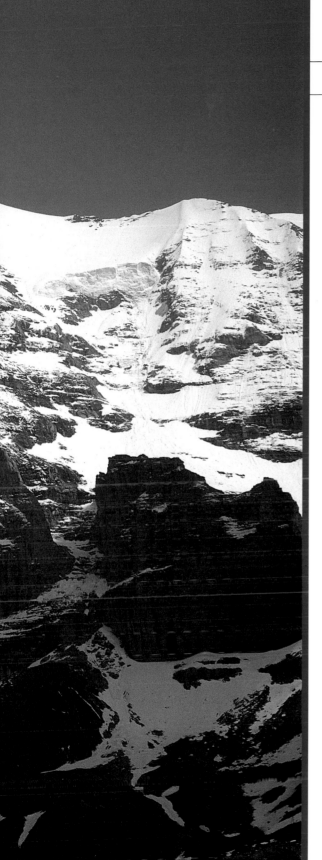

EIGER, NORTH FACE, HECKMAIR ROUTE

1938 – BERNESE ALPS

SUMMIT HEIGHT

3970m

HEIGHT OF FACE

c. 1800m (between 2200 and 3970m)

DIFFICULTIES

IV/V, often wet and icy; 50–55 degrees on the ice fields

TIME

10–20 hours in normal conditions

STARTING POINT

Alpiglen; or, better, Kleine Scheidegg (2061m); take the rack railway from Grindelwald.

OVERVIEW

The line climbed by the first climbers starts on the right-hand side of the concave face, makes a rising leftwards traverse to the left of the Roter Fluh to join the upper part of the Ramp and then moves back directly above the Ramp Ice Field into the middle of the face before trending left to the Summit Ice Field.

TIPS

The face is well-endowed with *in situ* pitons and the Swiss Air Rescue Service has shown remarkable skill in effecting rescues from the route. Nevertheless, on this huge face it is mountaineering skills that count for most: experience, confident and safe ropework and, above all, fitness. The route has several enjoyable sections of climbing and is nowhere unduly difficult but can become all but impossible when iced up. Due to the stonefall it is inadvisable to climb the ice fields during the afternoon. Safe bivouacs can be found on the Flat Iron or on the upper right-hand edge of the Ramp Ice Field. Should the weather deteriorate it is probably better to descend from any point up to the Ramp.

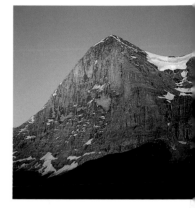

The Eigerwand in the evening light.

Anderl Heckmair, Ludwig Vörg, Fritz Kasparek and Heinrich Harrer made the first ascent of the North Face of the Eiger from 21 to 24 July 1938. It was a glorious moment in the history of mountaineering and a great sensation, since several climbers had previously perished on the Face.

'Neither the face nor the mountain look very nice. A steep pile of coal, but it is called the Eiger. I still believe that my life will certainly change if I do the Eigerwand.'

REINHARD KARL

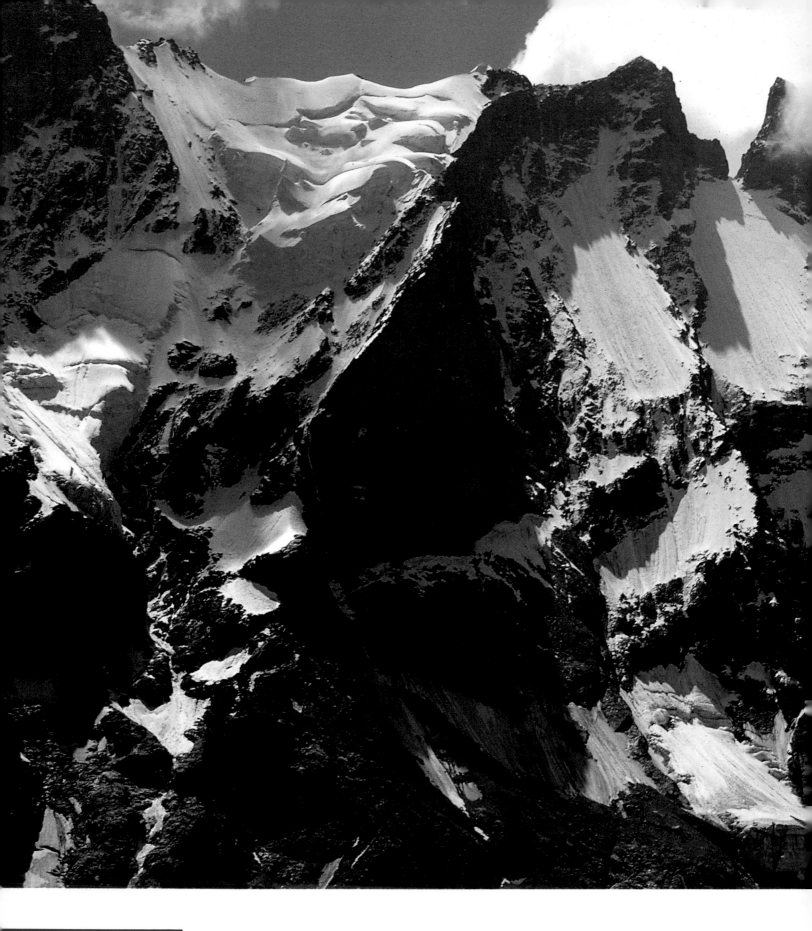

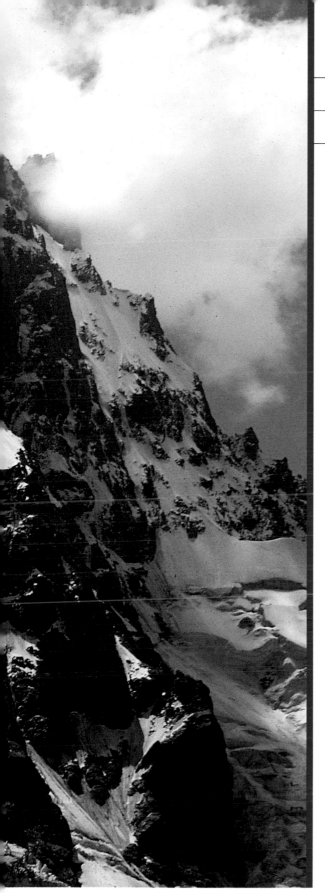

DYCH TAU, MAIN SUMMIT, NORTH-EAST FACE, CENTRAL BUTTRESS

1954 – CAUCASUS

SUMMIT HEIGHT

5200m

HEIGHT OF FACE

2000m+

DIFFICULTIES

Rock climbing to grade V and some aid (Russian 5B), steep ice and demanding mixed ground

TIME

26–30 hours in normal conditions

STARTING POINT

Bivouac on the right-hand lateral moraines of the Mischirgi Glacier; reached in 2 hours from the Besingi climbers' camp (25km on foot or by hire car from the village of Besingi).

OVERVIEW

There are three buttresses in the central part of the highest section of the Main Summit, North-East Face. The route takes a direct line up the central buttress, avoids the huge ice cliff above the top of the buttress on the right and climbs an ice slope to the summit ridge.

TIPS

The route is particularly susceptible to stonefall, particularly on the lower part. Several areas of loose rock.

'In the USSR, they had a completely different concept of big wall mountaineering. There, everything revolved around championships. According to their rules, each team received more points for new routes climbed in new areas. "Virgin" summits with steep faces thus became the dream of team captains and trainers in the USSR.'

REINHOLD MESSNER

The North-East Face of Dych Tau is the big face in the Caucasus. However, there are other rock and ice climbs that are just as impressive, high and difficult, like the big faces of the Besingi Wall or – pictured here – the Schchelda Wall near Uschba.

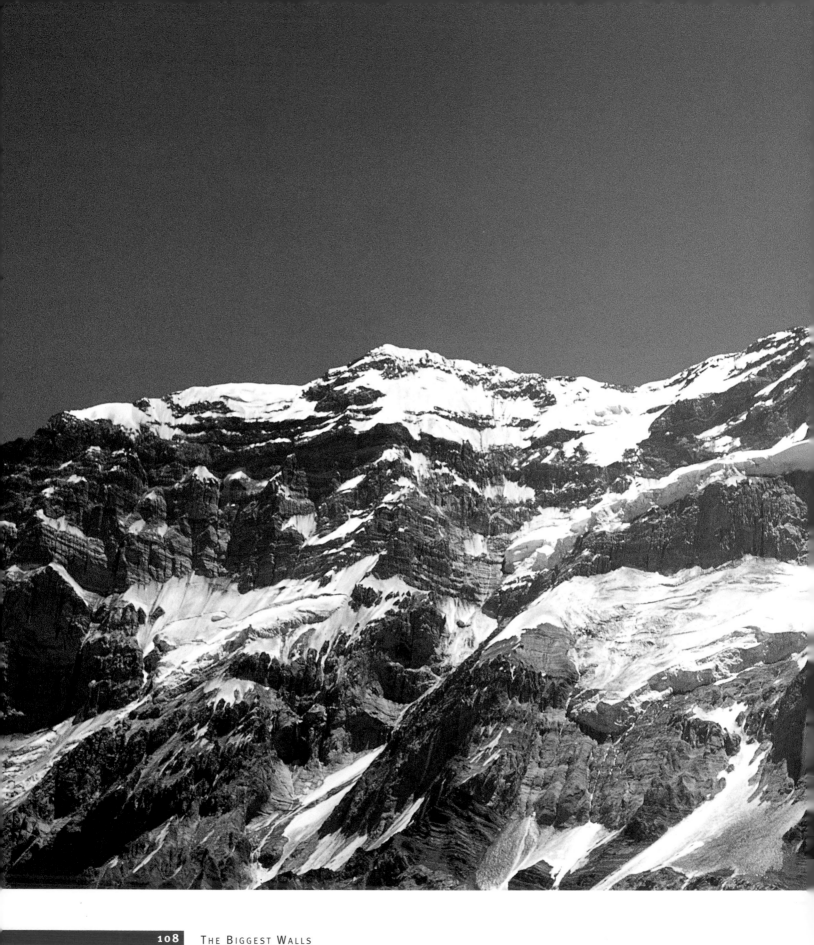

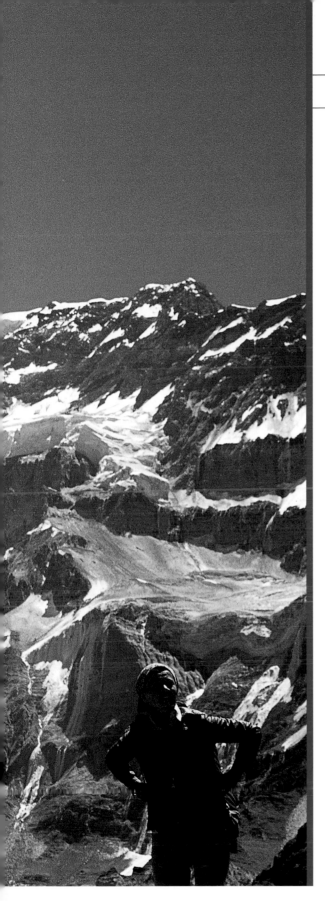

ACONCAGUA, SOUTH FACE, DIRETTISSIMA

1954/1974 CENTRAL ANDES

SUMMIT HEIGHT

6959m

HEIGHT OF FACE

c. 3000m (between 4000 and 6959m)

DIFFICULTIES

VI, very loose, ice to 90 degrees

TIME

2–3 weeks' acclimatization and preparation (fixing ropes); 2–4 days' climbing

STARTING POINT

Plaza de Francia or other places on the left edge of the uppermost part of the Horcones Glacier (c. 4100m), reached in 10–12 hours from Puente del Inca (Argentinia) via Confluencia.

OVERVIEW

The buttress leading to the summit, very prominent in its lower part, also leads in a direct line to the large glacial basin at two-thirds height. From here the route curves up and slightly leftwards to the summit.

TIPS

It is advisable to fix the first pillar to provide an escape route in the event of bad weather. Good sites for camps or bivouacs are found in the gullies above the big, loose pillar and on the large snow field beneath the summit headwall. Old fixed ropes are found everywhere on the route – take care!
For safety reasons, the only viable way of reaching the main summit is by the central buttress. On the headwall, the South Tyrol Route is preferable to the French Route, since it is shorter yet not significantly harder

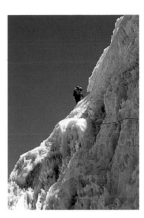

In the serac zone at 6000m on the South Face of Aconcagua.

'The French Route is the original route on the South Face and the best, too, if you start up the Slovenian variation and finish up the Messner Route.'

BARRY BLANCHARD

In addition to the three major lines, to date there are six variations, some of them very long, on the South Face of Aconcagua. The original route was first climbed in 1954 by A. Dagory, G. Poulet, E. Denis, R. Paragot, P. Lesueur and L. Bérardini.

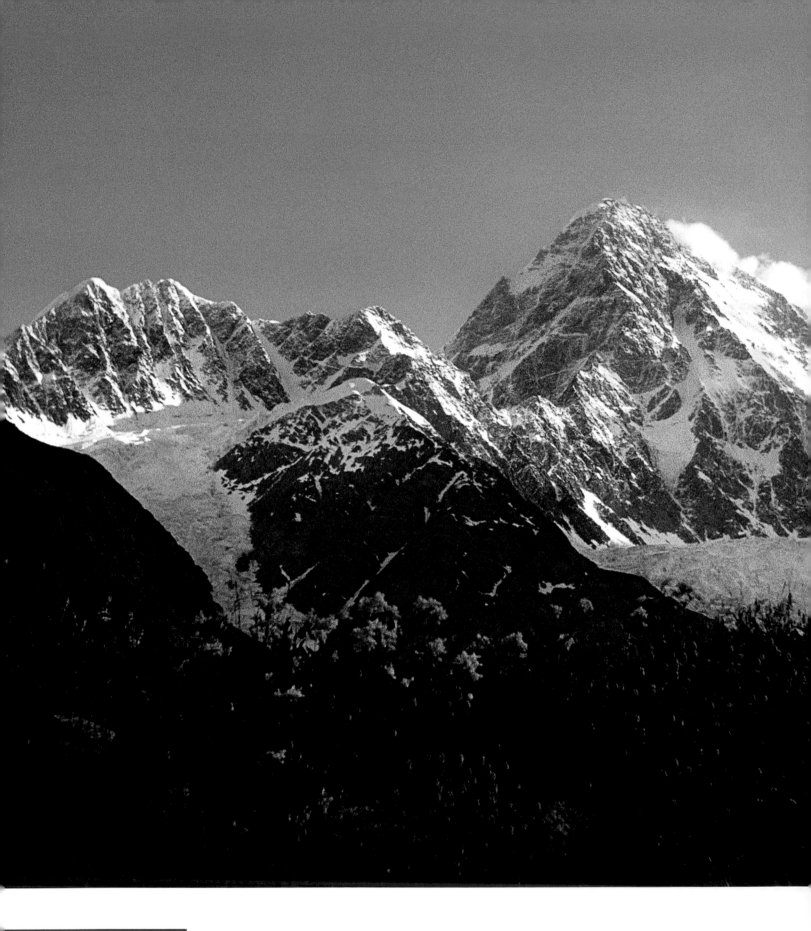

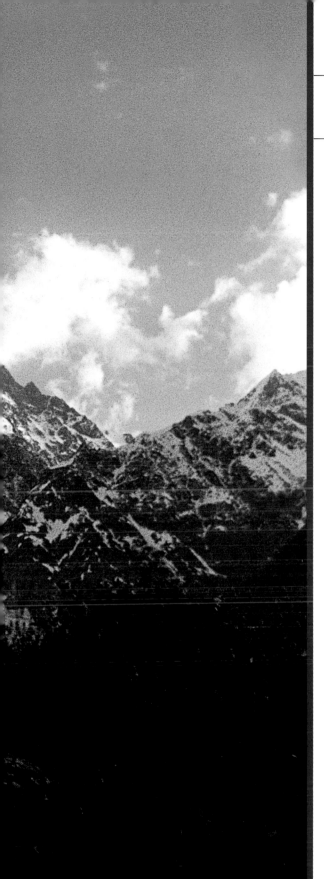

CHAPDARA, NORTH-WEST FACE

1965/1972 – FAN MOUNTAINS

BODCHONA, WEST FACE

1967 – FAN MOUNTAINS

Chapdara (5450m) and Bodchona (5138m) are located in the Fan Range, part of the Pamir Alai. The base camp and starting point on the Alaudinskie Lake at the confluence of the Arg and Ahbasoy rivers can be reached from Samarkand or from Dushanbe.

The North-West Face of Chapdara was first climbed in 1965 and given a Russian grade of 5B. In 1972 a difficult route up the centre of the 2100m face was climbed.

The West Face of Bodchona is about 1500m high, rising steeply above the Mutnye lakes and the Bodchona Glacier. First attempted in 1957 by Canadian climbers, it received its first ascent in 1967.

There are four ill-defined terraces on this red granite face. They provide the line of this in parts extremely difficult route, which is prone to stonefall and falling ice on its lower section. Reaching the first terrace is particularly challenging, as is the smooth section of face climbing above and a traverse beneath a cornice on the upper section of the face that is very poorly protected, if at all.

The first ascent was done with five bivouacs and the team reached the South Ridge after the fourth terrace, climbing this to the summit. They bivouacked again on the descent of the North-West Ridge.

In 1971 and 1972 two even harder routes were done on the West Face of the Bodchona.

The great routes climbed by Soviet climbers in areas like the Pamirs, Tien Shan and Caucasus went largely unnoticed in the West. In spite of their modest equipment, the Soviets were for a time the leading exponents of big wall mountaineering.

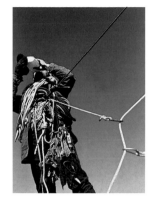

A heavy rack of gear on the North-West Face of Chapdara.

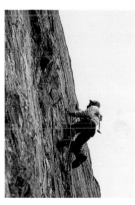

Difficult climbing on the West Face of the Bodchona.

In the Fan Range and in the Pamir area itself there are a number of 'big walls'; shown here is the South-East Face of Komakademiya Peak.

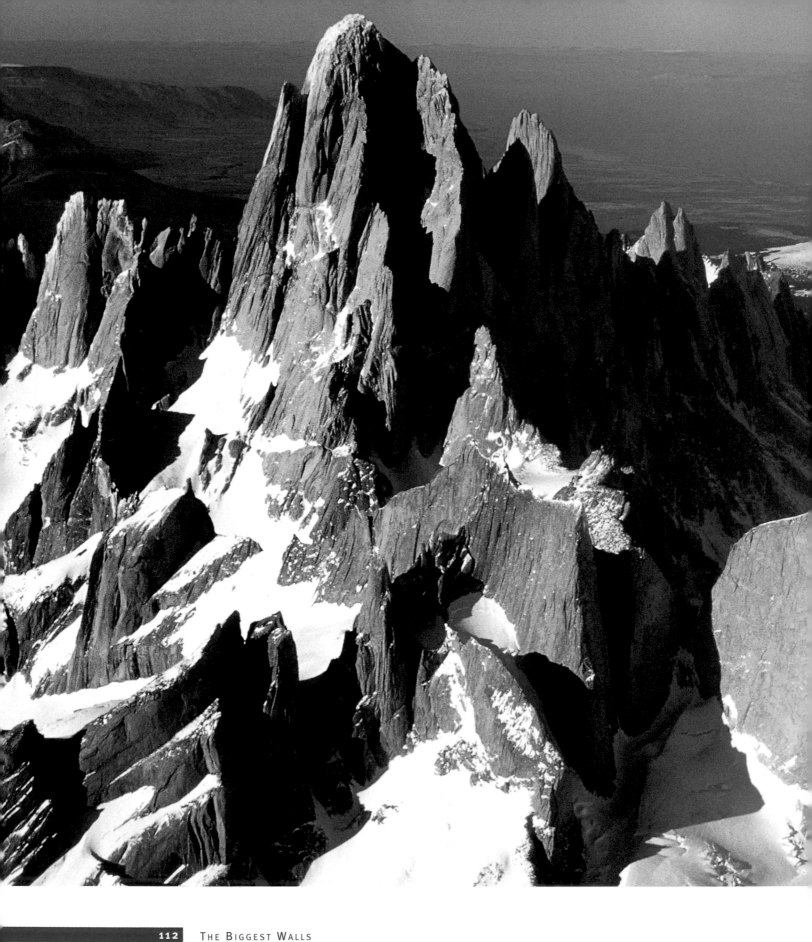

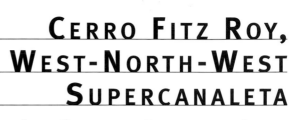

CERRO FITZ ROY, WEST-NORTH-WEST SUPERCANALETA

1965 – SOUTHERN PATAGONIAN ANDES

SUMMIT HEIGHT

3441m

HEIGHT OF FACE

c. 1300m (from 1750 to 3050m)

DIFFICULTIES

Extremely difficult ice and rock climbing (ED–)

TIME

One day walk in; 1–2 days' climbing

STARTING POINT

Bivouac at the foot of the face (Fitz Roy Norte Glacier), reached from the Hosteria Fitz Roy (road from Chaltén) via the base camp at Rio Blanco.

OVERVIEW

The Supercanaleta takes a line between the North-West and West ridges to join the long South-West (Summit) Ridge.

TIPS

The first ascent was done in Alpine style and took a total of three days up and down. Nowadays the route has less snow and is more dangerous.

'The Supercanaleta is the only route on Fitz Roy where fixed ropes have not been used, either on the first ascent or on subsequent repeat ascents. It is therefore the only one where to date every ascent has been accomplished in Alpine style.'

GINO BUSCAINI/
SILVIA METZELTIN,
1987

Cerro Fitz Roy from the north-west with the Supercanaleta clearly visible. It was first climbed in January 1965 by the Argentinians Carlos Comesaña and José Luis Fonrouge.

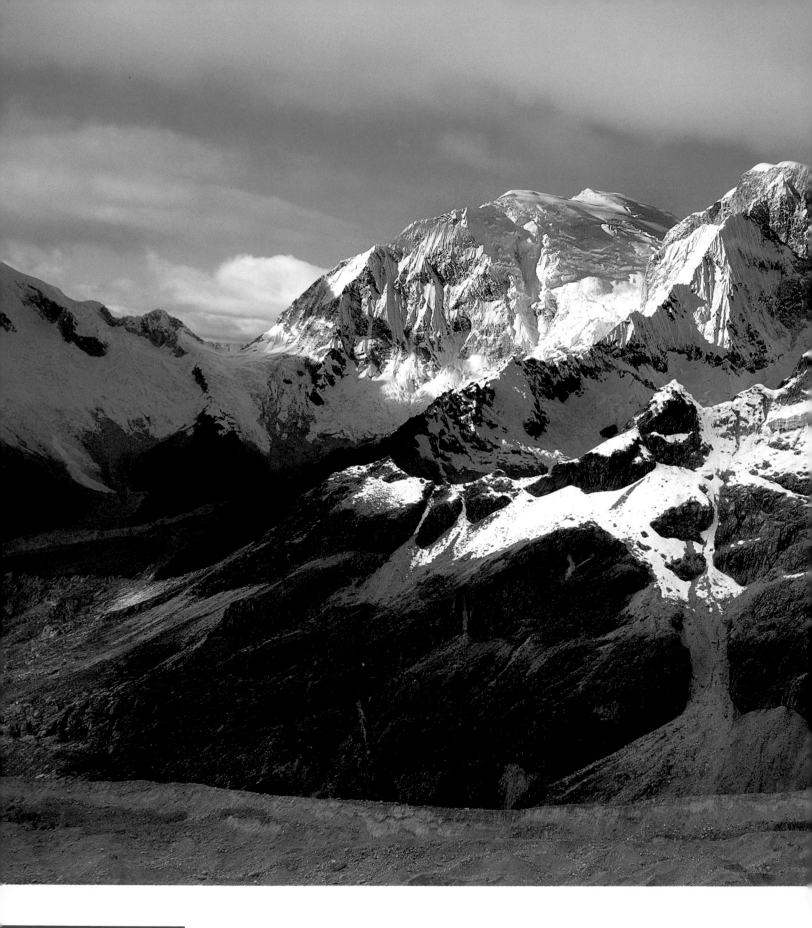

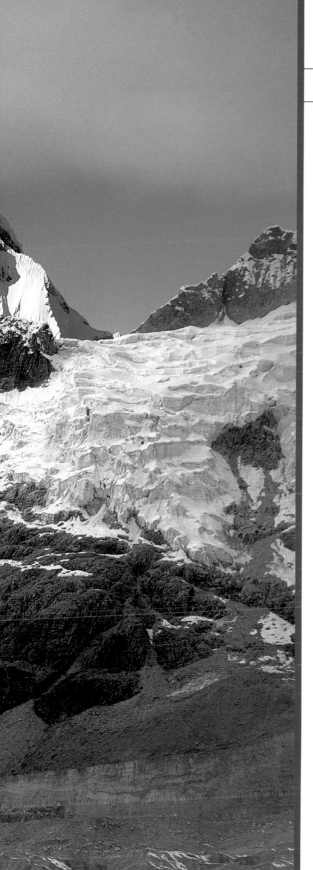

HUASCARÁN-NORTE, NORTH FACE

1966 – CORDILLERA BLANCA

SUMMIT HEIGHT

6650m

HEIGHT OF FACE

c. 1500m (between 5150 and 6650m)

DIFFICULTIES

Rock to V+/VI, hard mixed, ice to 60 degrees

TIME

2–3 weeks' acclimatization; 4–5 days' climbing

STARTING POINT

Base camp on the Llanganuco Glacier beneath the North Face, reached from the Llanganuco Lakes (roadhead from Yungay).

OVERVIEW

The route takes the prominent spur and buttress on the right-hand section of the face. The actual buttress begins with an obvious loose, steep wall – the so-called 'Pear' – which is nowadays usually avoided by climbing steep ice on the right. The upper section of the route leads leftwards into the centre of the face and then climbs the partially overhanging final wall to the summit ice cap, which is followed to the top.

TIPS

The first ascent team climbed this route in classic expedition style despite the constant danger of stonefall. They established two camps on the face and prepared the route with fixed ropes. One of the climbers was killed by stonefall whilst decending the fixed ropes. All of the North Face routes have since been climbed in Alpine style.

Further big faces in the Cordillera Blanca: Huascarán Sur, East Face (1200m); Huantsan, North Face (1400m); Chacraraju Este, East Face (1000m); Huandoy Sur, North-East Face (1000m); Ranrapalca, South-West Face (1000m); Chacraraju, West Face (950m).

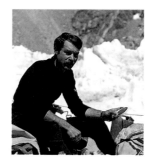

Renato Casarotto, solo ascentionist of a great face route on Huascarán.

'Afterwards, we all agreed that we had just undertaken one of the most demanding climbs we had ever done, comparable in difficulty to the hardest mixed routes in the Alps – but longer.'

ADRIAN BURGESS,
AFTER THE SECOND
ASCENT

The French Route – it takes a line up the right-hand side of the big rock face – is relatively safe from stone fall and has thus become something of a classic. The lead team of Robert Paragot, Robert Jacob, Claude Jaccoux and Dominique Leprince-Ringuet reached the summit on 10 July 1966, followed one day later by Lucien Bérardini, Georges Payot and Yannick Seigneur.

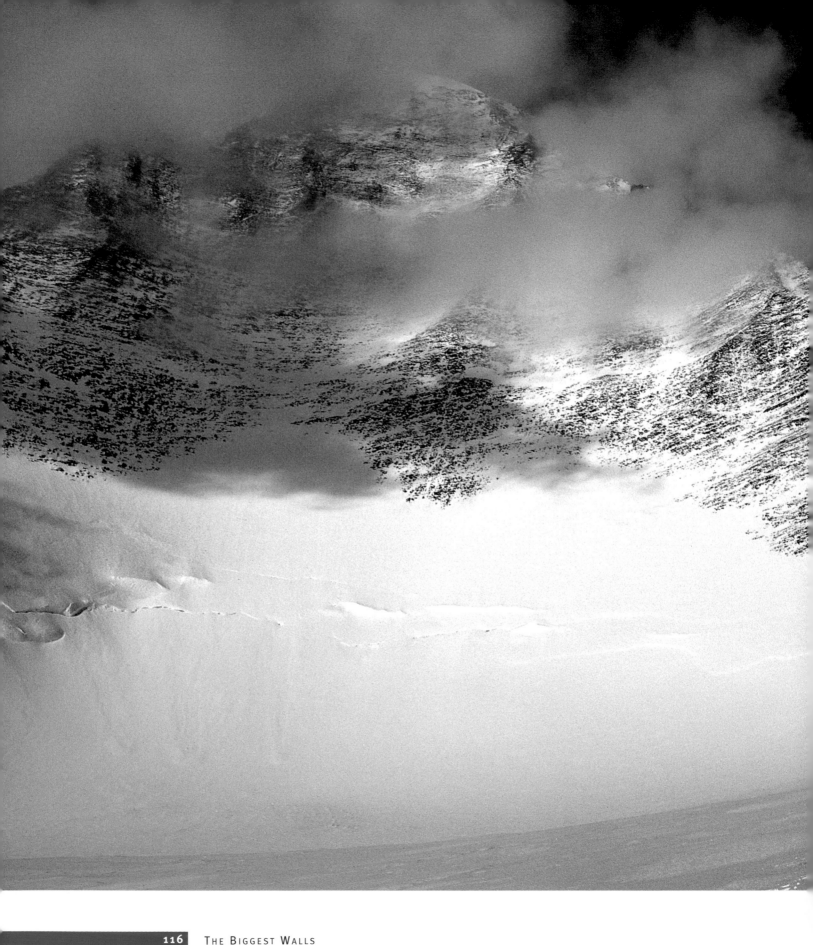

THE BIGGEST WALLS

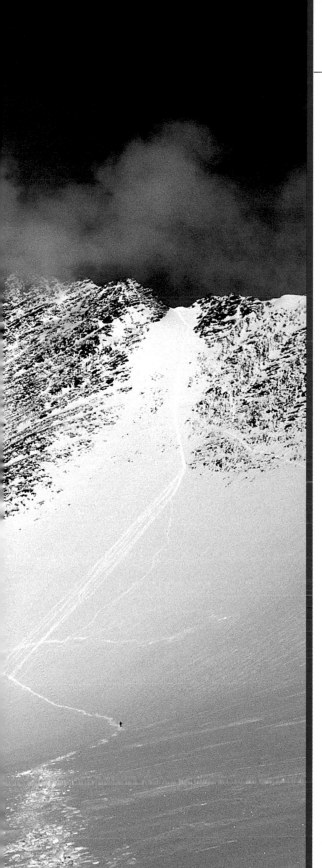

MOUNT TYREE

1967 – ANTARCTICA

SUMMIT HEIGHT

4827m

HEIGHT OF FACE

c. 2500m (between 2300 and 4827m)

DIFFICULTIES

Ice couloirs and slopes; demanding climbing (IV/V) on the North-West Ridge with some loose rock and mixed ground

TIME

After preparation (establishment of high camps), 3–4 days' climbing

STARTING POINT

Base camp (*c.* 2300m) below Mount Gardner, reached from the Nimitz Glacier (accessible only by plane from Chile via Patriot Hills).

OVERVIEW

The route takes a 1200m couloir to the plateau of Mount Gardner, then descends to the col between this peak and Mount Tyree (Gardner-Tyree Col). From the col, the first section of the 3.5km plus North-West Ridge of Mount Tyree is avoided on its north side before moving back onto the ridge and finally climbing the exposed upper section of the South Face to the summit.

TIPS

Mount Tyree is the second highest mountain in the Antarctic. The first climbers placed two high camps, one below the summit of Mount Gardner and a second at the col.

There are also some great routes on the 2000m West Face of Mount Vinson.

'Very remote, mixed climbing, bigger than the East Face of Monte Rosa.'

EKKERT GUNDELACH

Members of the American Antarctic Mountaineering Expedition John Evans and Barry Corbet reached the summit on 6 January 1967. The South Face was climbed by Erhard Loretan and a direct route added by Conrad Anker in the 1990s.

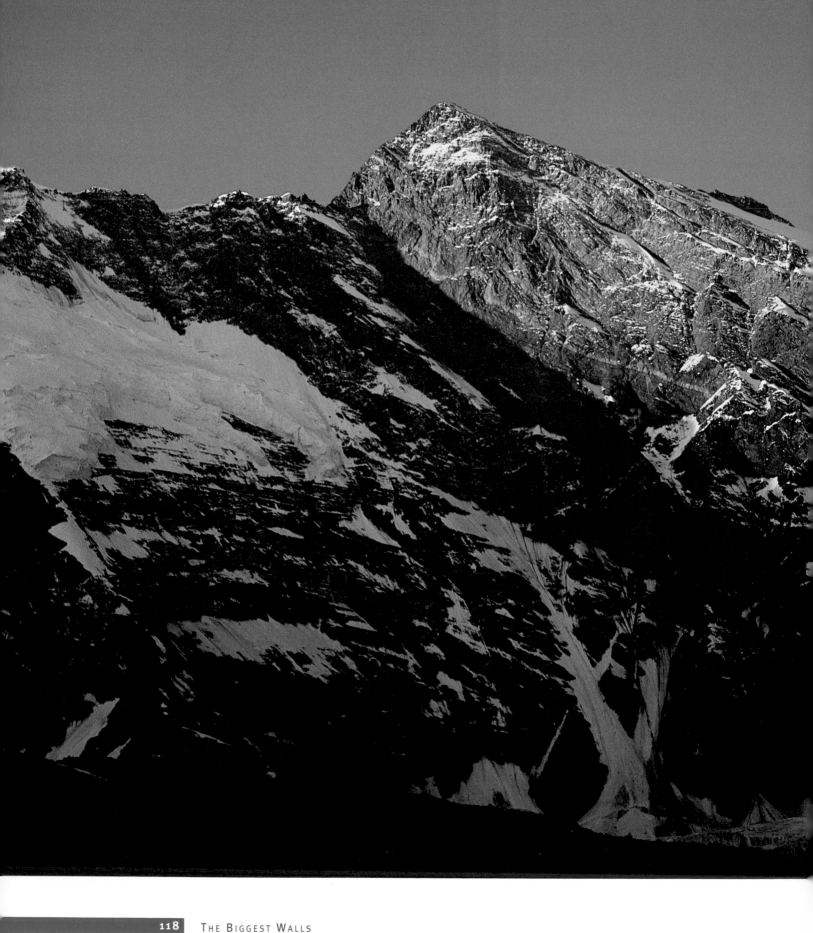

THE BIGGEST WALLS

PEAK COMMUNISM, SOUTH FACE, MYSLOVSKY ROUTE

1968 – PAMIRS

SUMMIT HEIGHT

7495m

HEIGHT OF FACE

c. 2900m (between 4600 and 7495m)

DIFFICULTIES

Extreme rock climbing, steep ice (Russian grade 6A)

TIME

After fixing some of the lower section of the face the first ascent team required 9 days to complete the climb

STARTING POINT

Base camp on the Belyaev Glacier; accessible by helicopter from Tashkent or Dushanbe to the Garmo Glacier, which is followed on foot to reach the Belyaev Glacier.

OVERVIEW

The route climbs the vertical belt of rock on the central right-hand (south-west) part of the face and then takes a rising leftwards line to the summit ridge.

TIPS

On the first ascent, fixed ropes were used on the difficult sections of the lower part of the face. Up to 6000m there is extreme danger from stonefall.

Further big faces in the High Pamirs: Pik Ahmadi Donish, South Face (2500m); Pik Engels, North-East Face (2200m); Pik Kommissarov, South Face (2200m), plus several other 2000m (e.g. Pik Korshenewskaja, West Face).

'As in other sporting disciplines, titles like "Master of Sports" were bestowed upon mountaineers in the USSR. The most coveted title was the "Snow Leopard", which was viewed as the ultimate accolade by high altitude mountaineers in the eastern block countries.'

SEBASTIAN HÖLZL

The first route on the extreme right-hand (south-west) side of the face was climbed in 1968 by E. Myslovsky, V. Gluhov, V. Ivanov and A. Ovchinnikov. Further, more difficult, lines on Peak Communism were found in 1973 and 1981, two of them on the central part of the face.

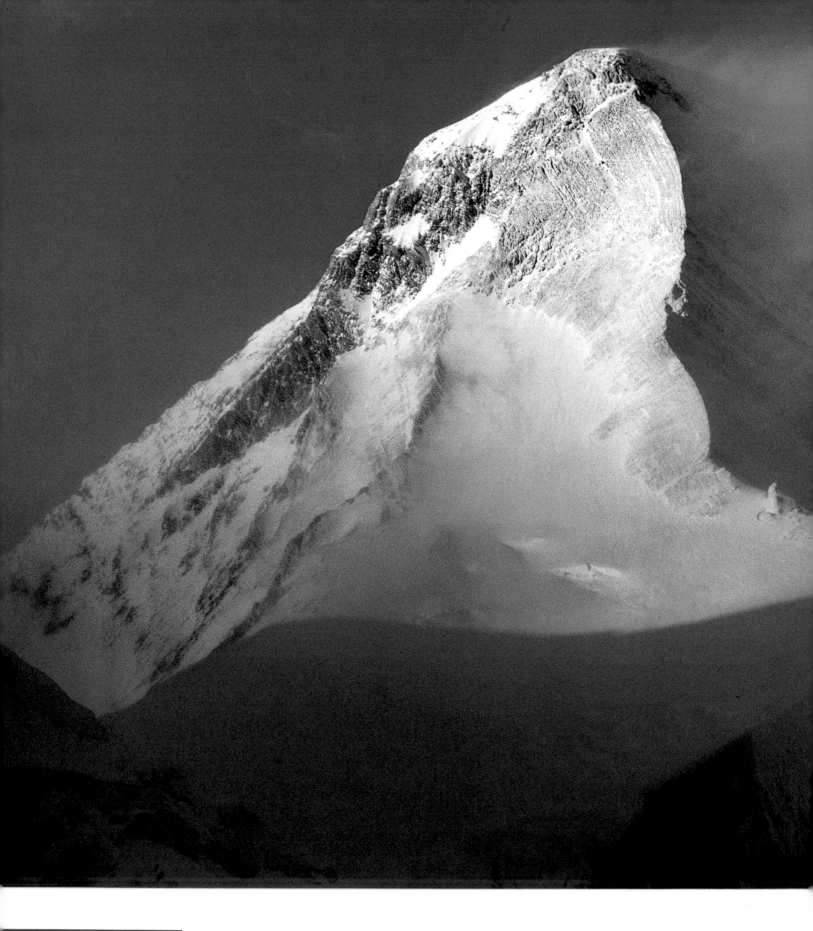

Khan Tengri, North Face

1970/1974 – Tien Shan

Summit Height

7010m

Height of Face

c. 2800m (between 4200 and 7010m)

Difficulties

6A (Russian grading) for the first route up the eastern part of the North Face; 6B for the Direct Route with its slabs and monolithic steep sections

Time

Several days for the eastern route; 6–9 days for the routes on the central section of the face

Starting Point

Base camp (*c.* 4200m) on the North Inylchek Glacier; by road from Almaty to Bayankol and then by helicopter.

Overview

The 1970 route climbs the long buttress on the left-hand side of the face to join the summit ridge; the two 1974 routes take almost parallel lines up the central part of the North Face.

Tips

In recent years a large base camp has been established at the foot of the Khan Tengri Face, complete with kitchen, first-aid post and logistical support. The normal route on Khan Tengri has been pre-prepared and fixed for group ascents. The North Face on the other hand – impressively steep and beautifully shaped – is only rarely attempted even though there are half a dozen routes on it.

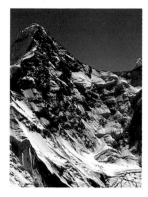

The 2800m-high North Face of Khan Tengri.

'From the bottom of the Bayumkol Valley we spied a huge, wide mass of mountain from whose snow-clad shoulder, a little way below the summit ridge, a vertical face almost 2000m in height dropped sheer to the valley below.'

Gottfried Merzbacher, 1902

The summit pyramid of Khan Tengri viewed from the west. The first route on the face was climbed by O. Hudyakov, R. Ivanov, L. Kabelsky, Y. Manshin and V. Yushkevich in 1970; the Myslovsky Route, and in particular the Studenin Route, first done in 1974, take very steep and direct lines.

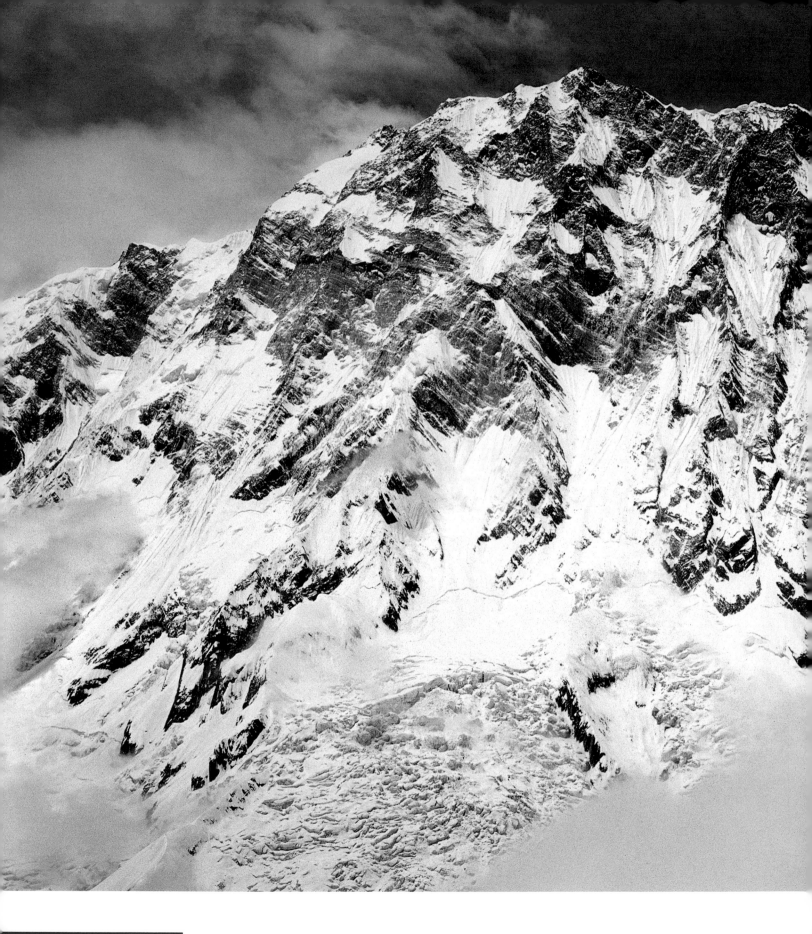

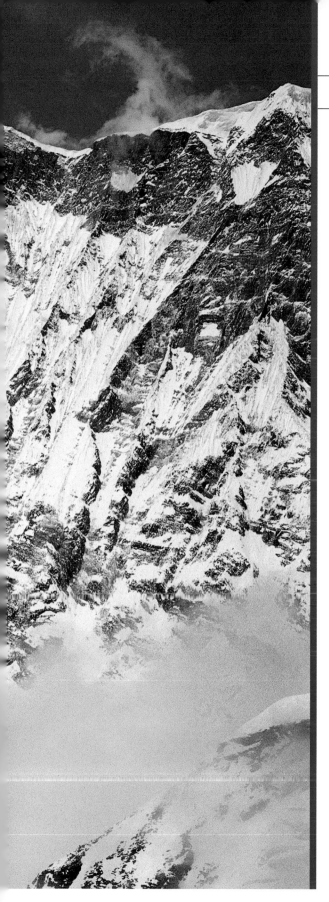

Annapurna I, South Face, Bonington Route

1970 – Nepal Himalaya

Summit Height

8091m

Height of Face

3200m (between 4900 and 8091m)

Difficulties

Sections of vertical rock (V and harder), very difficult ice ridge, steep ice traverses

Time

4–6 weeks' acclimatization and preparation (establishment of camps and fixed ropes on the face); 7–8 days' climbing

Starting Point

Base camp (4095m) on the lower northern slopes of Hiunchuli, reached by trekkers' path from Suikhet (road from Pokhara) via Dhampus, Landrung, Ghandrung and through the Modi Khola valley.

Overview

The left-hand (west) part of the South Face has three prominent buttresses. The route climbed by the first ascent team takes the left-hand buttress

Tips

The British expedition placed six camps on the face and used a total of 4500m of fixed rope. One of the members of the team perished in an avalanche at the end of the expedition.

Despite the extreme difficulties the Bonington Route sees frequent repeat ascents. The other routes on the South Face are more dangerous.

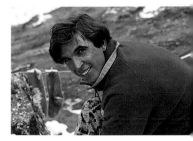

Enric Lucas, who accomplished his own route on the South Face of Annapurna.

'Looking down the South Face, I felt dizzy. The fact that the colossal leaning chunks of rock perched there had not collapsed seemed to defy Nature's laws. I saw with horror where Whillans and Haston had come up in 1970. A steep and seemingly bottomless precipice!'

Reinhold Messner

The Bonington Route takes the buttress in the middle part of the left-hand half of the photo. Don Whillans and Dougal Haston summitted on 27 May 1970, climbing from the top camp on the face. Ian Clough died in an avalanche below Camp III during the last phase of the expedition.

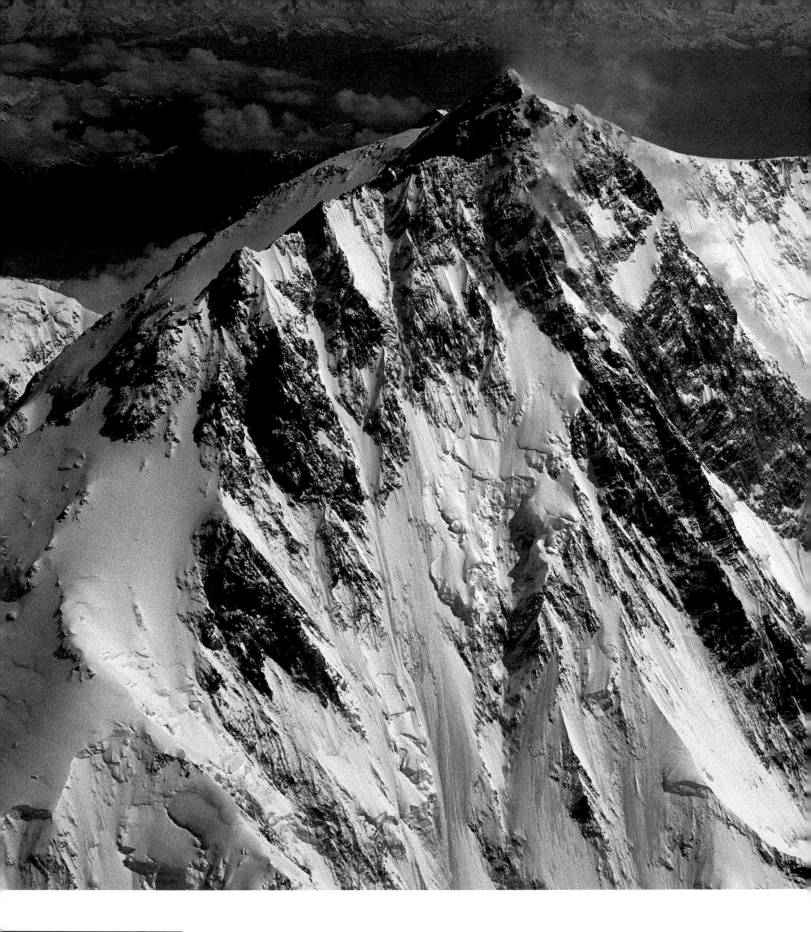

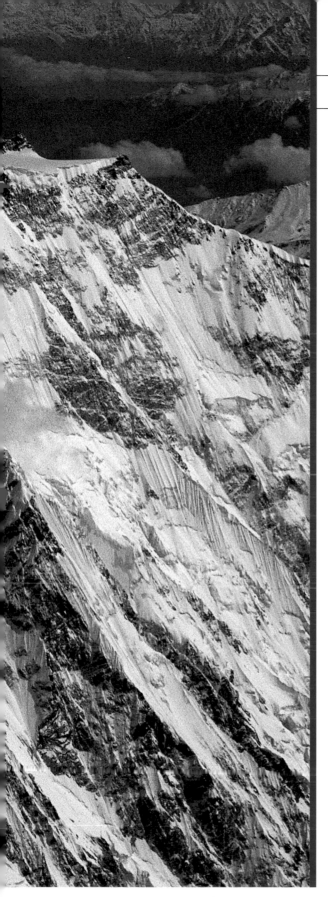

NANGA PARBAT, SOUTH FACE, CENTRAL BUTTRESS

1970 – KASHMIR HIMALAYA

SUMMIT HEIGHT

8125m

HEIGHT OF FACE

c. 4500m (between 3650 and 8125m)

DIFFICULTIES

II–IV, mostly iced up; ice to 90 degrees

TIME

4–6 weeks' acclimatization and preparation (establishment of camps and fixed ropes on the face); 5–8 days for the route

STARTING POINT

Tap Alpe (3560m); reached from Gilgit (Pakistan) via the Indus, Astor and Rupal valleys (Karakorum Highway, Jeep track, via ferrata).

OVERVIEW

The route mainly follows the middle buttress system, reached from the right above the first rock band. In the summit area it uses the gully to the right of the edge of the buttress.

TIPS

There are several good sites for camps. Retreat is dangerous when it is snowing, so it is advisable to cache sufficient provisions at the middle camps on the face. It is best to place the camp for the summit push just below the Merkl Couloir. The equipment carried should be suitable for medium grade rock climbing and extremely difficult ice. The ideal times for an ascent are the months of May and September.

'The descent becomes a tragedy. The older brother looks for the best possibilities. He finds a way through the two big serac zones. The brothers climb down blank ice, until they reach the upper rocks of the Mummery Rib. This they then descend.'

HORST HÖFLER

The fourth expedition to the Rupal Face (centre picture) of Nanga Parbat brought the long-awaited success. On 27 June 1970 South Tyroleans Reinhold and Günther Messner reached the summit, followed on 28 June 1970 by the North Tyrol man Felix Kuen and the German Peter Scholz, climbing from the highest camp on the Rupal Face. The four climbers' ascent was the first of this face, the biggest big wall in the world.

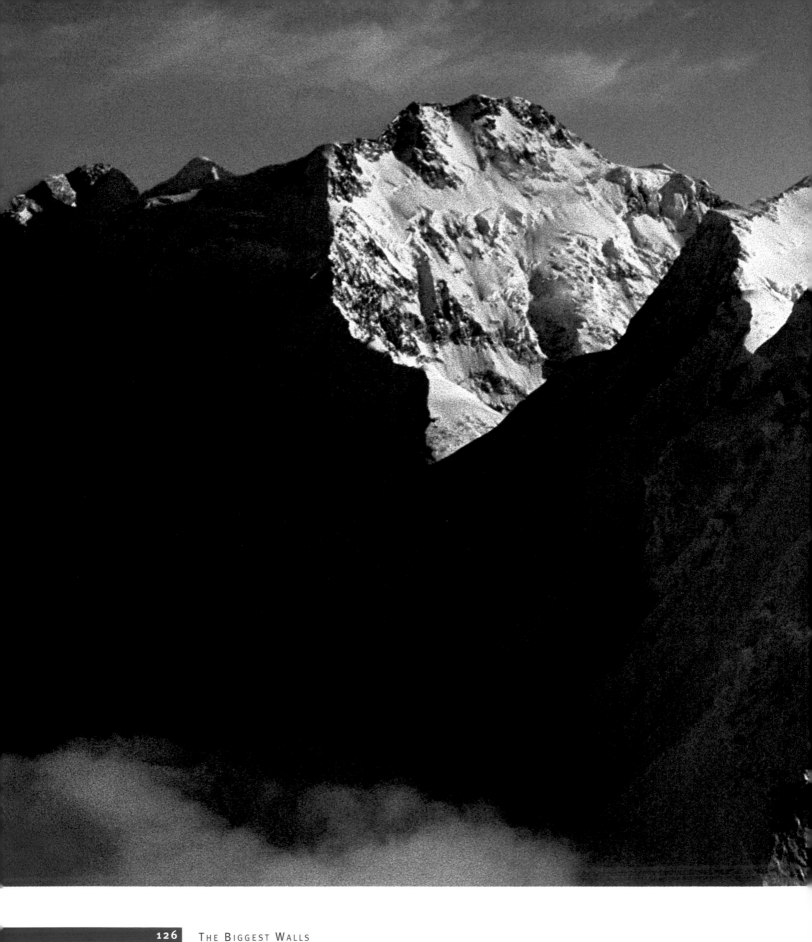

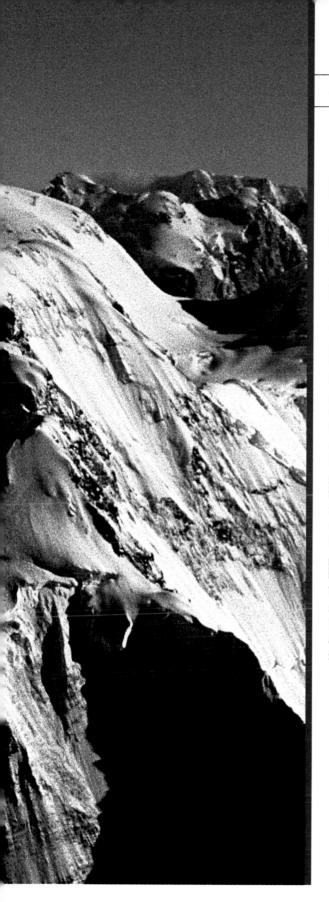

PIK PRZHEVALSKY, NORTH-EAST FACE

1974 – TIEN SHAN

SUMMIT HEIGHT

6350m

HEIGHT OF FACE

c. 2000m (between 4350 and 6350m)

DIFFICULTIES

Extremely diffcult (5B) route; mixed climbing, some of it on slate slabs that will not readily accept pitons

TIME

2–3 weeks' acclimatization; 5–6 days' climbing

STARTING POINT

Upper North Inylchek Glacier; Base Camp at 4200m; by road from Almaty to Bayankol and then by helicopter.

OVERVIEW

Climb an ice cliff to reach the foot of the face; mixed climbing (slate/ice/snow) leads to the big, triangular headwall, which is climbed to the summit.

TIPS

When the first ascent was made, the route was still relatively safe from objective dangers; the bivouacs are almost all poor, however. The first ascent team took nine days, three of which they spent on the headwall.

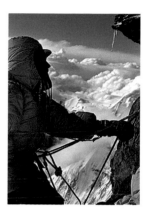

Belay on the North-East Face of Pik Przhevalsky.

'Viewed from the north, Pik Przhevalsky, crowned by a cap of snow, looks massive. The mountain is famous everywhere. It even appeared on maps published before the Russian Revolution. Soviet cartographers gave it the name of the celebrated traveller N.M. Przhevalsky.'

VICTOR SEDELNIKOV

The successful Soviet expedition team, which also included Victor Sedelnikov, reached the summit on 26 August 1974.

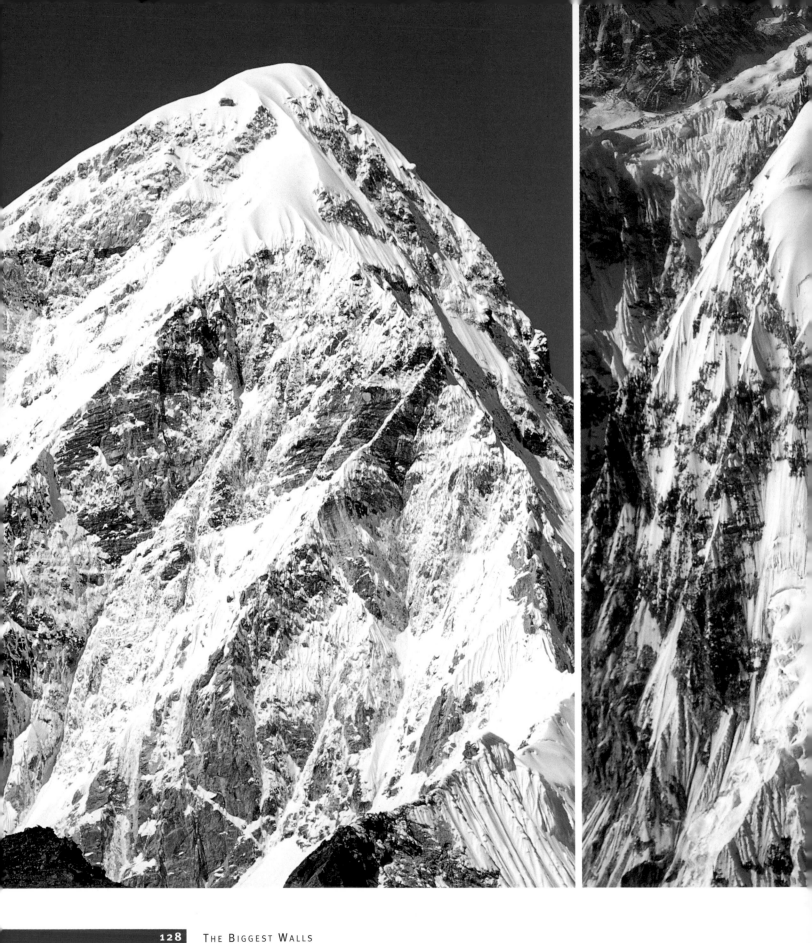

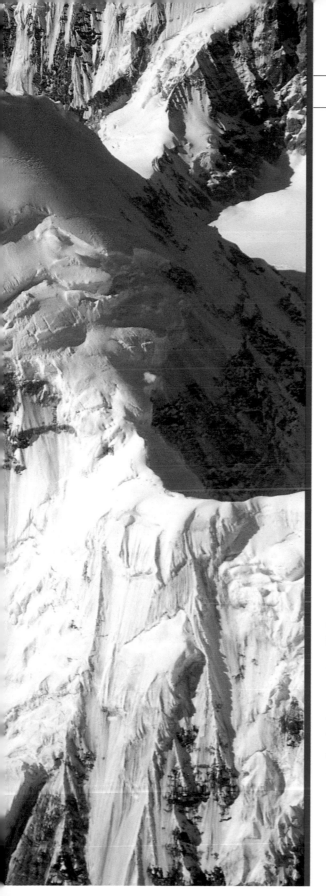

PUMORI, SOUTH-WEST BUTTRESS

1974 – NEPAL HIMALAYA

SUMMIT HEIGHT

7145m

HEIGHT OF FACE

A good 1550m (between 5600 and 7145m)

DIFFICULTIES

The French climbers who made the second ascent compared the rock climbing to that of the Innominata Ridge on Mont Blanc (D), and the ice to that of the North Face of the Courtes

TIME

Approx. 3 weeks' acclimatization; 3–4 days' climbing

STARTING POINT

Base camp (c. 5350m) beneath the South Face; from Lukla (airfield) via Namche Bazar, Pangpoche, Pheriche, Dugla, Lobuche and the Khumbu Glacier (identical approach to Everest base camp).

OVERVIEW

The South Face of Pumori has three huge and prominent buttresses. The route takes the right-hand of these buttresses, avoiding the lower section by climbing a couloir to the right.

TIPS

No details are known of the Japanese first ascent. The second ascent team encountered bad weather and spent weeks working to establish three camps on the face before making the final ascent in just three days. The third party of the second ascent team was last seen about 150m below the summit. All efforts to find any trace of the two climbers have so far remained unsuccessful.

'That first encounter with Pumori is probably more or less the same for every aspirant ... One sees the mountain, the "virgin jewel of the Khumbu", as Marcel Kurz called it, for the first time when Everest, wrapped in its perpetual toga of clouds, the savage peak of Lhotse and the Nuptse Wall have long since become a part of the daily secenery. ... We were alarmed; our Sherpas were too. Pumori had never played a part in the plans of the previous expeditions that they had come here with ... "You'll never get up it!", they said.'

GERHARD LENSER,
*ERSTERSTEIGER DES
PUMORI 1962*

Two views of the South Face of Pumori. There are now many routes on this face, all of them are big challenges but all can be climbed Alpine style.

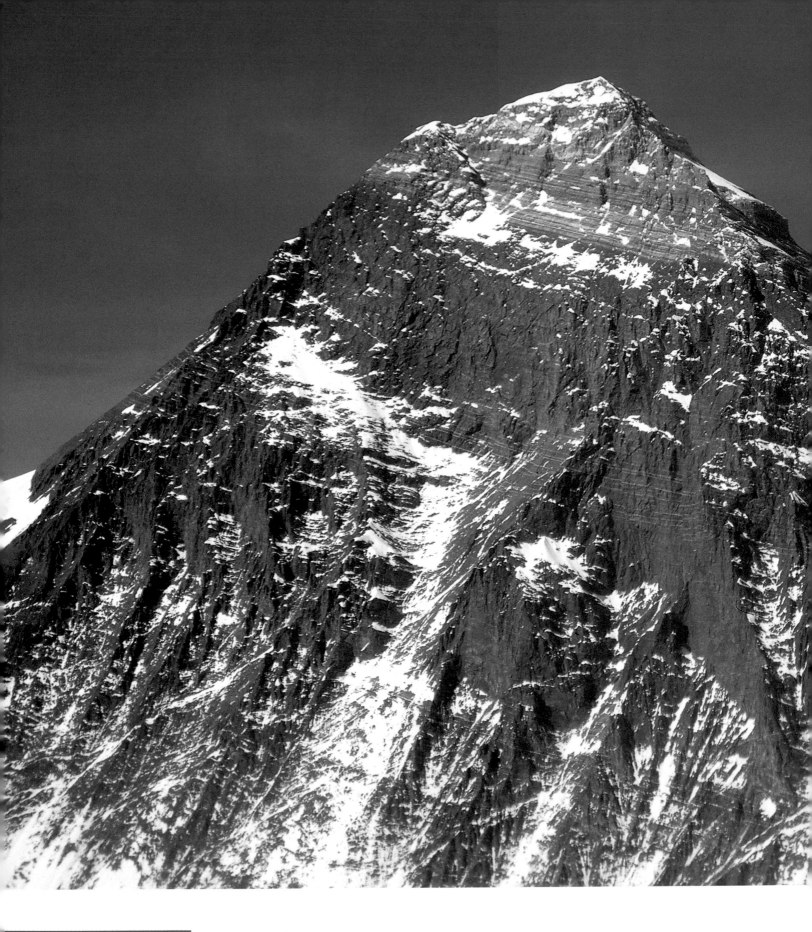

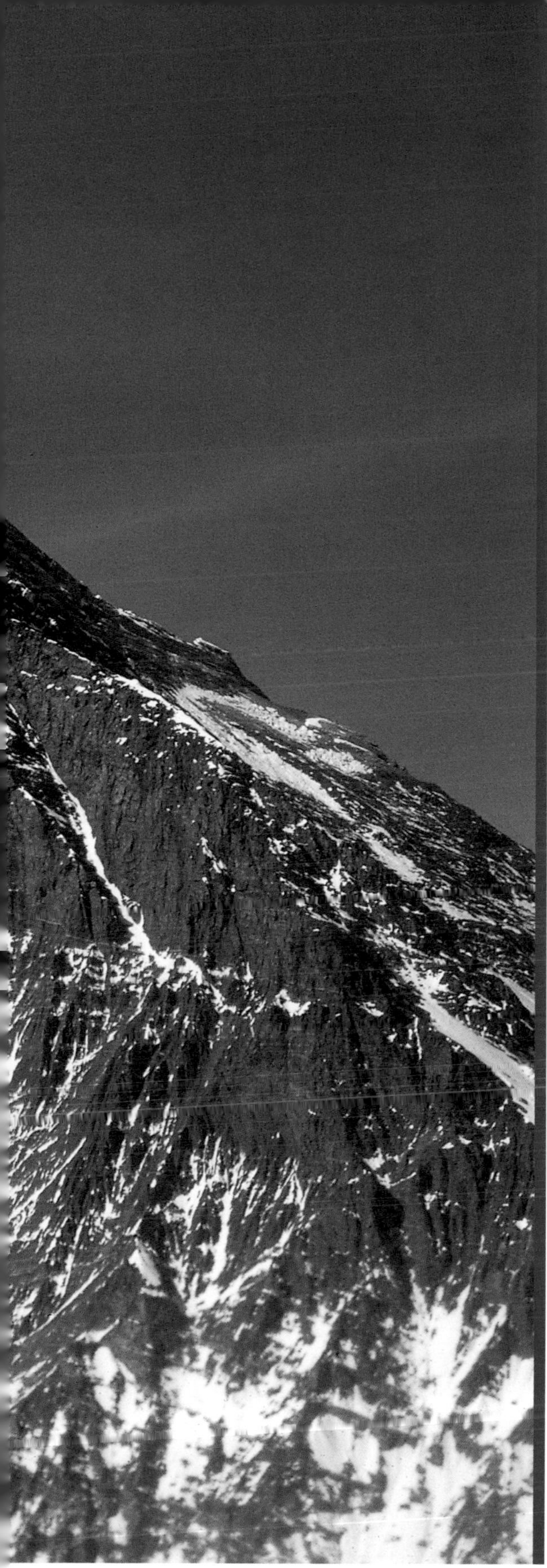

MOUNT EVEREST, SOUTH-WEST FACE, BRITISH ROUTE

1975 – NEPAL HIMALAYA

SUMMIT HEIGHT

8848m

HEIGHT OF FACE

A little over 2000m (between 6700 and 8751m)

DIFFICULTIES

Steep ice fields, couloirs and ramps and demanding mixed climbing; 20m rock step in the gully below the South Summit, usually iced up

TIME

4–6 weeks' acclimatization and preparation (establishment of camps and fixed ropes on the face); 6–7 days' climbing

STARTING POINT

Western Cwm, advanced base camp (Camp II) at about 6600m; reached from Everest Base Camp (5200m, approached from Lukla via Namche Bazar, Pangpoche, Pheriche, Dugla, Lobuche and the Khumbu Glacier) through the dangerous Khumbu Icefall.

OVERVIEW

The route goes up slightly to the right of the middle of the face, trends back into the centre ('Great Central Gully'), climbing ice fields to half height before going up and left towards the lowest part of the rock band, which is climbed on the left by a hidden ice couloir. Above the rock band it takes a rising rightwards line up a long snowfield and climbs a rightwards slanting gully to the South Summit. Over the Hillary Step to the summit of Everest.

'It would seem that, under such conditions, when you push yourself to the absolute limit and at the same time reduce your intake of oxygen, water and food, you are able somehow to activate hidden reserves in order to stay alive; not only reserves of energy, but reserves at a deeper level.'

DOUG SCOTT

Doug Scott and Dougal Haston reached the summit of Everest on 24 September 1975; two days later Peter Boardman and Sherpa Pertemba also completed their ascent. Mick Burke, who they met during their descent just below the highest point on Earth, did not return.

The 'Soviet Route' on the South Buttress (far left of picture) is a harder proposition than the Bonington (British) Route and joins the West Ridge just to the left of the summit.

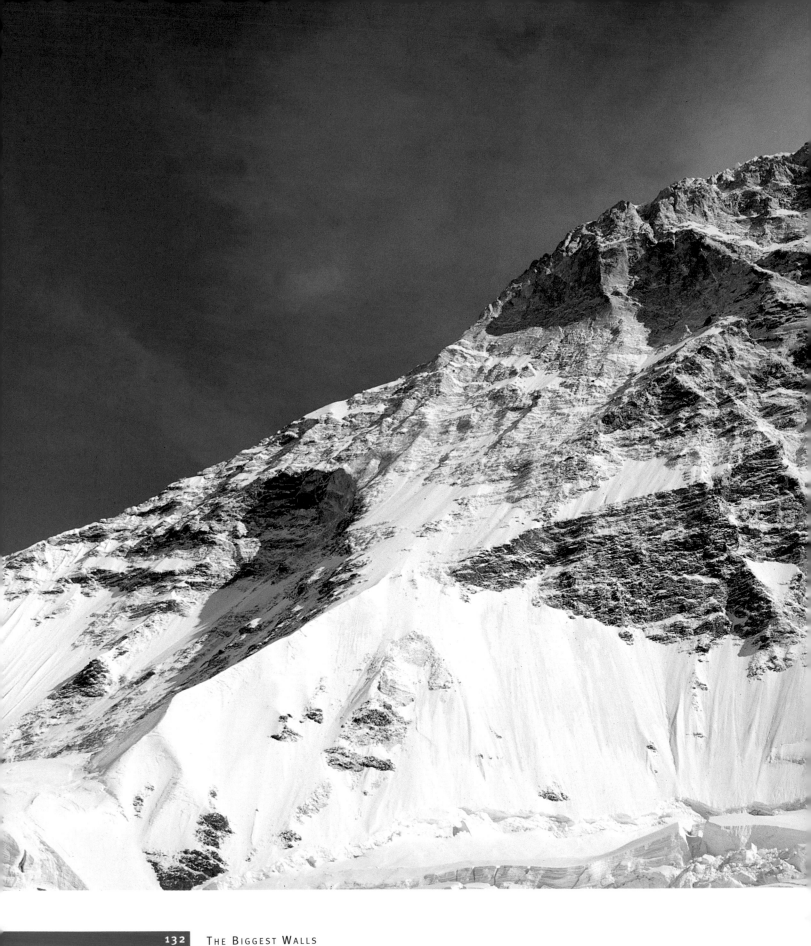

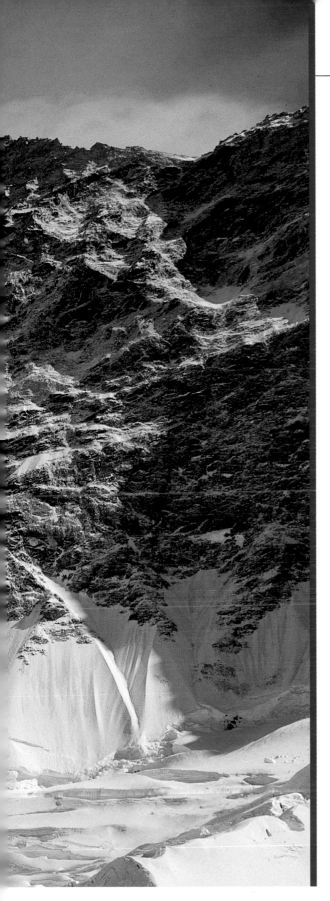

MAKALU, SOUTH FACE

1975 – NEPAL HIMALAYA

SUMMIT HEIGHT

8463m

HEIGHT OF FACE

Over 3100m (between 5100 and 8250m)

DIFFICULTIES

Rock to V, ice to 70 degrees

TIME

4–6 weeks' acclimatization and preparation (establishment of camps and fixed ropes on the face); 7–8 days' climbing

STARTING POINT

Makalu base camp (4850m); approach from Tumlingtar (airfield) via Khadbari, the Barun La and Shershon.

OVERVIEW

Climbs the rock pillar at the foot of the face. Then diagonally left across the glacier on the steep part of the South Face and up a very steep ice wall to gain mixed ground to the left of the summit fall line. Traverse right to reach the summit headwall.

TIPS

The face is prone to ice fall in parts and was first climbed in classic expedition style with five high camps (three of them on the steep part of the face). Preparations (establishing the camps, fixing the route to 7500m) took 18 days, with the final ascent from base camp to summit requiring a futher 8 days. One member of the summit team climbed without a mask from about 8050m. Pierre Bèghin's direct route to the right and the South-West Buttress to the right of the Kunaver Route are among the most beautiful climbs in the Himalayas.

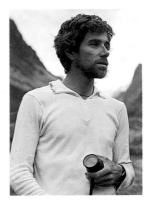

Pierre Béghin, who soloed the Direct Route on the South Face of Makalu.

'The 1975 Makalu Expedition finally brought success for the Slovenians, who were rapidly establishing their position in world mountaineering. Seven climbers reached the summit and descended again unharmed.'

VIKTOR GROŠELJ

Seven members of Aleš Kunaver's Makalu South Face Expedition 1975 reached the summit: Stane Belak and Manfreda Marjan on 6 October, Janko Ažman and Jernej Zaplotnik on 8 October, Viki Grošelj and Ivan Kotnik on 10 October and Janez Dovžan on 11 October.

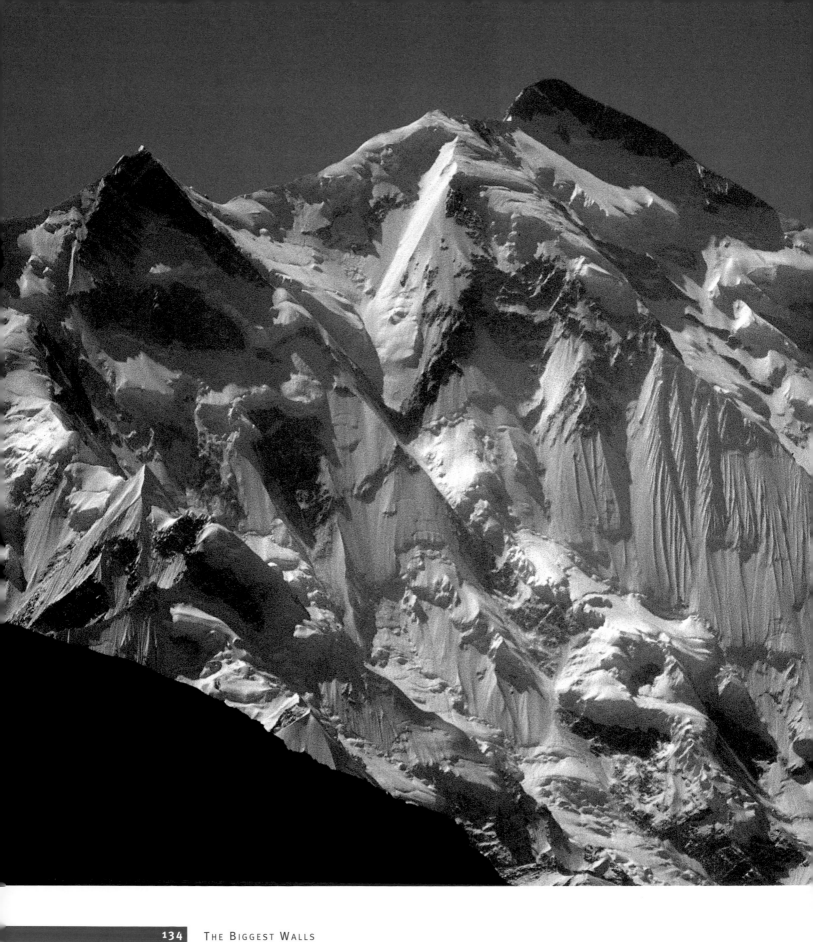

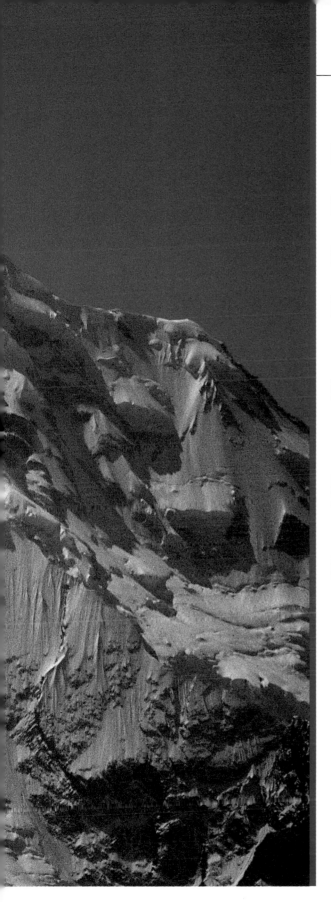

RAKAPOSHI, NORTH RIDGE

1978 – KARAKORUM

SUMMIT HEIGHT

7788m

HEIGHT OF FACE

c. 3400m (from 4400 to 7788m)

DIFFICULTIES

Rock to V+/A2, ice to 70 degrees

TIME

5–6 weeks' acclimatization and preparation (establishment of camps and fixed ropes on the face); 6–7 days' climbing

STARTING POINT

Base camp (c. 3650m) on the Ghulmet Glacier; approach from the Hunza Valley (Karakorum-Highway) via Ghulmet and through the valley of the same name.

OVERVIEW

The mighty northern aspect of Rakaposhi is dominated by the buttress-like North Ridge. The west side of the ridge is reached by a steep ice couloir.

TIPS

On the first ascent, six camps were placed on the ridge and much of the route was secured with fixed ropes. It is very exposed in parts, heavily corniced and prone to avalanches. The whole flank of the mountain offers splendid, but dangerous, big face routes.

'Just one hour later we look up again at the gleaming silver heights and recognize on the North Buttress the objective of our efforts, as it soars steeply upwards. We are enthralled by our plan to attempt this Himalayan giant by such a direttissima – but are also mightily impressed by the technical difficulties that lie before us.'

KARL M.
HERRLIGKOFFER

The North Ridge of Rakaposhi (North Buttress centre picture) was attempted by, among others, a Herrligkoffer expedition before a Japanese team finally met with success. On 2 August 1978, expedition leader Eiho Ohtani and Matsushi Yamashita reached the summit.

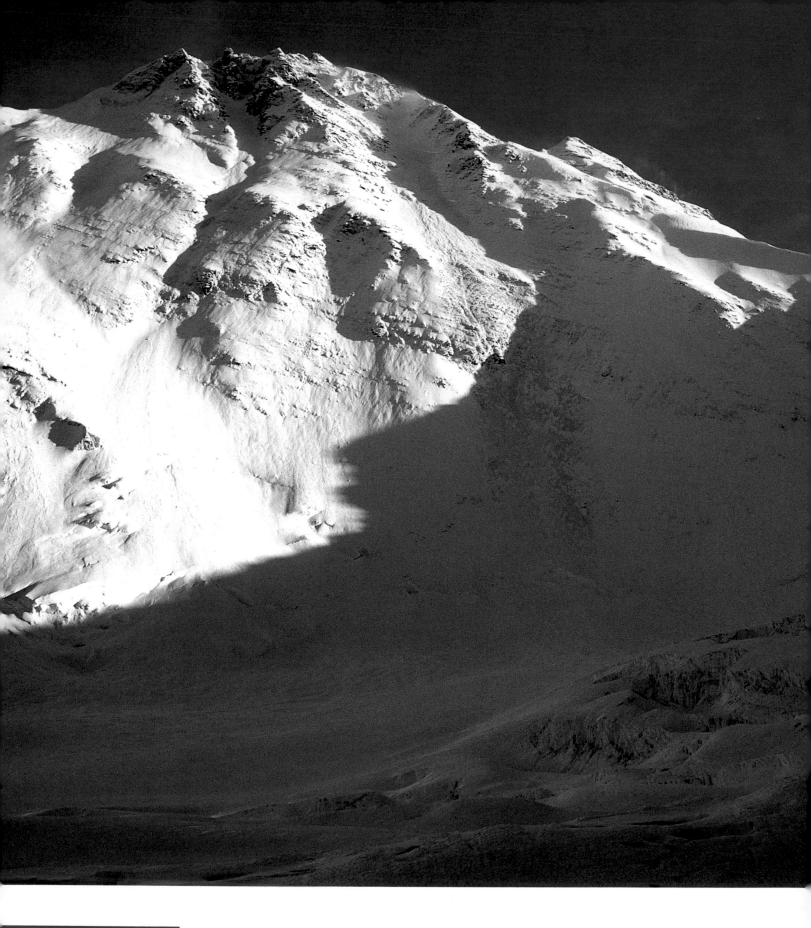

MOUNT EVEREST, NORTH-EAST FACE/ NORTH FACE

1980 – TIBET HIMALAYA

SUMMIT HEIGHT

8848m

HEIGHT OF FACE

c. 2700m (between 6150 and 8848m)

DIFFICULTIES (NORTH FACE)

Steep ice and strenuous snowfields, difficult mixed climbing, loose rock

TIME (NORTH FACE)

5–6 weeks' acclimatization and preparation (establishment of camps and fixed ropes on the face); 5–6 days' climbing

STARTING POINT (NORTH FACE)

Camp on the West Rongbuk Glacier, approach from Tingri (coming from Nepal) or from Shigatse (Tibet) via the Rongbuk Monastery; the road from the monastery is drivable by Jeep and leads for a further 5km up the valley to near the snout of the Rongbuk Glacier (c. 5150m, base camp area).

OVERVIEW (NORTH FACE)

The North Face, with its steep ice slope and rock band above, towers above the upper basin of the West Rongbuk Glacier. The rock band is split by a deep gully in its central part; this provides the line of the route. Above this, steep snow slopes and two further, smaller, rock bands lead to the Hornbein Couloir, which gives access to the summit pyramid.

TIPS (NORTH FACE)

There is serious danger of avalanches and stonefall on the route. Between this, the Japanese Route, and the Grand Couloir (Australian Route) further routes are possible on the face, all of them extremely difficult.

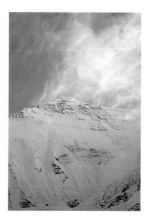

The North Face of Mount Everest.

'I took my heart in both hands and climbed on through this revolting filth, until I was almost at the top.'

ANDY HENDERSON, ONE OF THE FIRST ASCENT TEAMS OF THE AUSTRALIAN ROUTE

Success was achieved for a Japanese expedition on a direct line up the North Face in 1980. Four years later an Australian team climbed a route to the left of the Japanese Route, which takes the Norton Couloir on its upper section. Andy Henderson, Tim Macartney-Snape and Greg Mortimer summitted. Meanwhile, the North-East Face (big photo) has also been climbed.

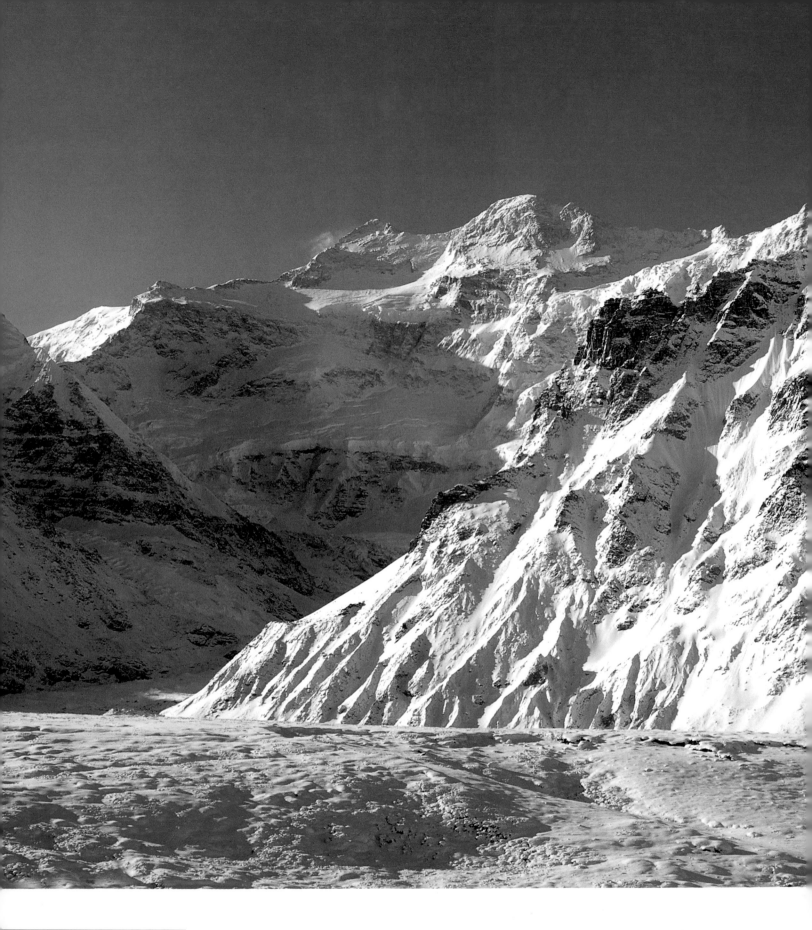

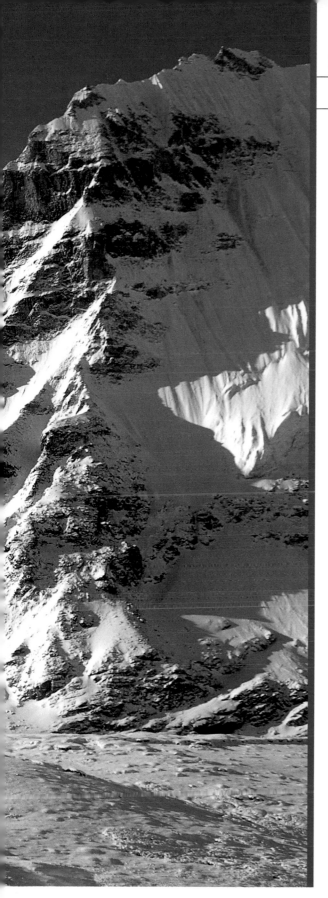

KANGCHENJUNGA, NORTH FACE, JAPANESE ROUTE

1980 – NEPAL HIMALAYA

SUMMIT HEIGHT

8598m

HEIGHT OF FACE

c. 3100m (between 5500 and 8598m)

DIFFICULTIES

In parts vertical serac barriers; the rock band between 7300 and 7900m gives difficult climbing

TIME

4–6 weeks' acclimatization and preparation (establishment of camps and fixed ropes on the face); 5–6 days' climbing

STARTING POINT

Base camp at Pangpema (c. 5500m) on the lateral moraines on the orographic right hand side of the Kangchenjunga Glacier, approached from Taplejung (airfield) via Taplechok, Kambachen and Lhonak.

OVERVIEW

The route avoids the fall line from the summit by a leftwards curving line, climbing serac and rock barriers and tackling the big rock band on the left-hand part of the face at its lowest point. Above this is the steep summit headwall with its two ice fields. All the other routes on the North Face can be considered as variations on the North Ridge or the Japanese Route.

TIPS

The first ascent team placed four camps on the face and used 2700m of fixed ropes.

'The North-West Face of Kang-chenjunga might have been designed specifically to repel mountaineers. It is structured in a horseshoe of three tiers of gigantic shelves, separated by cliffs of ice ...'

PETER BOARDMAN

During the course of the 1980 Japanese North Face Expedition, which was led by Masatsugu Konishi and proceded without the use of bottled oxygen, four members of the team reached the summit on 14 May 1980, amongst them Sherpa Ang Phurba. On 17 May a further four climbers summitted, amongst them the Sherpas Pemba Tsering and Dawa Norbu, who had broken trail through knee-deep snow.

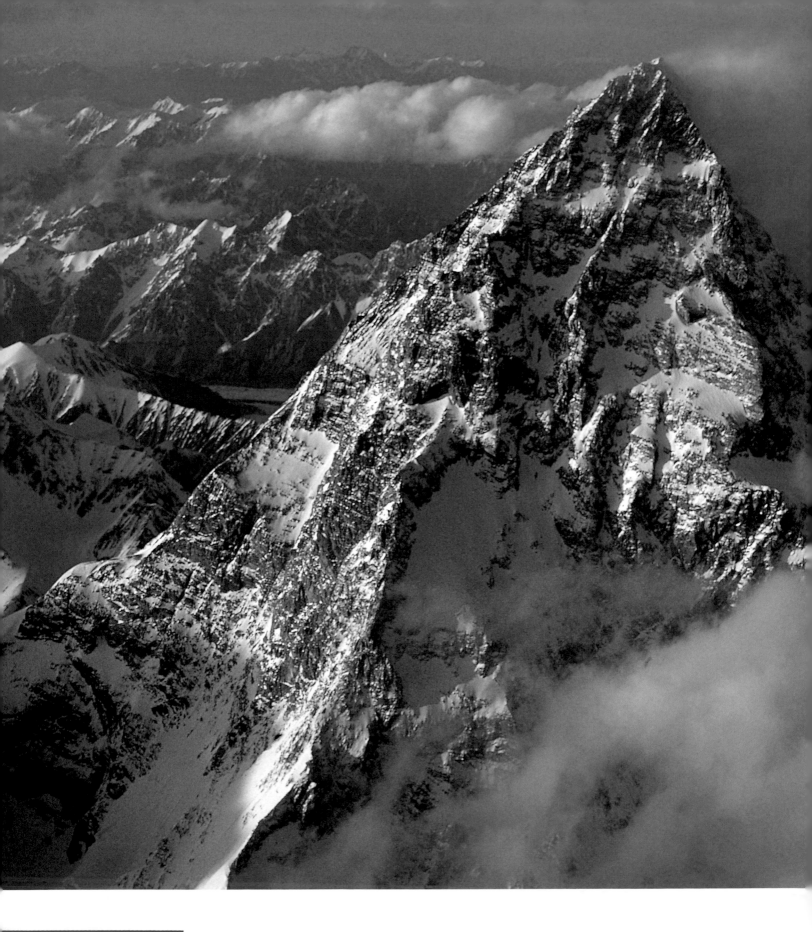

K2, WEST FACE

1981 – KARAKORUM

SUMMIT HEIGHT

8611m

HEIGHT OF FACE

c. 2700m (from 5500 to 8200m)

DIFFICULTIES

Difficult sections of rock climbing and steep ice fields; hard mixed climbing on the summit headwall

TIME

4–6 weeks' acclimatization and preparation (establishment of camps and fixed ropes on the face); 6–7 days' climbing

STARTING POINT

Base camp (c. 5350m) on the Savoia Glacier, approached from Askole (rough, Jeep track as far as Askole) via Paiju, Liligo, Urdokas, Baltoro Glacier, Concordia.

OVERVIEW

The route climbs a broad ice gully to the West Ridge before moving right until below the huge summit headwall. The left-hand side of the headwall is split by a Y-shaped couloir. Climb the trunk of the Y and the right-hand branch to reach the terraced wall above and trend rightwards up this to join the South-West Ridge.

TIPS

On the first ascent, five camps and 5500m of fixed rope were used on the face. The summit team bivouacked twice above Camp V (c. 8050m): at about 8500m on the ascent and again at about 8200m on the descent.

'They were exhausted [the successful K2 West Face summit team] but on 10 August they returned to Base Camp. Their return coincided with a break in the good weather that had made the climb possible and it then snowed continuously for seven days.'

TERUDO MATSUURA

Two participants of the K2 West Face Expedition, under the leadership of Terudo Matsuura – Eiho Ohtani (who had already been successful on the North Ridge of Rakaposhi) and Pakistani Nazir Ahmad Sabir – reached the summit on 7 August 1981.

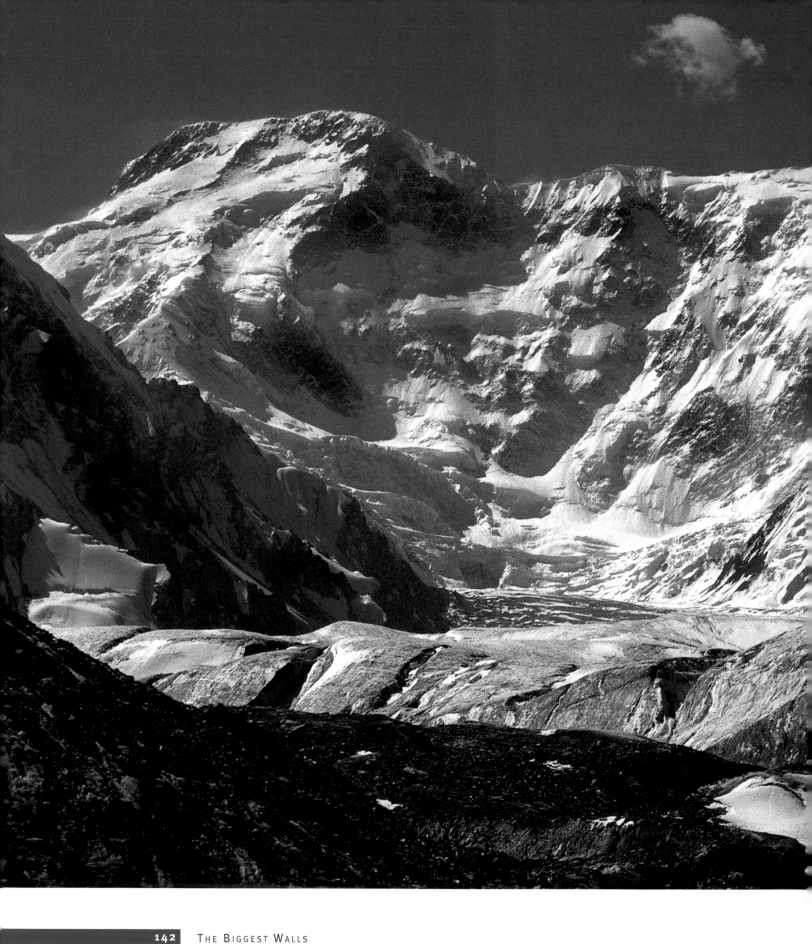

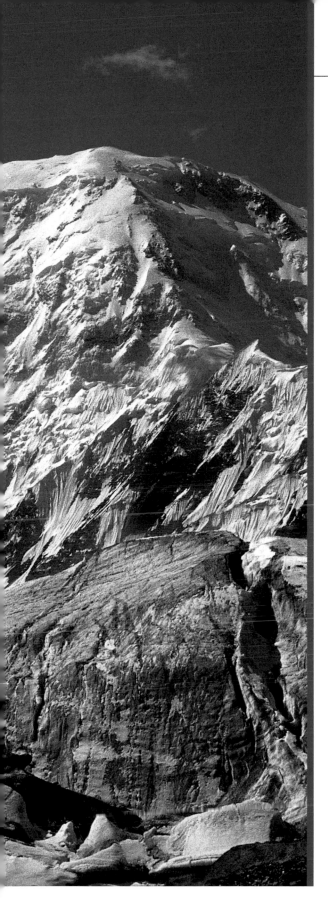

PIK POBJEDA, NORTH FACE

1982 – TIEN SHAN

SUMMIT HEIGHT

7439m

HEIGHT OF FACE

c. 3300m (from 4150 to 7439m)

DIFFICULTIES

6A (Russian grade), serac cliffs, steep ice slopes

TIME

4–5 weeks' acclimatization; 3–8 days' climbing

STARTING POINT

Zvezdochka Glacier; approach from base camp at approx. 4000m on the South Inylchek Glacier, which can be reached by helicopter from Bayankol (road from Almaty).

OVERVIEW

The route avoids the seracs and takes a line between huge steep walls on the right and a spur on the left to the summit.

TIPS

There is a high risk of avalanche on the lower section of the route. The first ascent team was caught in an avalanche on the traverse to the 'Dollar'. They survived as they were able to hang on to the fixed ropes.

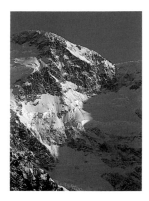

The North Face of Pik Pobjeda.

'After many attempts had ended in tragedy, in 1956 Abalakow became the first climber to reach the summit. Due to the changeable weather, the sudden drops in temperature, the storms and the length of the route, this mountain is an exceptionally difficult one to climb.'

ALFRED ZÄNGERLE

'Soviet mountaineers were successful on this big face in 1982.'

REINHOLD MESSNER

In 1982 V. Smirnov, Y. Moiseev, V. Suviga, V. Halitov and V. Shkarban became the first climbers to do the 3km-high face of Pik Pobjeda (left of picture).

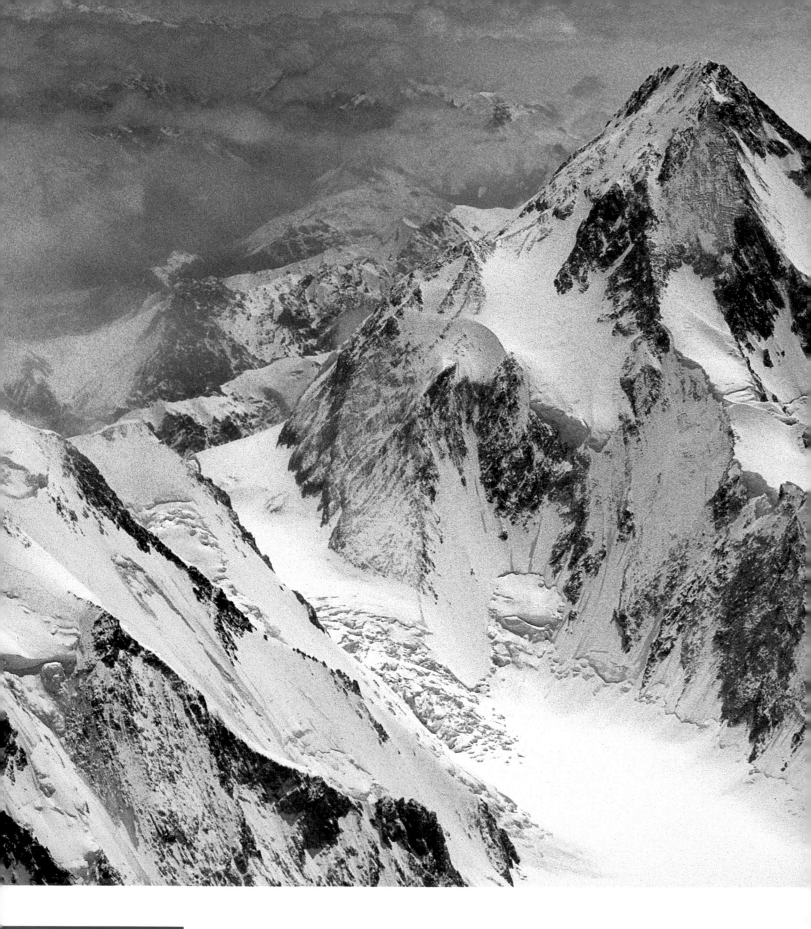

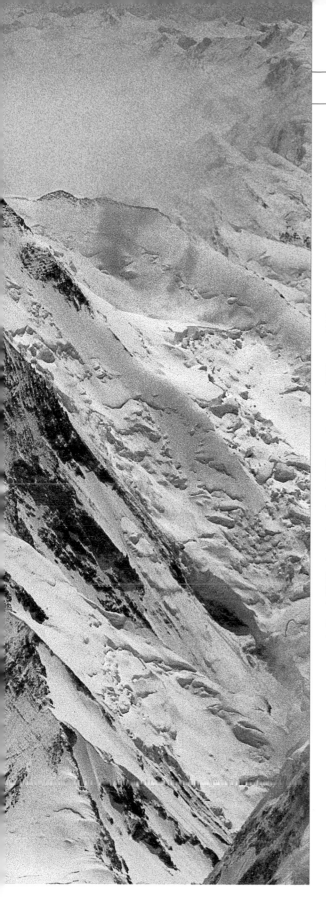

GASHERBRUM I, SOUTH-WEST FACE

1983 – KARAKORUM

SUMMIT HEIGHT

8068m

HEIGHT OF FACE

c. 2500m (from 5550 to 8068m)

DIFFICULTIES

Rock to grade V, difficult mixed climbing even on the summit headwall, steep ice slopes and seracs

TIME

4–5 weeks' acclimatization; 4 days' climbing

STARTING POINT

Base camp at approx. 5100m on the Abruzzi Glacier; approach from Askole (rough Jeep track as far as Askole) via Paiju, Liligo, Urdokas, Baltoro Glacier, Concordia and the Upper Baltoro Glacier.

OVERVIEW

The route takes a diagonal line from the bottom left to top right of the face, starting up ice slopes to gain a rock rib and following this into the central part of the face, finally climbing to the right of the summit fall line to join the South Ridge.

TIPS

There is a high risk of avalanche on the initial part of the climb. The first ascent team bivouacked three times on the face.

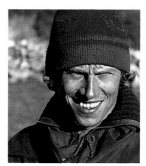

Nejc Zaplotnik, who climbed the ridge between the two faces.

'It became clear to me that "Alpine style" was the high art of mountaineering, not only from the sporting aspect, but also from a human perspective. Choose your companions carefully – casual acquaintances are of no use here.'

VOYTEK KURTYKA

The North-West Face of Gasherbrum (right of centre) and the South-West Face (right). On 22 July 1983, climbing Alpine style, Jerzy Kukuczka and Voytek Kurtyka had just a few pitches on the face left to climb when Kurtyka lost a crampon on the summit rocks of the South-West Face. They climbed back down to their last bivouac. The next morning Kukuczka found the crampon and the two men reached the summit of Hidden Peak via the South Ridge.

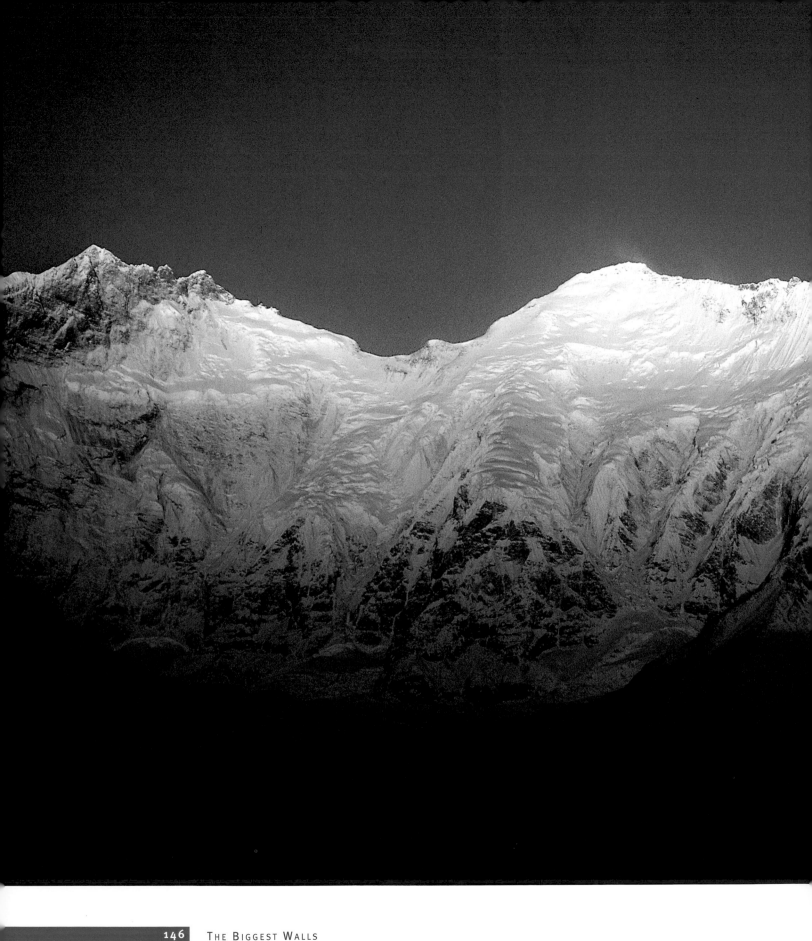

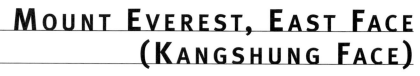

MOUNT EVEREST, EAST FACE (KANGSHUNG FACE)

1983 – TIBET HIMALAYA

SUMMIT HEIGHT

8848m

HEIGHT OF FACE

c. 3300m (between 5200 and 8475m)

DIFFICULTIES

Extremely difficult climbing (some aid), knife-edge snow ridge on the rock buttress (the 250m head-wall is overhanging), serac zone and strenuous snow slopes above

TIME

Up to 6 weeks' acclimatization and preparation (establishment of camps and fixed ropes on the face); 8–10 days' climbing

STARTING POINT

Base camp (c. 5180m) on the Kangshung Glacier (Tibet); approach from Kharta (roadhead) through the Kama Valley.

OVERVIEW

To the left (south) of the summit fall line, there is a 1200m cliff at the foot of the East Face; this is the most difficult section of the entire route. Above this, steep snow slopes interrupted by seracs lead up to the South-East Ridge.

The second route (climbed by Stephen Venables) goes left to the South Col.

TIPS

The first ascent was accomplished in classic expedition style with three camps, fixed ropes and a gear winch on the 1200m rock buttress (danger from stonefall here) and a further three camps on the snow slope (high risk of avalanche).

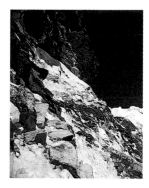

Ed Webster (centre of picture) on the Kangshung Face.

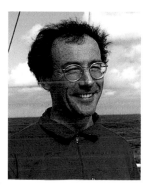

British climber Stephen Venables achieved fame with his climb to the summit of Mount Everest.

After weeks of laying seige to the huge and technically difficult Kangshung Face (the route takes the bulwark of rock to the left of centre), Carlos Buhler, Kim Momb and Louis Reichardt reached the summit of Mount Everest on 7 October 1983, followed on 9 October by Jay Cassel, George Lowe and Dan Reid. Stephen Venables found a new line further to the left.

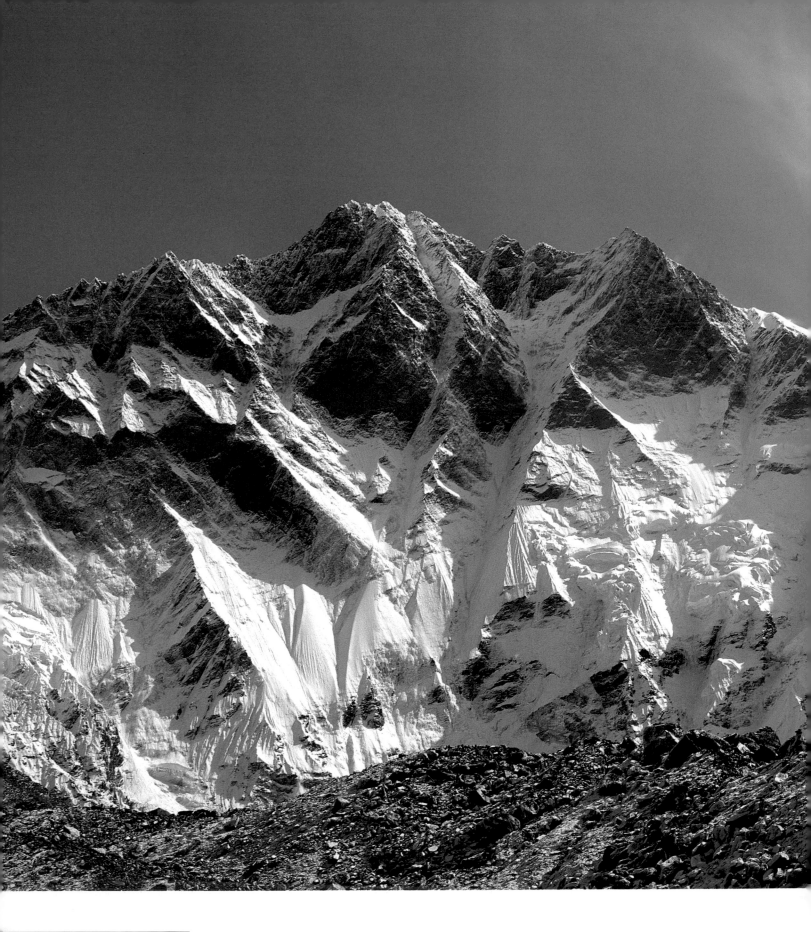

LHOTSE SHAR, SOUTH FACE

1984 – NEPAL HIMALAYA

SUMMIT HEIGHT

8400m

HEIGHT OF FACE

3000m (between 5400 and 8400m)

DIFFICULTIES

Rock climbing to V+, ice to 60 degrees and difficult mixed climbing

TIME

4–6 weeks' acclimatization and preparation (establishment of camps and fixed ropes on the face); 5–8 days' climbing

STARTING POINT

Base camp (at approx. 5250m) on the Lhotse Glacier, approach from Lukla (airfield) via Namche Bazar, Pangpoche, Dingpoche and Chukhung.

OVERVIEW

The route goes up the left-hand part of the face, taking a huge, icy buttress and a steep ice arête to beneath the triangular summit headwall. This is avoided on the left. Mixed ground on the south-west side leads to the summit.

TIPS

High risk of avalanche on the middle part of the face. On the first ascent the climbing was made more difficult by the daily falls of snow; six camps and 5000m of fixed ropes were used on the face.

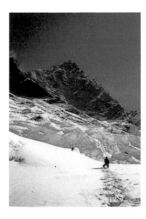

Beneath the huge summit pyramid.

'I had never climbed a whole mountain "à cheval" before. I was forced to stay in this position, there was no chance of standing up straight. The edge of the arête is too narrow, the snow too rotten.'

SEPP MAYERL,
ON THE FIRST ASCENT
OF LHOTSE SHAR

Ivan Gálvy led the successful Czech expedition to the South Face of Lhotse Shar (right of centre). On 21 May 1984 Peter Božik, Josef Rakoncaj and Jaromìr Stejskal reached the summit.

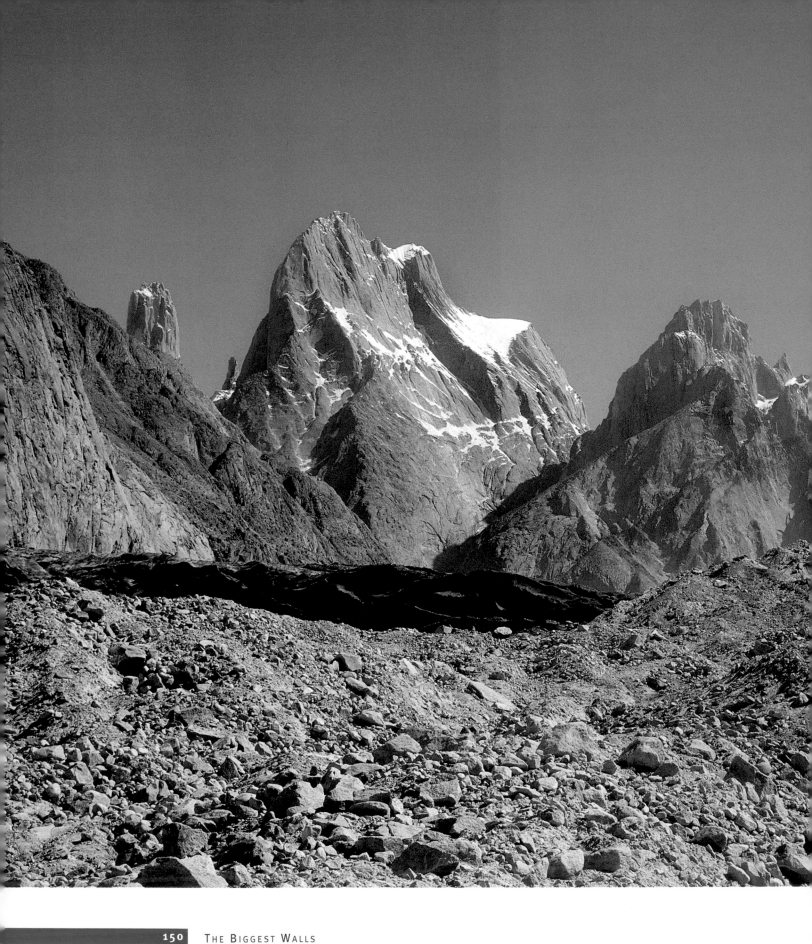

GREAT TRANGO TOWER, NORTH-EAST BUTTRESS, NORWEGIAN ROUTE

1984 – KARAKORUM

SUMMIT HEIGHT

6239m

HEIGHT OF FACE

c. 2000m (buttress height c. 1500m)

DIFFICULTIES

A4/VII, dangerous snow ridge and difficult mixed climbing in the summit area

TIME

3–4 weeks' acclimatization and preparation (transport of equipment); approx. 20 days' climbing (Big Wall system)

STARTING POINT

Base camp (c. 4200m) on the western edge of the Dunge Glacier, approach from Askole (rough Jeep track to here) via Paiju and Liligo.

OVERVIEW

The route follows a logical line up crack systems near the edge of the buttress. A heavily corniced snow ridge at two-thirds height leads to the upper, and most difficult, section of the buttress.

TIPS

There is a high risk of stonefall and icefall in the couloir leading to the buttress. The first climbers of the buttress died on the descent.

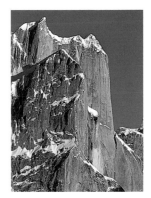

Compact granite on the Great Trango Tower. To the right is the Norwegian Pillar.

'This arête makes such a powerful impression on us that I gradually become the unwilling plaything of my emotions.'

BERND ARNOLD

The Trango Towers (left). In the summer of 1984, after 23 days' climbing, the Norwegians Hans-Christian Doseth – who had previously soloed a new route on the famous Troll Wall (Romsdal/Norway) – and Fin Daehli finally completed their hard new route on the North-East Buttress of the Great Trango Tower. They were unable to report on their climb, however, since both climbers were killed on the descent.

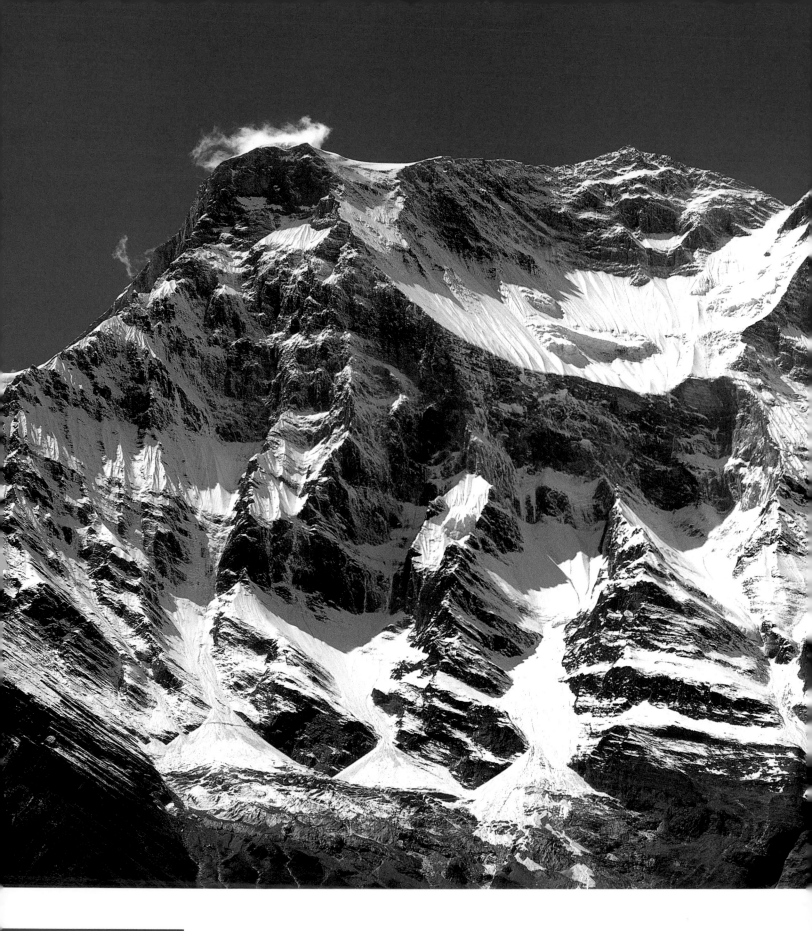

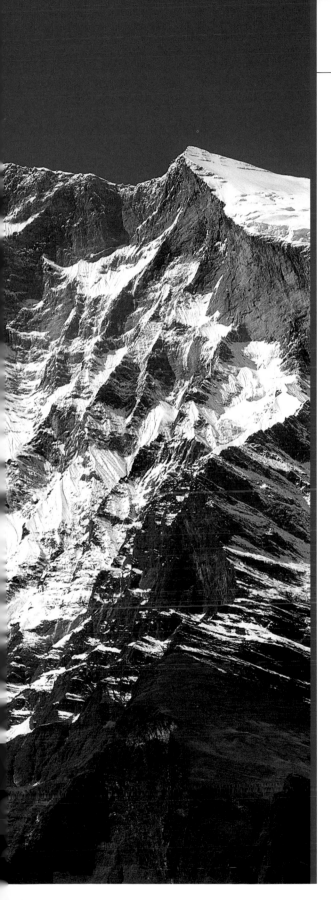

DHAULAGIRI I, WEST FACE

1984 – NEPAL HIMALAYA

SUMMIT HEIGHT

8167m

HEIGHT OF FACE

A good 4300m (between 3800 and 8167m)

DIFFICULTIES

Rock to IV, ice to 80 degrees

TIME

4–6 weeks' preparation (acclimatization and establishment of camps and fixed ropes on the face); 6–7 days' climbing

STARTING POINT

Base camp (3700m) below the West Face, approach from Baglung (airfield) via Beni, Bhimogaon, Maragaon and Dobang.

OVERVIEW

Above the extremely steep grass slopes (to 70 degrees) the West Face has three prominent spurs leading to a steep band of cliffs. The route goes left to the northernmost spur and climbs an avalanche-prone gully to gain a buttress which bounds this rock band on the left. Straight up the buttress and through the serac band to gain a steep ice wall which leads onto the North-West Ridge.

TIPS

The first ascent team placed five camps on the face. Between 5200 and 6600m there is an extremely high risk of avalanche and falling chunks of ice.

Between the South-West Buttress (Japanese Route) and the North Face there are half a dozen routes that – like the West Face of Manaslu – end on the summit plateau and are extremely dangerous.

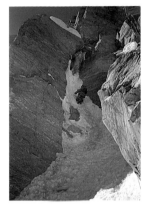

At 6200m on the right-hand buttress of the West Face.

'While traversing across the couloir the fixed rope started a rock fall. Although I knew from reports by the Safety Committee of the German Alpine Club that a Czechoslovakian climbing helmet had a very high impact strength, I wondered if the same thing applied to my back and my shoulders.'

JIŘI NOVÁK

The 23 October 1984 brought success for Jiři Novák's expedition to the West Face of Dhaulagiri, as Jan Šimon, Karel Jakeš and Jaromír Stejskal reached the summit.

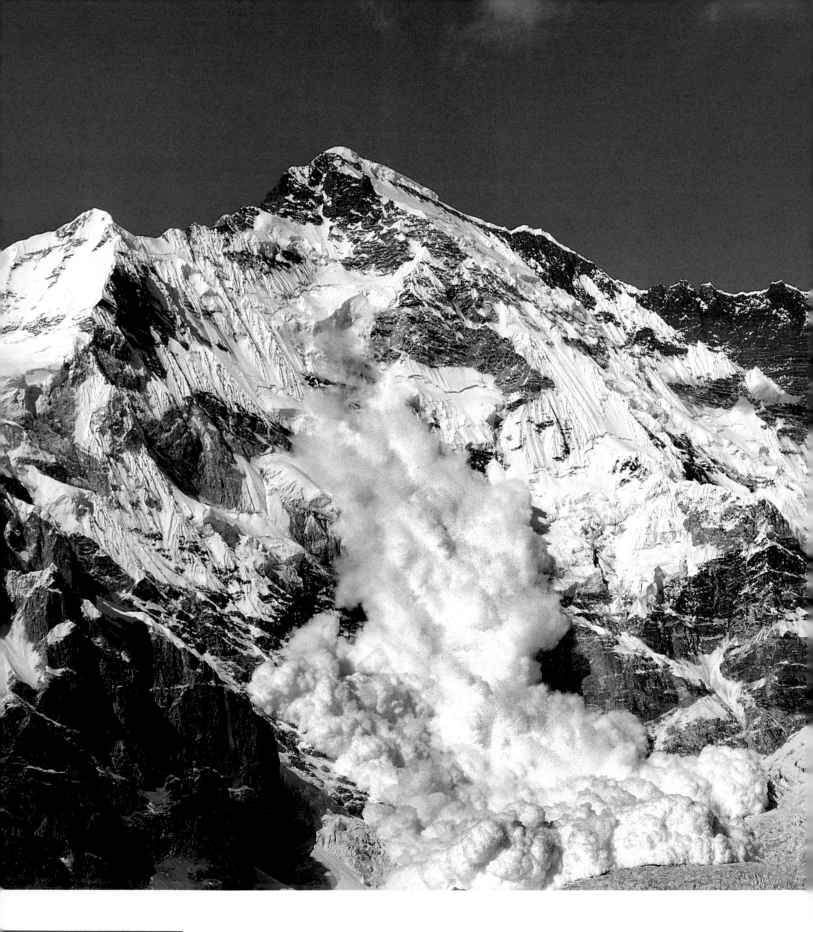

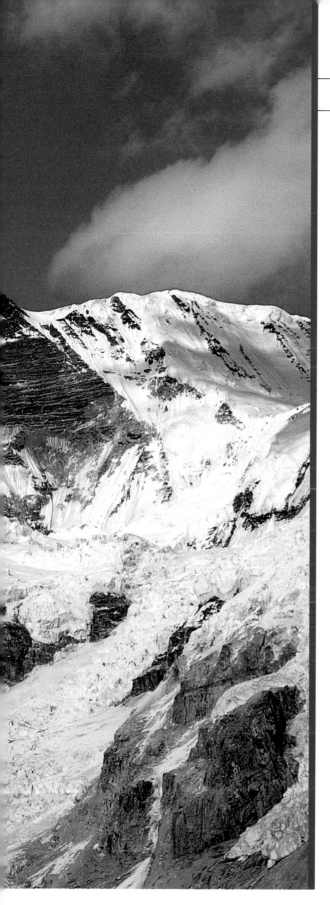

CHO OYU, SOUTH-EAST BUTTRESS

1985 – NEPAL HIMALAYA

SUMMIT HEIGHT

8201m

HEIGHT OF FACE

2800m (between 5400 and 8201m)

DIFFICULTIES

Extremely demanding rock and ice climbing; rock bands alternating with steep ice gullies; fluted ice walls and serac zones

TIME

4–5 weeks' acclimatization and preparation (establishment of camps and fixed ropes on the face); 5–7 days' climbing

STARTING POINT

Base camp on the Lungsampa Galcier, approach from Lukla (airstrip) via Namche Bazar, Dule and through the Gokyo valley.

OVERVIEW

The South-East Buttress divides the South-East and South-West Faces. The route takes a line up rock walls, mixed ground and steep ice slopes, starting to the left of the buttress and finally climbing the left-hand side of the South-East Face to the summit.

TIPS

There is a significant threat from seracs, stonefall and falling ice on the route. On the first ascent, four camps were placed on the face and fixed ropes were destroyed by stonefall. The first ascent of the South-East Buttress was accomplished in winter and was also the first winter ascent of Cho Oyu.

The South-East Face of Cho Oyu (Koblmüller/ Furtner) is another of the great Himalayan faces but here the avalanche danger is exceptional. Reinhard Karl lost his life on this route in 1982 when caught in an ice avalanche.

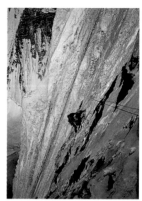

On the South-East Face of Cho Oyu.

'Jurek Kukuczka openly admitted the fact that, for him, mountaineering was a sport, by which he meant the arena, the competition. He actively sought heated public debate. He wanted to win.'

VOYTEK KURTYKA

A team of top Polish mountaineers achieved success on the difficult and dangerous South-East Buttress of Cho Oyu (takes a diagonal line up and left from the centre of picture) when, on 11 February 1985, Maciej Berbeka and Maciej Pawlikowski reached the summit, followed on 15 February by Jerzy Kukuczka and Andrzej Heinrich.

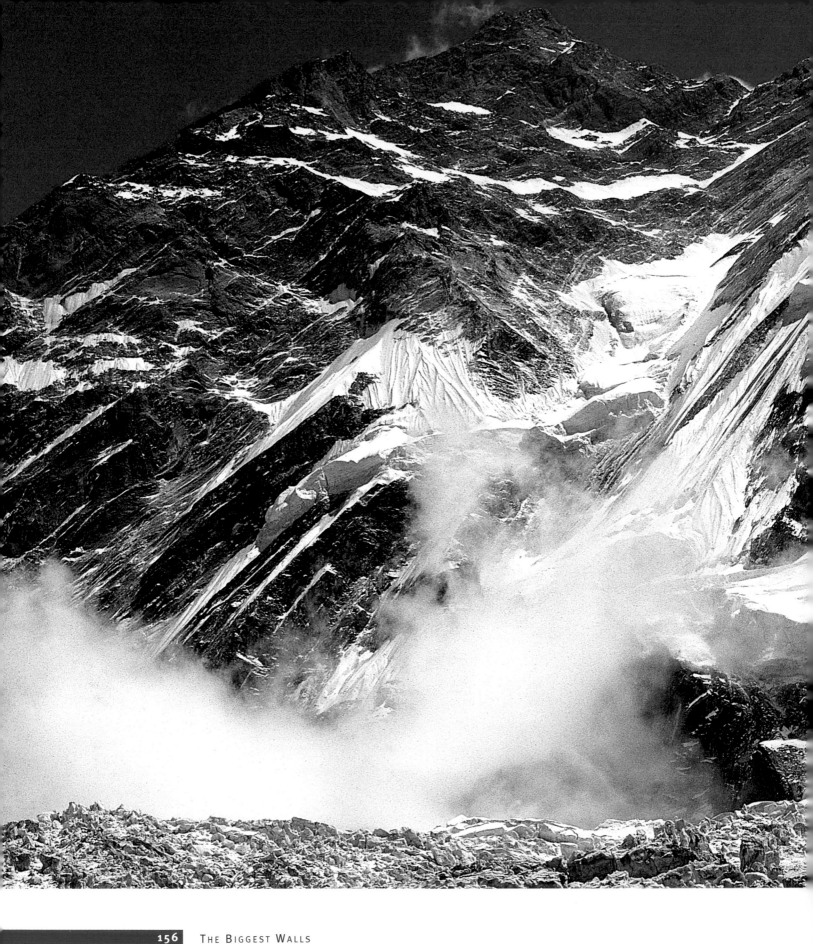

THE BIGGEST WALLS

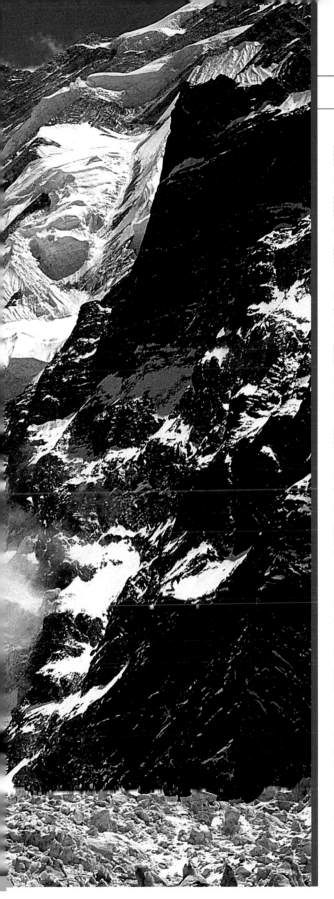

ANNAPURNA I, NORTH-WEST FACE

1985 – NEPAL HIMALAYA

SUMMIT HEIGHT

8091m

HEIGHT OF FACE

c. 3000m (between 5000 and 8000m)

DIFFICULTIES

Extreme mixed climbing, difficult friction climbing on a smooth rock band at about 6500m, sections of vertical ice; long, exposed summit ridge with loose rock

TIME

4–6 weeks' acclimatization and preparation (establishment of Camp I at the foot of the face and Camp II at about 6000m); 4–5 days' climbing

STARTING POINT

Base camp (*c.* 4100m) in the upper Miristi Khola, reached from Pokhara over the Gore Pani Pass and via Chitre, Tatopani (Kali Gandaki valley), Dana and the rock spur of the Thulo Begin.

OVERVIEW

The route goes up the concave depression to the right of the summit fall line. It leads up rightwards beneath the prominent, slanting terraces, above the big serac band into the centre of the depression and then trends rightwards across slabs and ice fields to join the summit ridge; then leftwards up the ridge to the main summit of Annapurna I.

TIPS

On the first ascent the face was climbed Alpine-style from 6000m. The route is threatened by seracs and very prone to avalanches after falls of snow. In the event that the descent of the North-West Face should prove too risky, it is advisable to study carefully the routes on the North Flank (French Route, Dutch Route). The base camp on the north side of Annapurna can be easily reached from the North-West Face base camp.

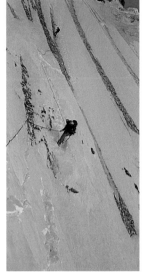

On the initial pitches of the face.

'With what assuredness Hans now led the glassy smooth wall of ice directly above the bivouac tent – and in these below zero temperatures! He pranced up the vertical ice. It was so absurd that I could not even shake my head.'

REINHOLD MESSNER

The North-West Face of Annapurna I. In 1985 Hans Kammerlander and Reinhold Messner climbed this great concave face to summit the mountain. The North-West Face Direct has often been attempted and ranks amongst the last great problems on the eight-thousanders.

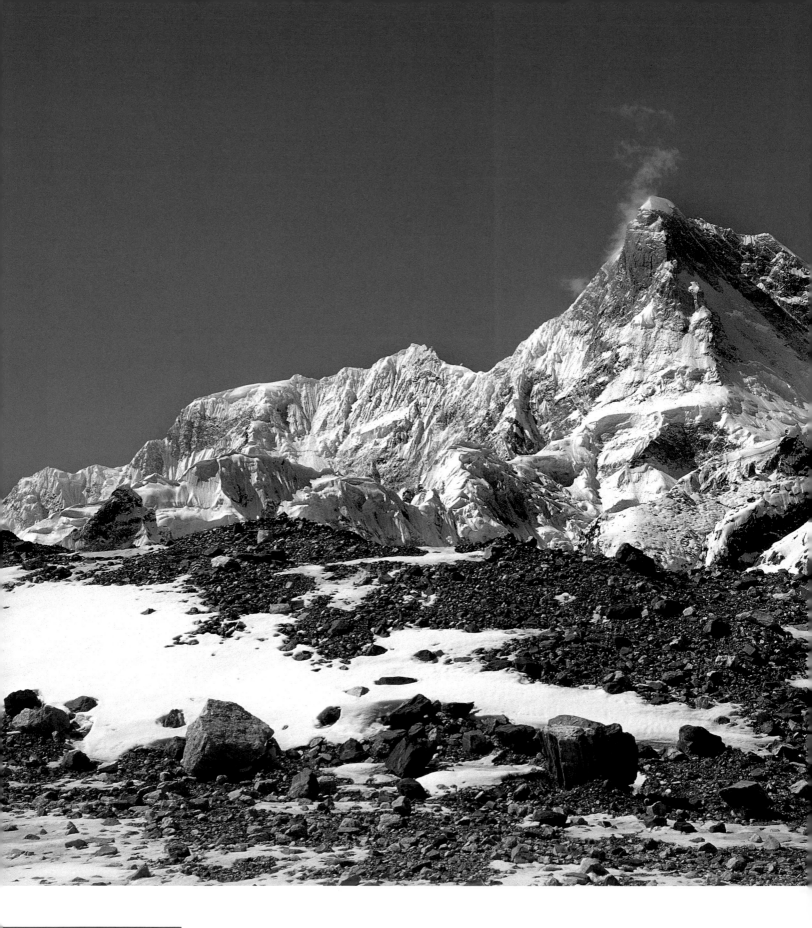

THE BIGGEST WALLS

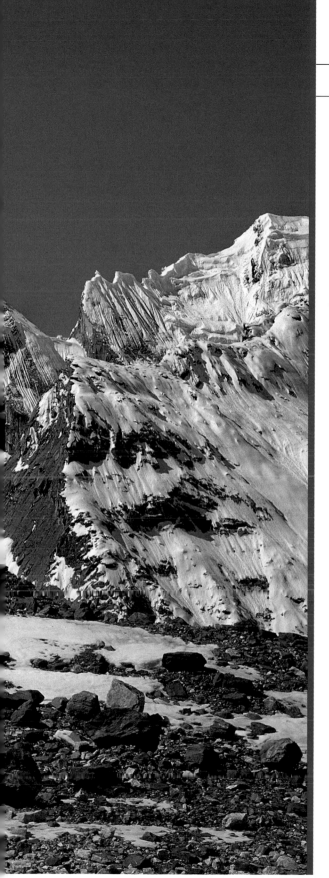

MASHERBRUM, NORTH-WEST FACE

1985 – KARAKORUM

SUMMIT HEIGHT

7824m

HEIGHT OF FACE

c. 3400m (between 4400 and 7824m)

DIFFICULTIES

Rock to VI–, ice to 85 degrees (one section of 90 degrees), hard mixed ground; long ridge section, heavily corniced

TIME

Approx. 4 weeks' acclimatization and preparation (establishment of camps and fixed ropes on the face); 4–5 days' climbing

STARTING POINT

Base camp (4300m) on the Mandu Glacier, approach from Askole (rough Jeep track to here) via Paiju, Liligo and braching off south from the Baltoro Glacier after Urdokas.

OVERVIEW

The route starts up a 1200m buttress on the left-hand side of the face and then climbs an easy-angled ridge to gain the final wall, where a huge groove system leads to the top.

TIPS

On the first and second ascent (accomplished almost simultaneously), four camps were placed and fixed ropes used on the face. On the lower third of the face in particular there is great danger from seracs and avalanches.

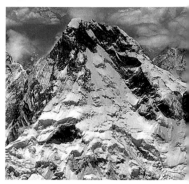

Masherbrum from the North-West.

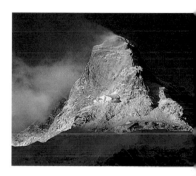

Masherbrum – beautiful, but dangerous.

'The sheer enormity of this vertical landscape overwhelms us.'

ROBERT RENZLER

In 1985 the North-West Face of Masherbrum (right of centre) was the objective of two separate expeditions. On 23 July, all ten participants of a Japanese undertaking (leader: Shin Kashu) reached the summit. Fifteen hours later, Austrians Robert Renzler, Andi Orgler and Michael Larcher also topped out on the North-West Face. The expeditions operated independently of each other.

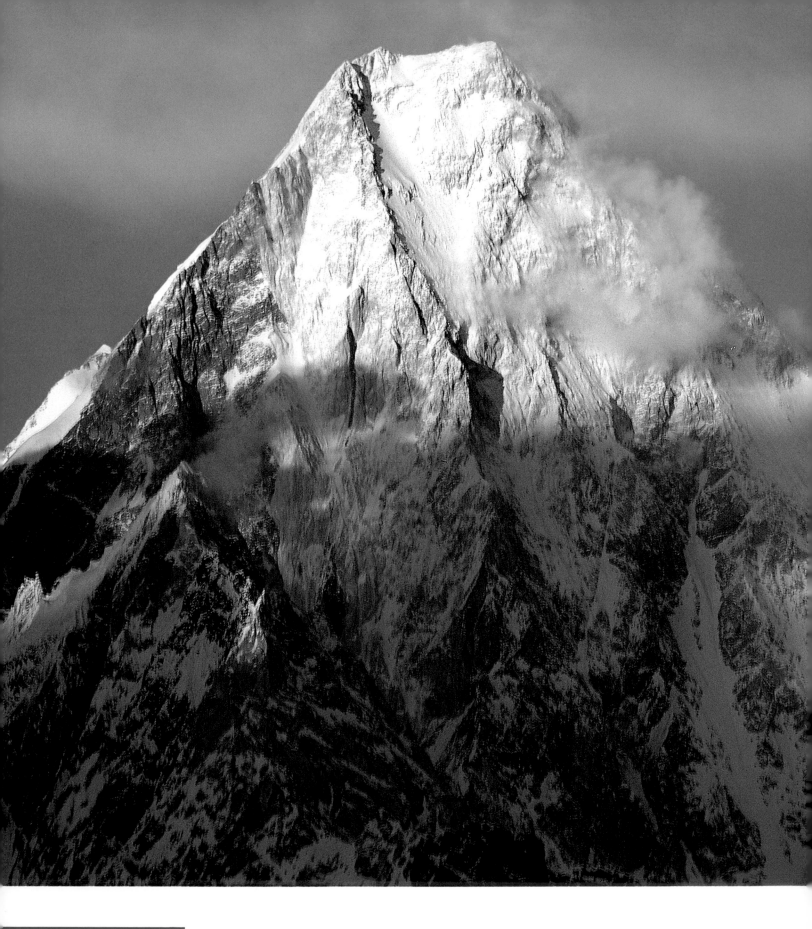

GASHERBRUM IV, WEST FACE

1985 – KARAKORUM

SUMMIT HEIGHT

7925m

HEIGHT OF FACE

c. 2300m (from 5600 to 7900m)

DIFFICULTIES

Rock to V, extremely hard mixed climbing, long sections of ice

TIME

4–5 weeks' acclimatization; 5–6 days' climbing

STARTING POINT

Base camp on the western Baltoro Glacier, approach from Askole (rough Jeep track to here) via Paiju, Liligo, Urdokas, Baltoro Glacier and Concordia.

OVERVIEW

The route climbs the big snow/ice couloir on the right-hand part of the face and then slants up and left to the top of the buttress bounding this on the left. From here it takes a diagonal leftwards line to the first (false) summit.

A second West Face route (the Korean Route) takes the nicely shaped face further to the left.

TIPS

The two climbers who made the first ascent climbed their route in Alpine style with eight bivouacs on the face (poor bivouac sites). The rock varies from extremely brittle to compact zones of marble. The climbing is, in parts, unprotected and protection is at best difficult to arrange. The first ascent team left the route just short of the false summit and descended by the North Ridge to the small cache of food and drink they had placed at 7100m.

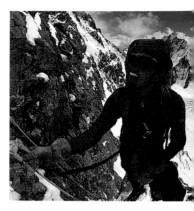

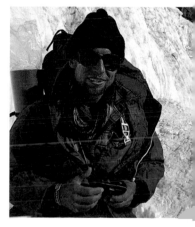

Robert Schauer (top) and Voytek Kurtyka,

'We didn't conquer Gasherbrum IV; it conquered us.'

ROBERT SCHAUER

Wojciech (Voytek) Kurtyka and Robert Schauer made an Alpine-style ascent of the 'Shining Wall' of Gasherbrum IV between 13 and 20 July 1985. The climb still ranks as one of the outstanding achievements in Big Wall mountaineering.

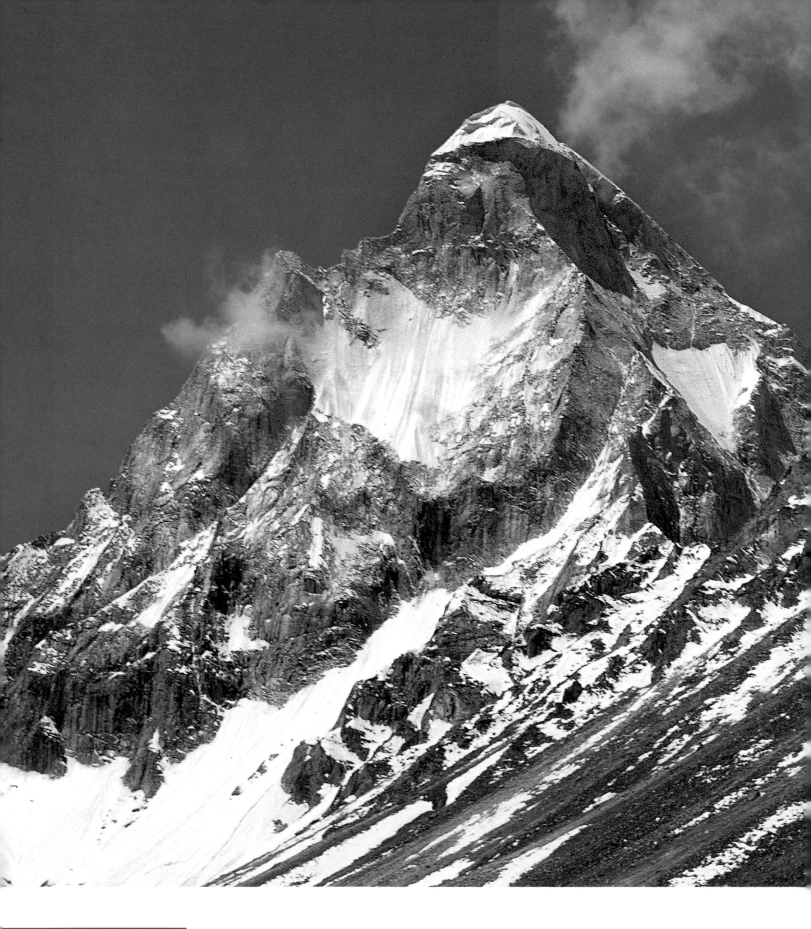

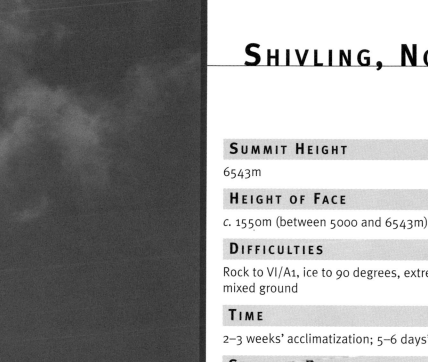

SHIVLING, NORTH-EAST FACE

1986 – GARHWAL-HIMALAYA

SUMMIT HEIGHT

6543m

HEIGHT OF FACE

c. 1550m (between 5000 and 6543m)

DIFFICULTIES

Rock to VI/A1, ice to 90 degrees, extremely difficult mixed ground

TIME

2–3 weeks' acclimatization; 5–6 days' climbing

STARTING POINT

Base camp at Tapovan (c. 4200m), approach from Gangotri (roadhead) along the Ganges and across the Gangotri Glacier.

OVERVIEW

The right-hand section of the North-East Face is split by an ice couloir that is wide at the bottom. The route climbs out of this up a steep rock wall and then the mixed ground above to the big ice cliff in the middle of the face. Climb this to reach the vertical summit headwall and continue over the ice cap to the North-East Summit.

TIPS

The first ascent team climbed this avalanche-prone face over 8 days and in poor conditions. There are similar, and harder, objectives to be found in the Garhwal Himalaya, both on Shivling and on other mountains such as Changabang or Bhagirathi.

'Shivling is one of the most impressive peaks in the Himalaya. The beautiful north-eastern aspect with the Chaturangi Glacier reminds me a lot of the Matterhorn. The summit rises 2000m above the glacier and is difficult to reach from all sides.'

DOUG SCOTT

In June 1986, after eight days' climbing on the technically very difficult North-East Face (left of centre), the Italians Enrico Rosso, Paolo Bernascone and Fabrizio Manoni emerged onto the summit.

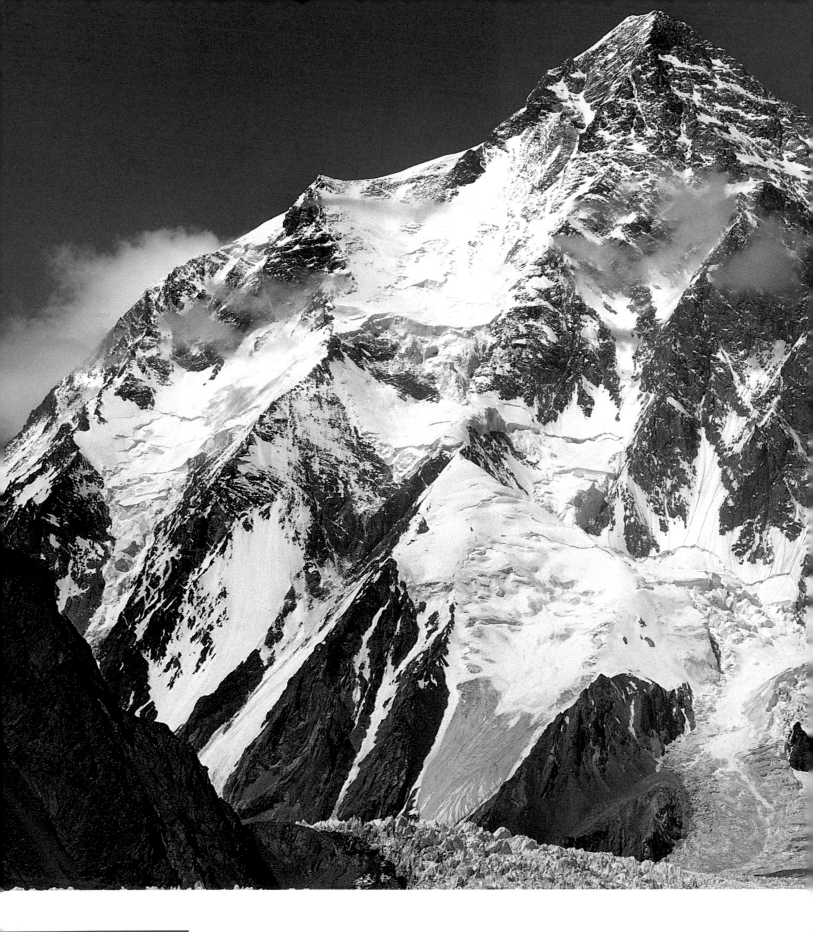

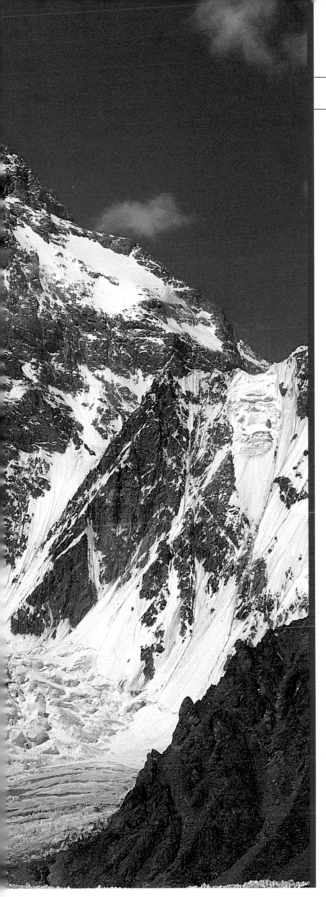

K2, SOUTH FACE, KUKUCZKA ROUTE

1986 – KARAKORUM

SUMMIT HEIGHT

8611m

HEIGHT OF FACE

c. 3100m (from 5300 to c. 8400m)

DIFFICULTIES

Ice to 55 degrees and difficult mixed climbing; the crux section (to V+) is located on the uppermost section of the face, above 8200m

TIME

4–6 weeks' acclimatization and preparation; 6–7 days' climbing

STARTING POINT

Base camp (5070m) on the middle moraines of the Godwin Austen Glacier, approach from Askole (rough jeep track to here) via Paiju, Liligo, Urdokas, Baltoro Glacier and Concordia.

OVERVIEW

The lower part of the route climbs the prominent ice spur east of the Filippi Glacier and continues just left of the huge serac cliffs to reach the ice wall and a sickle-shaped couloir. Up the couloir to its end and a junction with the Abruzzi Route at about 8400m.

TIPS

On the first ascent, two camps and a gear dump were placed on the face, to a height of 7400m and several sections of the route were fixed. The two men then spent 6 days and three tent bivouacs on the upper part of the face, joining the Normal Route and following this to the summit. After two further bivouacs one of the pair fell to his death on the Abruzzi Route.

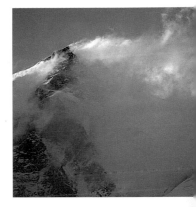

Storm on K2.

'Astonishingly enough, Kukuczka was neither egocentric nor vain and lost none of his natural pleasantness when he became internationally famous. On the other hand I did find the thoughtless way he made accusations annoying.'

VOYTEK KURTYKA

After almost one week of very hard climbing on the 3000m-plus South Face of K2 (centre of picture), Jerzy Kukuczka and Tadeusz Piotrowski finally reached the summit in the evening of 8 July 1986.

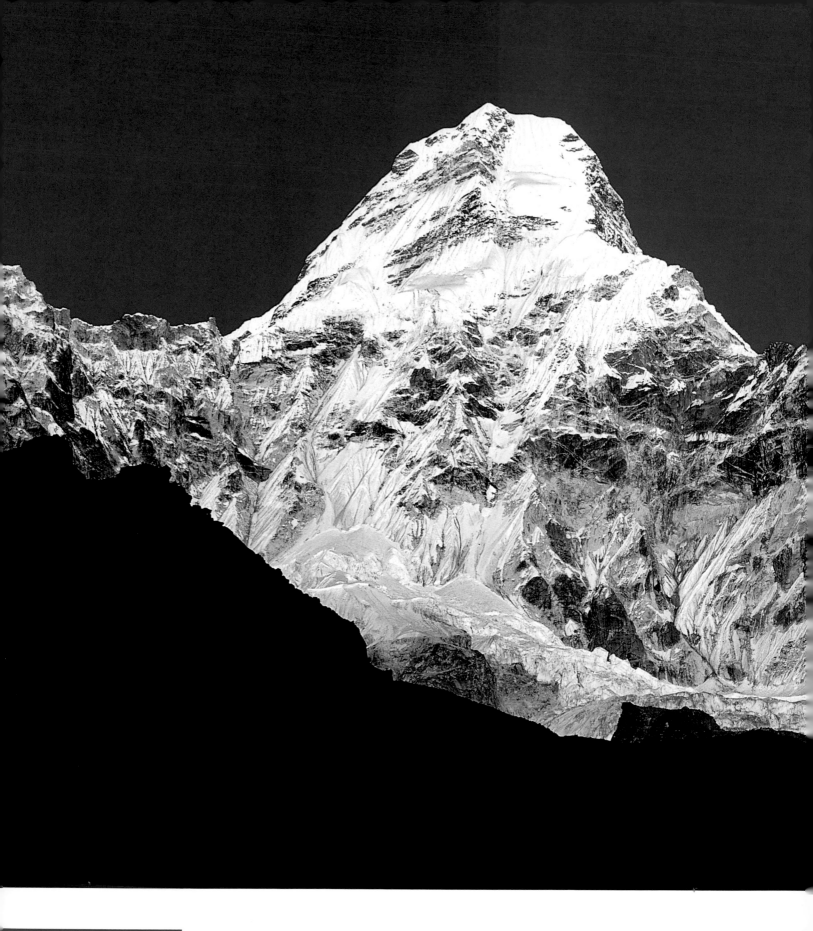

THE BIGGEST WALLS

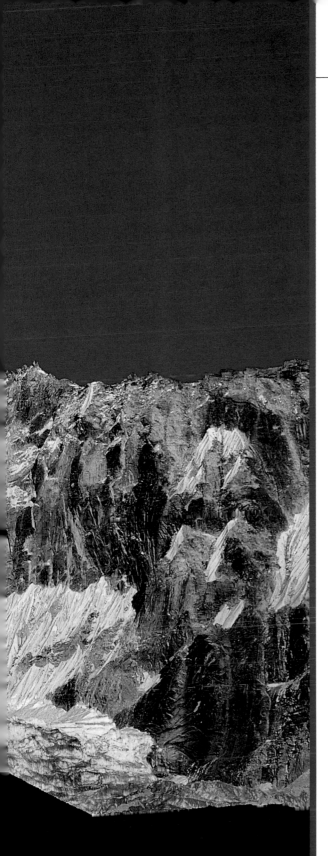

AMA DABLAM, WEST FACE

1986 – NEPAL HIMALAYA

SUMMIT HEIGHT

6828m

HEIGHT OF FACE

over 1400m (between 5400 and 6828m)

DIFFICULTIES

Rock to IV+, ice to 80 degrees

TIME

3–4 weeks' acclimatization; 3–4 days' climbing

STARTING POINT

Bivouac (c. 5300m) on an island of rock on the Mingbo Glacier; approach from Lukla (airfield) via Namche Bazar, Pangpoche and Lhabarma.

OVERVIEW

The route climbs the centre of the face direct. The lower part takes the steep ice slopes and mixed ground straight up between the huge, flanking rock barriers. On the upper section it takes a direct line left of the prominent ice cliff (the notorious 'Medallion' that gives the mountain its name) and up the final ice wall to join the summit ridge.

TIPS

There is a risk of ice avalanches and stonefall on the route. During a first ascent attempt in 1979 one of the team of four, climbing as two ropes of two, was killed by an ice avalanche. The three survivors were rescued from the face by Reinhold Messner and Oswald Oelz.

The first ascent was accomplished solo, over two days, with one bivouac on the face and a second on the summit.

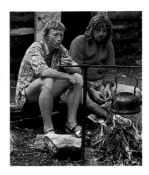

Josef Nežerka and Miroslav Šmid.

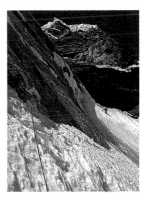

On the West Face of Ama Dablam.

'Reinhold hurried on ahead, placing protection at critical points and constantly shouting at me to climb faster.'

OSWALD OELZ

In 1986, the leader of a Czech/Swiss expedition, Miroslav Šmid, soloed the ideal line on the dangerous West face of Ama Dablam.

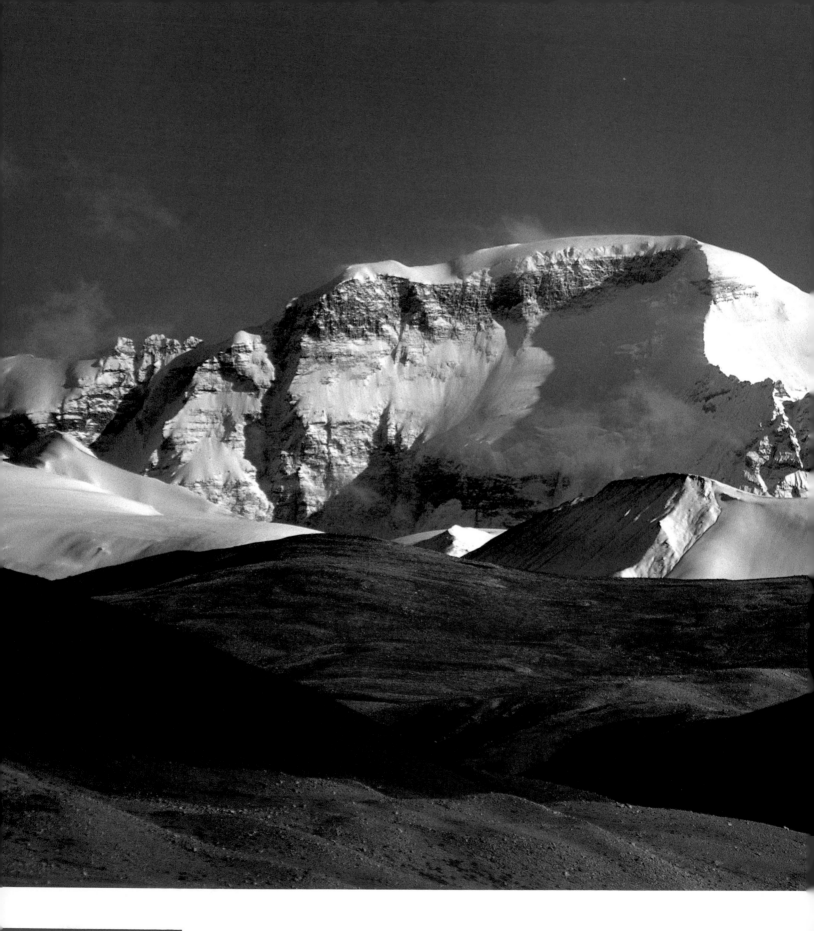

CHO OYU, NORTH FACE

1988 – TIBET HIMALAYA

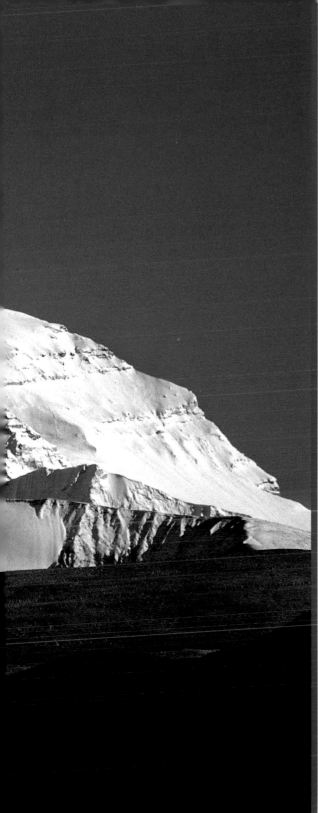

SUMMIT HEIGHT

8201m

HEIGHT OF FACE

2000m (between 6200 and 8201m)

DIFFICULTIES

Extremely hard mixed climbing on the lower and uppermost part of the face (vertical crux section exiting the couloir at approx. 8140m), ice to 60 degrees

TIME

3–4 weeks' acclimatization and preparation (establishment of camps and on the face); 3–4 days' climbing

STARTING POINT

Base camp on the Balung Glacier, approach from Balung (via Tingri).

OVERVIEW

The route takes a line on the right-hand side of the face, to the right of the dangerous band of seracs that bars the way to the upper part of the North Face. The first 300m take the mixed ground on left-hand side of the initial wall (to the right of the central hanging glacier). Then diagonally right to the big ice wall, trending leftwards up this, passing the huge serac band on the right to gain the steep summit wall (variation on the right).

It might be possible to climb a route up the central rocky section of the face; this would be extremely hard.

TIPS

The first climbers to succeed placed two camps on the face. Similar big-face routes exist on Gyachung Khang and on Cho Oyu.

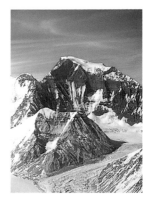

Gyachung Khang from the east.

'The face is four kilometres wide and more than 2000m high, hidden behind smaller summits that rise up in front of it.'

ROMAN ROBAS

Slovenian climbers celebrated success on the North Face of Cho Oyu in 1988 when all seven expedition members reached the summit. On 2 November Iztok Tomazin summited, climbing solo from Camp III (7200m), followed on 5 November by Viki Grošelj and Jože Rozman, on 8 November by Marko Prezelj and Rado Nadvesnik and on 9 November by Blaž Jereb and Roman Robas.

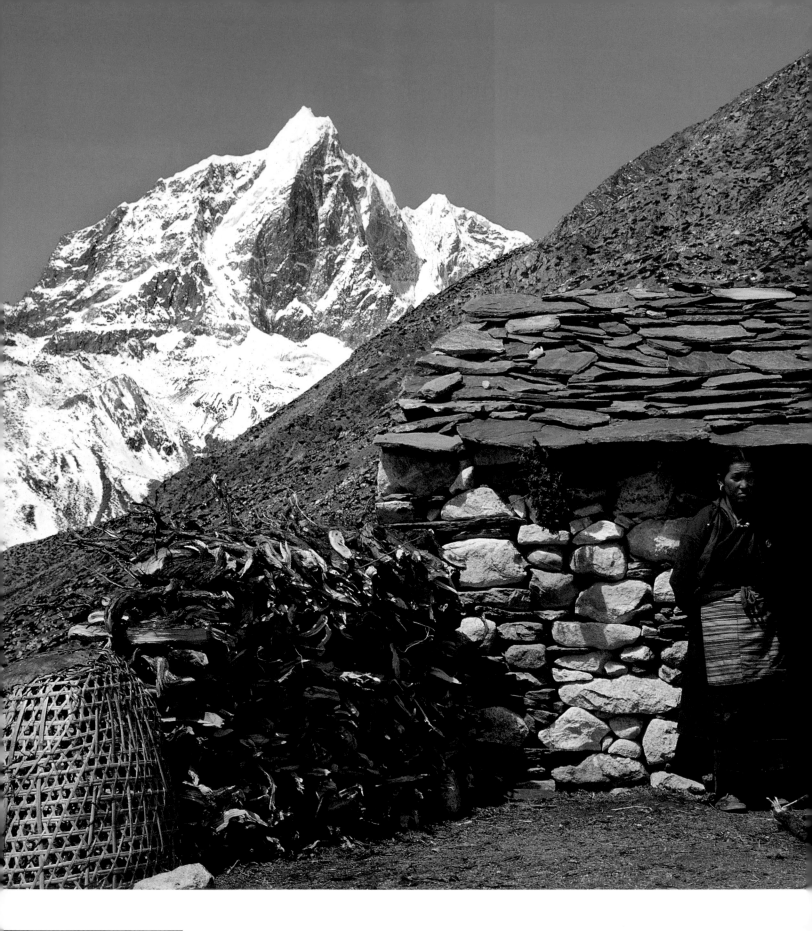

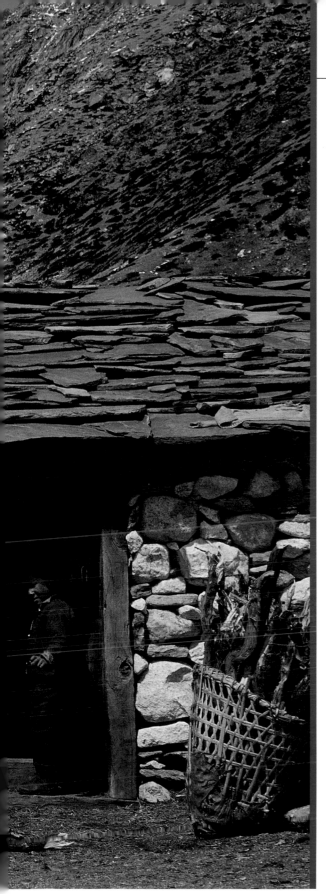

TABOCHE, EAST FACE

1989 – NEPAL HIMALAYA

SUMMIT HEIGHT

6542m

HEIGHT OF FACE

c. 1250m

DIFFICULTIES

VII/A3 and extremely difficult mixed climbing

TIME

2–3 weeks' acclimatization; 5–6 days' climbing

STARTING POINT

Base camp on the Taboche Glacier at approx. 5100m, approach from Lukla (airfield) via Namche Bazar, Pangpoche and Samdrang.

OVERVIEW

The route follows a natural direct line up the central part of the face, climbing compact rock buttresses, groove systems and gullies. The first 450m are purely rock, followed by mixed ground and an ice chimney to finish. A similarly difficult (ED+) route was established in 1995 to the right of the East Face, climbing the North-East Buttress above the prominent steep ramp.

TIPS

The first ascent was made in winter with only two hours of sunlight per day and took 8½ days in all.

'In 1995 Mick Fowler and Pat Littlejohn spent seven days on their superb new line to the right of the original East Face Route. Their most spectacular bivouac was spent in a 70cm-wide ice tube, which they christened "The Torture Tube"'

HORST HÖFLER

Taboche, with the East Face shown. Jeff Lowe and John Roskelley climbed an outstanding new line up the centre of this face in the winter of 1989. After eight and a half bitterly cold days and nights they finally topped out on 15 February.

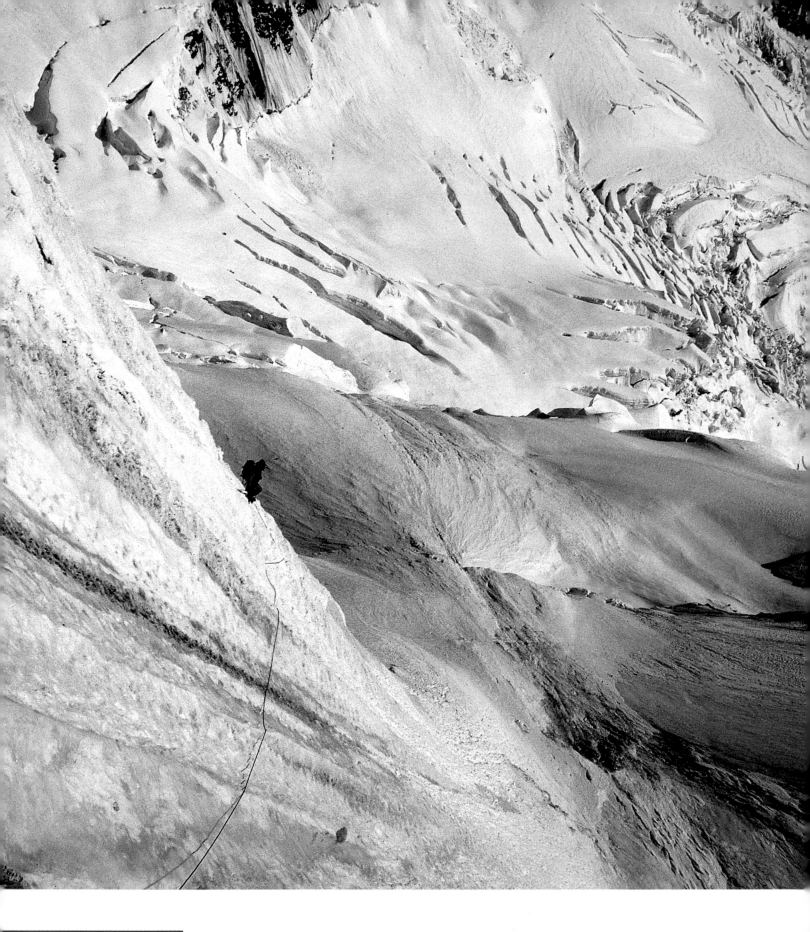

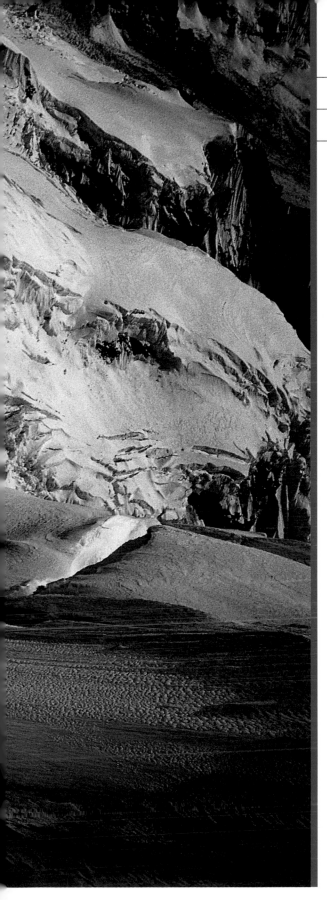

CHO OYU, SOUTH-EAST FACE AND SOUTH-WEST FACE

1990 – NEPAL HIMALAYA

SUMMIT HEIGHT

8201m

HEIGHT OF FACE

c. 2000m (between 6100 and 8100m)

DIFFICULTIES (SOUTH-WEST FACE)

Rock to grade IV, ice to 60 degrees

TIME (SOUTH-WEST FACE)

3–4 weeks' acclimatization; 2–3 days' climbing

STARTING POINT (SOUTH-WEST FACE)

Base camp (c. 5700m) on the Gyabrag Glacier, easily approached either from the south (old Normal Route; from Thame) or the north (Tingri).

OVERVIEW (SOUTH-WEST FACE)

The route starts up a big ice couloir on the right-hand part of the face, before taking a more or less direct line through the rock band and ice fields and finally moving out right to join the South-West Ridge some 100m below the summit.

TIPS (SOUTH-WEST FACE)

The first ascent was accomplished in Alpine style over two days with a bivouac at 8150m. This route and a second route on the South-West Face are classic climbs and are best done Alpine style. The South-East Face was climbed in 1978 by Edi Koblmüller and Alois Furtner. The avalanche danger is extreme.

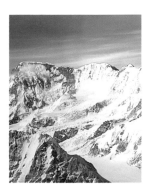

Cho Oyu South-East Face.

'I had intended to rest for two or three hours until the moon came out but I was sleepy and it was a nice night so I sat back comfortably in my 'snow deck chair' and slept. The next day, extremely dehydrated, I descended to the foot of the face.'

VOYTEK KURTYKA

On the steep South-East Face of Cho Oyu. Climbing through the night of 19 September 1990, and summiting the following day, Voytek Kurtyka, Erhard Loretan and Jean Troillet did the central line on the South-West Face. They bivouacked at 8150m on the South-West Ridge.

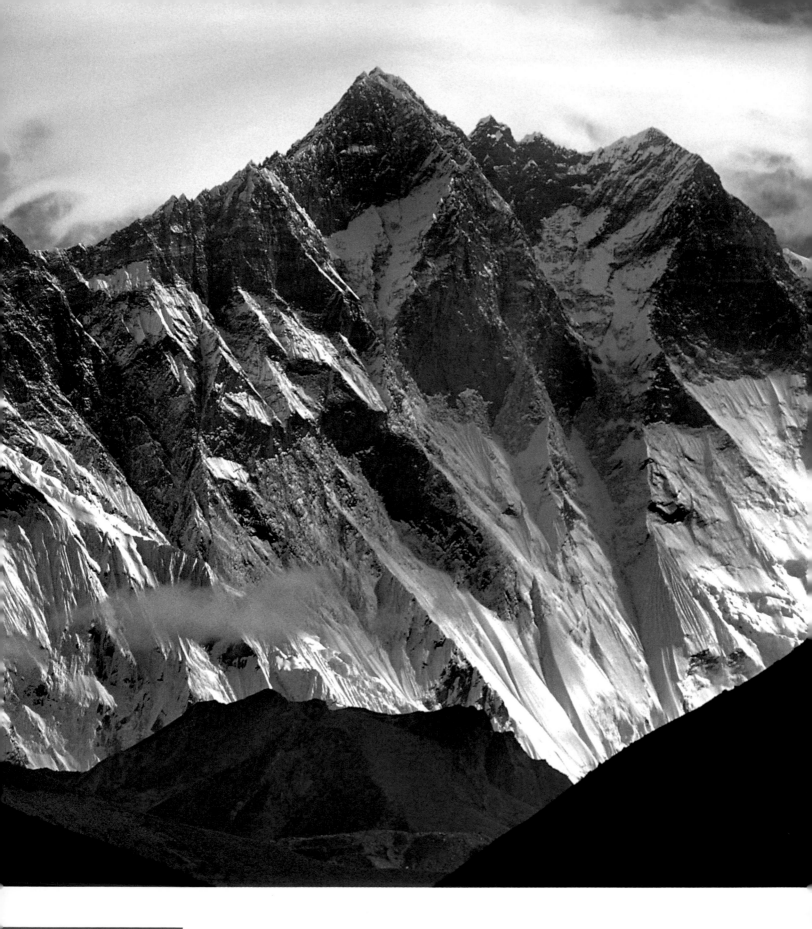

THE BIGGEST WALLS

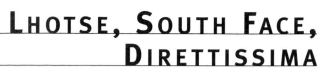

LHOTSE, SOUTH FACE, DIRETTISSIMA

1990 – NEPAL HIMALAYA

SUMMIT HEIGHT

8516m

HEIGHT OF FACE

c. 3200m (from 5300 to 8516m)

DIFFICULTIES

Rock to VI, very steep ice slopes, extremely difficult summit ridge

TIME

4–6 weeks' acclimatization and preparation (establishment of camps and fixed ropes on the face); 7–8 days' climbing

STARTING POINT

Base camp (approx. 5250m) on the Lhotse Glacier, approach from Lukla (airfield) via Namche Bazar, Pangpoche, Dingpoche and Chhukhung.

OVERVIEW

The route generally follows the summit fall line, taking a series of increasingly steep ice slopes and mixed ground to beneath the huge, central cliff on the upper part of the face. The Yugoslavian Route avoids this on the left, while the 'Direttissima' goes up to its right, climbing a huge groove system to the ridge and along this to the summit.

TIPS

There is a serious danger of avalanches as far as the steep cliff in the centre of the face and the hard rock climbing sections are, as a rule, covered in ice. The main difficulties lie between 7400m and the summit. The first ascent team placed six camps on the face and fixed ropes on most of the route. The summit team spent six days at over 8000m.

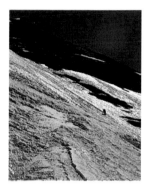

On the South Face of Lhotse.

'Jurek Kukuczka died in 1989 on the South Face of Lhotse. He came off, the rope broke and he fell more than 1000m down the face.'

VOYTEK KURTYKA

In 1990 Aleksander Shevchenko led a Soviet expedition of twenty climbers to the South Face of Lhotse. Their Direttissima (left of centre) finally solved the greatest outstanding Himalayan big wall problem of the 1980s. On 16 October, Sergej Bershov and Vladimir Karatayev reached the summit from Camp VI.

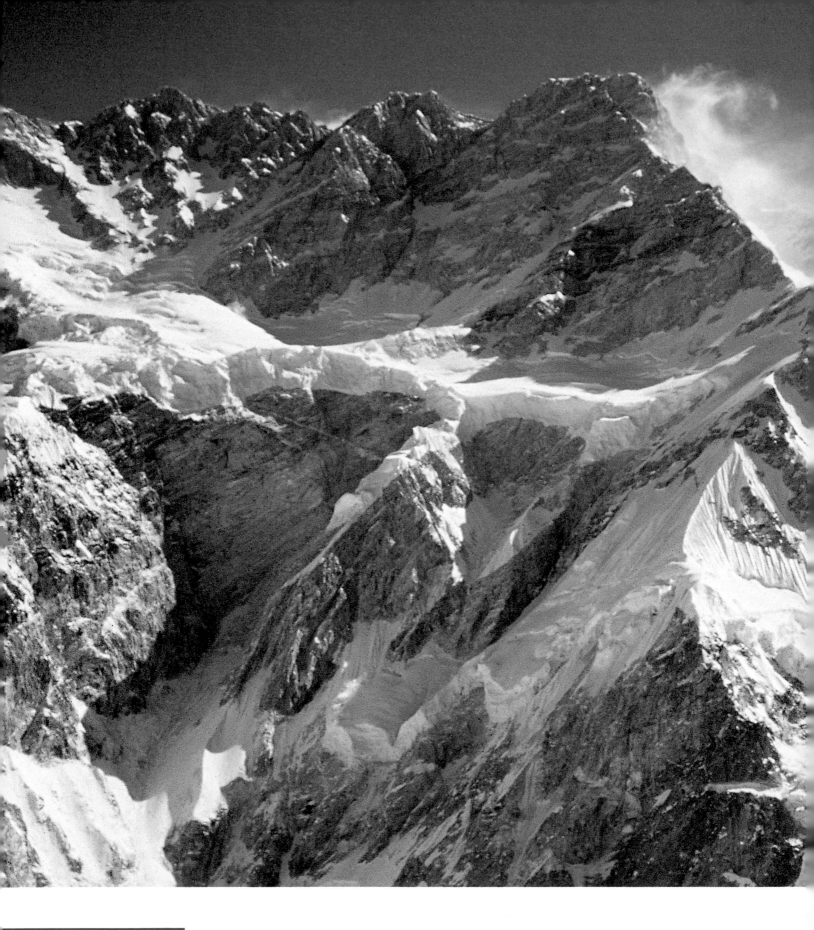

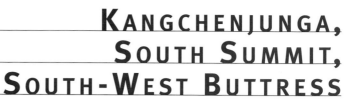

KANGCHENJUNGA, SOUTH SUMMIT, SOUTH-WEST BUTTRESS

1991 – NEPAL HIMALAYA

SUMMIT HEIGHT

8476m

HEIGHT OF FACE

c. 2900m (from 5550 to 8476m)

DIFFICULTIES

VI/A1 on rock and 80 degree ice; V and 60 degrees +
on the upper section of the buttress

TIME

4–6 weeks' acclimatization (one member of the first
ascent team climbed the 7350m Talung Peak); 5–7
days' climbing

STARTING POINT

Base camp (c. 5100m) on the Yalung Glacier,
approach from Taplejung (airfield) via Taplechok,
Chairam, Lapsang (Simbua Khola), the high mountain
pastures of Ramser and Tso Camp (4740m).

OVERVIEW

Viewed from the Yalung-Gletscher, the South-West
Buttress of the South Summit appears as the right-
hand bounding edge of the mighty Kangchenjunga
Flank. The route takes a rising rightwards line,
crossing the features described by G.O. Dyhrenfurth
as the 'eastern bulwark' and the 'hog's back' to gain
the very steep upper half of the buttress.

TIPS

The first ascent was made Alpine style with four
bivouacs in a small tent.

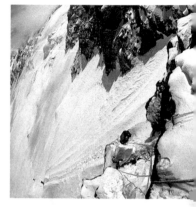

On the North Face of
Kangchenjunga.

'During the descent
it got dark. We had
only one head
torch. At 7900m, we
left the Polish
Route and turned
our attention to a
couloir between the
Middle and South
Summits.'

ANDREJ ŠTREMFELJ

Kangchenjunga, South
Summit, South-West Buttress.
This superb route was the 1991
objective of a Slovenian
expedition under Tone Škarja.
Marko Prezelj and Andrej
Štremfelj made the first ascent
between 26 and 29 April in
Alpine style.

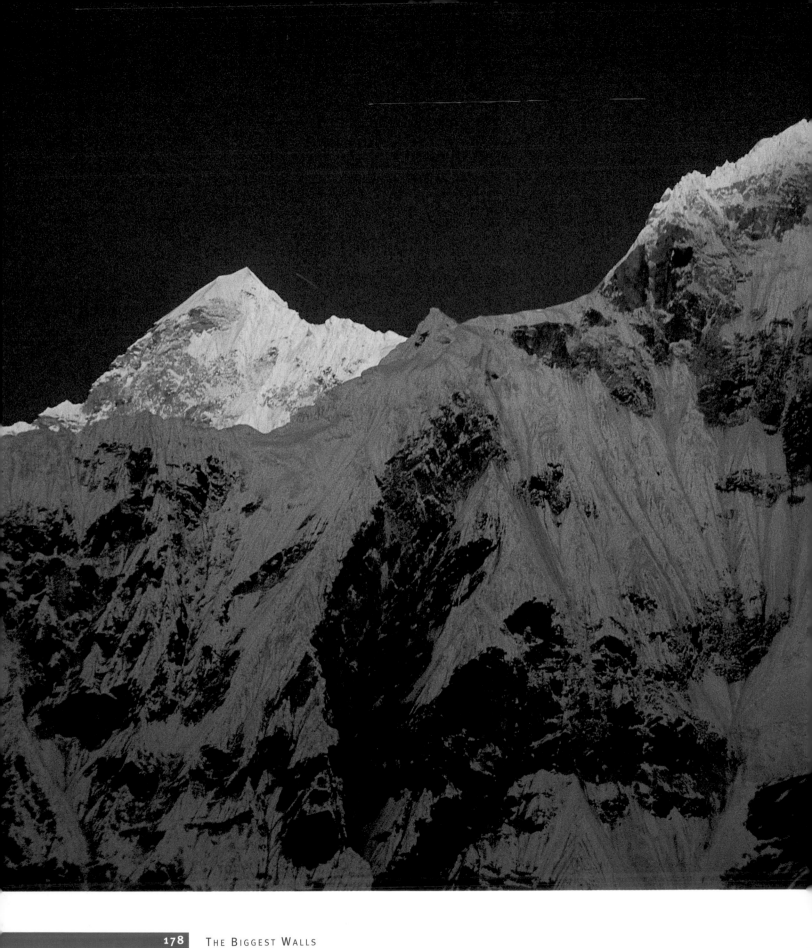

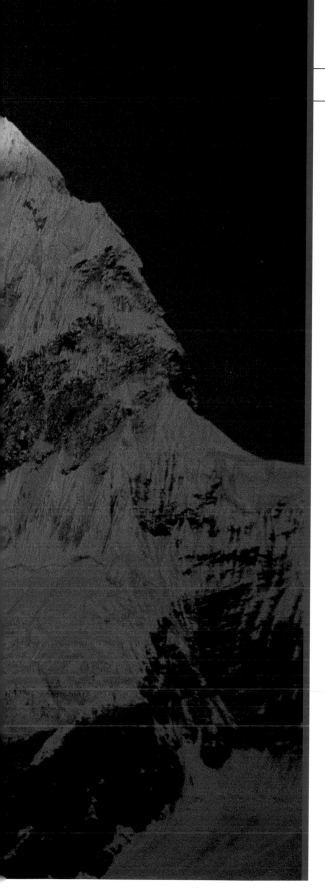

JANNU, EAST SUMMIT, EAST FACE

1991 – NEPAL HIMALAYA

SUMMIT HEIGHT

7468m

HEIGHT OF FACE

c. 2000m (from 5500 to 7468m)

DIFFICULTIES

Isolated sections of VII (one of them at about 7000m), several pitches of V, VI, VI+; extremely hard mixed climbing, ice to 90/95 degrees

TIME

3–4 weeks' acclimatization; 3–4 days' climbing

STARTING POINT

Camp (at about 5400m) on the eastern Kumbhakarna (Jannu) Glacier, approach from Taplejung (airfield) via Taplechok, Chairam, Lapsang (Simbua Khola), the high mountain pastures of Ramser Tso Camp (4740m) and the Kanch Base Camp (*c.* 5100m).

OVERVIEW

Starting on the left-hand side of the face, the route breaks through the lower rock bands at their weakest point and then goes up diagonally rightwards between two belts of cliffs to gain the centre of the face. From here it trends up and diagonally left to join the South-East Ridge.

TIPS

The two-man first ascent team climbed the face – which, in parts, has a very high risk of avalanche – Alpine style to about 80m (7050m) below the South-East Ridge, where a snowstorm and avalanches meant they were unable to continue. However, the face itself was climbed.

There are similar big face climbs on the twin Jannu summits, north and east.

'At six o'clock in the evening we were back at the ice cave in which we had spent our first bivouac. We rested until 11 o'clock and then continued our descent through the night. At 6 o'clock in the morning we found ourselves at the foot of the face.'

BOJAN POČKAR

During the 1991 Slovenian Kangchenjunga Expedition, which made the first ascent of the South Summit, South-West Buttress Route, Vanja Furlan and Bojan Počkar also added the first ascent of the extremely hard East Face of Jannu's East Summit, which they achieved over several days from 28 April to 1 May, climbing Alpine style to an altitude of 7050m.

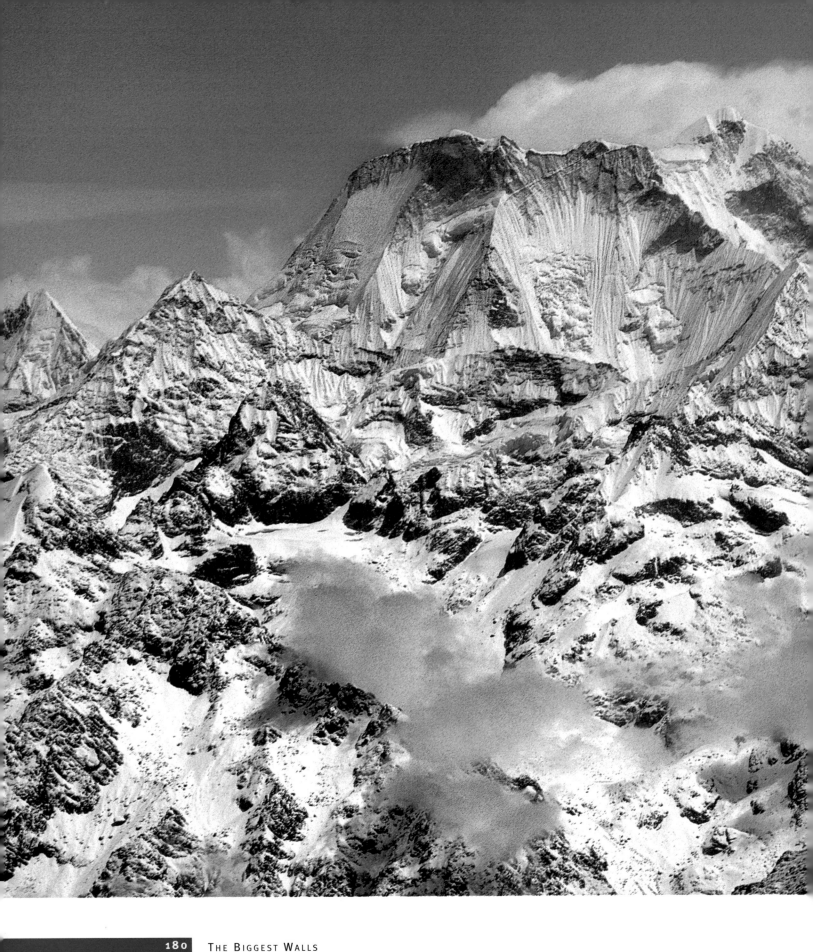

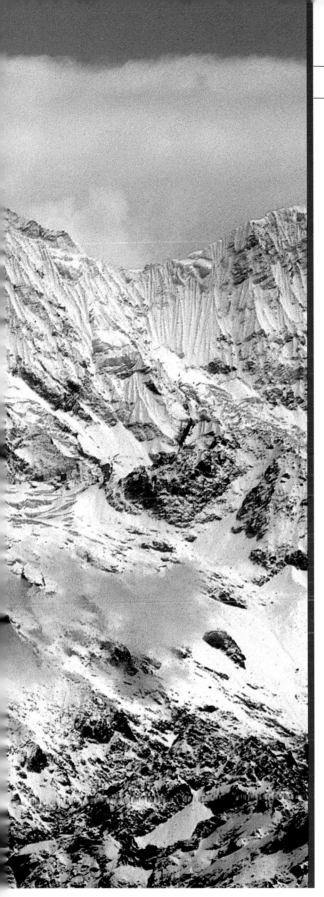

Menlungtse, Main Summit, North-East Face

1992 – Tibetan Himalaya

Summit Height

7181m

Height of Face

2000m (between 5150 and 7181m)

Difficulties

TD (ice to 75 degrees)

Time

2–3 weeks' acclimatization; 2–3 days' climbing

Starting Point

Advanced base camp at *c.* 5100m on the Drogpa Nagtsang Glacier; approach from Tingri over the Fushi La and via Chang bu Jiang (Jeep track to here), Tombu (4200m) and Palbugthang (4600m, base camp).

Overview

This pure ice route takes a line to the left of the central rock wall to join the steep summit ridge.

Tips

The first ascent was accomplished Alpine style with one bivouac on the face. The team took 15½ hours for the ascent and 11½ hours to descend by the same route. After new snowfall there is a serious avalanche risk.

On Menlungtse, on Gaurishankar (Rolwaling Himalaya) and on many other seven-thousanders – and on 6000m peaks like Thalay Sagar (Garhwal Himalaya) – there are still numerous extreme big faces to be discovered and climbed.

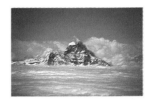

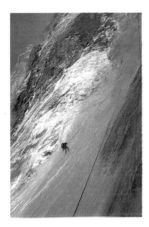

On Thalay Sagar.

The impressive massif of Menlungtse. The South-East Face of the main summit (right of centre) was climbed on 22/23 October 1992 by Slovenians Marko Prezelj and Andrej Štremfelj.

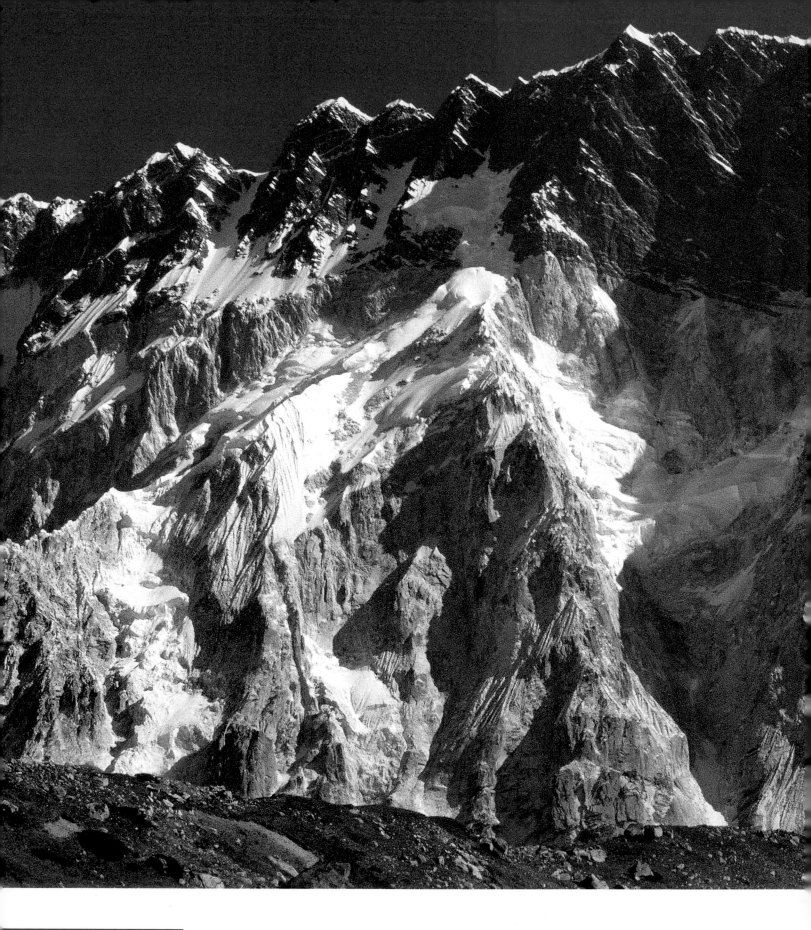

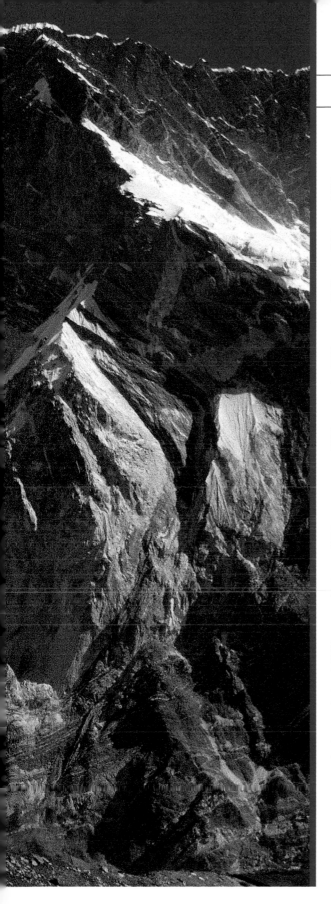

NUPTSE, EAST SUMMIT, SOUTH-EAST BUTTRESS

1995 – NEPAL HIMALAYA

SUMMIT HEIGHT

7804m

HEIGHT OF FACE

c. 2500m (between 5300 and 7804m)

DIFFICULTIES

Rock to VII+/A2, ice to 85 degrees, difficult mixed climbing

TIME

4–5 weeks' acclimatization and preparation (establishment of camps and fixed ropes on the face); 5–6 days' climbing

STARTING POINT

Base camp (5200m) on the western lateral moraines of the Lhotse-Nup Glacier; approach from Lukla (airfield) via Namche Bazar, Pangpoche, Dingpoche and Chhukhung.

OVERVIEW

On the wide South Face of Nuptse there is a strikingly prominent leaning pillar in the central section of the face, which provides the line of the route. From the top of the pillar, easier-angled yet more difficult mixed ground leads to the summit.

TIPS

The top of the pillar has been reached by several expeditions, but none has yet completed the route to the summit.

The 4km wide South Face between the West Summit of Nuptse and Lhotse holds dozens of possible new routes.

'Suddenly the curtain parted and we stared upwards in disbelief. There, where we had expected to see the sky, was our summit! When we had finally completed our first reality check and a sober analysis of the actual conditions on the pillar we were all suffering from stiff necks.'

WOLFGANG POHL

This 2500m-plus route (centre of picture) to the East Summit of Nuptse has been attempted by several teams, amongst them a German expedition including Robert Jasper and lead by Hans Kammerlander. Although the buttress itself has been climbed several times, to date no one has summited the route.

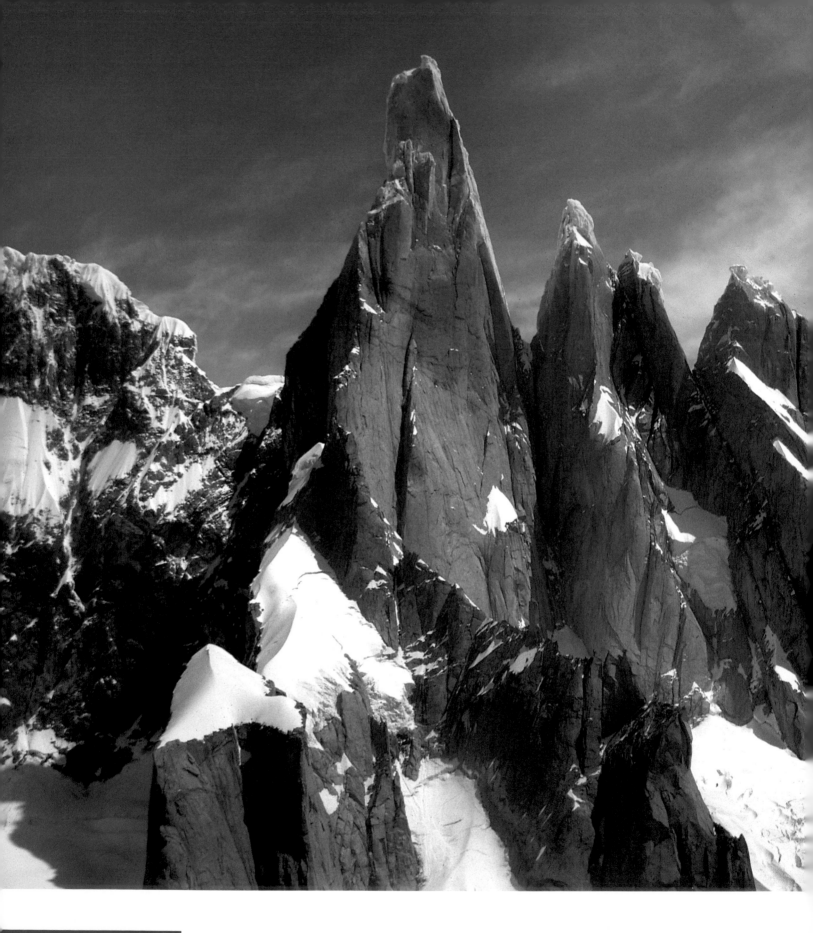

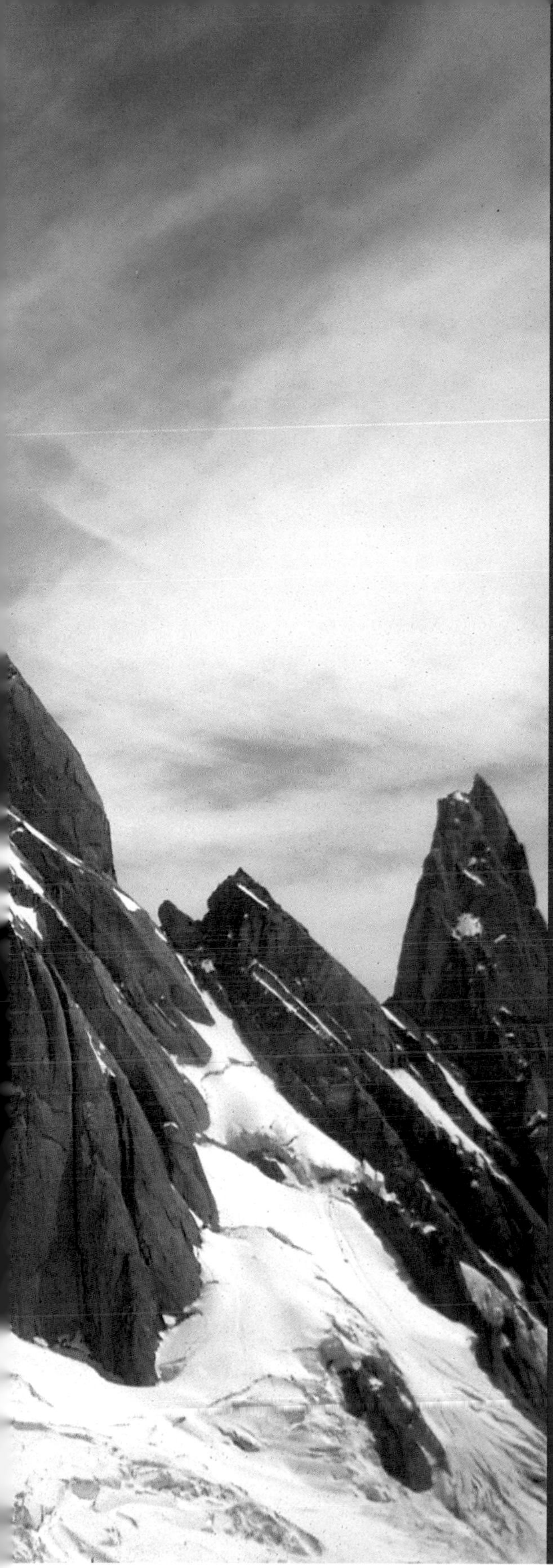

CERRO TORRE, INFINITO SOUTH

1995 – SOUTHERN PATAGONIAN ANDES

SUMMIT HEIGHT

3128m

HEIGHT OF FACE

c. 1350m (from 1780 to 3128m)

DIFFICULTIES

A4/VII

TIME

15–25 days, using the Big Wall system

STARTING POINT

Torre Glacier; approach from Chaltén via the Hosteria Fitz Roy (roadhead) and the Laguna Torre.

OVERVIEW

The 'Infinito Sud' is the South Face Direttissima and takes a line between the Slovenian Routes of 1988 (left) and 1994 (right).

TIPS

The first ascent team spent 24 days on the wall, using an aluminium bivi box as a 'mobile camp'. The summit ice mushroom could not be climbed. Descent was made via the 1970 Maestri Bolt Route.

Due to the weather conditions, all of the routes on Cerro Torre, particularly those on the south and east of the mountain are serious Big Wall undertakings.

'The big problem on Cerro Torre is the storms. Every big face there should really be measured twice.'

REINHOLD MESSNER

'If the storm would only abate we could then reach the summit. But the mountain answers our gentle request with a windy belch.'

REINHARD KARL

Over a period of 23 days, from 4 to 26 November 1995, Ermanno Salvaterra, Piergiorgio Vidi and Roberto Manni climbed their ideal line on the South Face (left of the sunlit wall) of Cerro Torre.

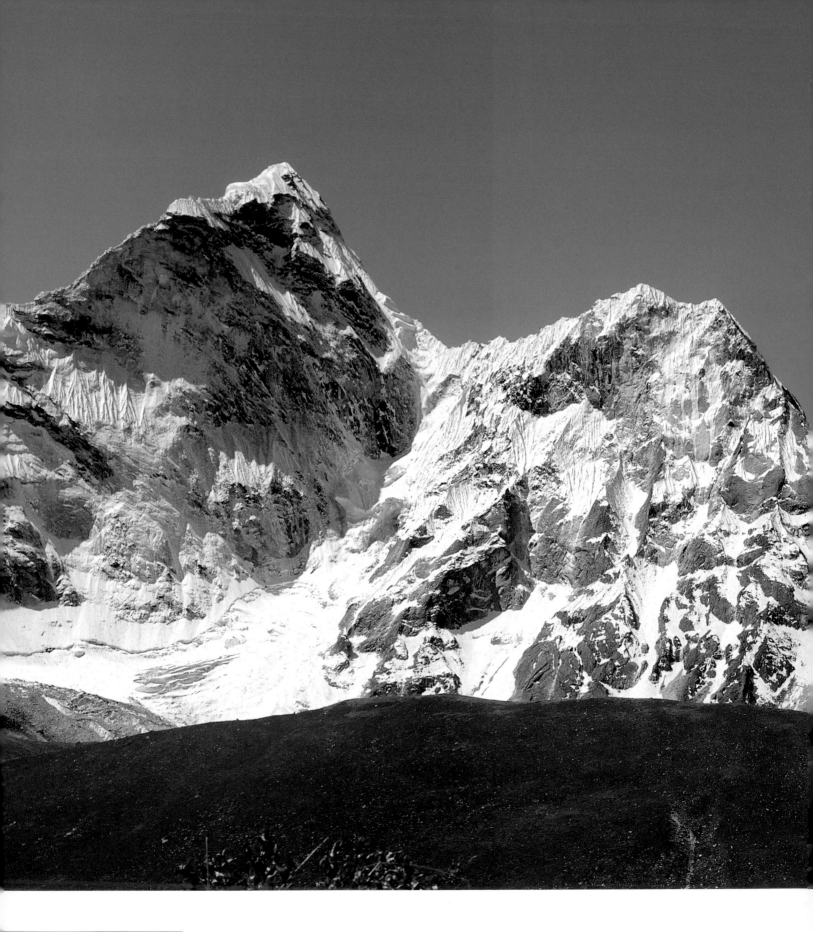

Ama Dablam,
North-West Face

1996 – Nepal Himalaya

Summit Height
6828m

Height of Face
1650m (between 5180 and 6828m)

Difficulties
Rock to VI/A2, ice to 90 degrees

Time
3–4 weeks' acclimatization; 5–6 days' climbing

Starting Point
Base camp on the Duwo Glacier, approach from Lukla (airfield) via Namche Bazar, Pangpoche and Duwo.

Overview
The route climbs a hanging glacier to the left of the huge band of seracs to gain the face proper, which begins with a high rock band. This is breached at its 'weakest point' before a long rightwards traverse leads onto the central ice field. The rock band above is climbed at the point where the ice reaches furthest up the cliff. Trend right across an ice field towards the summit fall line and climb mixed ground to the ridge.

Tips
After one failed attempt, the two-man first ascent team climbed the face Alpine style over five days. The lower part of the face is threatened by seracs and there is considerable danger of avalanches. The rock on the second rock band is loose.

Ama Dablam from the north.

'A few metres above the stance I pulled off a rock the size of a rucksack and together, in splendid harmony, we flew down the face. ... Tomaz was able to hold my fall.'

Vanja Furlan

The Slovenians Vanja Furlan und Tomaž Humar made the first ascent of the 1650m high, extremely difficult West Face of Ama Dablam (left of picture) from 30 April to 4 May 1996, in Alpine style. They dedicated their route to the passionate Big Wall climber Stane Belak, who made the first ascents of the South Face of Makalu and the right-hand side of the South Face of Dhaulagiri and lost his life in December 1995 in the Julian Alps.

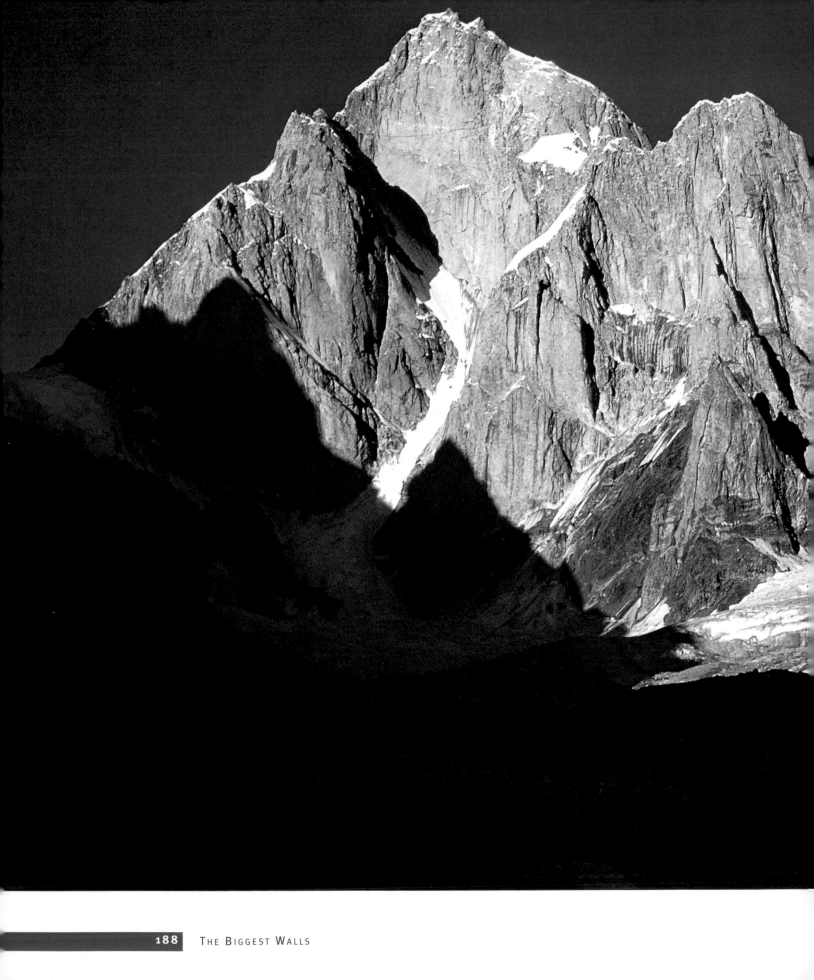

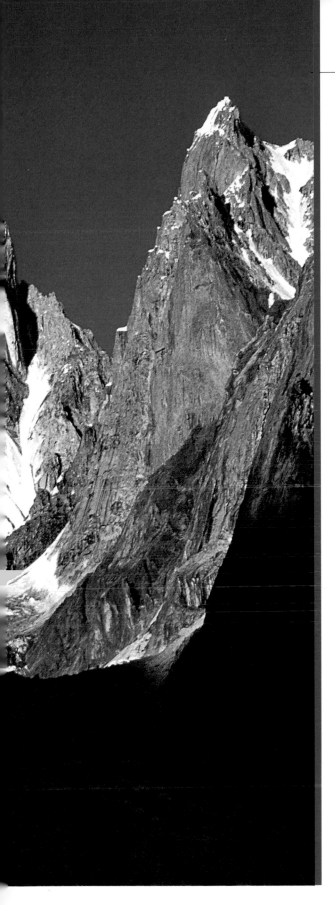

LATOK II, WEST FACE

1997 – KARAKORUM

SUMMIT HEIGHT

7108m

HEIGHT OF FACE

c. 2100m (between 5000 and 7108m)

DIFFICULTIES

A3/VII, ice to 55 degrees, difficult mixed ground near the top of the route

TIME

5–6 days, after acclimatization and transport of equipment up the ice couloir to the start of the 1000m 'Big Wall'

STARTING POINT

Advanced base camp at the foot of the wall (c. 4900m). Base camp (c. 4400m) is located in a grassy hollow between moraines at the confluence of the Uzun Brakk Glacier and the nameless glacier that comes down from the West Face of Latok II. (From Askole – rough Jeep track to here – follow the Braldu River and go 30km up the Biafo Glacier.)

OVERVIEW

The route climbs the c. 1000m ice couloir to the foot of the actual West Face. From here it takes a line more or less up the centre of the face on compact granite. Higher up, thin cracks lead to the mixed ground of the exit pitches.

TIPS

The ice couloir is under constant threat from seracs, stonefall and avalanches and can only be justifiably climbed at night. Fixed ropes were used on the first ascent, both in the couloir and on a large part of the Big Wall itself.

On the neighbouring Ogre, which has only ever been climbed once, there are a number of Big Wall problems waiting to be solved.

'We have done it, as a team. All four of us together on the summit. Toni, Conrad, Thomas and me. The summit is just a small, flat pile of snow at a height of 7108m but it is more, much more than that. For us the summit means the end of a desire that had captivated us for years.'

ALEXANDER HUBER

Alexander and Thomas Huber, Toni Gutsch and the leading US mountaineer Conrad Anker climbed a direct line on the West Face of Latok II. All four climbers summited on 19 July 1997.

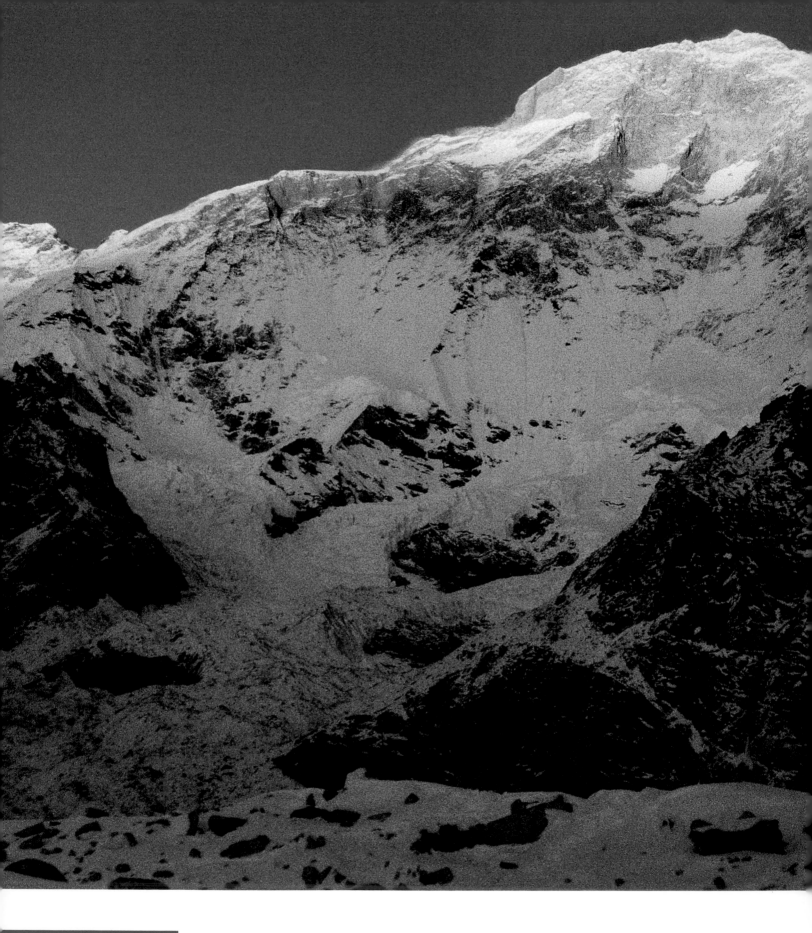

MAKALU, WEST FACE

1997 – NEPAL HIMALAYA

SUMMIT HEIGHT

8463m

HEIGHT OF FACE

c. 2650m (between 5800 and 8463m)

DIFFICULTIES

Extremely difficult route with big ice fields (to 55 degrees), hard mixed climbing and an almost vertical rock pillar

TIME

4–6 weeks' acclimatization and preparation (establishment of camps and fixed ropes on the face); 4–8 days' climbing

STARTING POINT

Makalu Base Camp (4850m), approached from Tumlingtar (airfield) via Khadbari, the Barun La and Shershon.

OVERVIEW

The route starts roughly in the centre of the face and climbs a steep hanging glacier before taking a rising rightwards line up ice fields and mixed ground to gain the left-hand (northern) cliffs of the West Buttress. Continue just left of the buttress, moving right onto the top of the buttress before the overhanging central summit headwall. Then up the South Ridge to the summit.

TIPS

On the first ascent, a camp was placed at 7300m on the face. From here, the team bivouacked several times before reaching the top of the West Buttress. About 250m below the summit one of the members of the expedition died of exhaustion; three days later, another was killed by a falling rock during the descent.

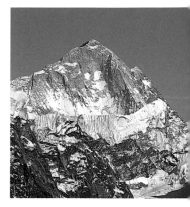

The West Face of Makalu.

'The most memorable moment was when Alexej shouted down that the face was done.'

NIKOLAI JILINE

The new line on the West Face of Makalu to the left of the West Buttress was 'the best of '97'. This technically demanding route was the work of a Russian expedition under the leadership of Sergej Efimov. Five members of the six-man team reached the summit on 21 May: Alexej Bolotov, Yuri Ermatchek, Nikolai Jiline, Dmitri Pavlenko and Igor Bugachevski. They rated the route as 'the most difficult climb of their lives'. Salavat Habibulin died of exhaustion about 250m short of the summit. Bugachevski was killed by stonefall on the descent.

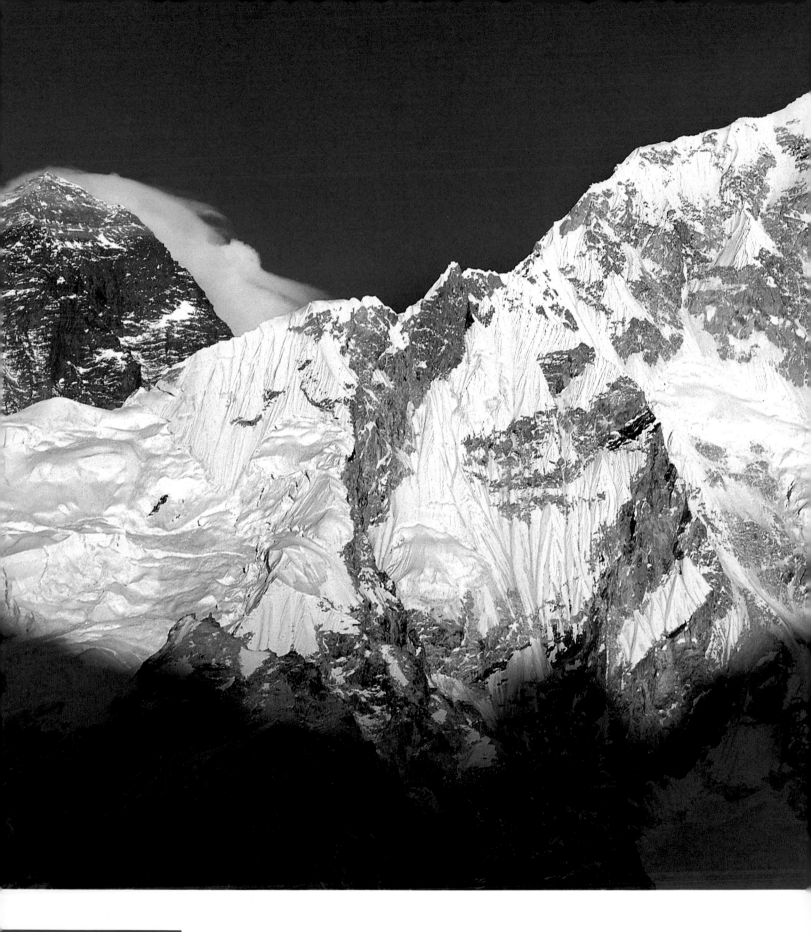

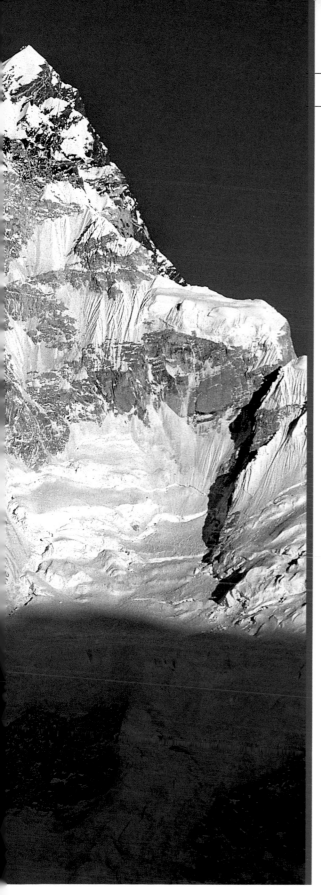

NUPTSE, NORTH-WEST SUMMIT, WEST FACE

1997 – NEPAL HIMALAYA

SUMMIT HEIGHT

7742m

HEIGHT OF FACE

Over 2500m (from 5200 to 7742m)

DIFFICULTIES

Rock to VI, ice to 80 degrees, extremely hard mixed climbing

TIME

Approx. 4 weeks' acclimatization; 5–6 days' climbing

STARTING POINT

Glacier camp beneath the West Face; approach from Lukla (airfield) via Namche Bazar, Pangpoche, Pheriche, Dugla, Lobuche and the Khumbu Glacier.

OVERVIEW

To gain the actual face, an extremely steep serac band is crossed on its far left-hand side. A steep ice wall is then climbed, direct at first, then rightwards. Cross two rock bands in the central part of the face, avoid the direct line on the summit head wall on the right and then straight up to the North-West Summit.

TIPS

The first ascent was done Alpine style, with four bivouacs in a small bivi tent. There is extreme danger from falling chunks of ice in the serac zone at the foot of the face and the face itself is prone to avalanches and frequent stonefall. One of the first climbers slipped off close to the summit – presumably the high wind caused him to lose his balance – and fell to his death down the South Face.

'My head tells me I should keep going but my body reacts slowly and loses strength rapidly. A horrible feeling! Automatically, I place my ice tools and crampons in the hard ice, powered only by the instinct to survive.'

TOMAŽ HUMAR

Tomaž Humar and Janez Jeglič made an Alpine-style ascent of the extremely difficult 2500m West Face of the North-West Summit of Nuptse from 27 to 31 October. Jeglič had gone on ahead a short way below the top, reached the summit at 1.00pm and waved. A short while later Humar reached the highest point but failed to meet up with his partner. He could see his footsteps on the south side of the ridge, caught a very brief glimpse of Jeglič, shouted to him and watched carefully. The wind was blowing in gusts as Humar reached the last of his partners tracks. He saw only the radio and heard that it was still turned on. Jeglič had gone.

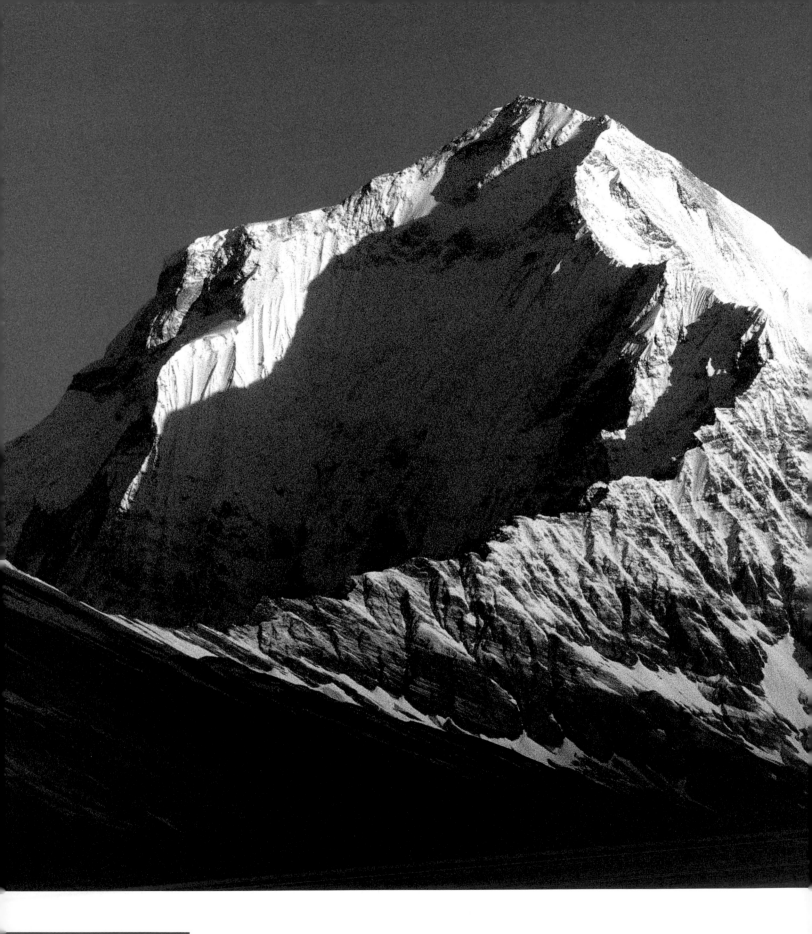

DHAULAGIRI I, SOUTH FACE, HUMAR ROUTE

1999 – NEPAL HIMALAYA

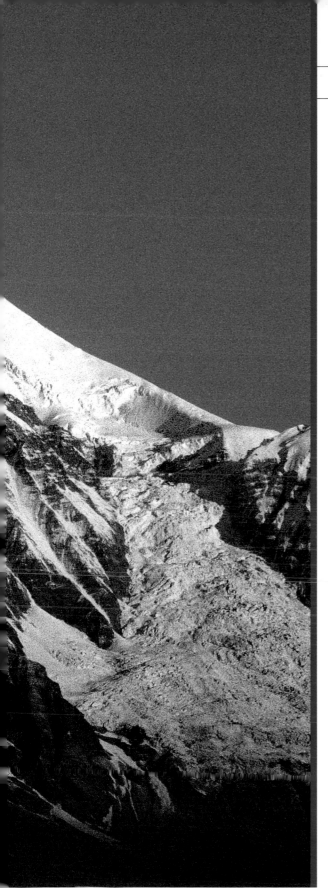

SUMMIT HEIGHT

8167m

HEIGHT OF FACE

c. 4200m (between 3800 and 8000m)

DIFFICULTIES

To M ('mixed') 7+, rock to VII and ice to 90 degrees; extremely hard mixed climbing, even at 7600m

TIME

4–6 weeks' acclimatization; 7–10 days' climbing

STARTING POINT

Base camp is approached either by helicopter or on foot from the Kali Gandaki through a very dangerous gorge.

OVERVIEW

The route takes a line to the right of the central couloir, climbing two rock buttresses and trending right up the huge, very steep ice wall to the top.

TIPS

There is a serious danger of stonefall and falling ice on the route. On the first ascent the route was soloed in eight days by Tomaz Humar, who then traversed from the exit pitch on the South-East Ridge across the East Face (narrow at this point) to the Normal Route (North-East Buttress) and descended this.

The extent to which Slovenian mountaineers have dominated big wall mountaineering over the last decade is illustrated by their impressive routes on the South-West Face of Shisha Pangma (2150m, 1989), the South-East Face of Api (2600m), the North-West Face of Dolaye (2500m), the South Face of Nampa (1950m, all 1996) and the North Face of Gyachung Khang (1999).

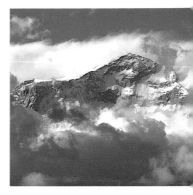

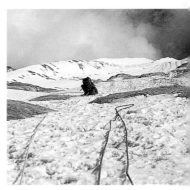

Belak's attempt on the South Face.

'The water froze against my body, cracking with every move I made.'

TOMAŽ HUMAR

Tomaž Humar, currently one of the most successful mountaineers in the world, is credited with finding the best solution so far to the South Face of Dhaulagiri I with his eight-day solo ascent accomplished from 26 October to 2 November 1999. A huge achievement and the latest milestone in Big Wall mountaineering.

Mount McKinley (Denali), East Face

Alaska

Summit Height

6195m

Height of Face

Over 2000m

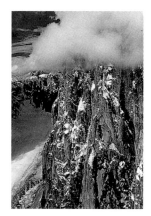

Big Wall on Mount Dickey.

The ice-plastered East Face of the highest mountain of the North American continent is still unclimbed and is, perhaps, the greatest remaining big mountain face in the western hemisphere. It is entirely possible that US climbers will find a solution to it. In recent years they have produced a series of top-flight climbers for whom big-wall mountaineering is becoming more and more popular. There is another big wall on Mount McKinley (Denali) in addition to this face: the South Face.

One of the famous lines is the Cassin Pillar (1961). Even harder are the American Route (1967) and the Czech Direct (1984).

Apart from the routes on Denali, the big walls of Mount Foraker (5303m), Mount Huntington (3731m) or Mount Hunter (4442m) also offer ample opportunities for multi-day (or even multi-week) climbs of the highest standards.

Mount Logan (5959m), the highest mountain in Canada, has one of the highest big walls in the world with its 4000m South Face. Between 1965 and 1979 'some of the best routes in North America' (Chic Scott) were added to its buttresses and ridges. Since the face is also several kilometres wide, there are still numerous possibilities for new routes. Similar scope exists on other mountains in the St Elias region. The fifty-pitch routes on the walls and buttresses of Mount Kennedy, for example, have occupied top climbers for many weeks and months (e.g. North Buttress, 1968, 56 pitches, VI/A3).

It is not only in the Himalayas, then, but in the 'New World' too, that huge possibilities still exist for generations of climbers to push back the frontiers of big wall mountaineering – and that in a remote and wilderness setting.

> **'All of my future climbs will be directed towards the greatest possible challenges: summits that can only be reached by climbing devilishly dangerous big walls.'**
>
> Tomaž Humar

On Mount McKinley in Alaska: not only the freezing cold of the arctic north, but midnight sun too.

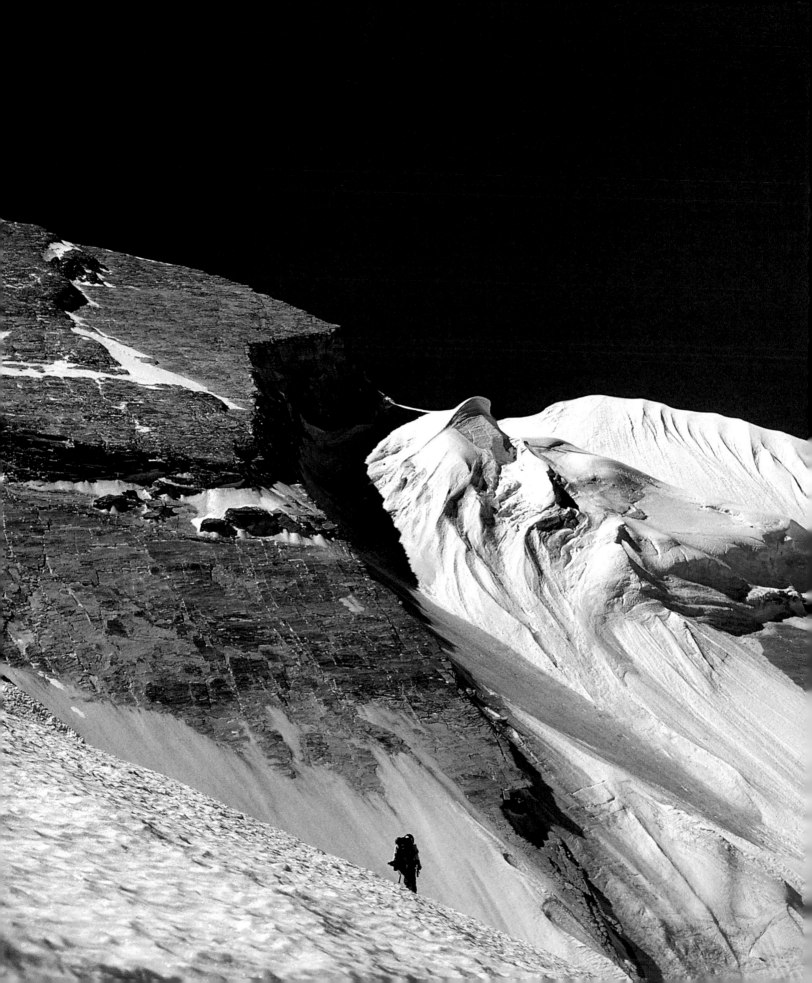

EXPEDITIONS 2000

The times when expeditions were organized and financed by the state or by some club or other do not appear to be over yet. As in the past there are still some individual expedition managers who set up expeditions using contracts with industry and the press, through fund-raising and political contacts, and then invite leading mountaineers to join them. But nowadays the more normal way is for a group of friends to set off to a particular destination abroad or to use the services of a commercial expedition. The many different groups then assemble at Base Camp and set off up the mountain in single file. But they do not venture onto the Big Walls. It is not necessarily the case that such a mammoth expedition has more chance of success than a small group. This way of doing things merely makes it easier to get to altitude – and thus into the danger zone.

On the Big Walls things are the same as they have always been. A group of friends set themselves the objective of a difficult and high climb on one of the mountains of the world, and plans for years in advance. The preparations are comprehensive, the acquisition of equipment costs money and not every participant has holiday entitlement at the desired time. But fortunately half a dozen expedition members can make use of the cheap charter flights and once there, specialist tour operators are available to organize the transport to Base Camp.

But then, on the mountain, the disagreements soon begin. Almost always. If indeed there are no differences of opinion during the expedition, then neither will there be any friction afterwards. If differences do emerge, however, neither expedition contracts nor keeping silent will cause them simply to disappear from the world. Fundamental differences of opinion are at the heart of every expedition. If one were to delete these differences in opinion from the reports presented afterwards, they would give a distorted or even dishonest picture of events. It would be ridiculous to instruct a court of law to investigate what happened, for example, below the summit of the South Face of Aconcagua. Outsiders would be in no position to reconstruct events, nor to empathize and certainly not to examine or to judge.

For these reasons, I rejected the idea of participant contracts for all the trips that I organized and to this day have never regretted the decision. Perhaps I chose my climbing companions with too little care, but our anarchic approach did work. The responsibility I took upon myself as 'expedition leader' on a dozen Big Walls induced me to proceed slowly and with caution and to take over the lead at critical points during the climb.

I do not think much of authoritarian expedition leadership, particularly when the leader of the team is not chosen by the team members as a result of his mountaineering experience, his ability and his organizational skills.

(facing page): On the central part of the North-West Face of Annapurna.

(bottom): The unclimbed faces of the Himalaya, the Karakorum and the Pamirs are more numerous than those that have been climbed. There are plenty of challenging objectives – the real challenge lies in the creative solutions to these problems.

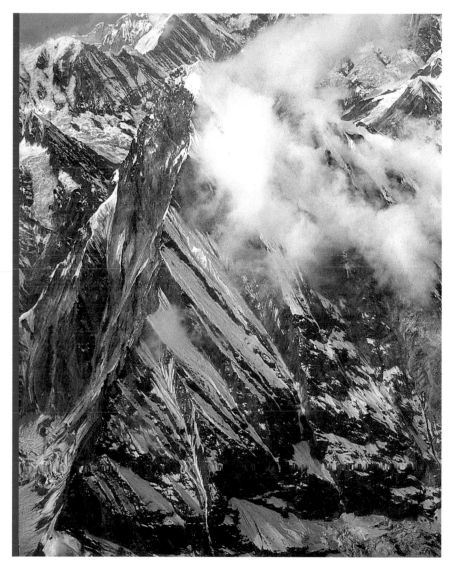

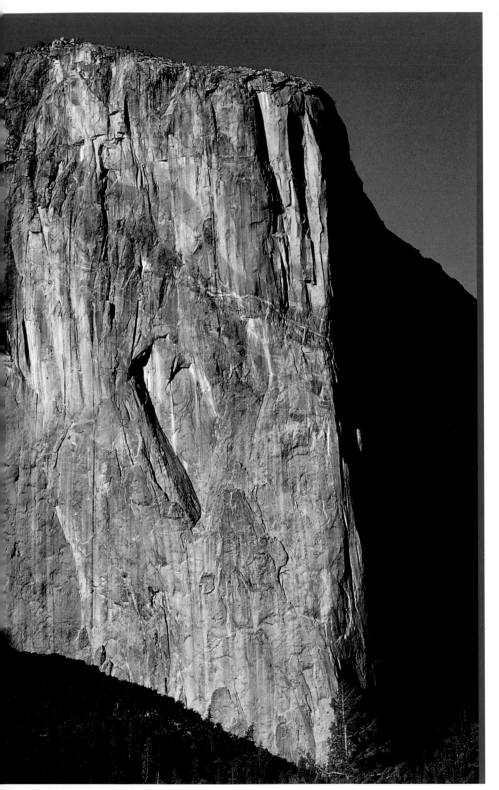

Yes, there are still 'last problems', and there will continue to be. What does not seem possible today will be attempted tomorrow and done the next day.

But even the Big Walls that have already been climbed usually retain their charismatic aura. To repeat these routes remains a challenge; whether and how often a route is climbed is a criteria for its flair. How many of the Big Walls have received few or no repeat attempts? Even the East Face of Monte Rosa, a 'problem' since the beginnings of modern mountaineering, is and remains a great route, just like the Eigerwand and the South Face of Makalu, even though these latter two do place considerably higher demands on the climber. And the central section of the Rupal Face has not been repeated since 1970!

When Tomaž Humar soloed the South Face of Dhaulagiri, all he wanted to do was to get up it. His route never became fashionable, no more so than the West Face of Makalu, the North Face of Jannu or the West Face of Gasherbrum IV would become world famous.

The other Big Walls are a different matter. These routes, although technically far more difficult than anything climbed on the Big Faces, are much safer and shorter. Nowadays, such vertical rock climbing can be well organized with Portaledges and Cliff-hangers.

The highest of these Big Walls in the world on the Great Trango Tower in the Karakorum was climbed for the first time in 1999 and will soon be a classic. When it was first climbed there were already three teams on the mountain at the same time, one Russian, one from the USA (Lowe, Ogden, Synnott) and an international group with Gabor Berecz, Oskar Nadasdi and Thomas Tivadar. This second team arrived too late to secure the first ascent, which it had been in planning for a long time. The Americans had already climbed a series of dihedrals – a logical line – when Tivadar arrived at Base Camp. He and his partner found another route 'Lost Butterfly', almost 2000m of vertical rock, difficulty level A4+, free climbing 5.10 (VII), a total of forty-five rope lengths. When the Americans had finished their route Tivadar followed it for a further ten pitches.

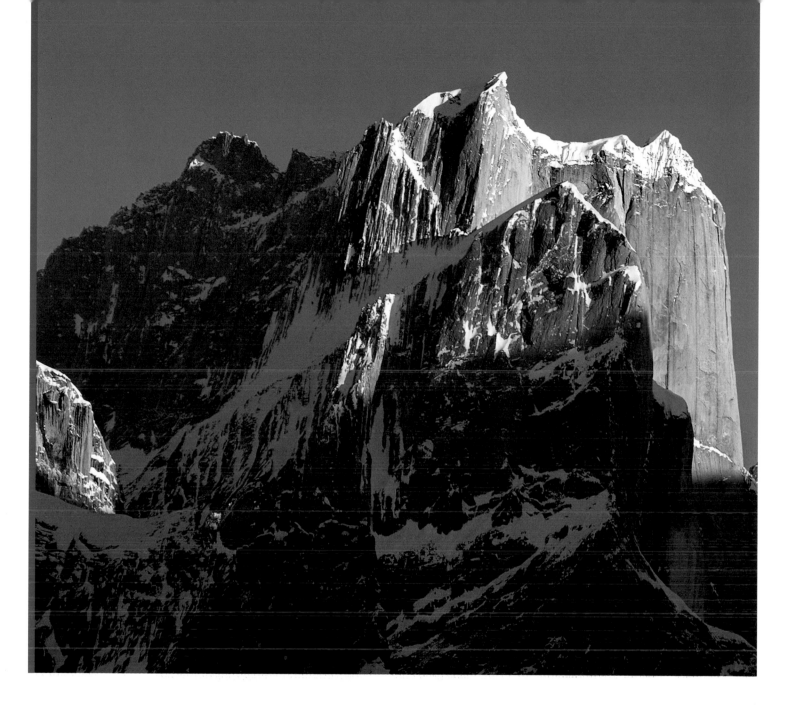

These are the new dimensions! Respect is due. Nevertheless, Big Walls of this type are climbed all over the world – on Baffin Island, in Antarctica, in the Pamir and in Patagonia. But only a few dare to venture onto the true Big Walls, the 'Great Faces'.

These Big Walls are the mixed climbing test pieces which share the common attributes of steepness, difficulty and danger – the East Face of Gasherbrum I, the direct West Face of Makalu, the giant wall on Namcha Barwa or the South-West Buttress of Annapurna IV, to name but a few. They are the essence of the challenge. There are hundreds more, perhaps not all as high as the South Face of Dhaulagiri but many are steeper, more difficult, more dangerous – like for example the North-East Wall of the Arwa Tower in the Garhwal Himalaya.

One thing is certain: such problems, if they should ever be solved, will be avoided, just like the main route on the North-West Face of the Kleine Civetta in the Dolomites, a climb that, almost 100 years after the first ascent, can still be a nail-biting experience for even the best climbers today.

Big Wall climbing, whether practised on El Capitan (facing page) or on the Trango Towers (above) is in no way identical to Big Wall mountaineering, even though the two systems do overlap nowadays.

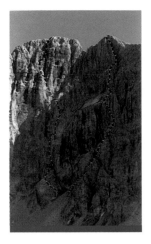

The twin summits of the Civetta with the Solleder Route on the left and the Haupt Route on the right.

'After its first ascent this route offered one of the most important rock climbing trips around. After the other great faces in the Civetta group had been climbed this ascent lost a lot of its significance. As far as the line is concerned it is ideal, yet the rock is very friable in parts and particularly on the lower two thirds of the wall there is great danger from stonefall.'

TONI HIEBELER

The future began almost eighty years ago on the Civetta Wall, fifty years ago on the South Face of Aconcagua and only yesterday on the White Wall of Dhaula. In the mid-sixties, the central Civetta Wall was still considered to be the 'wall of walls', at least in the Dolomites. The rock face above Lake Alleghe was stylized by Domenico Rudatis, with considerable use of hyperbole, as 'the kingdom of the sixth grade' and is much more than merely a series of dolomite limestone towers piled vertically above one another. The stonefall, the rock, which in many parts is wet and/or friable, and the 'Cristallo', the heart-shaped ice field to the upper right of the middle of the wall give it a serious feel. The sunny South Face of the Marmolada may be broader and more compact, but it is less dismissing. The North face of Monte Agnér is higher, but not so secretive. Even now, when walls four times as high have been climbed on the eight-thousanders and when neither the ascents nor the number of fatalities on the Eigerwand are counted any longer, the Civetta Wall still hides a puzzle: the mountaineering masterpiece of one Oswald Gabriel Haupt.

His direct route on the North Wall of the Kleine Civetta has never been repeated as a complete rock route and is obviously every bit as difficult as the other two classic routes that climb the central section of the face, the 'Solleder' and the 'Philipp-Flamm'.

In the summer of 1967 I climbed a route to the main summit of the Civetta with Sepp Mayerl, Heini Holzer and Renato Reali. It was a logical line because it lent itself to free-climbing, and went up between these existing lines, using the last section of the Solleder route before topping out. Our 'variation start' is more direct and safer as far as stonefall is concerned but the climbing is not more difficult. Although is it no easier than the Philipp-Flamm dihedral further left, the line it takes is not so modern in concept.

Like Walter Philipp ten years earlier, in those days I was of the opinion that 'modern alpinism needed the impetus of the free-climbing style' and thus I free-climbed exclusively.

The route climbed by Walter Philipp and Dieter Flamm over three days in 1957, taking the striking dihedral system to the left of the central section of the face, was both model and stimulus to me at one and the same time. I knew Philipp's route and shared his opinion: 'True to the motto "artists work without a safety net", the two young climbers climb the dihedral with inadequate protection from just three bolts in 30m, at a consistent level of difficulty of V or VI, right up to a point beneath the large roof. The next morning, after bivouacking, they manage to overcome this section in free-climbing style, safeguarded only by the three pegs on the belay.'

Philipp's dream was to come true: 'To be able to do a route one day on which free climbing, which in certain circles was really scorned, could achieve new acclaim'.

Walter Philipp could have been the spiritual relation of Emil Solleder. 'I had never before seen a wall such as this in the Alps'. This exclamation by Solleder showed at the same time his respect and his enthusiasm for the Civetta Wall.

Hans Fiechtl had warned Solleder against making his attempt: 'You should keep you hands off this face. The terrible stonefall, the amount of ice and the endless wall – Preuss, Dibona, Innerkofler and a whole row of Englishmen with really important guides have stood in vain before it.' He wanted to attempt it nevertheless. 'The lower section in particular looks hopeless', Solleder realized at the start of the climb.

After an attempt with Lettenbauer and Gaberl as a trio, with Lettenbauer leading the difficult starting traverse, on 7 August 1925 Solleder and Lettenbauer set off again. They mastered the central section of the wall beneath the main summit with only a dozen intermediate pegs and in just one day! Solleder, who this time led the whole climb, used only one climbing 'trick' to overcome a section of the face that was 'impossible' to free climb when, hardly a rope length beneath the gully, it took a big, fat ring peg to succeed. Inclined somewhat downwards, but hammered into the rock right up to the ring, it was the only way of attacking this section of the route. It was the first time that the wall had refused to succumb to pure climbing techniques, and it came at one of the most exposed points on the climb.

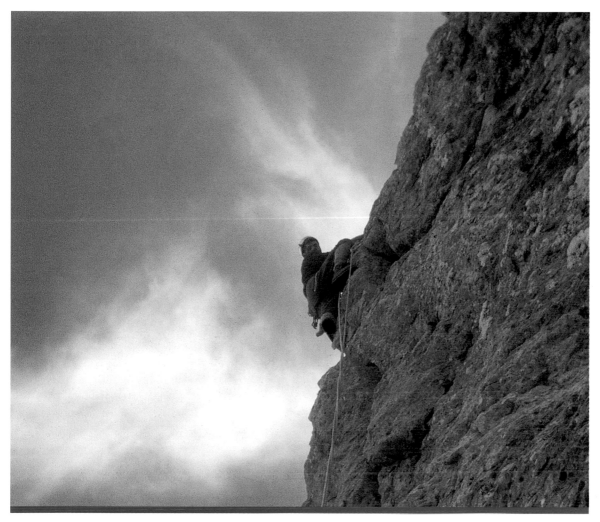

'In February 1993, Georg Kronthaler and Nicholas Mailänder successfully completed the first winter ascent of the "Haupt-Lömpel" on the Kleine Civetta.'

HORST HÖFLER

'"That Haupt must have been a cheeky scoundrel" Georg says whilst I, securely protected with a wire wedge, cheat my way up via a filigreed slab in the lower VI degree of difficulty.'

NICHOLAS MAILÄNDER

The Solleder route on the Civetta was to become the yardstick for the climbing art of a young generation of rock acrobats who a few years later were looking for new routes on the Civetta.

For half a century it was a must for every ambitious Dolomite climber. It is therefore understandable that the classic 'Solleder' should have eclipsed the old Haupt route on the right section of the face and all but erased it from the Alpine journals and yearbooks. It would be a mistake, however, if the climber Haupt was also to be forgotten. On the contrary G. Haupt belongs amongst the most significant mountaineers in the history of Alpine climbing.

On 30 July 1920 Oswald Gabriel Haupt and Karl Lömpel had found a direct route on the North Face of the Kleine Civetta which Haupt described precisely for the high mountain climber 'Purtscheller/Hess': 38 rope lengths, 1000m difference in altitude, in parts extremely difficult crack,

chimney and wall climbing. The 'Solleder' (1400m) is shorter than the 'Haupt' (1500m).

The difficulties are about the same, although the 'Solleder' has more climbing at grade VI, a level of difficulty which had just previously been defined as the limit of what it was possible to climb.

After only two repeats, with variations, during the past eighty years (Vittorio Ratti and Luigi Esposito in 1937 and Giuliano de Marchi and Alessandro Masucci in 1985) one should consider that with the 'Haupt-Lömpel' route the first grade VI in climbing history had been achieved back in 1910, and also that Oswald Gabriel Haupt should be recognized as an important character in alpinism. Climbing history does not have to be re-written; it just needs a correction.

In 1910, the most difficult of the great Dolomite routes were the Einser North Face (first ascent 18 July 1910) in the Sexten Dolomites and the South-West Face of the Croz dell'Altissimo (first ascent

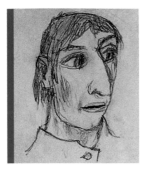

Oswald Gabriel Haupt.
Portrait by Peter Fellin.

'When our aneroid
showed 2500m – we
were about 100
metres below the
ice field and still
had 700 or 800
metres left to climb
– we began to have
considerable
doubts because of
the deterioration in
the weather. Since
we had yet to make
a decision to tackle
the strikingly big
black chimneys, we
decided to stop for
a break in a small
cave and to observe
the weather. Then
we decided to make
our retreat.

PAUL HÜBEL, 1907

16 August 1910 with Angelo Dibona and Luigi Rizzi as mountain guides and Guido and Max Meyer as paying guests). A year later Preuss and Relly were successful in the first repeat of this bold Brenta Tour, which approaches the VI level on one section. Preuss, a measure for the level the art of climbing had achieved at that time, was unable to attempt the Haupt-Lömpel route on the Kleine Civetta and so a direct comparison was not possible.

Haupt did, however, manage to repeat another Dibona route, the North-West Buttress on the Langkofel (first climbed on 19 July 1911 by Dibona, Rizzi and the Mayer brothers), a route which those who climbed it first had rated as probably the most difficult climb in the Dolomites, more difficult than their route on the Croz dell'Altissimo. They had tricked their way up the crux section of the Langkofel summit tower using a lasso method. Only a month later (19 August 1911) Haupt and Flum made the second ascent, taking a more difficult, more direct route on the lower section and with Haupt leading the crux of the Dibona route on the summit tower free.

Back to the Direttissima on the Kleine Civetta. Even by today's standards, the 'Haupt-Lömpel' is a modern mountaineering route. There is no doubt that pre- 1910 no other route existed which was so difficult, so long and so demanding.

Only after the First World War were new routes achieved in the Dolomites which could be considered counterparts to the 'Haupt-Lömpel': the North Face of Agnér 'first climbed in 1921 by Jori/Andreoletti/Zanutti), the Pelmo North Wall (1924, Simon/Rossi), the North Face of the Furchetta (1925, Solleder/Wiessener) and the North-West Face of the Civetta (1925, Solleder/Lettenbauer).

In my 'storm and stress' days I repeated half a dozen Haupt routes in the Dolomites. All of them impressed me because of their difficulty, their bold lines, and because there were hardly any pegs *in situ*. They were all undergraded. Only one was well known, the 'Kiene-Crack' on the Fünffinger Spitze. This route to the left of the 'Schmitt Chimney', also known as the 'Diagonal Crack' was climbed for the first time on 26 August 1912 by Haupt and Kiene. Today it is a fashionable route. Almost all the other Haupt routes – are there fifty or more? – are mentioned as notes in the margin or not mentioned at all. Just like Haupt's name in the Alpine history books.

So who was this Dieter Oswald Haupt?

Hans Kiene, from Bozen, has left us a short biography of his friend and climbing companion in his work *Erschliessung der Dolomiten* ('Dolomiten', 1949) which allows us to draw a few conclusions about the life of the best Dolomite climber before the First World War.

Oswald Gabriel Haupt was a gym teacher who came to the Dolomites to go mountaineering in the summers between 1905 and 1913. This large athletic man climbed mainly with friends from Würzburg (Karl Lömpel for example) and a circle of friends of the Kiene brothers from Bozen. He was said to be a pure rock climber and must have cut quite an odd figure. Indeed, with his aquiline nose on his animal-like face, he was often said to have looked like a backwoodsman from the high Alpine pastures.

He was no intellectual and did not play a character.

He was one thing: an extreme individualist with a lot of energy and desire, who did what was important to him. He entertained friends with his humour and strangers he snubbed with his intelligence. As a climber he was careful, experienced and equipped with that pure instinct for sense of direction, rock and weather conditions, which makes the few geniuses amongst mountaineers stand out. They did not merely try to calculate what was still feasible, they went and did it.

In discussion Oswald Gabriel Haupt often took a radical stance and he did not take seriously those 'armchair fanatics' who merely wrote about climbing. It is no wonder that he argued with editors and specialist journals and that nobody else would publish him. That his importance as a creative Dolomite climber was not clear to anyone but a few friends has something to do with the courage of his convictions and his conception of himself which was often wrongly perceived as arrogance.

Oswald Gabriel Haupt, who usually climbed wearing old leather gloves and smoking a cigar, had the ability to shock nosy parkers, irritate know-alls and impress climbing partners.

Oswald Gabriel Haupt came to the Dolomites for the last time in 1913. For the third time, he climbed the Guglia di Brenta, which he had done in 1906 with Ferdinand Forcher-Mayr (later president of the South Tyrol Alpine Club). Then he took his

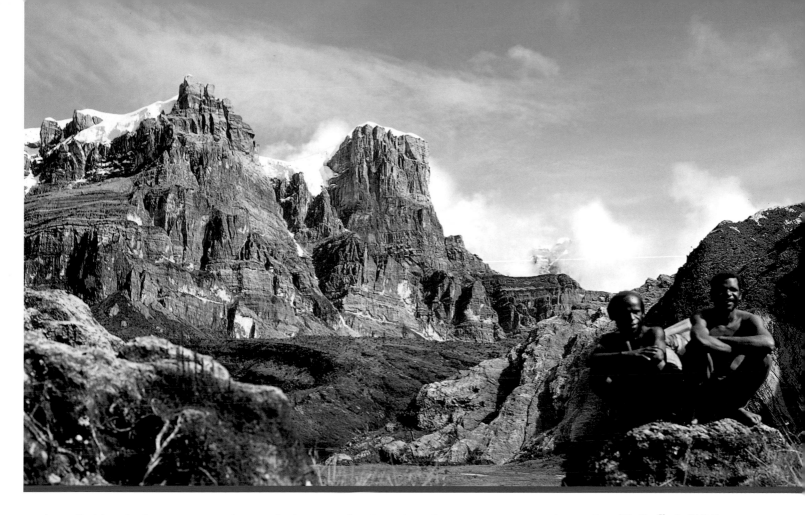

nephew climbing. During a storm, as they made the descent from Torre di Brenta, the latter suffered a fractured skull during a fall and died a few days later in the hospital in Bozen.

This affected Haupt so much that he gave up climbing. Only in 1917 did he begin to climb again – South Tyrol was inaccessible to him because of the war, so he went to the Kaiser, the Wetterstein and the Karwendel. He died on the North Face of the Kaltwasserspitze. Only in 1921 were his body and that of his climbing partner found on a ledge (a bivouac site?) – squashed by a mass of fallen rocks.

What happened to the 'Haupt-Lömpel' on the Kleine Civetta?

It sank more and more into oblivion. During Haupt's lifetime they made the 'mistake' of finishing the climb on a subsidiary summit and later on it was to be overshadowed by the 'Solleder'; this route, in turn, was eclipsed by the 'Philipp-Flamm'.

Now the wheel must have turned full circle if we are again to talk about 'honest' values.

The fact that the 'Kleine Civetta' (3207m), originally considered as the 'Southern Summit' is a few metres lower than the Main Summit (3220m) no longer counts.

Today on the Civetta there is no climb that is longer, more dangerous and more serious than the 'Haupt'. Nor, in the broadest sense of the word, is there a more difficult one. Yet nobody repeats it. At the height of summer there are often a dozen ropes a day on the 'Philipp-Flamm' which is protected with normal pegs and drilled bolts. It is the safest of the three old direct routes on the central section of the wall. The 'Solleder-Lettenbauer', which has also been over-pegged and thus devalued, is repeated less often. If the weather turns bad while you are on it, this can have worse consequences than on the 'Philipp-Flamm', which is protected by roofs and overhangs.

Thus, a re-evaluation of the grading system is once again needed! The length of the route, the availability or non-availability of protection of any kind, the difficulty of route finding must all be taken

Like the Civetta Wall, the Carstensz Mountains of New Guinea also have several big and seldom-climbed faces.

'To date, Oswald Gabriel Haupt has not received the accolades he deserved, yet now he can be considered as a "Big Wall Climber", more so than any other. As a man who pushed the limits of the possible, he even surpassed Paul Preuss.'

REINHOLD MESSNER

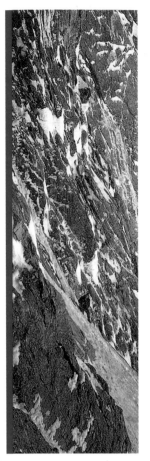

Big Wall mountaineering is also possible in less frequented regions. Forgotten, scorned and feared routes are the objectives of the true experts.

into account if we want to judge a route correctly. We must also consider the so-called 'objective dangers' – which, to be precise, are really subjective if, in addition to climbing ability, we consider instinct, geological knowledge and knowledge about the weather to be part of the mountaineer's capabilities. Also the feeling that the true artists do not merely have the feeling in their little finger, they have it in their head.

A mountaineer of Haupt's genius, who has left nothing behind for the researchers of Alpine history other than a few dozen first ascents, can today really only be judged with reference to these attributes.

For the doctor Giuliano De Marchi, who accompanied me to Makalu in 1986, there is no doubt that Oswald Gabriel Haupt was at least equal to Hans Dülfer in his skills as a pure climber. As a mountaineer he was far superior to him.

For me one thing is certain: Oswald Gabriel Haupt was the best climber of his time! Anyone who does not believe it should try to repeat his route on the Civetta. The friable rock, the wetness, the exposure and the lack of adequate protection mean that even today it is still a difficult repeat.

How great was his achievement then on this dangerous route, with the equipment of 1910, without a route description, without satellite weather reports, without the attendant possibility of helicopter rescue as a back up. The leading mountaineers before the First World War did not climb better than Wolfgang Güllich, to be sure, but they had developed instincts which allowed them to climb safely, even on the North Face of the Kleine Civetta, without good protection, something which I would not like to recommend that the climbing generation of today seek to emulate. It is rare even today that such routes are climbed, be it on Lobuje Peak, on the Great Trango Tower, or on the Ogre.

In 1910, in the heyday of O.G. Haupt, the use of pitons as a trick to effect upward progress was scorned; as a means of protection it was considered an exception. All other modern means of protecting a climb were then unknown. Thus climbers had developed skills to help them survive their dangerous game, skills which have become blunted or lost with the increase in safety equipment and climbing aids.

Overall, the 'Haupt Route' on the Civetta can by today's standards be graded higher than the 'Solleder' and this in turn is of a higher standard than the 'Philipp-Flamm'. This statement turns Alpine history upside down and poses many questions for the young climbing generation.

The danger which today we try to eliminate was and remains an essential and motivating element in alpinism. Since on an artificial climbing wall every danger can be eliminated in favour of increased difficulty and only athletic climbing ability counts, the trend for decades has been to make more and more climbing walls out of the mountains. The true boundary, however, the one that reveals our human limits, is not the tenth, eleventh or twelfth grade but the danger, the causes of which are founded in nature – in the nature of both man and mountain.

I have nothing against artificial climbing walls with screwed-on hand and footholds and intermediate protection points every metre. Yet I still fail to understand that rock should be drilled, filled and prepared in order for people to be happy on it. Since 'free climbers' have in many places started to introduce battery powered drills, quick drying adhesive and cement in order to place pegs and bolts, there now are too many people going to those places, even those places that only yesterday were the preserve of ravens, jackdaws and eagles, where rare lizards and geckos once had their hiding places.

Oswald Gabriel Haupt, this illustrious unknown man, was no modern climber; his way of life was post-modern. He accepted his limits. Anywhere he could not reach without artificial means he did not go. For him there were 'taboo zones'. He respected those rock walls which he could not overcome as impossible for him and therefore inaccessible. His ethic was dictated by the limits of man versus nature and as such his style can be recommended as being worthy of emulation.

Haupt himself did not do this. With his lifetime's achievement, he has left us a piece of art that can only truly be understood by those who love the Civetta Wall. But anyone who climbs by the principle 'enough is not enough' (this is the name given to one of the routes) will have to experience that those people who devastate these walls with their limitless use of technical aids will in the end be banished, driven from them by their own fear.

PERSPECTIVES

How many times have I flown over the Himalaya? This snowland is at its most impressive from a bird's-eye view. Seen from a plane the angles of the Great Walls seem to vary from second to second. After every slight tremor, or every time the aircraft banks, the wall appears to fall flat or to steepen. One moment Mount Everest will look smaller than Lhotse, then it is the other way around; the next, the South-West Face of Everest seems as vertical as the North Face of the Grosse Zinne, then it leans back again and once again hopes and dreams stir within me – hopes that this face could be climbed by two people in Alpine-style.

Meanwhile we have turned round – our flight time is coming to an end, and we glide off to the north west. A glance back reveals the north side of Everest to the Chinese – or more correctly, the Tibetan, side – not as steep as the south side, but this flank too is enormous.

And now we are really close to Cho Oyu, the summit like a giant ice-cream cone. To the left is the steep drop of the South-West Wall with its many gullies and icefields – and not without its dangers. To the right, the South Buttress, which rises diagonally from right to left and which involves mainly ice-climbing. Right of that again is a rather more gentle slope, mainly snow and rock but certainly with the threat of avalanche.

Just as I toyed for five years with the idea of climbing the South Face of Dhaulagiri South Wall so now I played with the idea of climbing the South Buttress of Cho Oyu. But this gigantic pillar 'would have to wait a while', as for a long time the Nepalese authorities refused to grant climbing permits for the mountain. And as long as there were no permits to be had, the buttress – which eventually fell to Polish mountaineers – could not be attempted.

Some of the summits that are spread out beneath me are still unclimbed. But far more than any one of these summits – summits on which no man has yet stood – I am looking at the whole landscape lying below me, as if there must somewhere be one valley, one mountain flank just for me. Suddenly a mountain emerges, the shape of which I like, and now I only have eyes for that one summit. I commit it to my memory. I do not know its name, but nevertheless I know I would like to climb it, or at least attempt it.

For me all these mountains belong to the world, in the same way as I belong to the world, together with the deserts, the rivers, the flowers and the trees. The mountains are neither good nor evil, they are neither my enemies nor my friends; they are simply there. And although there can be storms and avalanches there, the mountains are not malicious.

Harmony, the coexistence of all caution and danger, can only exist in mountaineering when the storms and the avalanches are accepted just as readily as the perfect shapes of these mountains we find so beautiful.

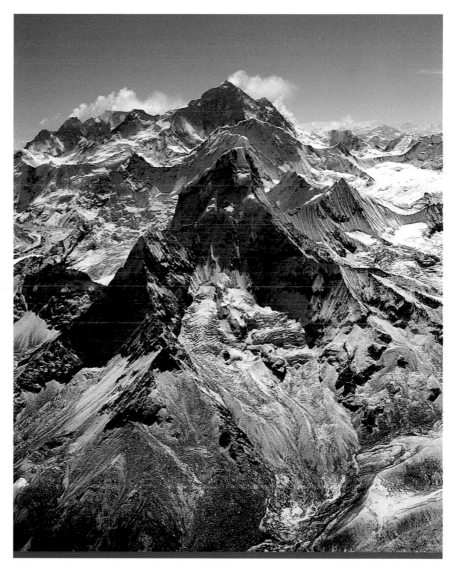

Ama Dablam (centre of picture) and Makalu (on the horizon) are amongst the most beautiful peaks in the Himalayas.

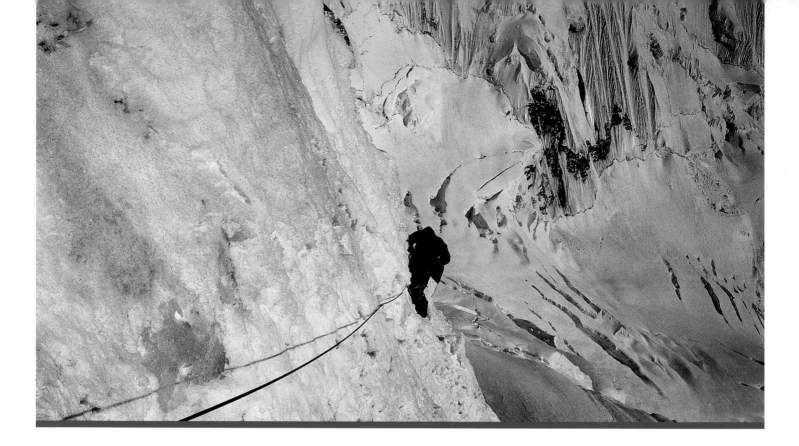

'In the Karakorum alone the great walls are so numerous that the life of one mountaineer is not long enough to study, let alone attempt, all of them. But in Alaska, in Canada, in Garhwal, in Sikkim and Kashmir too there are so many unexplored walls that the top climbers have no need to fear.'

REINHOLD MESSNER

The same fascination that radiates from these shapes also surrounds the unexplored faces. For me in even greater measure, as I view them from the extreme mountaineering perspective. I sense that a challenge is most intensive when the term 'impossible' hangs in the air, even though today in mountaineering nothing is really 'impossible' any more. Yes, by using every imaginable artificial aid any kind of difficulty can now be overcome, even if every danger cannot be averted. And this is where the act of 'pushing back the frontiers' begins. The word 'adventure' has become such an overexploited and devalued term that I no longer care to use it. Imagination plays as much a part in great mountaineering as courage, stamina, determination and enthusiasm.

Mountaineering will not only remain fascinating as long as there are unclimbed mountains and untouched flanks and faces. Mountaineering can still be interesting even when everything has been 'done', but only for those who are open to finding authentic new solutions, and who do so without technology and infrastructure.

After my flights around the Himalayas I am certain that for generations, probably for the duration of the existence of mountaineering, there will be untouched, unclimbed walls, for I have seen hundreds of such objectives. The South Face Direct to the summit of Dhaulagiri is one such challenge.

In the same way as our life is subject to a natural rhythm, so it is with climbing, with each individual route, with each attempt we make to achieve our secret goal or find something within ourselves. If we attempt to miss out a step, we are thrown off balance and the harmony of the process is disturbed.

So every ascent is preceded by the idea. Successes and defeats alternate in the same way as advance and retreat, expectation and disappointment. Viewed in this way every retreat is a necessary constituent of success, a window to a new horizon.

After a great summit success, when one is right there at the top, one can only come down again. And when one is right down at the bottom, once energy levels have been restored, one can climb up again. This interplay of forces eventually leads to true liberation.

Everyone is free to develop and nurture their own imagination, everyone is unique in character, and everyone can realize their own horizons. The things that find recognition with others are not the things that are really important in mountaineering, but the things that are important to oneself. Anyone who is involved in top-level alpinism must be prepared to accept that those same people who congratulate after a 'success' will be scornful after a 'defeat'.

Anyone who wishes to fulfil his dreams however, should not listen to others; he should not shy away from the risks linked with the realization of every dream; he must be prepared to give each one of his dreams a chance to succeed.

Anyone who attempts to orient himself according to the standards set by others can not strive to reach new horizons. What counts is to discover the standards within ourselves and not to let any outside ideas of what constitutes a worthy goal be forced upon us and above all to find the goal within ourselves. Only the courage to embrace new ideas and skills are the guarantees for the next step.

Jannu! All the face routes are still open projects.

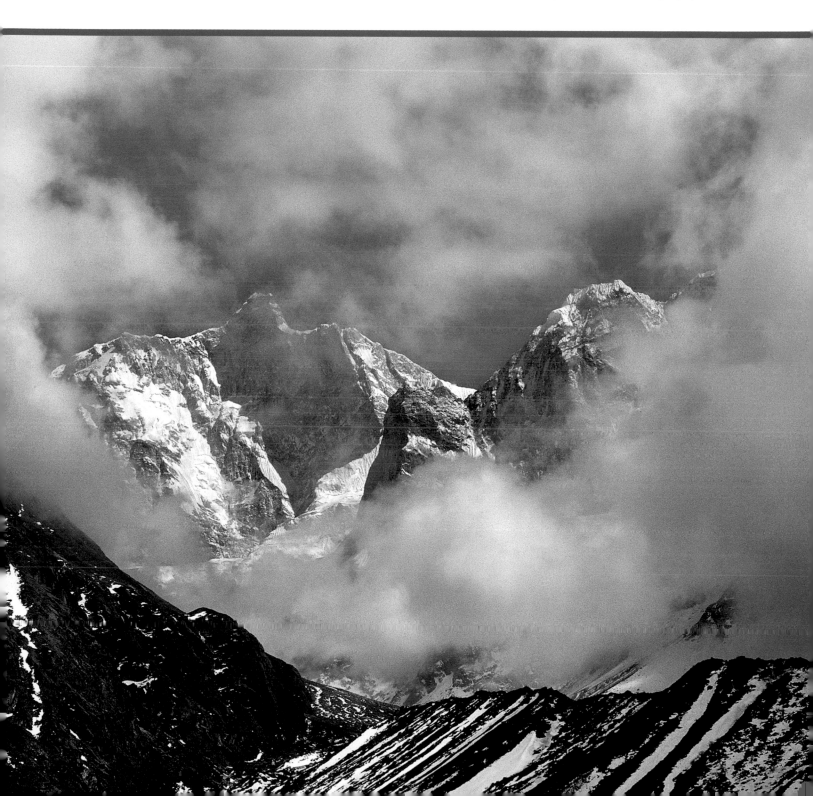

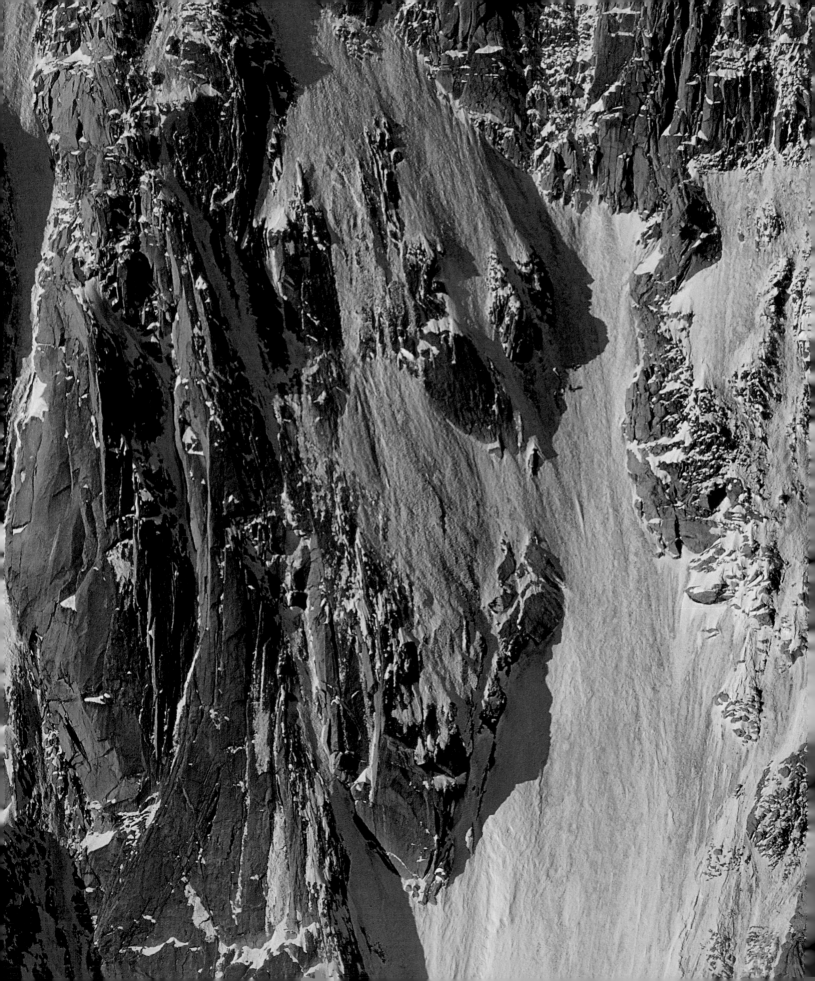

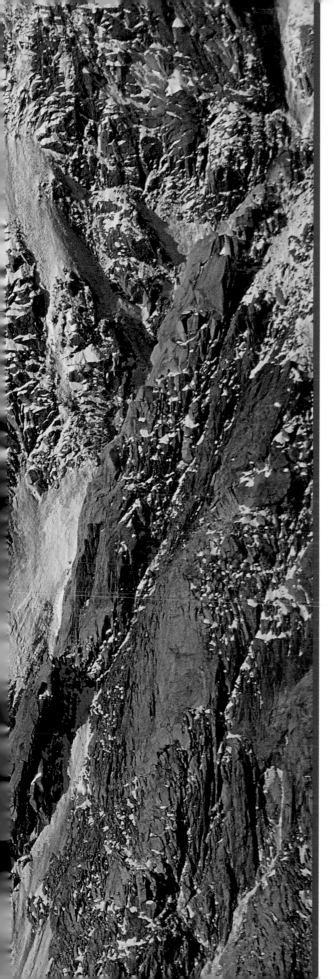

GREAT DAYS, GREAT WALLS

The Great Days is the title of the second book by Walter Bonatti in which he recounts his exploits on the North Face of the Eiger North Wall, the Walker Spur in winter and the Grand Pilier D'Angle. The book, and Bonnatti's mountaineering career, ends with a solo first ascent on the North Face of the Matterhorn in winter. That was in 1965.

Back then, this route of Bonatti's stood as a marker for the level that classic Alpine mountaineering had achieved, in much the same way that the East Face of Monte Rosa, the North West Face of the Civetta and the North Face of the Eiger had done in 1900, 1925 and 1950 respectively.

Walter Bonatti predicted the further development of mountaineering on the Big Walls. What he had achieved on the great walls of the Alps would find its continuation on the big faces of the eight-thousanders and by 1975 it was the South Face of Annapurna South Wall, the Rupal Flank and the South-West Face of Everest that were considered to be the new dimensions in classic mountaineering. The new ice-climbing techniques as well as the globalization of mountaineering then allowed for an enormous further advance in development.

Today, twenty-five years on, almost all the big faces of the eight thousanders have been climbed, while on the 6000 and 7000m peaks such difficult problems have been solved that we can now speak of a new quality of Big Wall Mountaineering. It is these new dimensions with which I am concerned in this book, and with the difficulties and dangers in such high and exposed circumstances that previous generations would not have dared to attempt.

What is transmitted to cosy living rooms at great expense via satellite does not show the ultimate achievements in Big Wall Mountaineering, even today. On the contrary, the more live reports we get from a mountain face, the more preparation has to be done in advance – whether on TV or on the Internet – and the greater the loss of exposure and commitment.

The ingredients of Big Wall Mountaineering remain the same: extreme difficulty, a face over 2000m high and, above all, that level of exposure that is so quickly lost when a TV crew assumes the role of passive observer. So, no aids, no communications, no bolts. No artificial oxygen either. The ABC of the king's discipline of our sport is indeed this easy to define!

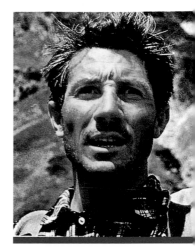

(top): Walter Bonatti, for two decades the most famous Italian mountaineer. A man of the Big Walls.

(facing page): Climbers (centre of picture) on the Grand Pilier d'Angle, Mont Blanc.

'In order to push further the boundaries in the world of the vertical I had to introduce a new dimension: high altitude! Thus one had to transfer to the Himalayas, what I had done in the Alps – extreme alpinism at a height of 8000m and Alpine style.'

WALTER BONATTI

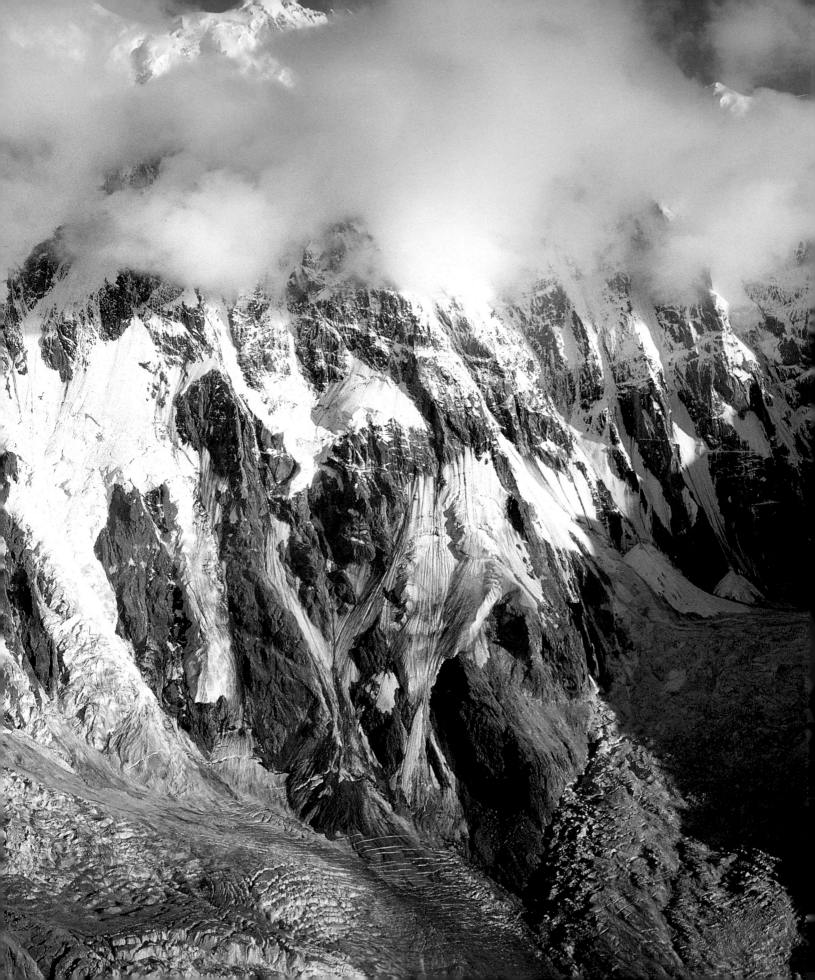

NEW HORIZONS

After reading this book, in which I write of the Big Walls of the Alps, the Andes and the Himalayas, the impression could be created I have tried to establish a set of standards valid for all time. Yet I did not intend to set any ultimate values, only new ones. I was interested first and foremost in extending the concept of the Big Walls. And in the same way as I have not relied upon values attributed to the mountains by others, I hope that the young mountaineering generation will not seek to adhere to my values. None of that which mountaineers have so far achieved would have been possible if it had not at some time been dreamt up by some individual or other, if someone had not used all the power of imagination and dared to go where no one had ever been before. The strength needed to fulfil a task can only develop from a strong idea.

The Mazeno Wall in the Nanga Parbat massif (facing page) and (below) Namcha Barwa (7782m) in Eastern Tibet. Both faces are as yet unclimbed.

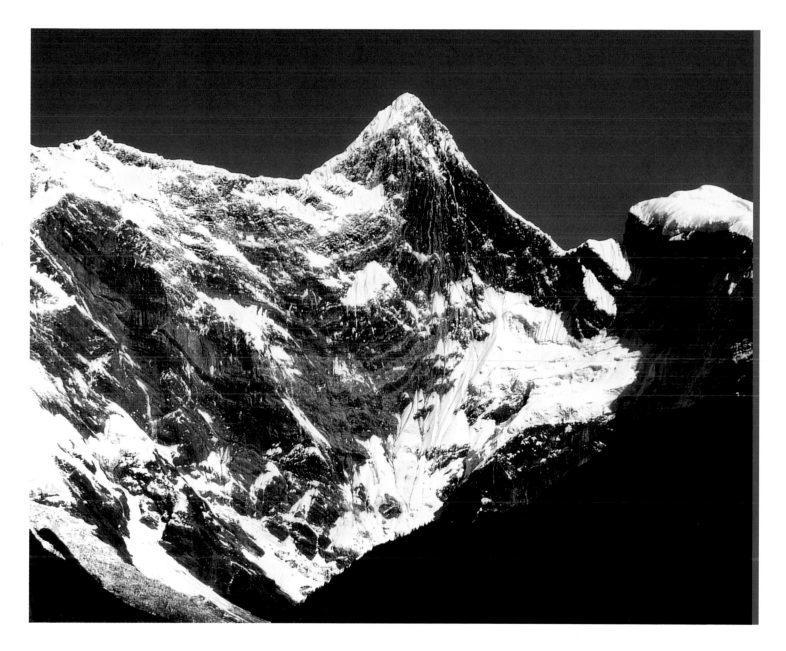

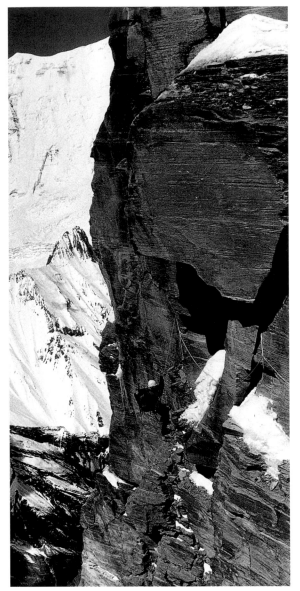

On the West Face of Dhaulagiri.

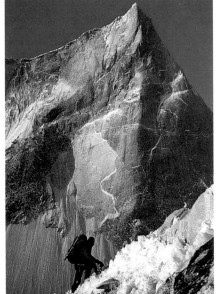

The North-East Face of the Arwa Tower.

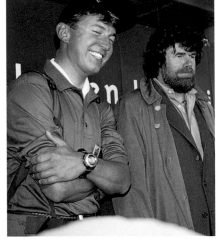

Tomaž Humar after his return from
Dhaulagiri with Reinhold Messner.

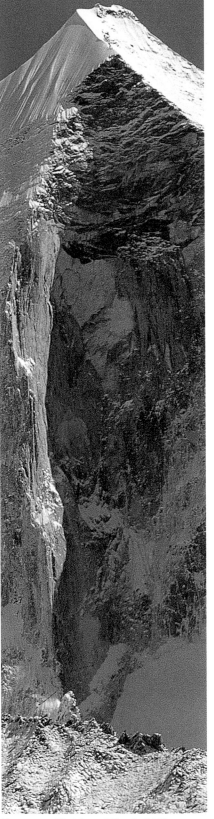

The concave West Face of Bhagirathi III.

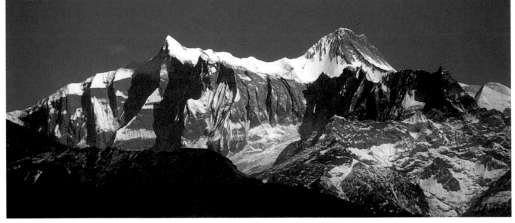

The Annapurnas, with the long sweep of the Annapurna IV face clearly visible.

Title of the original German edition:
Die Grossen Wände

© 2000 BLV Verlagsgesellschaft mbH, München/Germany

North American English language edition
first published in 2001 by
The Mountaineers Books
1001 SW Klickitat Way, Suite 201
Seattle, WA 98134

English translation © The Crowood Press Ltd 2001

Library of Congress Cataloging-in-Publication Data
A catalog record for this book is available at the Library of Congress.

ISBN 0-89886-844-0

Photo credits:
All photographs are taken from Reinhold Messner's archives, with the exception of:
Viki Grošelj: p. 2/3, p. 13, p. 95 top right, p. 96/97, p. 145 top right, p. 176/177, p. 195 bottom right.
Toni Gutsch: p. 8 bottom right
Horst Höfler: main title, p. 98/99, p. 114/115
Thomas Huber: p. 188/189
Archive Robert Jasper: p. 45
Pervez Khan: p. 78, p. 81, p. 124/125, p. 134/135, p. 140/141, p. 144/145, p. 159 top right.
Stane Klemenc: p. 24
Radovan Kuchař: p. 67
Michael Larcher: p. 159 top right.
Peter Mathis: p. 46 left, p. 50 left, p. 55 right, p. 63, p. 210/211
Jiři Novak: cover, p. 77 top right, p. 104/105, p. 133 top right, p. 148/149, p. 149 top right, p. 152/153, p. 153 top right, p. 167 top right, p. 168/169, p. 178/179
Tone Škanja: p. 87
Archive Jakob Tappeiner: p. 28, p. 102/103
Stephen Venables: p. 146/147, p. 147 top right.
Victor Zhak: p. 110/111

English text typeset by
D & N Publishing, Baydon, Marlborough, Wiltshire.

Printed and bound in Singapore by
Craft Print International Ltd

Title page: On the middle section of the East Face of the Watzmann.

Front endpaper: On Mount Everest; to the left, the South West Face.

Rear endpaper: View down the South Face of Dhaulagiri.

Pages 2–3: Two climbers on the 1988 Slovenian Cho Oyu North Face Expedition.

Pages 4–5: On the Welzenbach Couloir on the Rupal Face of Nanga Parbat; first ascent, 1970.

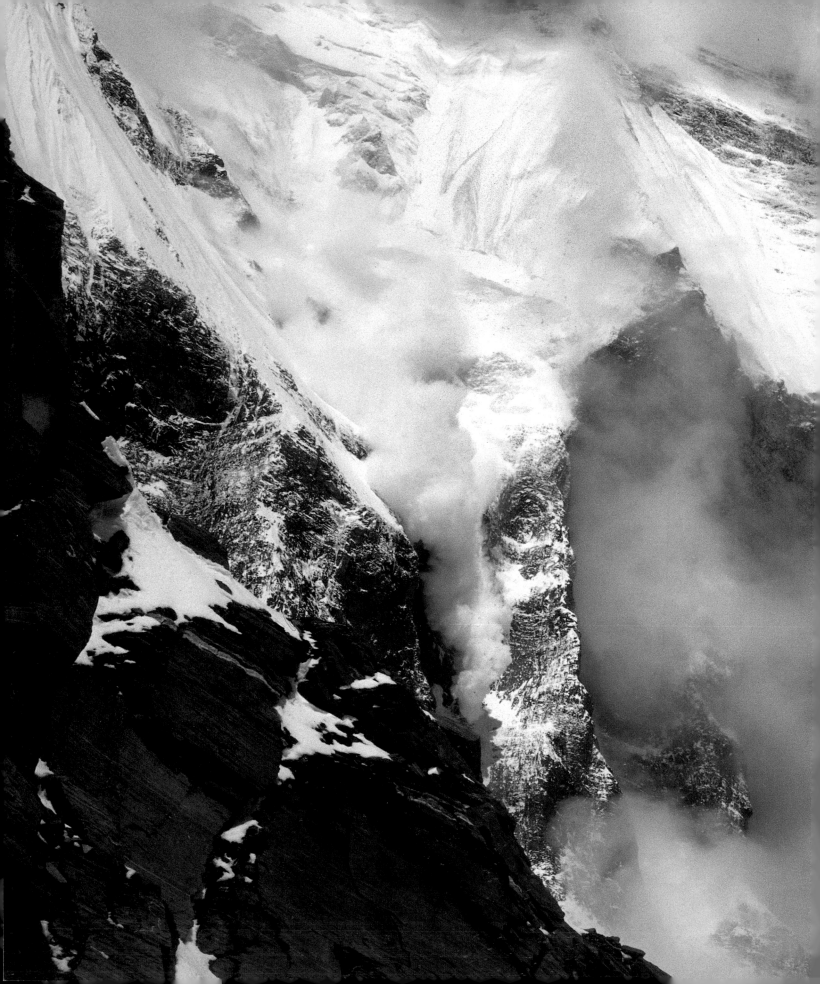

Fledge on a Ledge

AN URBAN FALCON STORY

Doug Chapman

ISBN 978-1-64300-641-3 (Hardcover)
ISBN 978-1-64300-642-0 (Digital)

Covenant Books, Inc.
11661 Hwy 707
Murrells Inlet, SC 29576
www.covenantbooks.com

Dedicated to my father Stan and my falcon friends especially Karen and Deb who made this journey fun.

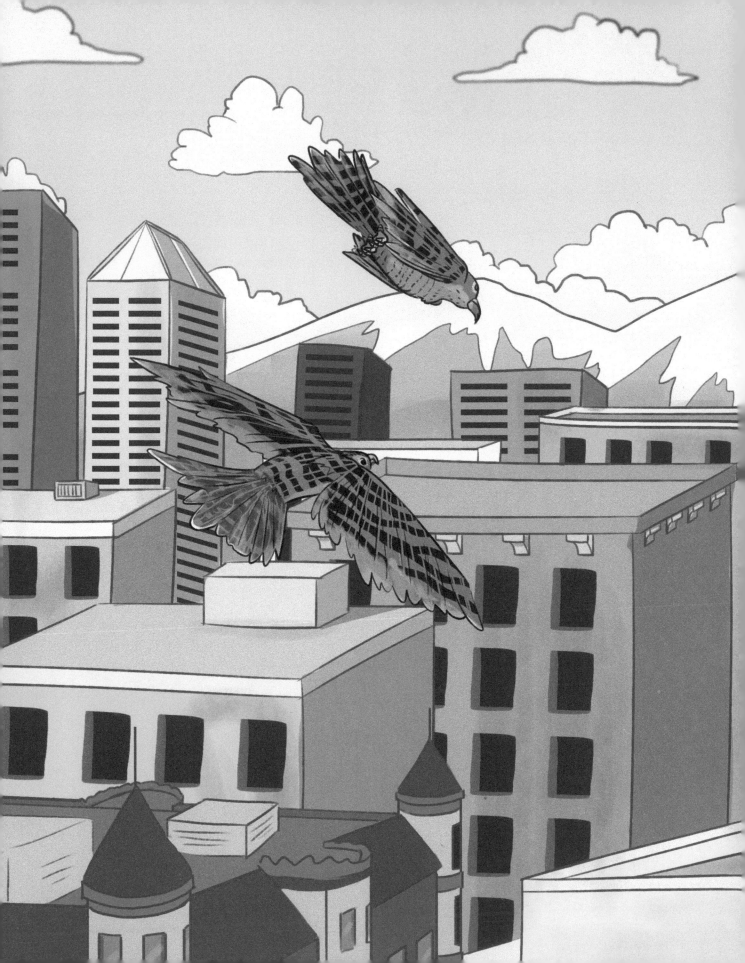

In downtown Boise all is right,
A pair of falcons catch my sight.

Finding food is their main chore,
the fastest bird swoops and soars.

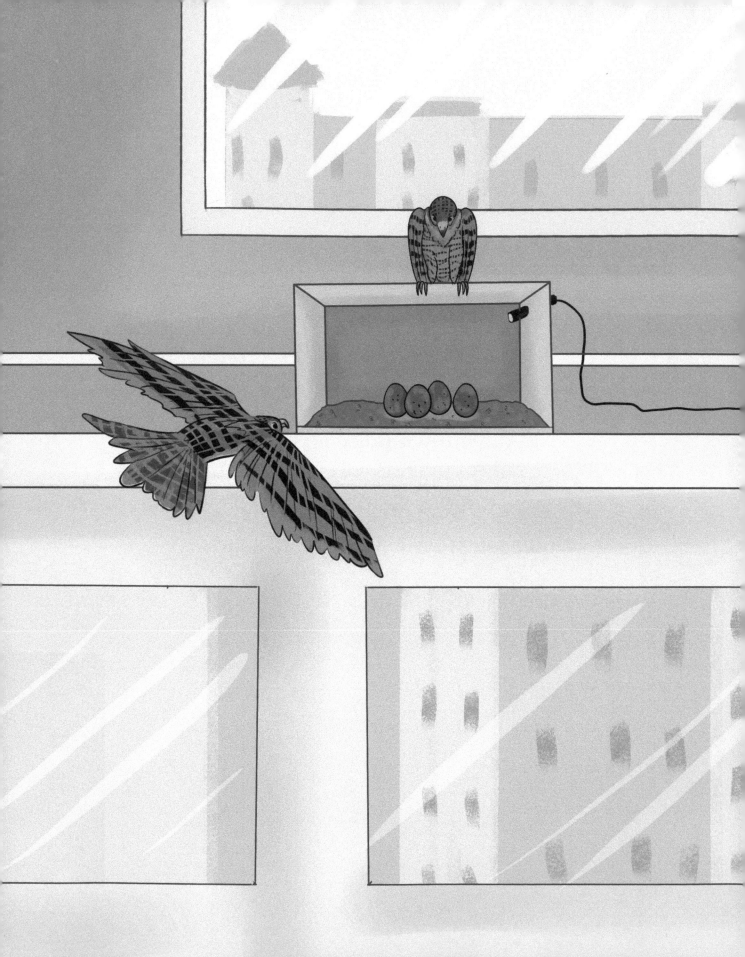

And on a ledge above the street,
a box is placed for them to meet.

And here four eggs were laid inside
the nest box less than three feet wide.

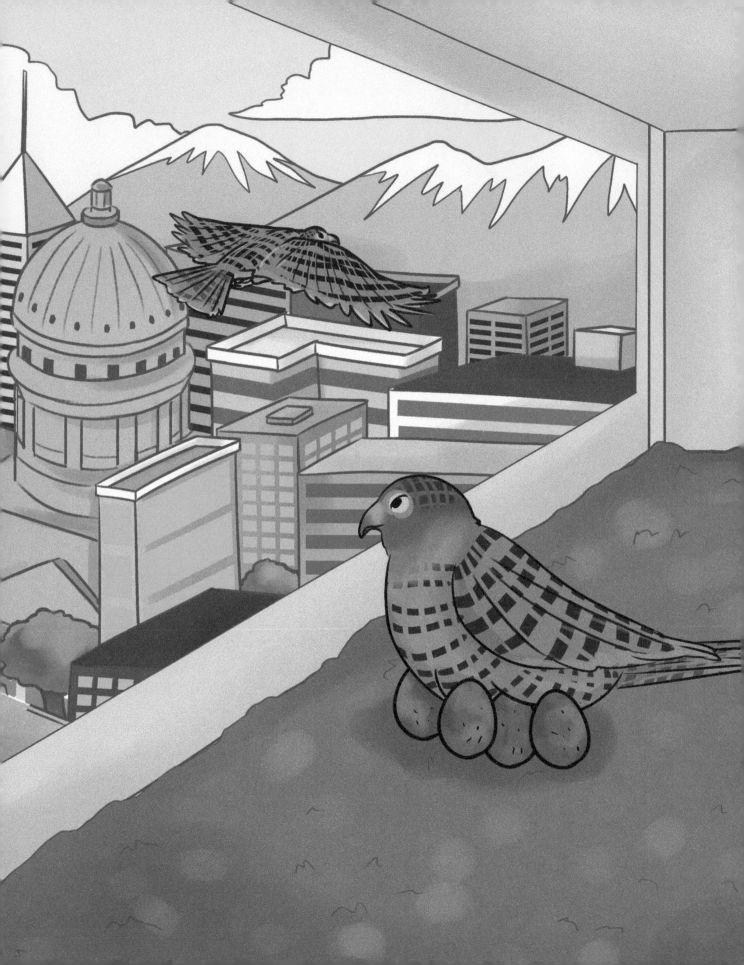

The Mom and Dad take turns to keep warm the eggs through wake and sleep.

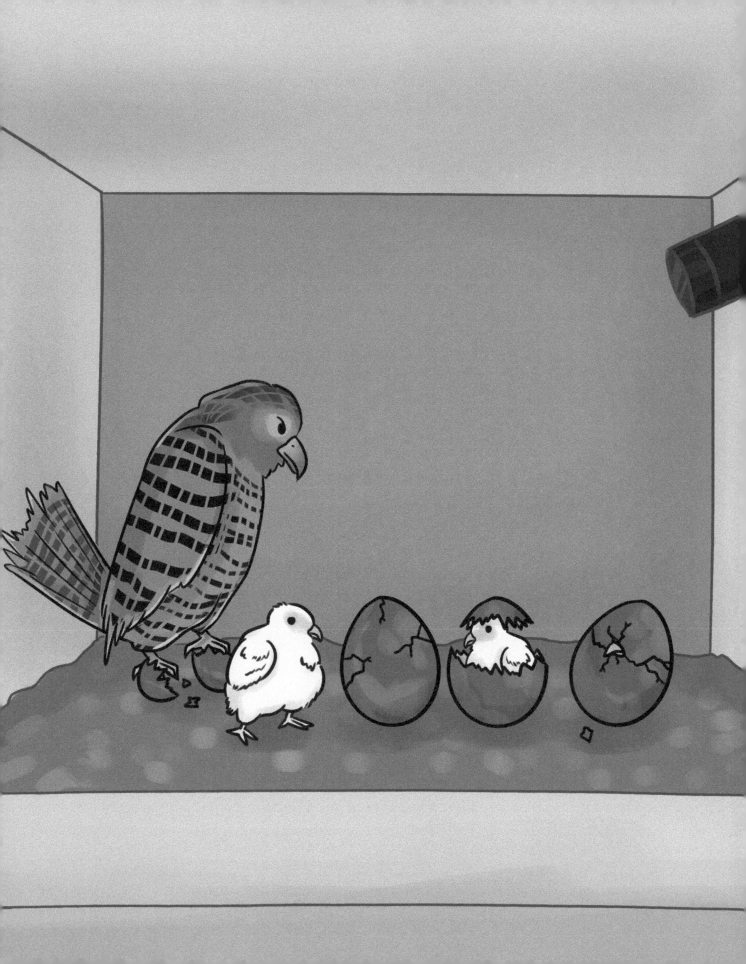

And four weeks later a little crack
a chick came out, one falcon hatched.

And soon three more had broken through
to see the world, bright and new.

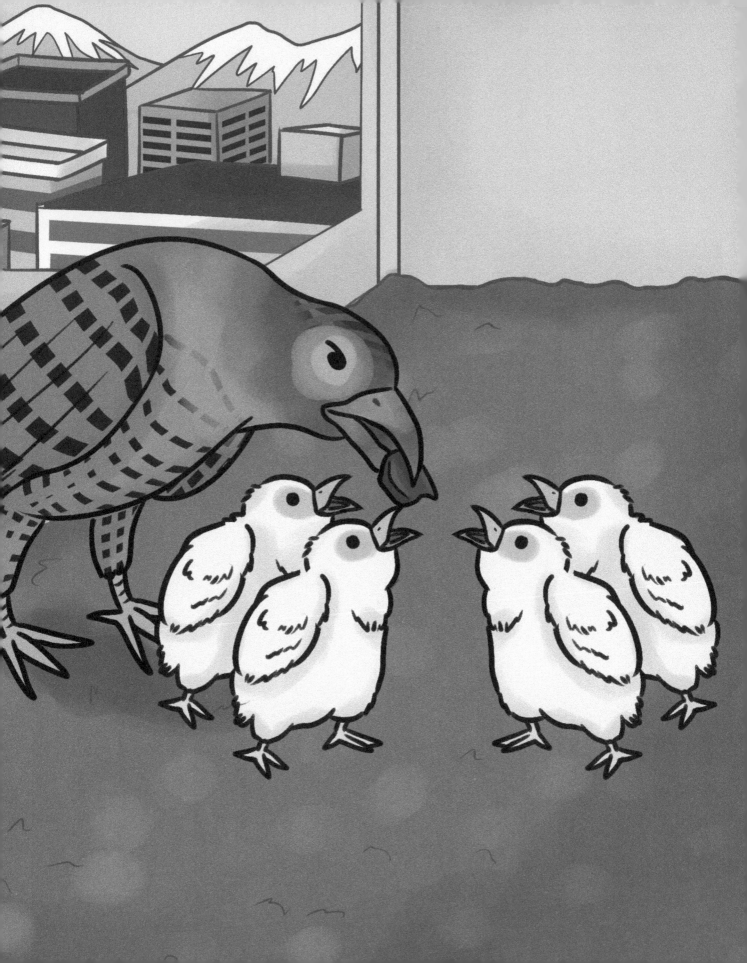

Both Mom and Dad brought food each day.
The chicks would eat and drift away.

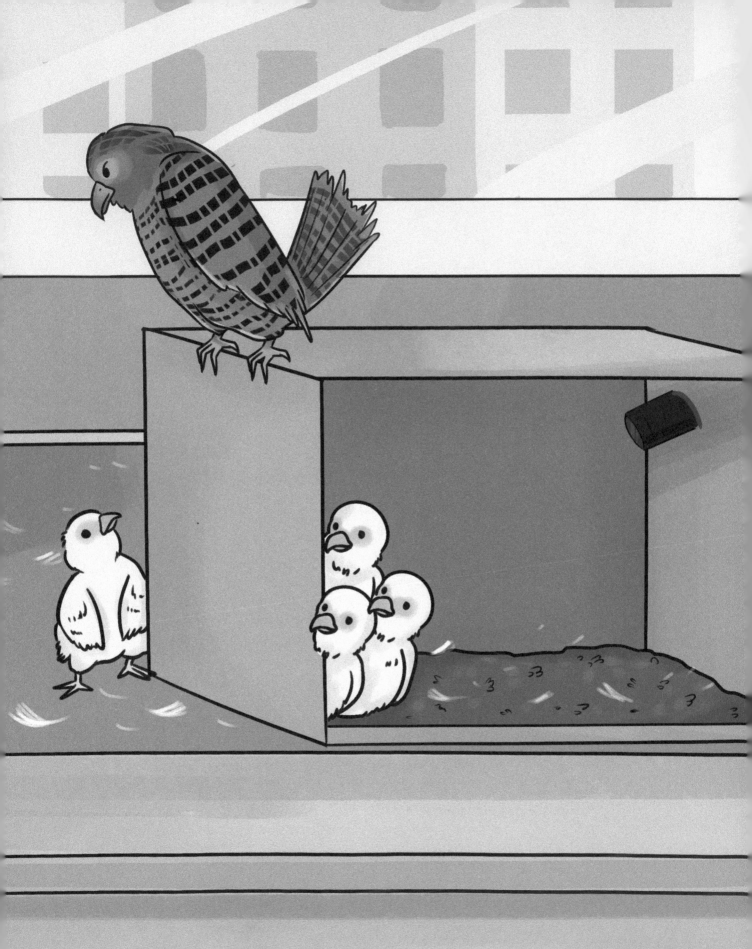

The first chick hatched began to roam.
Beyond the box; the great unknown.

Though Mom and Dad tried their best,
the oldest chick fell from the nest.

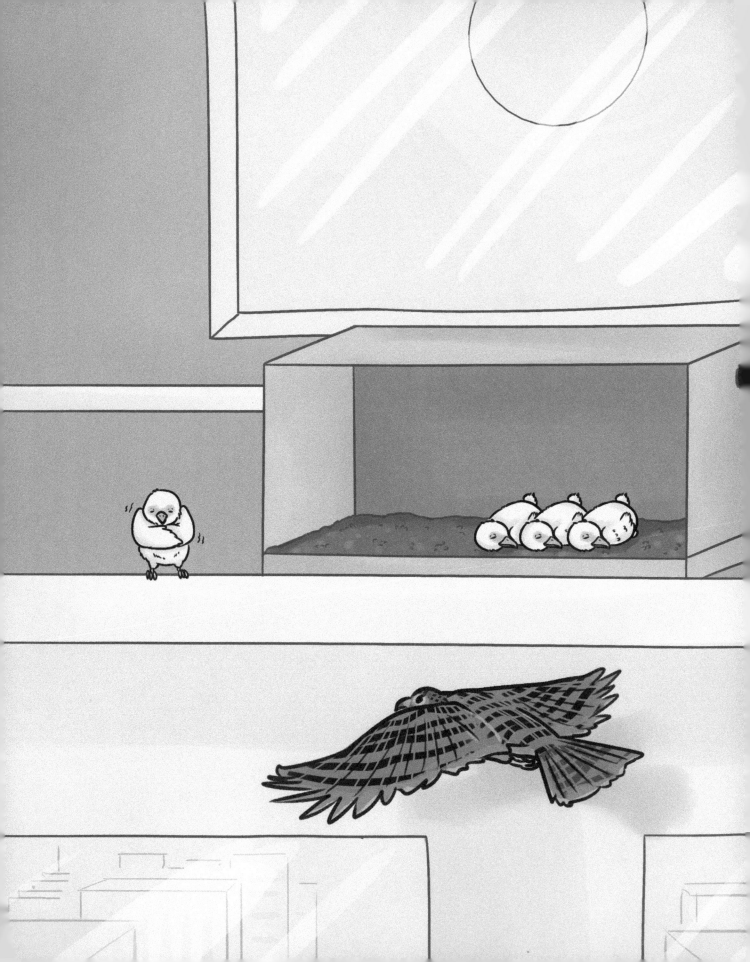

She landed hard upon the ledge
and shied away from the scary edge.

For one whole night she slept alone
in a corner, not far from home.

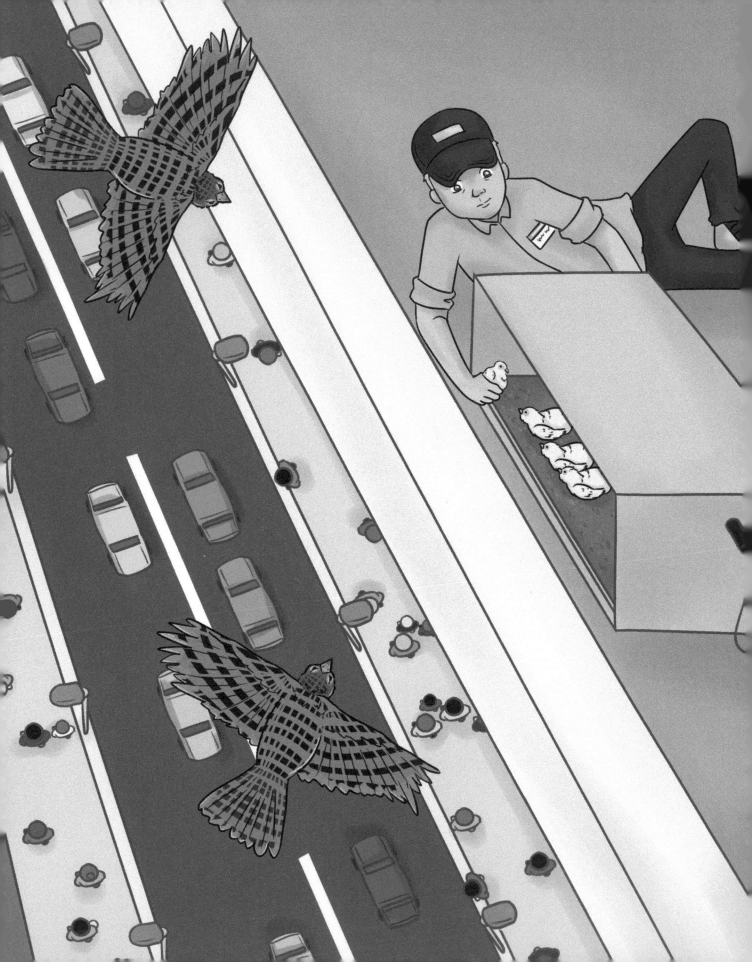

But Ranger Bruce had seen her fall
for a webcam was built into the wall.

And on the ledge, the ranger did creep
to place the chick back in her keep.

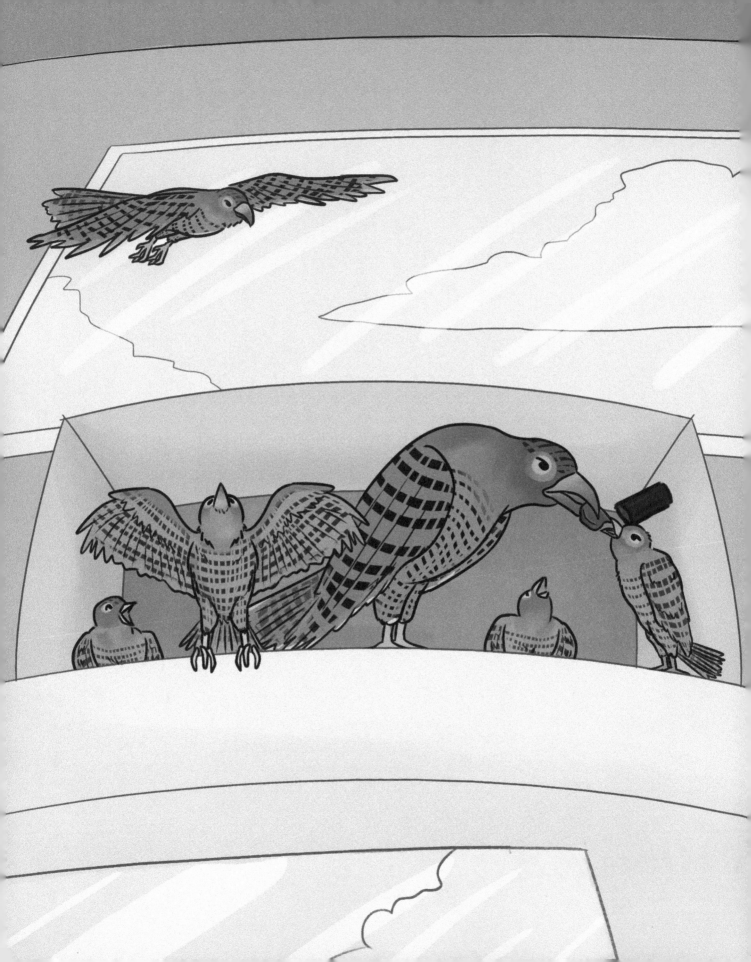

And so our little brood of falcons
ate and slept, grew feathers and talons.

They were quite ornery and fought for food,
as teenagers do they got attitude.

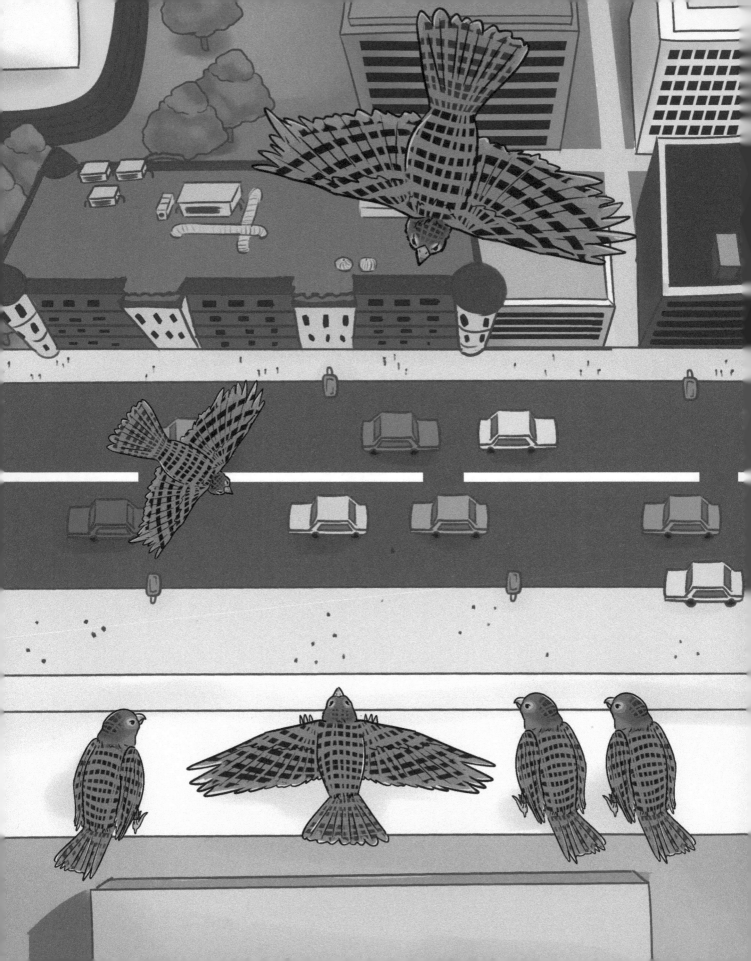

Older and bolder they left the nest
to explore the ledge, eat, and rest.

For flight was what they had in mind,
the streets below would not be kind.

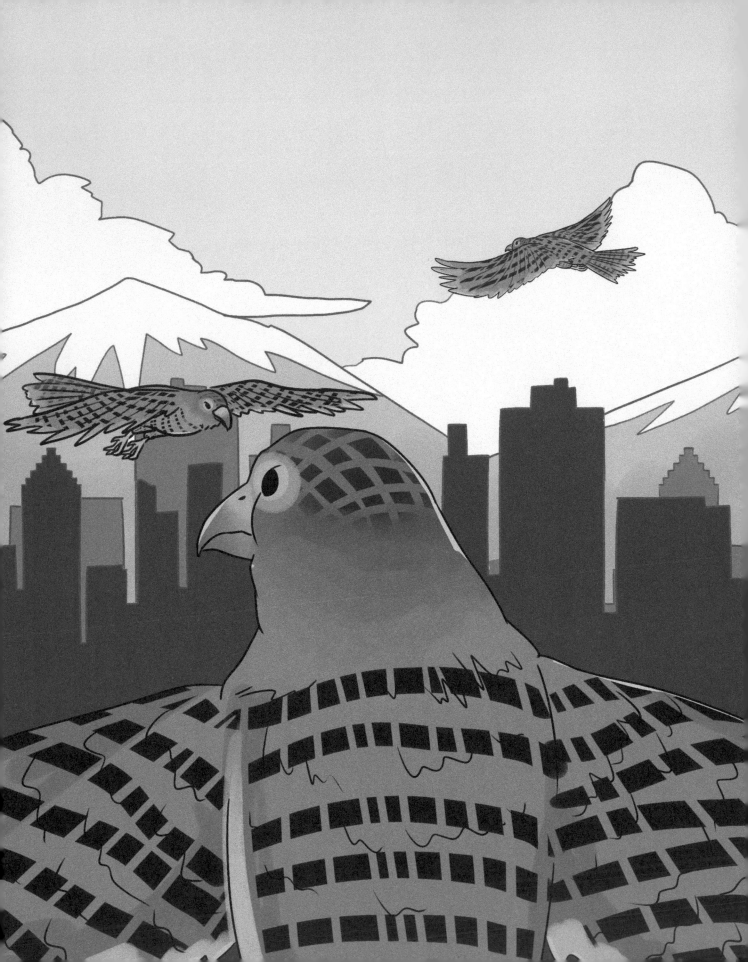

They flapped their wings and practiced launch
and scrambled fast when Mom brought lunch.

But one would be the first to try,
she had the courage, desire to fly.

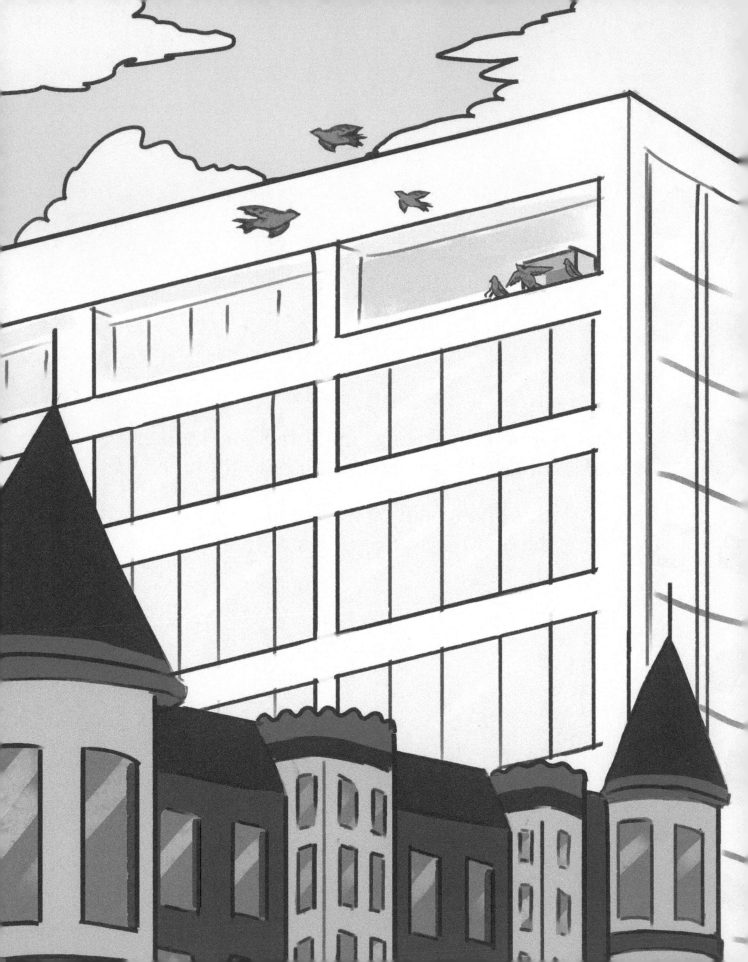

She ran and flapped and neared the edge.
She took off soaring, the first to fledge.

Brothers and sisters watched the sight.
Who would be next to take the flight?

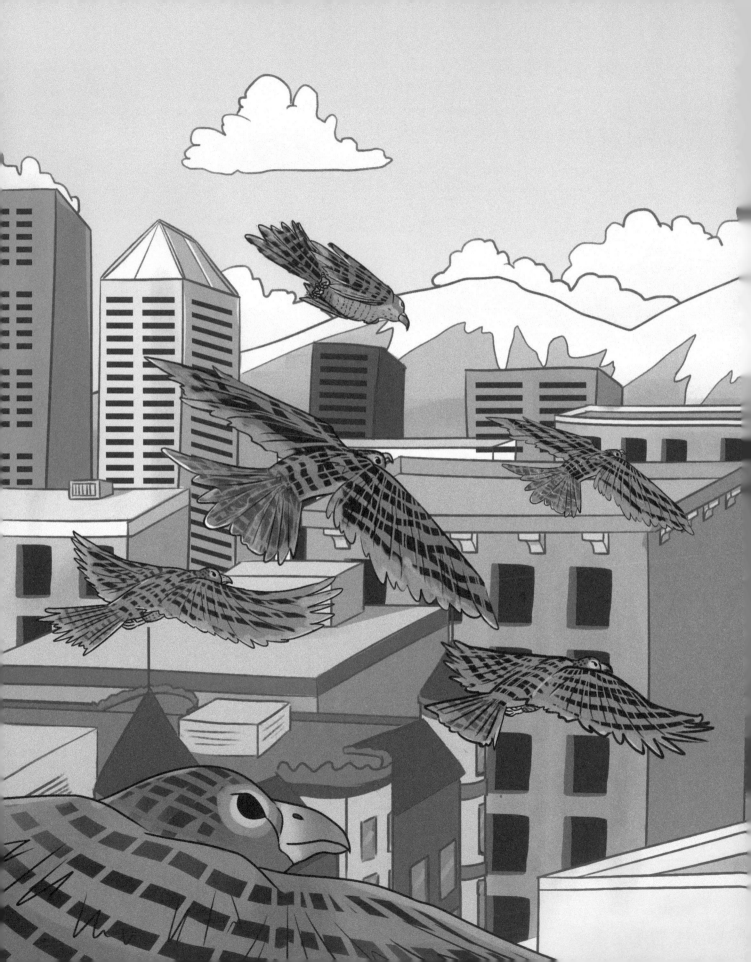

One by one they found their wings
and left the ledge to find new things.

They learned to hunt and eat their kill.
But flight by far was their main thrill.

The End

About the Author

Doug Chapman was raised on Orcas Island in Washington State where animals and nature were a part of everyday life. After moving to Boise, Idaho, Doug became involved with the Peregrine Fund, installing a webcam in a peregrine falcon nest box to the delight of children and adults worldwide.

CPSIA information can be obtained
at www.ICGtesting.com
Printed in the USA
LVHW071253250620
658981LV00024B/195

Sensing Spaces

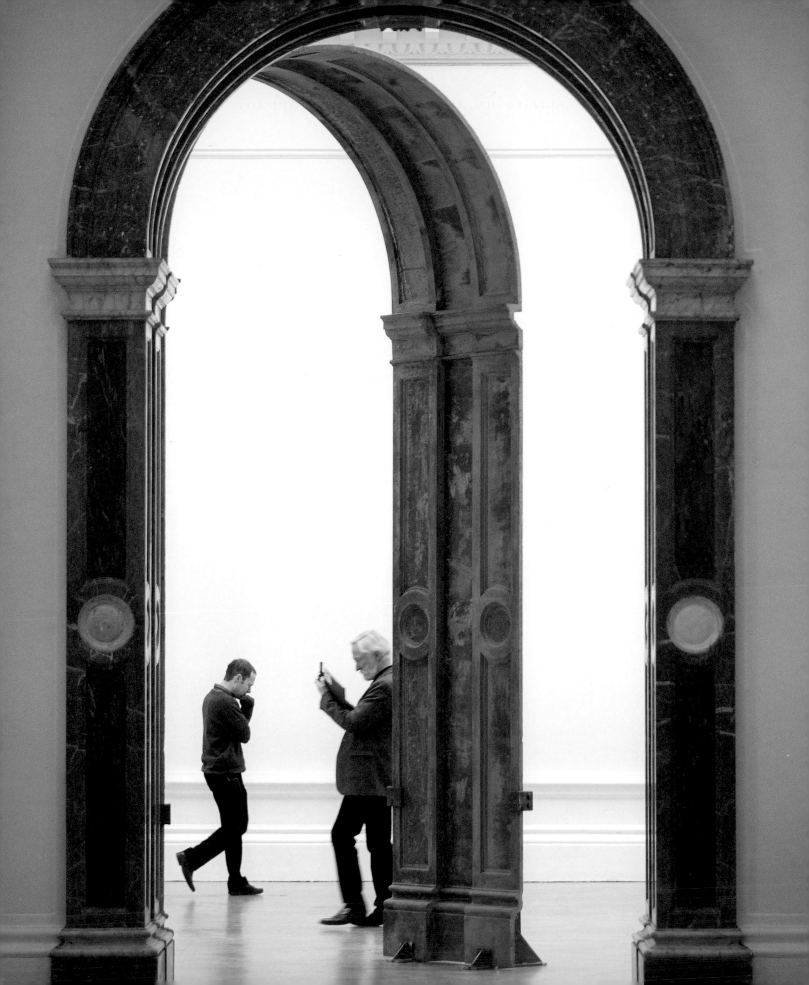

Sensing Spaces
Architecture
Reimagined

Royal
Academy
of Arts

First published
on the occasion
of the exhibition
'Sensing Spaces:
Architecture
Reimagined'

Royal Academy of Arts,
London
25 January – 6 April 2014

Supported by
Scott and Laura Malkin

Supported by

Supported by

ARAUCO.
Growing the Future

Exhibition Curators
Kate Goodwin
assisted by Sarah Lea

**Royal Academy
Exhibitions**
Director:
Kathleen Soriano
Natalie Gibbons
Katharine Oakes
Nicole Ruegsegger
Andrea Tarsia

**Royal Academy
Publications**
Beatrice Gullström
Alison Hissey
Elizabeth Horne
Carola Krueger
Peter Sawbridge
Nick Tite

Cover
Álvaro Siza, sketch of
Annenberg Courtyard
with installation

Catalogue
Project editors:
Vicky Wilson and
Tom Neville

Design:
Esterson Associates

Translation from
the Portuguese:
(Eduardo Souto de
Moura) Candida Wigan

Gallery plan:
Unlimited /
Patrick Morrissey

Colour origination:
DawkinsColour

Printed in Wales
by Gomer Press Ltd

Acknowledgements
An exhibition such
as this could not have
been achieved without
the advice, support
and encouragement
of many people.
For acting as critical
advisors, I would like
to thank:
Peter Buchanan
Peter Cook RA
Leon van Schaik
Philip Ursprung

And I extend my most
sincere thanks to the
following individuals;
some have offered
a valuable hour while
others have given
continuous support:
Erieta Attali
Eliza Bonham Carter
Iain Borden
Alexander Brodsky
Dominic Campbell
Peter Carl
Helen Castle
Emma Enderby
Michelle Fagan
Edward Farleigh
Sally Faulder
Kevin Fellingham
Adrian Forty
Piers Gough RA
Rob Gregory
Joseph Grima
Fiona Hannah
Niall Hobhouse

Owen Hopkins
Catherine Ince
Jessica Karlsen
Bea Kelleher
Julia Lampshire
Jules Lubbock
Georgina Mackie
Jennifer Maksymetz
Jeremy Melvin
Jay Merrick
Marco de Michelis
Tom Neville
Juhani Pallasmaa
Eric Parry RA
Michael Peszynski
Elisa Poli
James Putman
Peter Rich
Vicky Richardson
Jana Scholze
Beth Schneider
Alan Stanton RA
MaryAnne Stevens
Cassius Taylor-Smith
Abraham Thomas
Cecilia Treves
Paul Williams
Vicky Wilson
Peter Zumthor

Finally, for their
unending generosity
of spirit and their
inspirational work,
I would like to extend
my heartfelt thanks
to all the architects
involved and to those
in their offices who
have assisted us:

Grafton Architects:
Yvonne Farrell,
Shelley McNamara,
Gerard Carty, Philippe
O'Sullivan, James Rossa
O'Hare, Edwin Jebb
Kéré Architecture:
Diébédo Francis Kéré,
Dominique Mayer,
Daniela Gardeweg,
Pedro Montero
Gosalbez, Julia Phillips,
Jamie Keats, Claudia
Buhmann, Jerome Byron
Kengo Kuma
& Associates:
Kengo Kuma,
Ryuya Umezawa
Li Xiaodong Atelier:
Li Xiaodong, Liu
Shiqing, Li Kun, Wang
Xinyu, Chen Weixin
Pezo von
Ellrichshausen:
Mauricio Pezo and Sofia
von Ellrichshausen,
Yannic Calvez, Marta
Mato, Peter Weeber,
Marta Tonelli, Philip
Kempfer
Álvaro Siza
Souto Moura
Arquitectos:
Eduardo Souto de
Moura, Luisa Moura
with Carlos Sampaio
(Prégaia)

Kate Goodwin

Contents

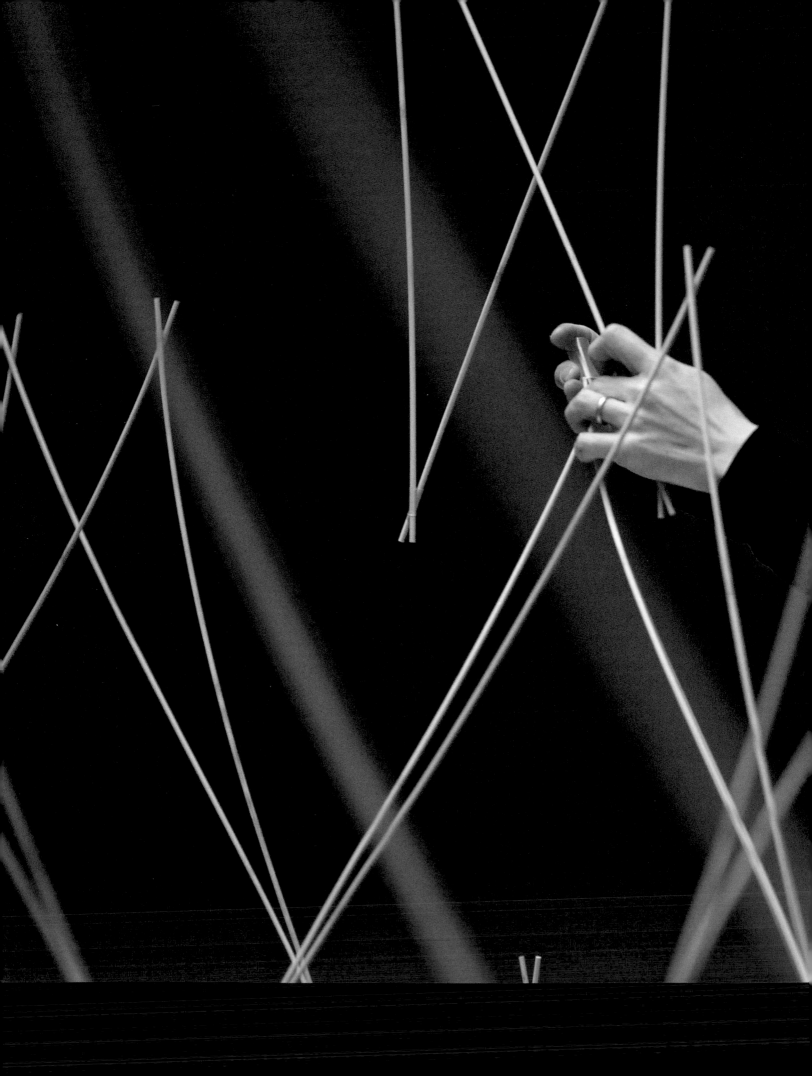

Installations

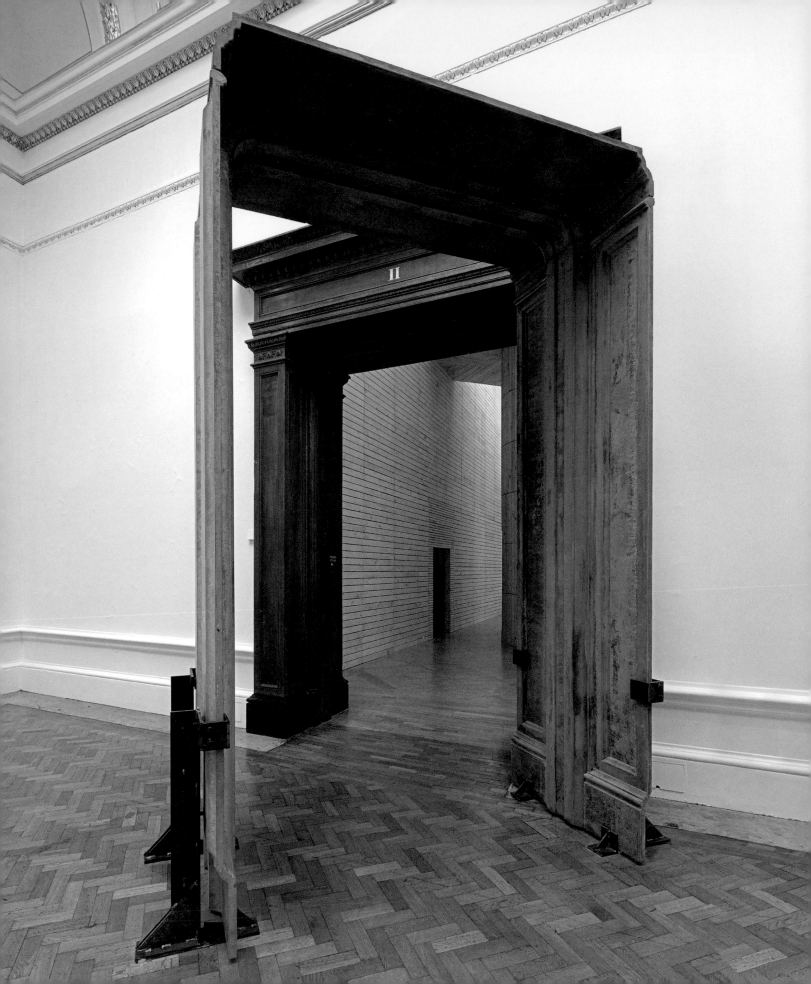

Gallery Plan

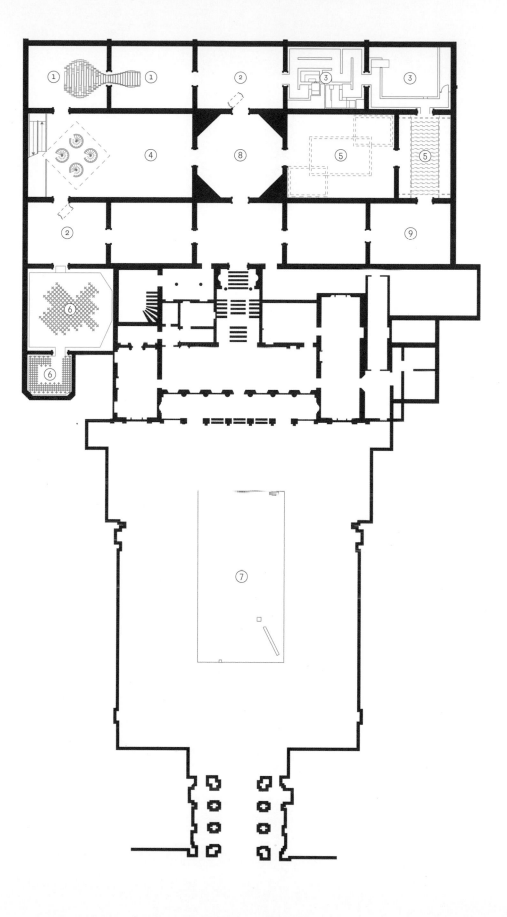

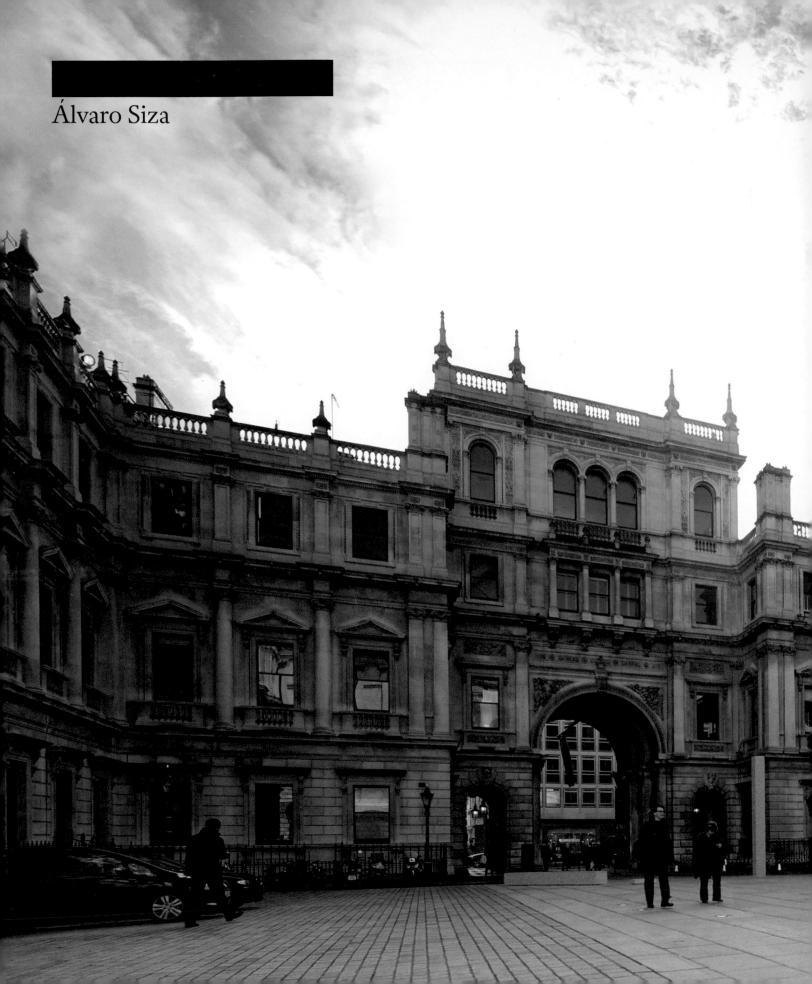

Álvaro Siza

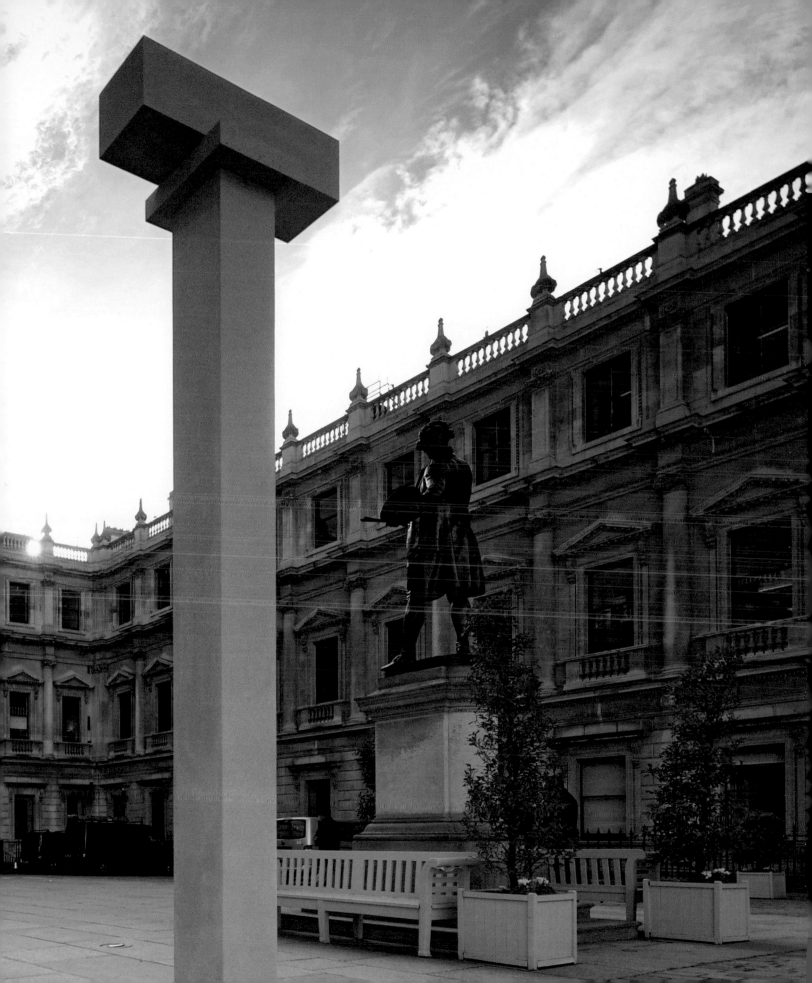

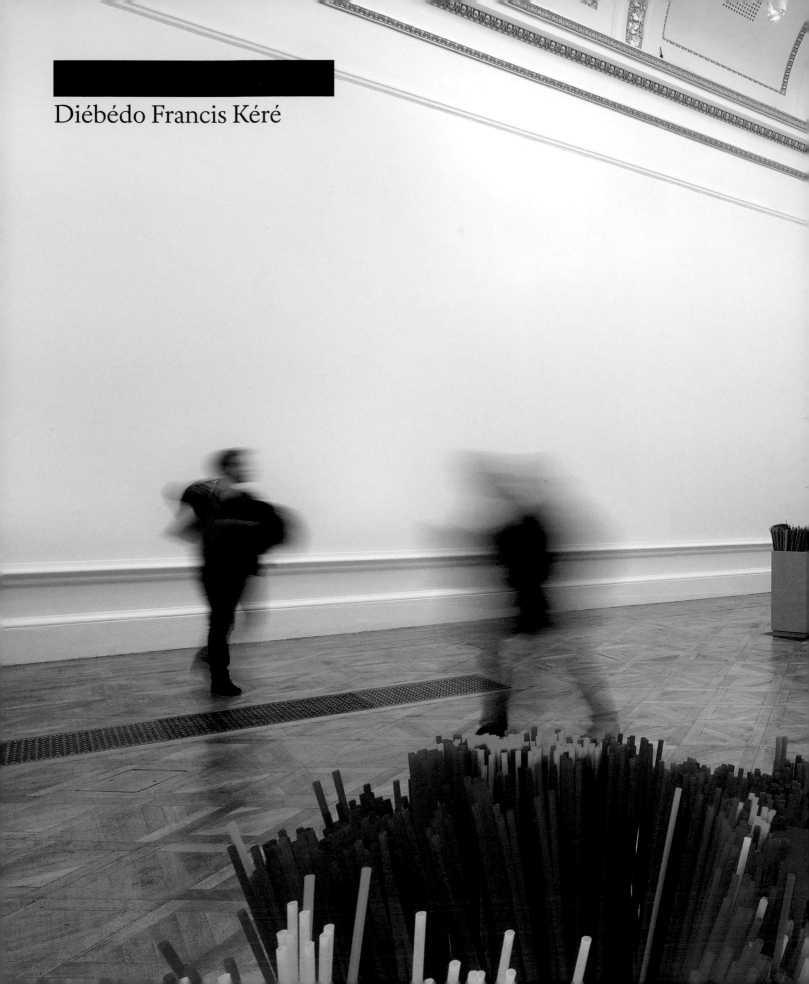

Diébédo Francis Kéré

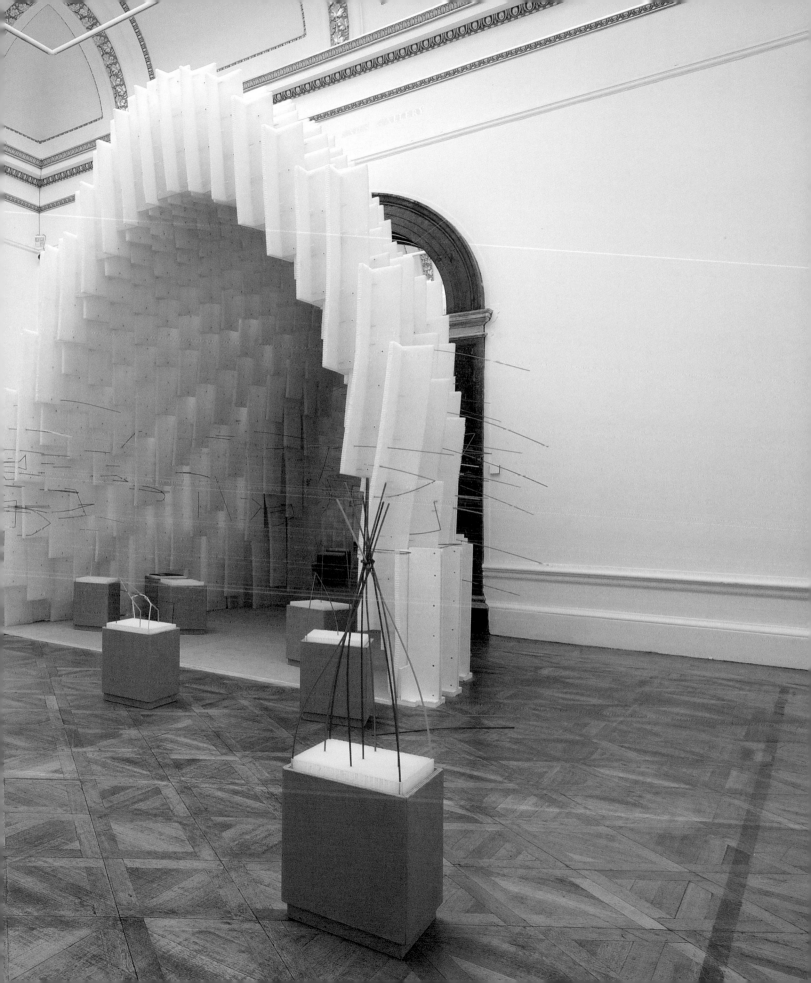

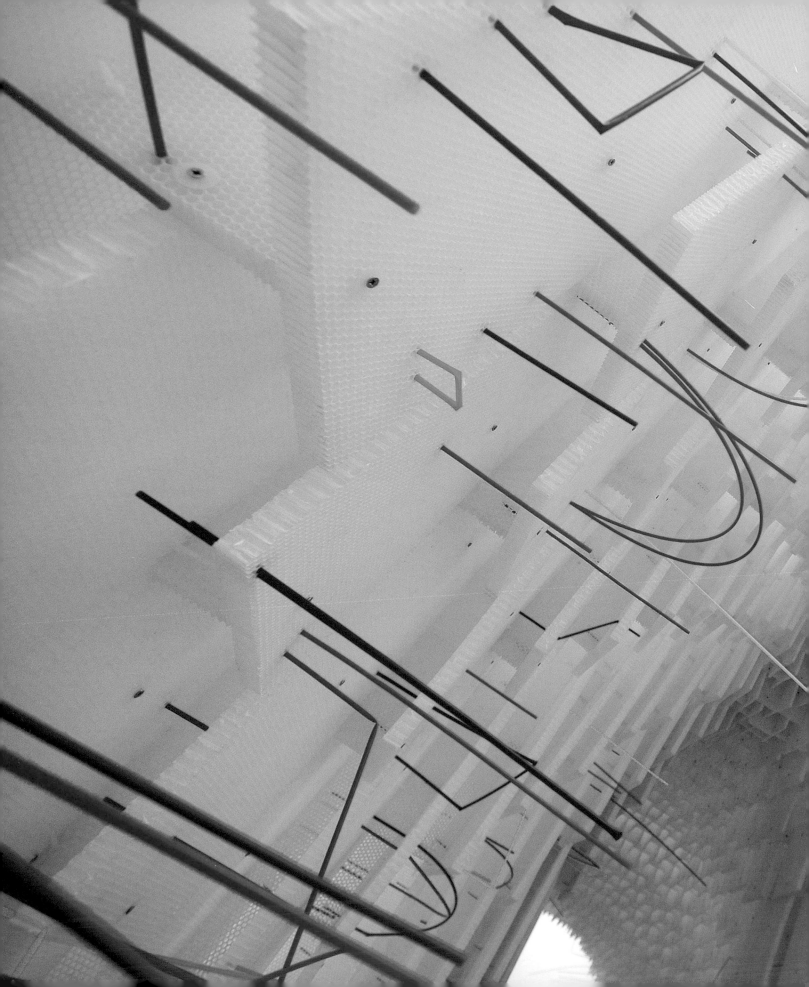

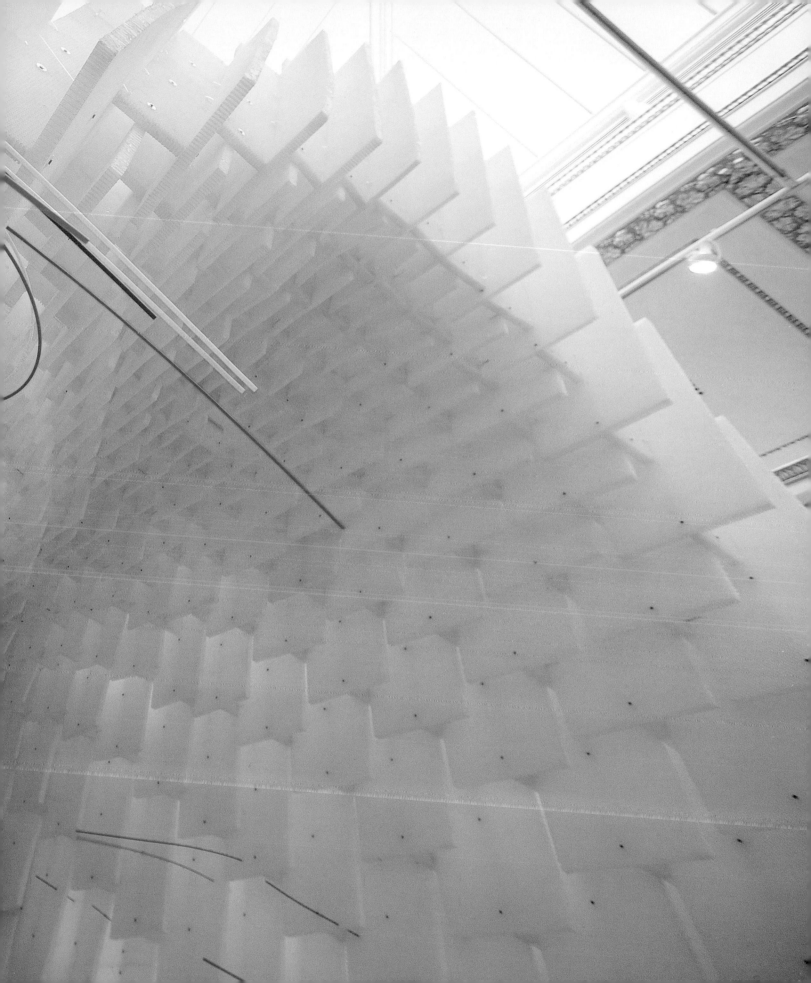

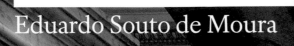

Eduardo Souto de Moura

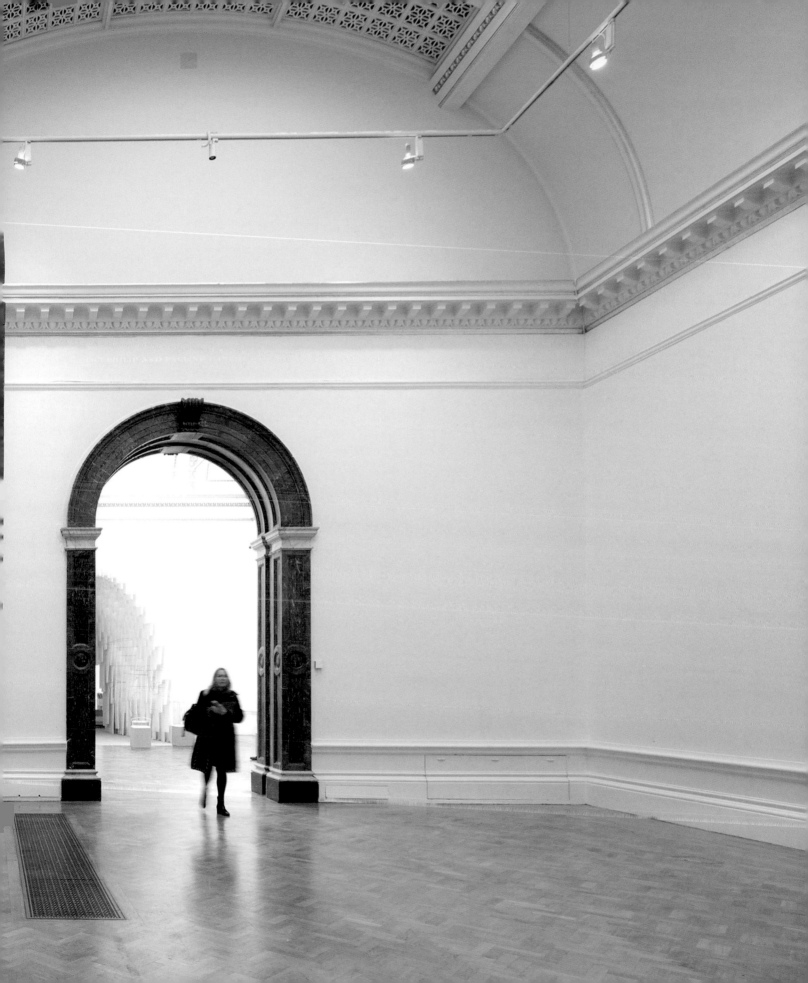

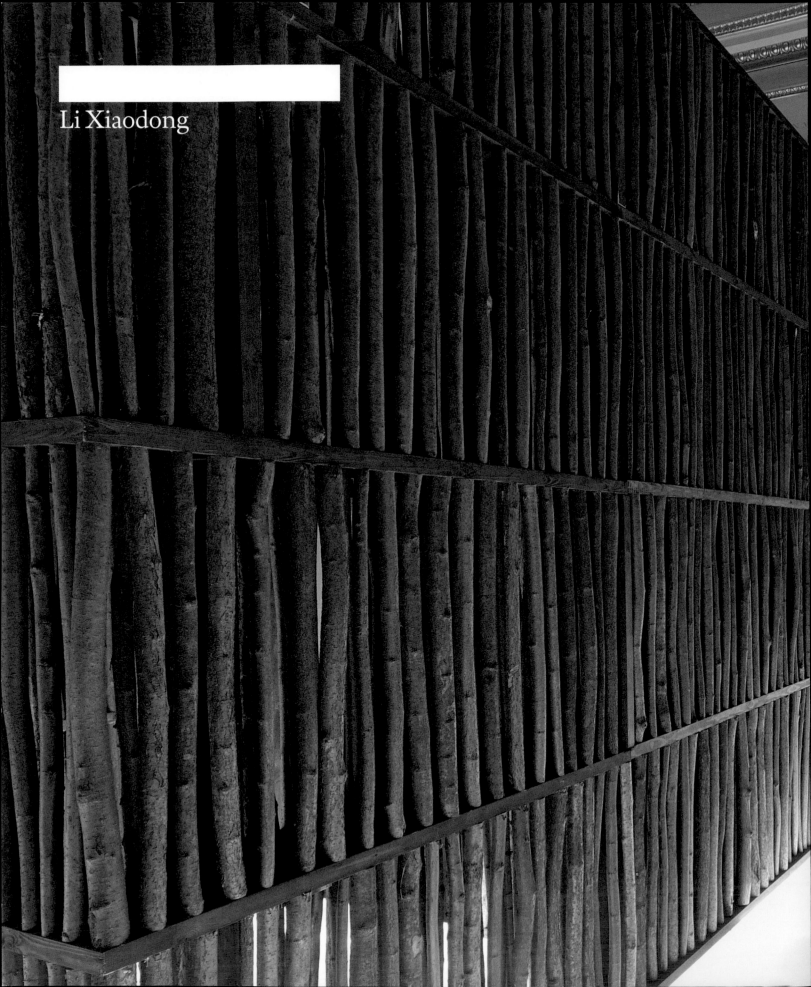

Li Xiaodong

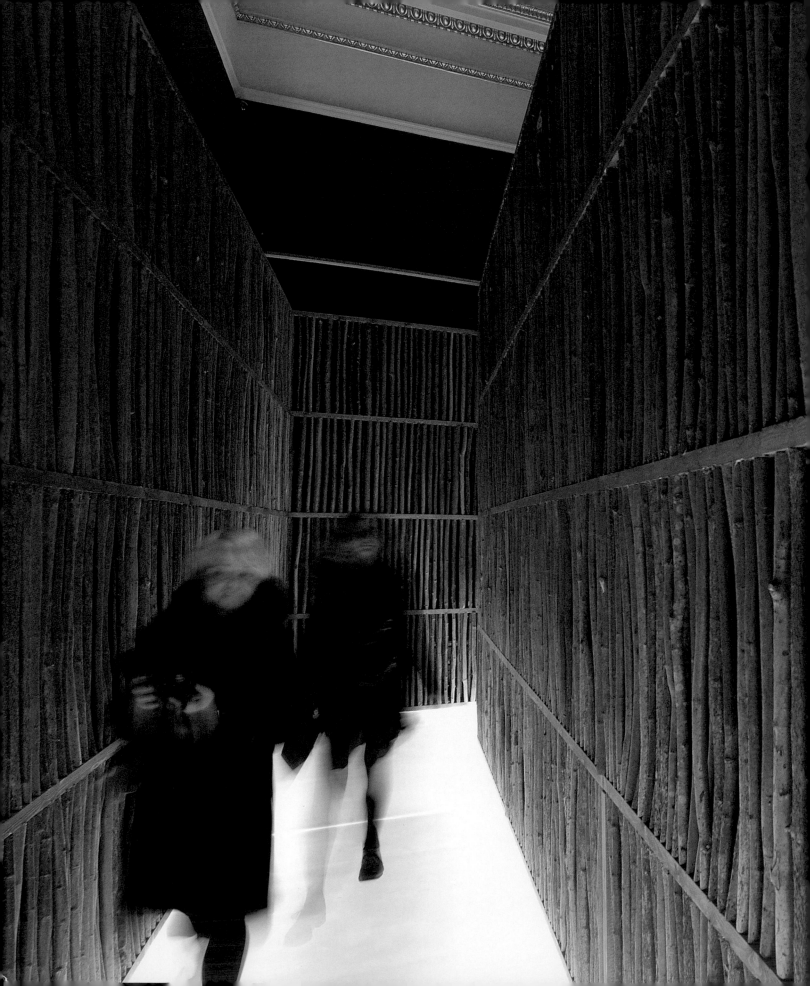

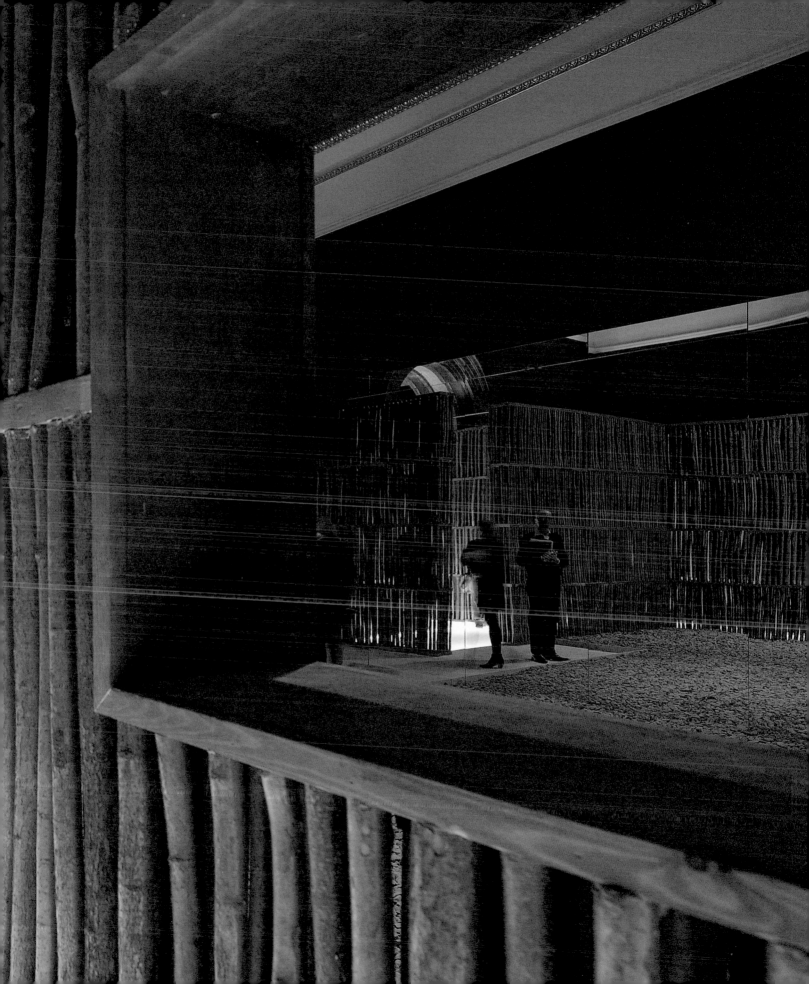

Pezo von Ellrichshausen

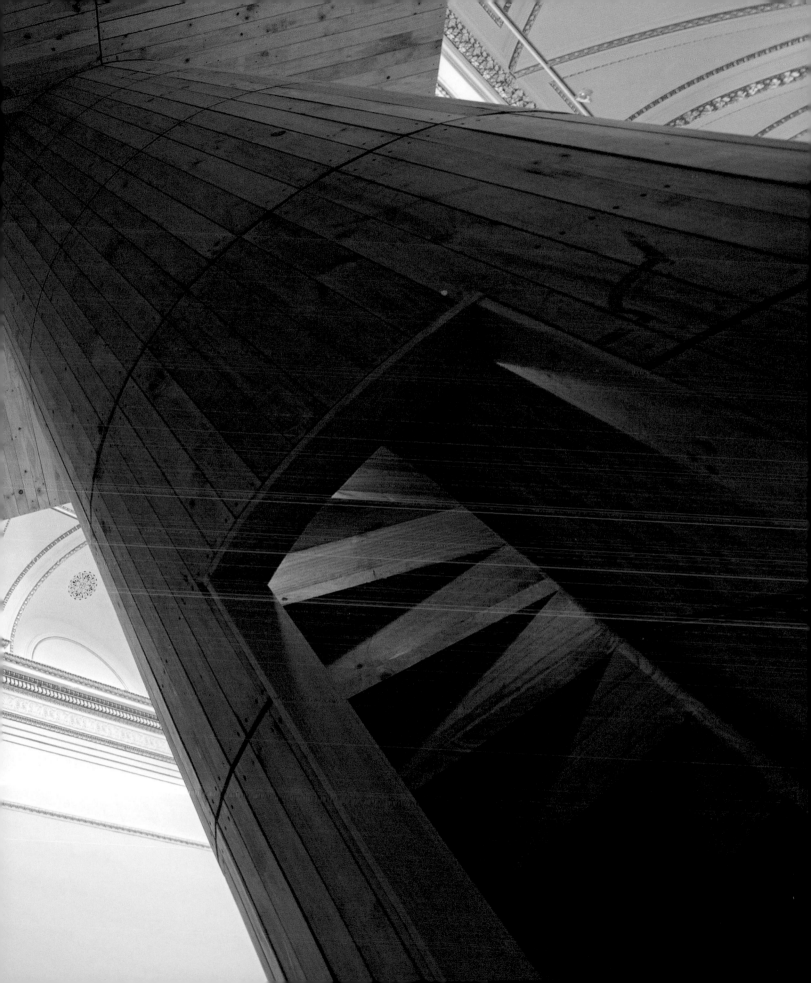

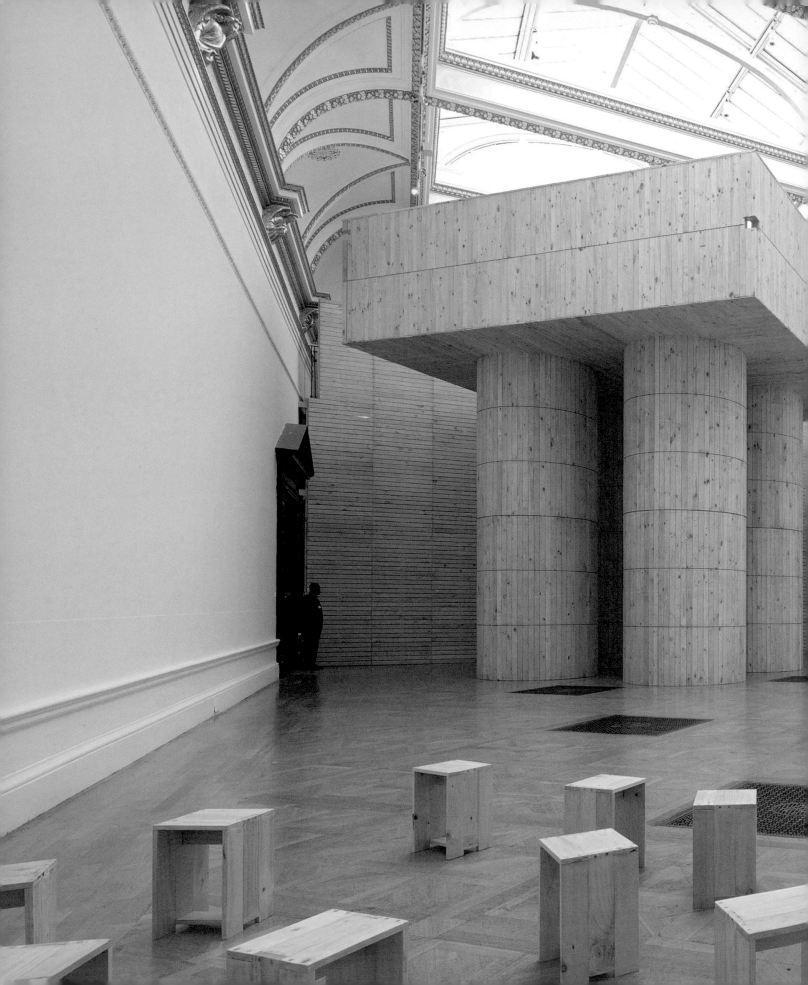

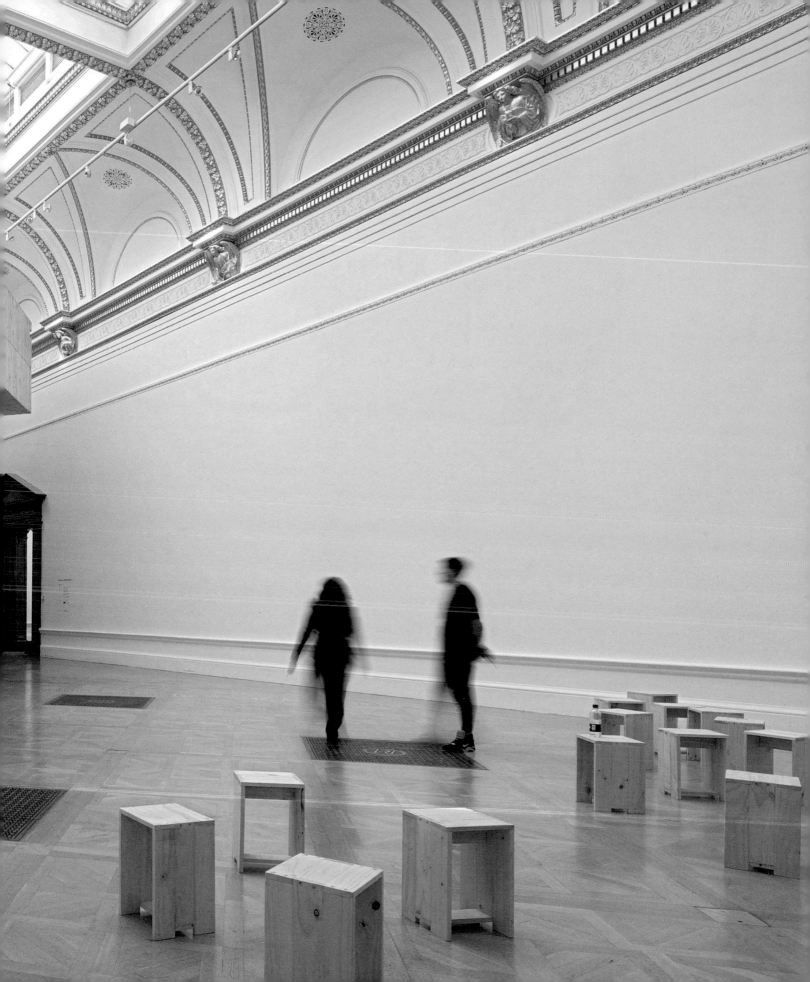

Grafton Architects

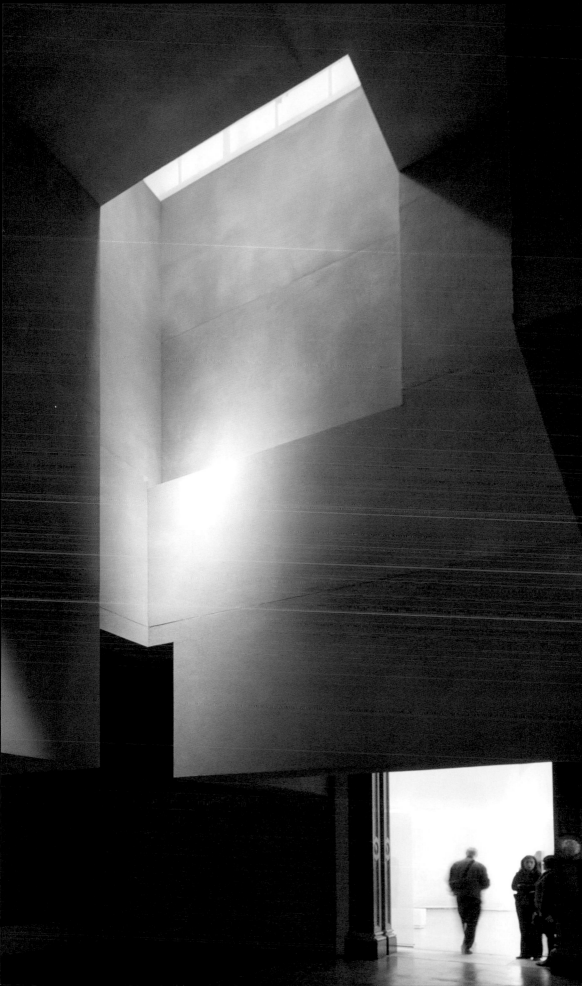

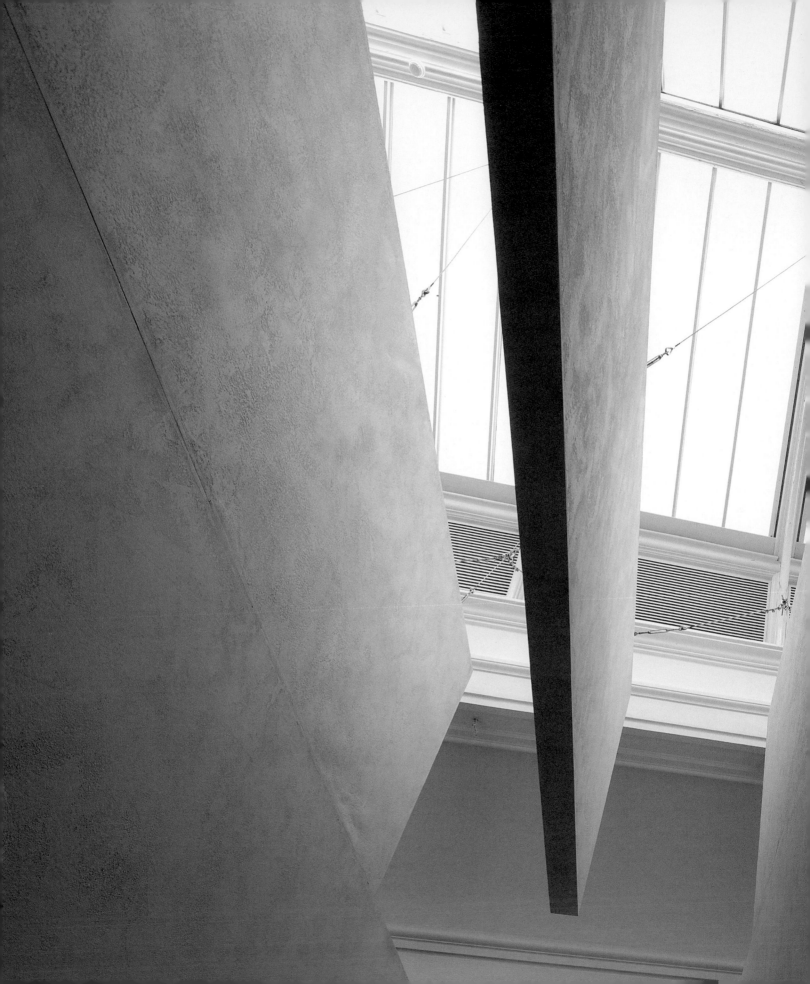

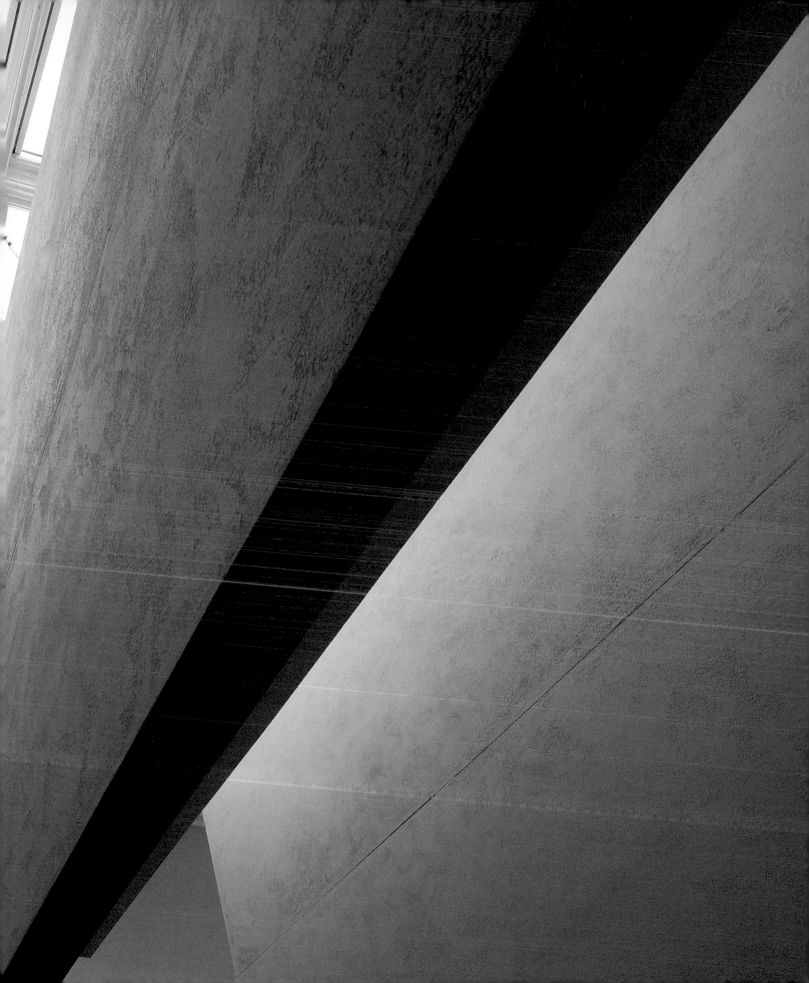

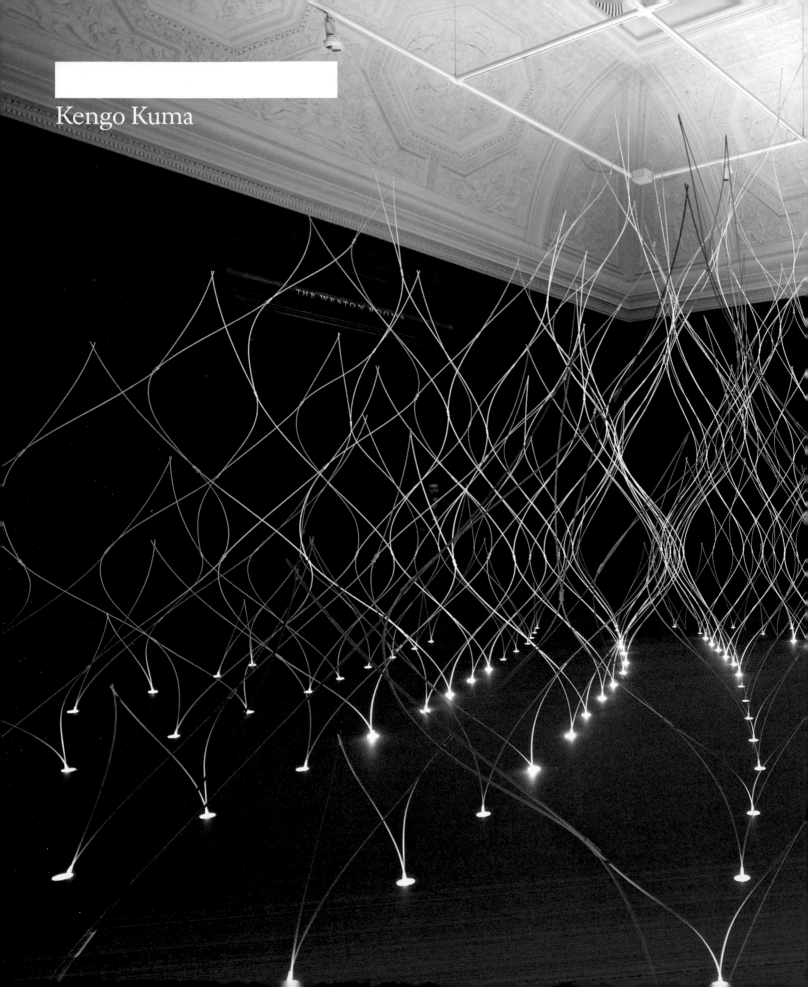

Kengo Kuma

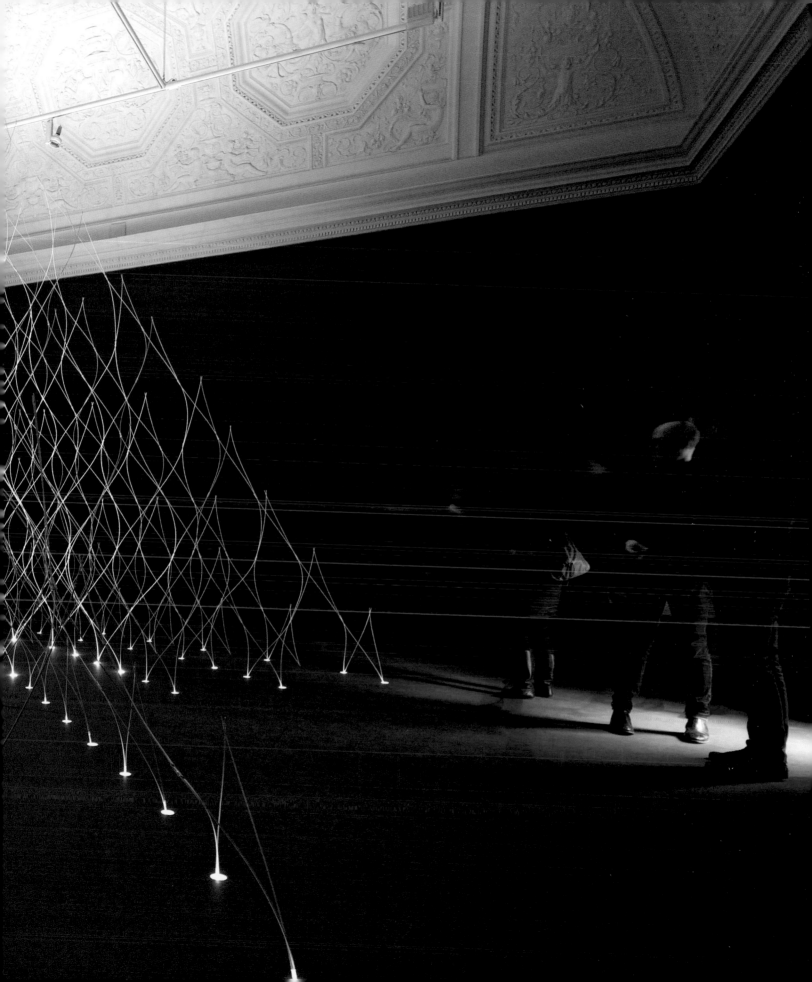

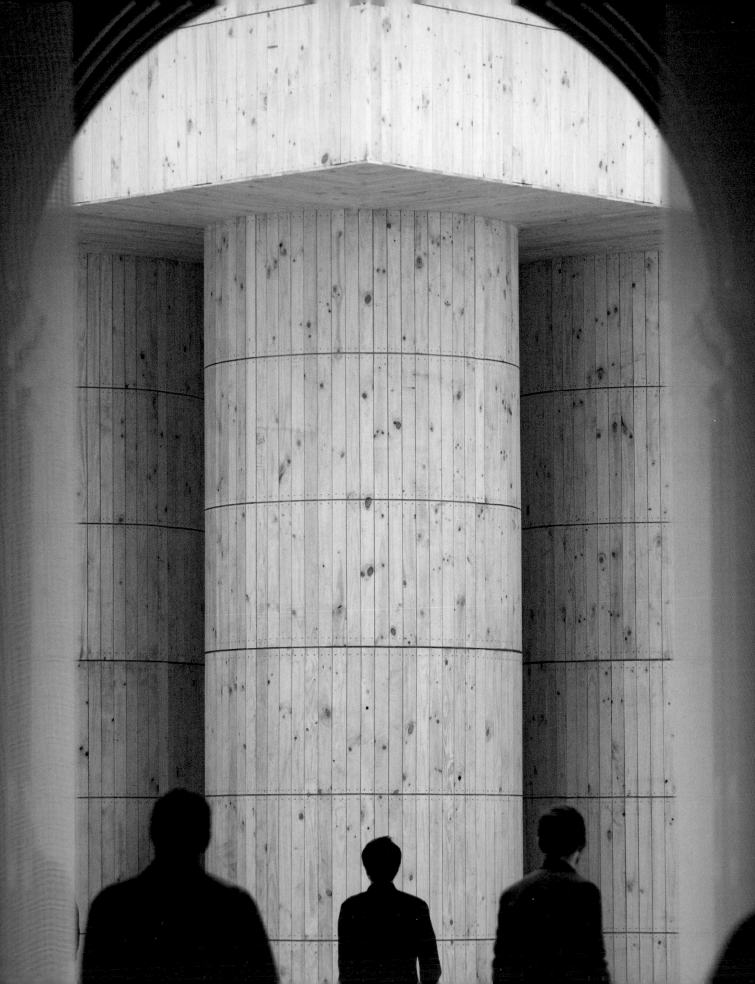

President's Foreword

Architecture has been part of the Royal Academy since the very beginning. Our first Treasurer, the architect Sir William Chambers RA, designed the majestic north block of Somerset House to be our first home. As the Academy grew in size, moving to the National Gallery and then in 1867 to our present home, Burlington House on Piccadilly, the buildings we have occupied have done much to shape us as an institution – and we have shaped and adapted them.

Our Main Galleries have been the site of many groundbreaking architecture exhibitions, among them 'New Architecture: Foster, Rogers, Stirling' (1986) and 'Living Bridges' (1996). 'Sensing Spaces: Architecture Reimagined', however, sets out to redefine what an architecture exhibition might be. Instead of displaying drawings, models and photographs to illustrate an architect's work and ideas, 'Sensing Spaces' offers visitors the opportunity to engage with architecture directly and to experience it through their bodies and senses.

In recent years much discussion on architecture has focused on economic, social or political issues, sometimes obscuring its cultural value and its capacity to offer transcendent experience. There is, therefore, no better moment – and no better place than the Royal Academy – for an exhibition devoted to architecture's sensory, experiential and emotive qualities. For 'Sensing Spaces', we have commissioned seven architects from around the world to create installations and environments in our Main Galleries. Individually and together, their work raises intriguing questions about the boundaries between art and architecture, the human qualities of space, and the role buildings play in shaping our lives.

The Royal Academy would not have been able to celebrate the value and significance of architecture without the passion and creativity of the architects involved, and we thank them and the members of their offices for their hard work and commitment. We also applaud Shizuka Harui and SHSH Architecture + Scenography for their design of the Wohl Central Hall and film room; Patrick Morrissey of Unlimited for his graphic design; and Candida Richardson for her evocative films.

With the support of Kathleen Soriano, our Director of Exhibitions, 'Sensing Spaces' has been proposed and curated by Kate Goodwin, the Drue Heinz Curator of Architecture at the Royal Academy, who has worked tirelessly to realise this groundbreaking project. The exhibition has drawn on the knowledge, skill and energies of many individuals among the RA staff including Sarah Lea, Nicole Ruegsegger, Natalie Gibbons, Katharine Oakes, Andrea Tarsia, and Philip Pearce and the RA's engineering team. Further thanks are due to Russell Schofield and Duncan Barton and their team at MDM Props Ltd, and to Ricardo Ballesta SPA, Pregaia, MER, Sykes, and MOMART.

The exhibition would not have been possible without the services of AKT II, Consulting Structural and Civil Engineers, specifically Hanif Kara, Ed Moseley, Daniel Bosia and David Illingworth, the in-kind support of Arauco, and the support of Christine Fu and Lesley Wong, Scott and Laura Malkin, the Chilean Ministry of Culture, the Embassy of Chile in the UK, Daiko and Yokoyama Bamboo Products Co. Ltd. We thank them all for their generosity.
Christopher Le Brun PRA,
President, Royal Academy of Arts

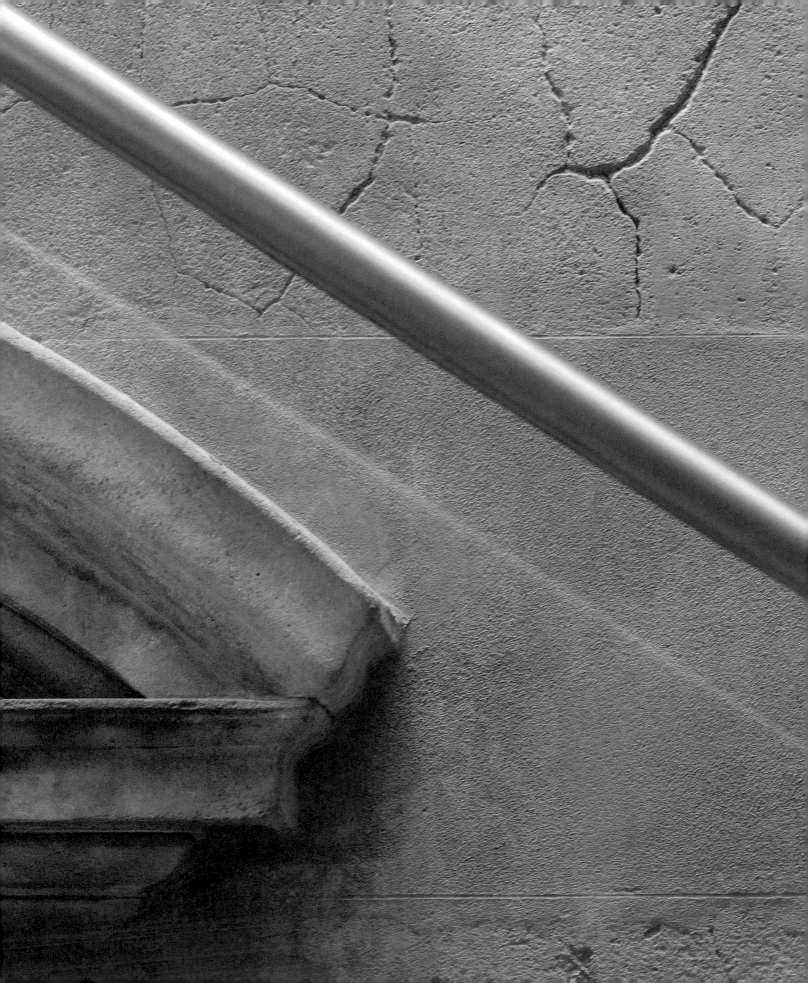

Curator's Preface
Kate Goodwin

In the memories I have of it, shaped as they were
by a child's understanding, it is not a building;
to my mind, it consists of discrete parts: here
a room, there a room, and here a stretch of
passageway that does not connect these two
rooms but is preserved in isolation, as a fragment.
In this way, it is all dispersed within me: the rooms,
the staircases that descend with such elaborate
ceremony, and other tight, spiral stairs where
one passed through the dark as the blood passes
through the veins; the rooms in the towers, the
balconies hung on high, the unexpected galleries
on to which one was thrust by a little door – all of
these things are still with me, and will never cease
to be in me.
Rainer Maria Rilke, *The Notebooks of Malte Laurids
Brigge*, 1910

Kate Goodwin is
Drue Heinz Curator
of Architecture
at the Royal
Academy of Arts

The task set by 'Sensing Spaces: Architecture
Reimagined' is far from simple: to evoke the
experience and power of architecture within
a traditional gallery environment, specifically
the grand Beaux-Arts spaces of the Royal Academy
of Arts. Exhibitions of architecture – consisting for
the most part of drawings, photographs and models
– often distance us from what we might experience
in direct contact with a building; here, instead,
we asked whether an exhibition could become
the means to highlight not merely the functional
or purely visual aspects of architecture but also
the sensation of inhabiting built space. Could an
exhibition be devised that would encourage visitors
to question their ideas about architecture and test
its capacity to move them? Could such an experience
awaken visitors' sensibilities to the spaces around
them, not only within but beyond the gallery walls?

When Burlington House became its new home
in 1867, the Royal Academy added to the back of
an eighteenth-century town palace a suite of grand
galleries designed for the display of works of art. This
is our site – an expression of the ambition and values
of its time and its creators. Over the past century and
a half, these galleries have been host to spectacular
exhibitions and occasions, continually transformed
by people and use. But how do these buildings
influence us, and what do they leave within us?

Our daily activities of working, sleeping or playing
mostly take place within, and interact with, some
form of architecture. Buildings are the ever-present
background to our lives. Today, they are created largely
as a practical and rational response to a brief, to the
demands and constraints of function and site, and

First we shape our buildings and afterwards our buildings shape us.
Winston Churchill

I haven't understood a bar of music in my life, but I have felt it.
Igor Stravinsky

as the shelter and container for what we do. How they might affect our senses and spirit is often a secondary consideration. But, arguably, much of the richness of architecture comes from the multifaceted way our senses respond to it, from the way it catches our imaginations, and from its emotional impact on us.

We all possess a dense layering of knowledge gleaned from experience, and architecture has been part of our physical and imaginative explorations of our spatial boundaries since birth. Although our awareness is not always active, particularly when the spaces around us are predefined and beyond our control, we regularly choose and transform the places we inhabit. Even as children, we make dens with proportions appropriate to our small size.

Such physical explorations of space are central to our understanding of architecture. We often have a visceral response to the built environment, perceived through the body and senses before it is rationalised by the mind. This response cannot be captured through a magazine cover or a single photographic image or text; we encounter a building in its setting, we move through it, we feel it, we inhabit it, alone or with others. Appreciation of its particularity may take time, discerned over the course of a day or through the changing seasons.

Being physically, emotionally and psychologically aware of the spaces that surround us and of our place within them could be described as having a sense of presence. It is not possible to pinpoint a single factor that evokes 'presence', and it is a challenge to describe. One can imagine that over almost two millennia, visitors to the Pantheon in Rome have felt the hairs on the back of their necks stand on end beneath the vast enclosing dome with its open oculus. Or one might feel 'present' in a more everyday setting or moment, such as running a hand over a banister for the thousandth time.

The heart of this exhibition is the interaction between three factors: the nature of physical spaces, our perception of them, and their evocative power. Seven architects from around the world – Grafton Architects (Ireland), Diébédo Francis Kéré (Burkina Faso and Germany), Kengo Kuma (Japan), Li Xiaodong (China), Pezo von Ellrichshausen (Chile) and Álvaro Siza and Eduardo Souto de Moura (Portugal) – have been invited to use the Royal Academy's galleries to test themselves and their discipline, to create unique spaces for an audience to experience. These architects have been selected because they distinctly engage with the ways architecture might move beyond practical and functional concerns to address the human spirit. Their buildings are strongly anchored in their

Without the senses we would have no true idea of space. And without writing we would have only a partial record of how individuals experience their own place in the world.
Diana Fuss, *The Sense of an Interior: Four Writers and the Rooms That Shaped Them*, 2004

A definition may be very exact, and yet go but a very little way towards informing us of the nature of the thing defined.
Edmund Burke, 'An Introduction on Taste' in *A Philosophical Enquiry into the Origin of Our Ideas of the Sublime and Beautiful*, 1759

contexts: from the physical urban and natural – landscapes in which they are located to the cultures and traditions that surround them. These architects use their appreciation of history to create buildings that acknowledge the past but are also highly meaningful within the present. They consider how people will inhabit their buildings, how the human body and senses will respond to their spaces. They do all this in sometimes shared and sometimes opposing ways, as the interviews in this catalogue and their installations reveal. And their different cultural, geographical and generational sensibilities bring a rich array of perspectives that encourage a broader understanding of architecture and what it can offer us.

As the following pages reflect, this exhibition has been conceived in a spirit of enquiry, begun through discussion and developed through the process of design with the architects. From the outset a direction and framework were established which deliberately resisted defining what the outcome could, should or would be. Each architect has worked with an open brief: to explore the potential of architecture, its relevance to people, the connections it evokes, and how one might convey these using architectural constructions within the traditional spaces of the Royal Academy. Each architect proposed initial ideas which then found a home in a particular place within the RA and evolved in response to their designated location, setting up dialogues with each other and between the existing and the new. The result might be seen as a series of moments or fragments that individually and collectively suggest something of the nature and potential of architecture. The installations may also be likened to a city, which gains its vitality and character from the ensemble as much as from its individual elements. And like a city, this exhibition needs people to bring it to life.

Architects have been invited to create the spaces for this exhibition, but this in no way implies that architecture is the sole territory of architects – on the contrary. Our responses to buildings or spaces are neither predefined by the architect nor inherent in the architecture itself. Although 'Sensing Spaces' explores each architect's intentions in the spaces they have created, it is equally concerned with what visitors discover by being open to the proposals architecture makes to us and to what it calls out from within us. As well as enabling us to find greater pleasure in the spaces we inhabit, this exhibition will perhaps heighten our awareness of the sensory realm of architecture and thereby encourage the creation of a more rewarding built environment.

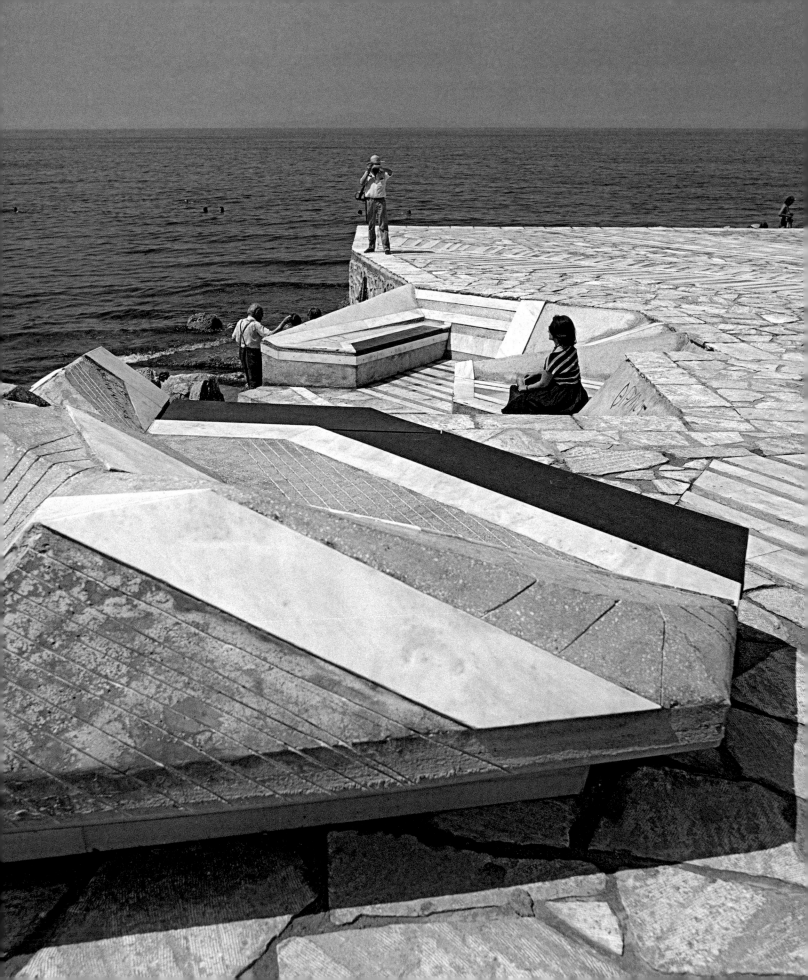

Presence: The Light Touch of Architecture
Philip Ursprung

1 (opposite) Nella Golanda, Flisvos Sculptured Quay, Palaio Faliro, near Athens, Greece (1986). Photograph by Dimitrios Kalapodas, 1987.

Philip Ursprung is Professor of History of Art and Architecture at the Institute for the History and Theory of Architecture, ETH Zurich

In spring 2013 I travelled to Athens with my students. Our hosts took us to the coast, showing us how unregulated expansion during the post-war building boom had cut off the city from the beach. We were heading towards the yacht harbour, planning to stop at Palaio Faliro to see the Flisvos Sculptured Quay by Greek artist Nella Golanda. Our hosts had chosen this project, completed in 1986, as a rare and successful example of how the beach can be made accessible.

I remember that we were walking along the shore, half paying attention to our guides, half absorbed by the beautiful view of the Mediterranean. Suddenly our pace slowed and we came to a halt. The students started to form little groups and chat together; some sat down, others took pictures, one even did a headstand. I enjoyed the warmth of the air, the fresh, salt smell of the sea, the intense blue of the sky. It took me a while to realise what had happened. We had reached our destination, the Flisvos Sculptured Quay, but our hosts had deliberately not announced it. Yet without any explanation or introduction we felt we had arrived at a very specific place. There was no need to hurry, no urge to move on. We were simply – present.

I started to look more carefully at the site. It was an inclined terrace, made of concrete faced with unevenly cut marble slabs in various colours, sloping gently towards the sea. There was no balustrade but I felt safe because the raw marble surface provided a good grip. I stood on solid ground, yet closer to the sea than on any other part of the promenade. It appeared as if one could simply take a run and leap into the water or even fly away towards the horizon.

On one side a niche had been carved out to form benches that were covered with stone and wood. On the other side a group of benches seemed to rise out of the massive terrace. These benches were arranged so people could sit close together and talk, despite the noise of the wind and sea. A few steps led down to a small sandy beach, both protected and framed by the quay.

We were immediately aware of the quality and beauty of this place, which stood in sharp contrast to the randomness of the many infrastructure buildings we had seen scattered along the coast. But we were also puzzled and so started to discuss what we saw. Was this architecture? Was it a sculpture? Was it a piece of infrastructure? Was it scenography? Was it landscape architecture? Was it a stage for a theatre, a viewing platform, a jetty, a pedestal, a fortification, an outdoor lounge? It was impossible to define the genre of the structure, and we even found it difficult to describe its size. But we felt that what was built related in a specific way to our bodies, that it produced a state of heightened attention to the here and now, and that it sharpened our appreciation of our surroundings.

Performative space

I had never been to the site before, and I had not known about Nella Golanda until I arrived in Greece. Nevertheless, I felt a kind of *déjà vu*. Where else had I experienced a comparable sense of my own presence within the built environment? The relationship between the artificial and the landscape, between small-scale and large-scale, between the carefully arranged, almost ornamental stone slabs

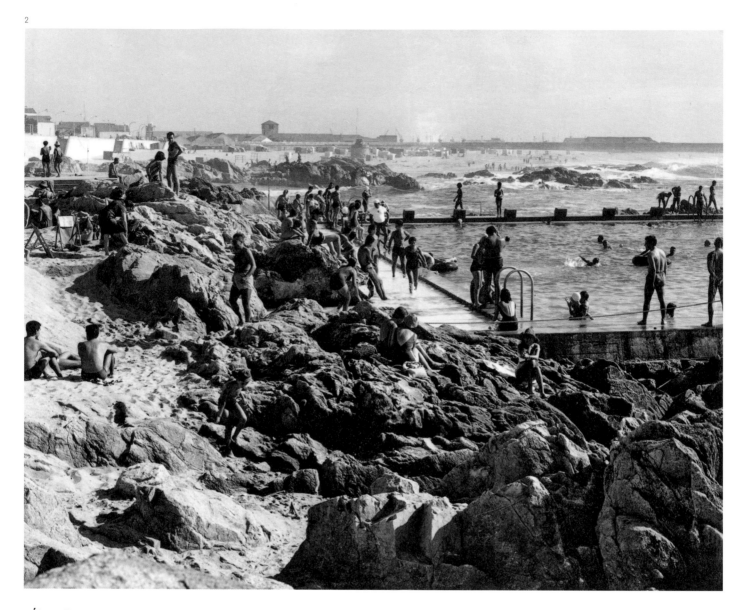

2 Álvaro Siza, public pool at Leça da Palmeira, near Porto, Portugal (1961–66). Photograph by A. Vieira, early 1960s.

and the overall structure reminded me of other places I had visited. As I walked around the quay, sensing the surface of the marble beneath my shoes, feeling the contrast between the rough concrete and the polished wood of the benches with my fingertips, I remembered a trip to the public pool of Leça da Palmeira, built near Porto by Álvaro Siza in the early 1960s. Some colleagues had taken me there two years ago on a sunny day in spring, when it was still too cold to swim. In Siza's pool, with its concrete terraces and stairs apparently directly added to or carved out of the rocks, I had felt both close to and protected from the Atlantic Ocean. The rocky shore and the concrete interventions were framing one another, so to speak. I had been fascinated by a similar conjunction when I visited the Municipal

Stadium at Braga (2003) by Eduardo Souto de Moura, where the rawness of the existing stone quarry forms a contrast with the elegant concrete structure of the stands. The oscillation between visual and tactile, and the path the architecture offers for visitors to follow – the sense of the theatrical – are crucial for both architects.

The merging of the painterly, sculptural, architectural and performative that I experienced at Palaio Faliro also reminded me of Gibellina Vecchia, where Italian artist Alberto Burri cast a concrete landscape over the ruins of a Sicilian village that had been destroyed by an earthquake. Famous in the 1950s and 1960s for large-format paintings with roughly treated surfaces including clay and cloth, Burri had raised the scale of painting to an

3

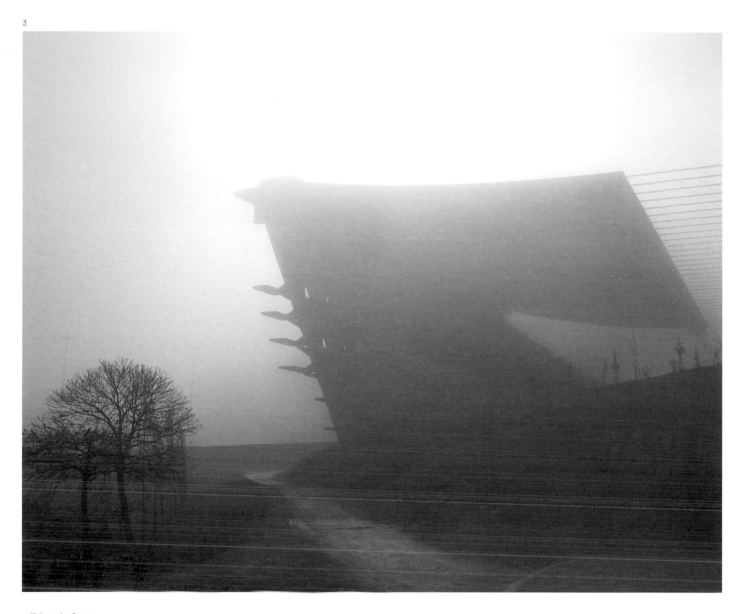

3 Eduardo Souto
de Moura, Braga
Municipal Stadium,
Portugal (2003).
Photograph by
Maria Manuel
Oliveira, 2004.

4 (overleaf) Alberto
Burri, 'Grande Cretto',
Gibellina Vecchia,
Sicily, Italy (1981).
Photograph
by Marcello
Paternostro, 2008.

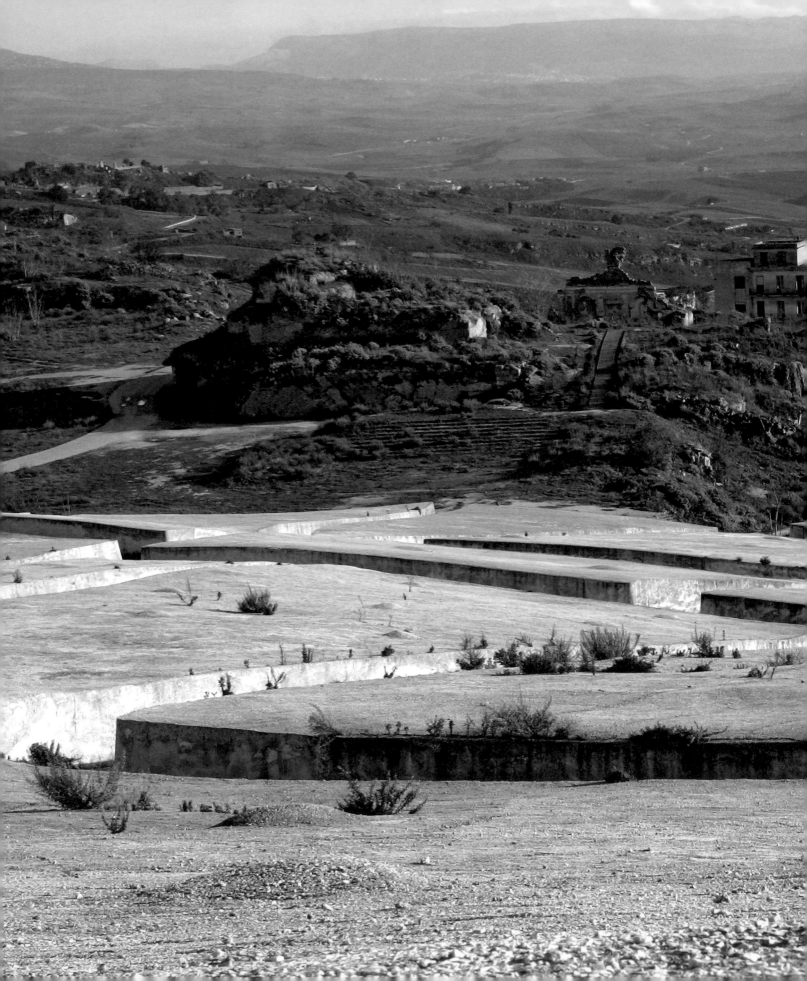

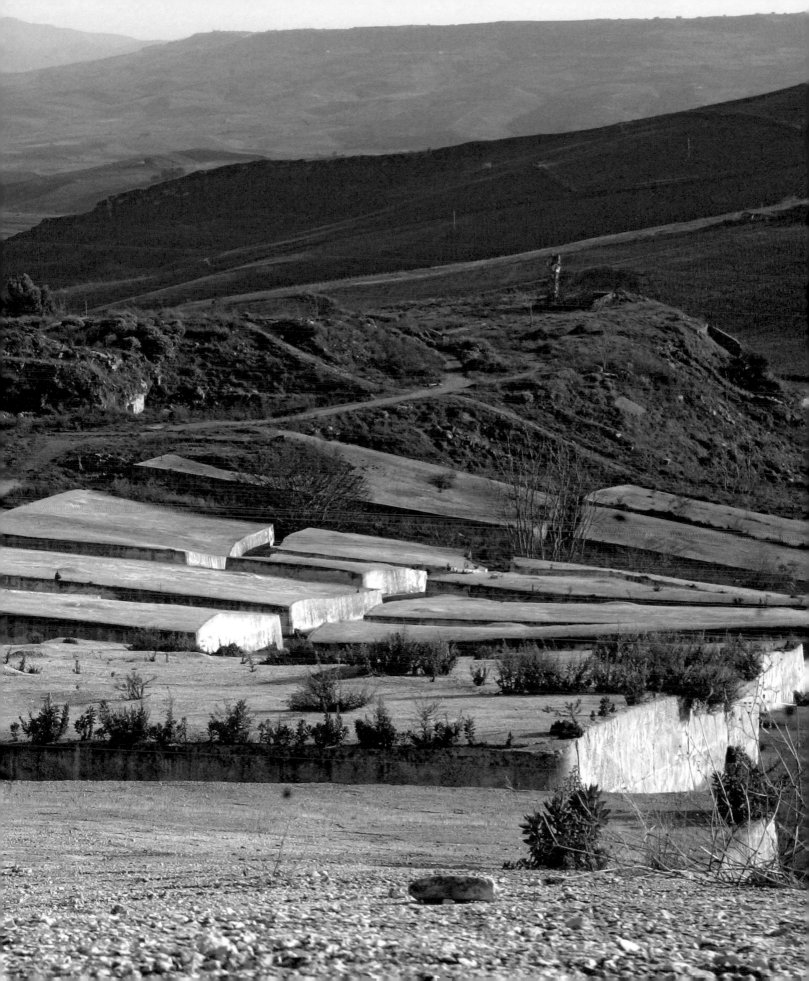

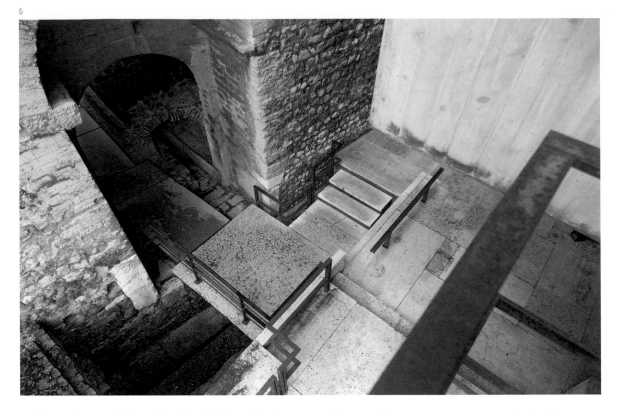

5 Carlo Scarpa,
Castelvecchio
Museum restoration,
Verona, Italy
(1959–73).
Photograph by Peter
Guthrie, 2013.

entire settlement. His work, *Grande Cretto* (1981), allowed visitors literally to sink into the surface of a very large painting, to disappear into the cracks, which functioned both as real paths and as traces of the artistic process. And finally, the nuances in material, texture and colour beneath my feet at Palaio Faliro also recalled the path of stone and concrete slabs leading through the halls of Carlo Scarpa's renovation of the Castelvecchio Museum in Verona, realised between the late 1950s and the mid-1970s. In this museum, Scarpa went further than any other architect at that time in his attempt to orchestrate the movements of the building's users. I felt free to roam there, yet safely guided by a spatial narrative that uses light and shadow, narrow and open spaces and a variety of materials to involve the museum-goer.

During our brief stay at the Flisvos Sculptured Quay we experienced a comparable mix of guidance and freedom to move. In some sense, we felt like dancers or actors on a stage, performing freely, without a plot or fixed choreography, led simply by our surroundings. Perhaps we were particularly sensitive to this performative aspect because we had visited the ruins of the Theatre of Dionysus Eleuthereus the day before. Located directly beneath the Athens Acropolis, the birthplace of European theatre combines the contours of the landscape with rows of stone seats, open towards the distant sea. The natural topography of the landscape and the artificial topology of the architecture enhance each other, as if the stone slabs were framing the grass-covered slope and the slope formed a background for the whiteness of the stone rows and the stage. It is tempting to imagine how, in antiquity, this setting converged with the narrative of the play, the movement of the actors and the expectations of the audience, who were empowered to decide which author won the prize. While we were wandering among the ruins, the French theoretician Henri Lefevbre came to mind. In his 1974 book *The Production of Space*, Lefevbre evokes a unity of space and time:

A Greek theatre presupposes tragedy and comedy, and by extension the presence of the city's people and their allegiance to their heroes and gods. In theatrical space, music, choruses, masks, tiering – all such elements converge with language and actors. A spatial action overcomes conflicts, at least momentarily, even though it does not resolve them; it opens a way from everyday concerns to collective joy.[1]

The association of the theatre, of a performing space, evoked other, less well-known images

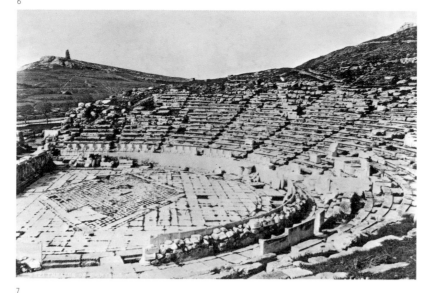

6 Theatre of Dionysus Eleuthereus, beneath the Acropolis in Athens, Greece (fifth century BCE). Photograph from c. 1930.

7 Adolphe Appia, a 'rhythmic space' designed to unify the elements of theatre and dance in music (1909).

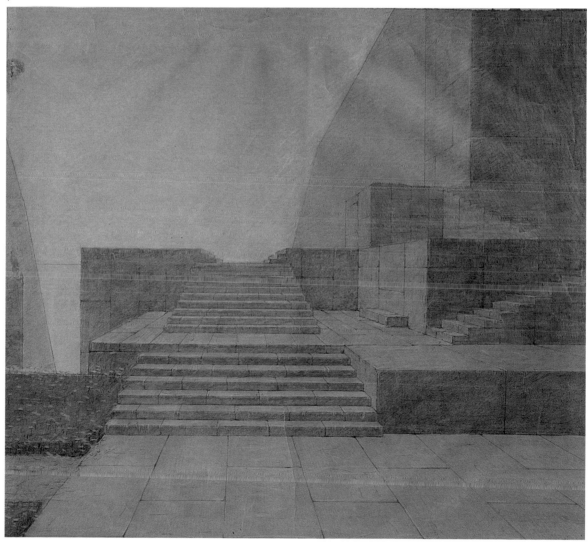

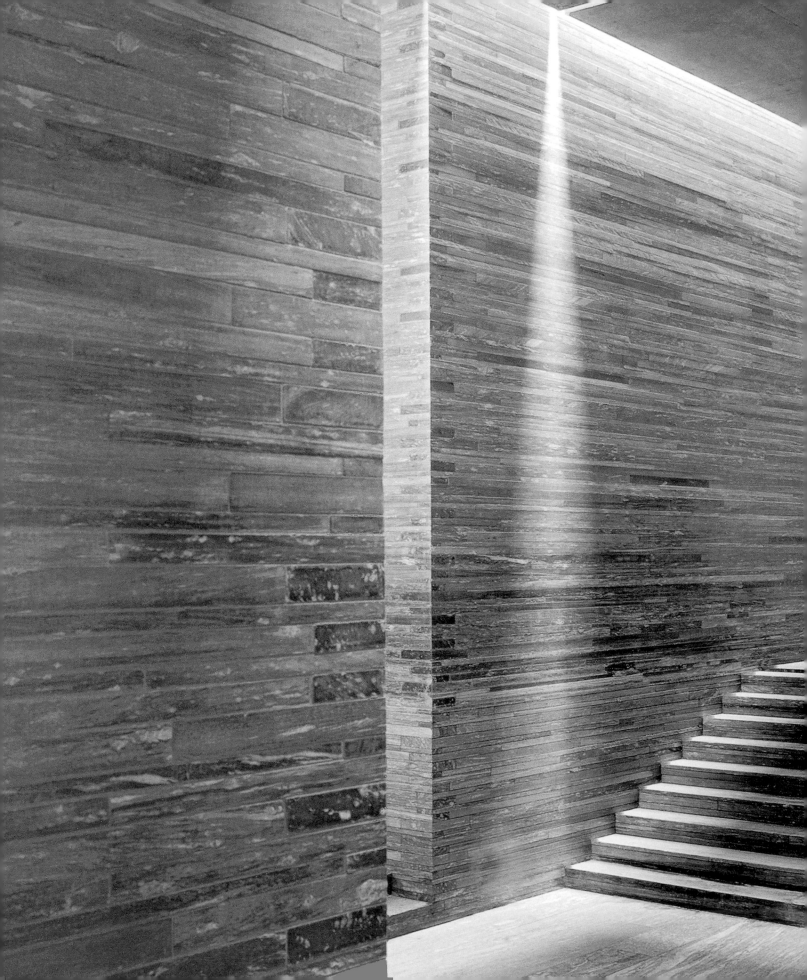

8 (opposite)
Peter Zumthor,
Thermal Baths,
Vals, Switzerland
(1996).
Photograph
by Hans Danuser,
2008.

made by the Swiss scenographer Adolphe Appia. Originally inspired by Richard Wagner's concept of the *Gesamtkunstwerk*, the total work of art, Appia revolutionised stage design in the early twentieth century. He replaced the illusionistic backdrops favoured by Wagner and most nineteenth-century directors with atmospheric stage sets that used monumental steps, ramps, platforms and curtains. Not painting, but architecture informed these designs; an overall atmosphere rather than specific pieces of scenery framed the performances, the intention being to create a sense of unity, to focus on light, sound and movement, and to heighten the audience's emotional involvement in the opera. Appia was interested in eurhythmics and developed a new approach to theatrical lighting, which he considered inseparable from the actors and the space. As he put it: 'Light has an almost miraculous flexibility... it can create shadows, make them living, and spread the harmony of their vibrations in space just as music does.' Appia literally set the stage for the experimental theatre of the second half of the twentieth century and in retrospect his projects seem to anticipate many spectacular atmospheric installations such as James Turrell's works with natural and artificial light, or the stage designs of Robert Wilson.

Atmosphere and aura

I am not referring to this Greek experience in order to highlight my own subjectivity. Rather, my reactions and those of my students are typical of a general trend in current architectural discussions, namely an interest in the way we as subjects relate to our built environment both physically and emotionally. There is a renewed interest in synaesthesia in art, architecture and design. It seems that we are becoming aware once more that the relationship between ourselves and buildings can no longer be merely visual. We want to be able to locate our bodies within the environment and we are interested in interaction, exchange, osmosis. We are not just a pair of eyes floating through space; we have bodies, senses, emotions, expectations and memories.

The monumental iconic buildings that dominated architectural discussion in the 1990s and 2000s, such as Frank Gehry's Guggenheim Museum in Bilbao (1997) or Norman Foster's 30 St Mary Axe, the 'Gherkin', in the City of London (2003), still make the headlines and are attractive to an ever increasing public. But the ideas they stand for have lost much of their appeal in recent years, at least in the United States, Europe and Japan.

The financial crisis, triggered by property bubbles in the United States, has highlighted the brutal contrast between the spectacular office towers of the financial industry and the fate of individual home-owners and tenants. Designed as landmarks on the skylines of big cities, commissioned both to attract capital and to express the power of investment, such buildings tend to increase the sense of alienation between people and the built environment. It is notable that since the Gulf area and Southeast Asian metropolises became studded with signature architecture, the wider public has tended to perceive such buildings as emblems of difference and exclusivity rather than proximity and community. Iconic buildings now seem to separate rather than to unite people.

It is therefore no wonder that, with the decline of star architecture, there has been a growing demand for buildings that act on various senses simultaneously, buildings that one can touch, smell or hear, that evoke mental images and resonate in one's memory. Could it be that this demand is compensation for the fact that many people consider the economic and political realms to be abstract, incomprehensible, beyond their own influence? Might the public need this reassurance in order to be confident of its own existence, in the same way as one occasionally twitches one's own arm to make sure one is not dreaming? Is this a reaction to counterbalance the individualisation and segregation that prevail in industrialised nations, or is it a regressive move back to the familiar? Whatever the reasons – and there are certainly contradictory motives for the trend towards the immediate and physical – it is no coincidence that some of the best of these new buildings stand not in the centres of megacities but in the provinces, far from airports and often in poor areas. Their budgets are usually tiny compared with the sums signature architecture requires. And their scale is closer to sculpture, fashion design or scenography than to the urban dimension.

Opened in 1996, during the heyday of signature architecture, Peter Zumthor's Thermal Baths in Vals are an exemplar of this trend. Their visual impact is striking, but even stronger is their impact on the other senses – such as the olfactory and the tactile – and people flock to the resort village in the Swiss Alps to experience the sensory effects the building produces. Those who have swum there will never forget the unexpected sight and smell of petals floating in the warm water of the flower pool, or how relaxing and inspiring it is to lie on a comfortable leather bench in a dimly lit chamber listening to musician Fritz Hauser's composition *Sounding Stones*. The entire complex recalls a cave cut into the rocks of the massif – hence its German name, Felsentherme – although the building is made out of concrete and the gneiss slabs with various grades of polishing are mere cladding, almost as in a stage set. The project is not about materials as such; it does not explore their 'essence' or 'nature', nor does it focus on their symbolic meaning or historical associations. Rather, these materials mediate between people who are relaxing or receiving treatment and their surroundings. The gneiss slabs on the walls and floors, the polished concrete, the leather seats and wooden benches, the bronze handrails and drinking cup in the dimly lit fountain room act as props, or tools, to enhance the contrasting experiences of coolness and heat and the slightly sulphurous taste of the water.

A more recent project by Zumthor goes even further in foregrounding a building's sensual qualities. The Bruder Klaus Feldkapelle (2007), a small chapel in a private field at Mechernich-Wachendorf, near Cologne, was commissioned by local farmers in honour of a patron saint. When I went to see it, I had to approach the monolithic concrete structure on foot, after wandering through the fields. Even for someone like myself, without religious faith, this slow approach through open meadows was an exciting experience. When I finally arrived at the building, I was confronted by a massive triangular concrete door. Its appearance and material made me expect a heavy mass, difficult to move, but when I took the handle it swung open more readily than I had anticipated. Simply by opening the door, I was involving myself in the choreography of the chapel, participating in its spatiality and materiality, literally activating the space.

Once inside, I was struck by the darkness and the smell of burnt wood. There is no artificial light, and daylight seems to percolate through an opening in the roof of the tipi-shaped structure and through a regular arrangement of glass tubes inserted into the concrete walls. The smell comes from the charred surface of the interior, which survives from burning the wooden struts that formed the framework. The concrete was poured and rammed in layers, which can still be distinguished on the façade, revealing the building process, while the lead floor has an uneven surface, a result of the pouring process and the heat that melted the metal. So the building carries the history of its own making, not as written information but in traces that anyone, specialist in architecture or not, can recognise.

How can we define this shift in perception, this tendency towards the synaesthetic? Although it seems quite obvious what is meant when people speak about the direct and unmediated perception of the built environment, the phenomenon is a challenge to theory. Much ink has flowed in attempting to describe this interrelation, and the multitude and vagueness of the terms in play indicate that a fundamental shift is taking place. One of the terms that has become popular in the realm of architecture is the notion of 'atmosphere', first theorised by German philosopher Gernot Böhme in the mid-1990s. Böhme wants to overcome the distance between the object and the viewer. For him, atmosphere is the 'common reality of the one who perceives and the object which is perceived'.[3] Furthermore, he pleads for an aesthetic practice that is not limited to art – traditionally the subject of aesthetic reflection – but which also includes 'design, scenography, advertisement, the production of musical atmospheres, cosmetics, interior design'.[4] Böhme's concept of atmosphere draws on what Walter Benjamin called the 'aura' in his famous essay 'The Work of Art in the Age of Mechanical Reproduction' (1936). Benjamin does not give a clear definition of what he means by aura. He uses an image, which has been quoted many times despite, or because of, its vagueness. In his words, the aura is the 'unique phenomenon of a distance, however close it may be. If, while resting on a summer afternoon, you follow with your eyes a mountain range on the horizon or a branch which casts its shadow over you, you experience the aura of those mountains, of that branch.'[5]

For our current discussion, it is particularly the oscillation between the near and far that is important. Aura, one could say, has to do with omitting a distance, and with involving other senses than the visual. The aura, in Benjamin's view, is lost when a work of art is mechanically reproduced. Of course, this idea has to be questioned today, when art and architecture are intrinsically linked to technical reproduction. Photography, film and video have long been established artistic genres. Although the result of mechanical reproduction, a photograph or a video installation is equal to – and not less 'auratic' than – a painting or sculpture, even if we know that other copies of it exist. The same goes for architecture: there would be little discourse about architecture without photography and video. Buildings are intrinsically tied to mechanical modes of production – about series, about repetition and reproduction. We are so used to seeing architecture by means of photography that we almost automatically look for the camera angle when we are confronted with a building.

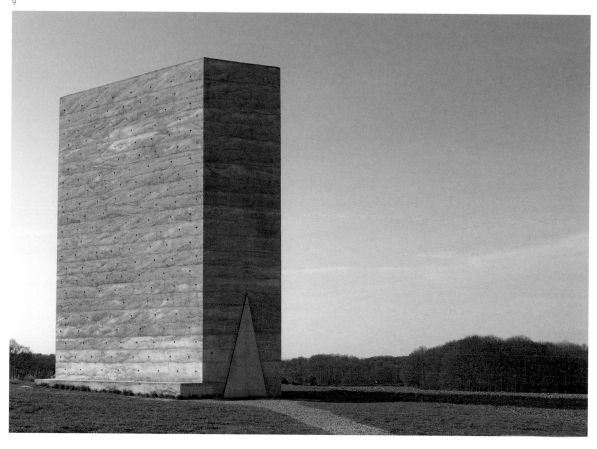

Immediacy and immersion are other terms used to describe this phenomenon. These terms are more often applied to art than to architecture. Installations by Olafur Eliasson, which embrace viewers in foggy environments as in *The Mediated Motion* in Zumthor's Bregenz Art Museum (2001) or the *Weather Project* at Tate Modern (2003), allow visitors to dive into atmospheric surroundings that are both detached from reality by the museum walls and 'real' because they actually affect the senses. People move around the work of art, can touch it, can interact with it to a point where they seem to change from the role of passive consumer to active participant. Of course, this participation is still controlled by the artist, but the need to keep moving, to find one's way through the fog, to reorient oneself, constantly sharpens the senses. Mainly in the realm of art, the notions of 'participation' and 'relational aesthetics' have become widely used during the last decade.

Among the many terms that feature in today's exploration of this issue, I find the concept of 'presence' particularly useful. It has been discussed in the last decade by various authors – and from various points of view. In their book *Empire* (2000), Michael Hardt and Antonio Negri outline the scenario of a worldwide realm in which an eternal present rules. In contrast to nineteenth-century imperialism, when individual nation states competed for territorial expansion, the empire Hardt and Negri describe is a new world order that presents 'its rule not as a transitory moment in the movement of history, but as a regime with no temporal boundaries and in this sense outside of history or at the end of history.'[6] According to the theoretician Hans Ulrich Gumbrecht, who deals with this issue in his books *Production of Presence: What Meaning Cannot Convey* (2004)[7] and *After 1945: Latency as Origin of the Present* (2013),[8] one of the reasons for the current interest in the present is the fact that our temporal horizon has narrowed. We are, so to speak, trapped in an eternal present, in which the dimensions of the past and the future are shrinking. To make a prognosis, to speculate about the future, has become extremely difficult, as has exploration of the past. We can no longer 'learn' from the past and project the lessons of history on to the future. The idea of progress, which marked the perception of time for inhabitants of industrialised nations since the Second World War, has come to an end. Of course, there is technological

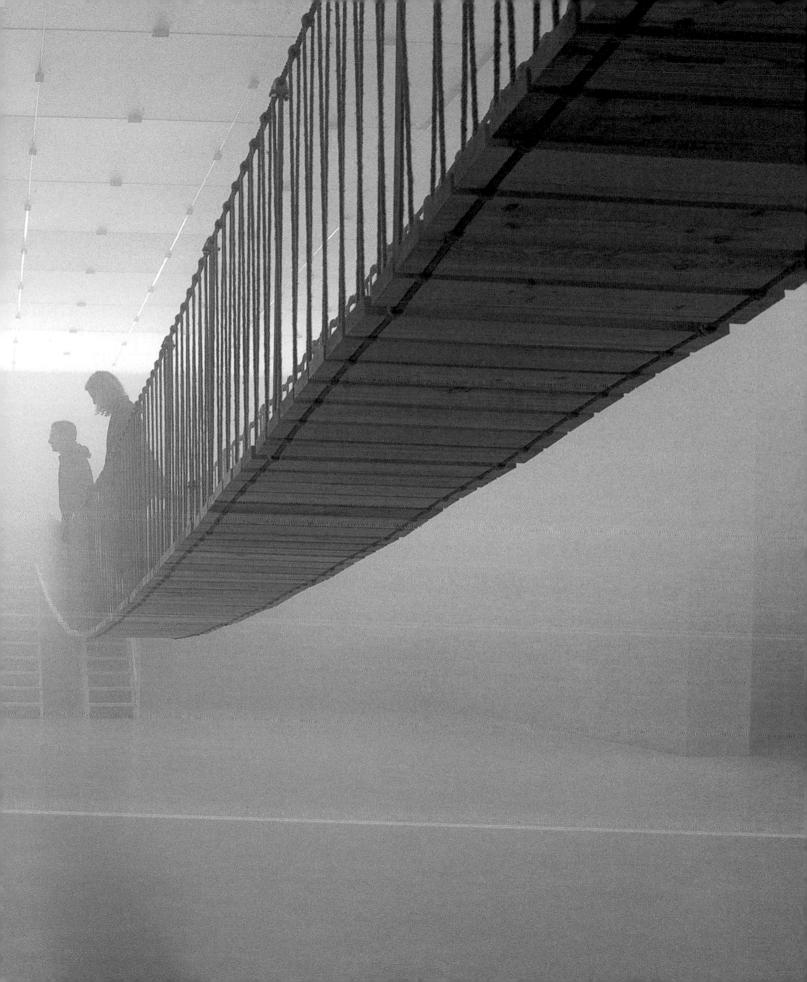

innovation, but it has become difficult to link this process to the individual subject. In the words of the French sociologist Alain Ehrenberg: 'We are changing, of course, but that does not necessarily mean we are progressing.'[9]

Paradoxically, the idea of the eternal present also implies that we feel disconnected from temporality, as if we have fallen out of time, as if the time we are living in is no longer ours. In a state of eternal present, everything extraordinary becomes rare and valuable. In consequence, the event turns into a cherished resource, into something desirable, because it makes us feel that we are participating in something important, that we are reconnected with temporality, that we are – present. No wonder the event is so popular, whether in the realm of entertainment, politics, lifestyle or architecture. What is valuable is the impression that one is connected to one's surroundings.

This desire to connect with one's surroundings is not new, of course. The longing for a supposedly intact, pre-industrial unity and coherence runs through the entire era of industrialisation. In the mid-nineteenth century, architects and theoreticians such as Gottfried Semper, Owen Jones and John Ruskin were influential advocates of a synthesis of the arts and among the harshest critics of the results of the division of labour. Towards the end of the century, Adolphe Appia, the Viennese Secessionists and the philosopher Henri Bergson called for a multi-sensory art and architecture. Bergson's book *Matter and Memory* (1896), with sales of several hundred thousand copies well into the 1940s, was adopted throughout the entire twentieth century, particularly after the renewed interest in Bergson initiated by Gilles Deleuze in the late 1960s. Many theorists focus on the role of the beholder and the way we experience our surroundings. Martin Heidegger's *Being and Time* (1927), John Dewey's *Art as Experience* (1934), Maurice Merleau-Ponty's *Phenomenology of Perception* (1945), Gaston Bachelard's *The Poetics of Space* (1958), Steen Eiler Rasmussen's *Experiencing Architecture* (1962) and Henri Lefebvre's *The Production of Space* (1974) are among the most influential examples of this line of thinking.

Gumbrecht gives a summary of the terms discussed above and defines the German concept of *Stimmung*, in the sense of 'mood' but also 'climate' or 'atmosphere', as a 'dimension of what can make the past present – immediately and intuitively present – to us'.[10] In his words:

What the metaphors 'climate' and 'atmosphere' share with the word *Stimmung* –

whose etymological root is *Stimme*, German for 'voice' – is that they suggest the presence of a material touch, typically a very light one, on the body of the (ap)perceiving party. Weather, sounds, and music all have a material yet invisible impact on us. *Stimmung* involves a sensation we associate with certain 'inner' feelings. Toni Morrison has described this aspect of *Stimmung* with the paradox of 'being touched as if from inside'.[11]

Approximation and exhibition

The concept of *Stimmung*, and particularly the metaphor of the 'light touch' evoked by Gumbrecht, provides another fruitful approach to the discussion of our relationship with architecture. It addresses the importance of physical sensation, but it also reminds us of the slight distance that remains between ourselves and our surroundings. It relates to the idea of approximation, of two phenomena being very close to each other but never identical, never completely united. It recalls what Benjamin writes when he talks about the aura of being both near *and* far. It recalls the difference from a merely visual relation. And it evokes the temporal aspect, the idea that the interrelation between subject and environment is a process, something that happens in both space and time and that therefore contains a historical dimension.

This might help us to understand Peter Zumthor's concept of presence. At a conference in Zurich in February 2013, in which Gumbrecht also participated, Zumthor said his goal was to produce the feeling of presence with his architecture, although he was aware this goal could not be achieved. He described what he meant by presence by evoking memories of himself running through a village as an eight-year-old boy, smelling fresh concrete: 'And when I think back, I think that was *pure presence* for me. Pure being. Intensity of the moment. And of course there is no meaning yet.'[12] This moment could not be repeated with the same intensity, but it could be evoked – not by showing the buildings and landscapes of his childhood, but in depicting contemporary landscapes and producing architecture. In his words: 'I would like to do buildings which do not mean anything. They just *are*. That is the greatest achievement for me.'[13]

It is obvious that the movement of the subject's body through space plays a role in this concept of presence, because it includes the performative aspect and the temporal dimension. Surroundings are constantly in a relationship with the human body – its size, its senses. Of course, since antiquity it has been commonplace to relate the human body to architecture and to conceive architectural elements as artefacts shaped after the human body, as anthropomorphic. But what is interesting within our context is the fact that our perception and our ability to relate our surroundings to our bodies seem to cause an interrelationship between an otherwise incoherent spatiality and temporality.

This anthropomorphic relationship is exactly what interests art historian Alina Payne when she describes the role of ornament in visual culture, stating that the '*tertium comparationis* that connects scale and sculpture (small or large, architectural or object-based) is the human body, which engages directly, physically and haptically, the three-dimensional world that surrounds it.'[14] Could it be that the current revival of architectural ornament – for example in the work of Herzog & de Meuron or Caruso St John, but also the interest that earlier exemplars, such as Carlo Scarpa, Richard Sullivan or Gottfried Semper, evoke today – is another symptom of the change taking place? Banned from the realm of architecture during most of the twentieth century, ornament is once more moving centre stage. Its present popularity is not only thanks to newly available tools, for instance lasers for cutting materials, but is also characteristic of a renewed interest in human scale, in elements that relate directly to our bodily experience, that allow us to identify and empathise with the very structure of architecture. We experienced this at Nella Golanda's Flisvos Sculptured Quay, where the stone slabs were arranged in an obviously ornamental way, care having been taken with the relationship between colours, textures and the size of each individual piece.

If the feeling of presence is a challenge to architecture, it is an even greater challenge to the exhibition of architecture. A wide gap exists between our daily experience of the built environment and the abstractions we are confronted with in architecture exhibitions in the guise of models, plans, photographs and descriptions. And it appears to be difficult to take the immediacy of life in the street – its noise, its smell, its pace and ever-changing atmosphere – across the institutional threshold of the museum and into a gallery space. Of course, it is a truism that architecture cannot be exhibited as such. To exhibit architecture is as much a challenge to the conventions of the genre as is exposure of art in the open, outside museum walls.

On the other hand, exhibitions are testing grounds, areas of experimentation. To use an exhibition not as a means to represent what we already know but as an opportunity to learn more about what we don't know opens up new terrain. Where, if not in the space of the exhibition, can one find better conditions to test a building's interaction with its users? Where is there more freedom to reshuffle the relations between different genres, and to move freely between architecture, sculpture and scenography? Asking how spatial artefacts affect the senses, how they interact with our bodies and allow us to see our environment in a new light, will also contribute to a better understanding of the function of architecture in our societies. If we are looking for an architecture that brings people together in space and time and goes beyond the iconic, the exhibition is a privileged medium for its development. It is here that approximation happens, and that presence, whatever its definition might be, can take place.

1 Henri Lefebvre, *The Production of Space*, translated from the French original of 1974 by Donald Nicholson-Smith, Oxford, 1991, p. 222

2 'Adolphe Appia, Actor, Space, Light, Painting' (1919), published in *Journal de Genève*, 23–24 January 1954; reprinted in Richard C. Beacham (ed.), *Adolphe Appia: Texts on Theatre*, London and New York, 1993, pp. 114–15, quoted on p. 114

3 Gernot Böhme, *Atmosphäre: Essays zur neuen Ästhetik*, Frankfurt am Main, 1995, p. 34; translation by Philip Ursprung

4 *Ibid.*, p. 35; translation by Philip Ursprung

5 Walter Benjamin, 'The Work of Art in the Age of Mechanical Reproduction' (originally published in 1936), in Walter Benjamin, *Illuminations: Essays and Reflections*, edited and with an introduction by Hannah Arendt, New York, 1968, pp. 217–52; quotation from pp. 224–25 (online: marxists.org/reference/subject/philosophy/works/ge/benjamin.htm)

6 Michael Hardt and Antonio Negri, *Empire*, Cambridge, Mass., 2000, pp. xiv–xv

7 Hans Ulrich Gumbrecht, *Production of Presence: What Meaning Cannot Convey*, Stanford, 2004

8 Hans Ulrich Gumbrecht, *After 1945: Latency as Origin of the Present*, Stanford, 2013

9 Alain Ehrenberg, *The Weariness of the Self: Diagnosing the History of Depression in the Contemporary Age*, Montreal and Kingston, 2009, p. 185

10 Hans Ulrich Gumbrecht, *After 1945: Latency as Origin of the Present*, op. cit., p. 24

11 *Ibid.*, p. 24

12 Peter Zumthor, oral presentation on the occasion of the conference 'Presence' at the Cabaret Voltaire, Zurich, 1 February 2013

13 Peter Zumthor, *ibid.*

14 Alina Payne, *From Ornament to Object: Genealogies of Architectural Modernism*, New Haven and London, 2012, p. 16

Architects

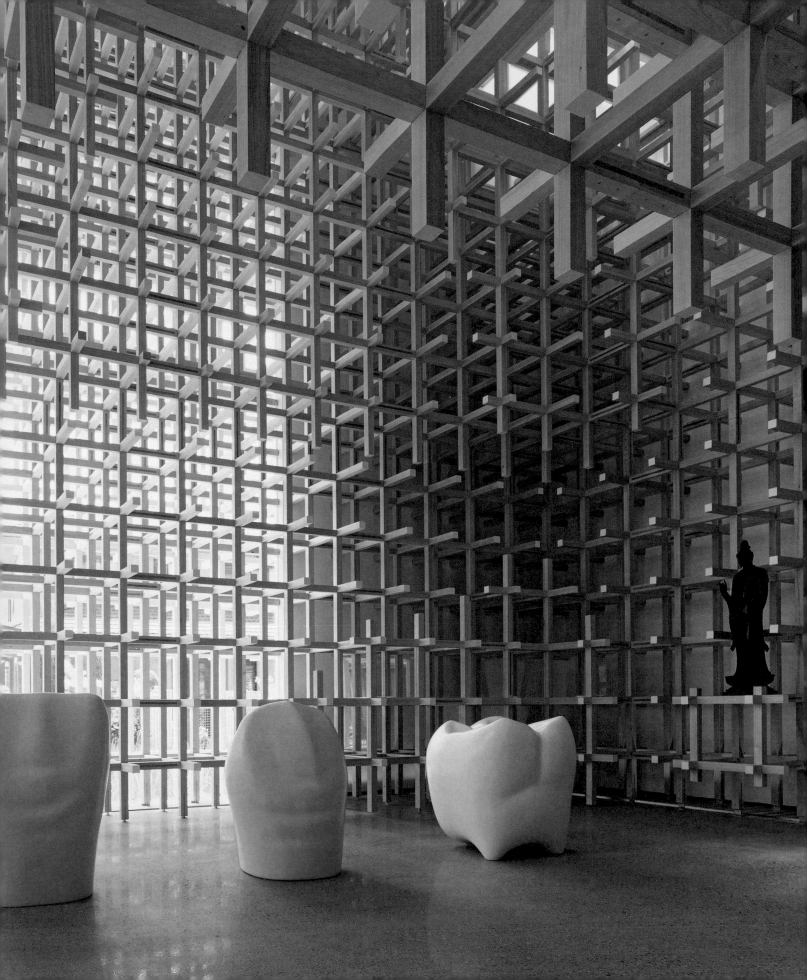

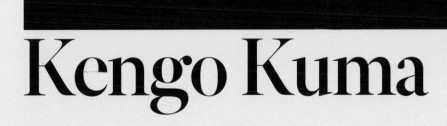

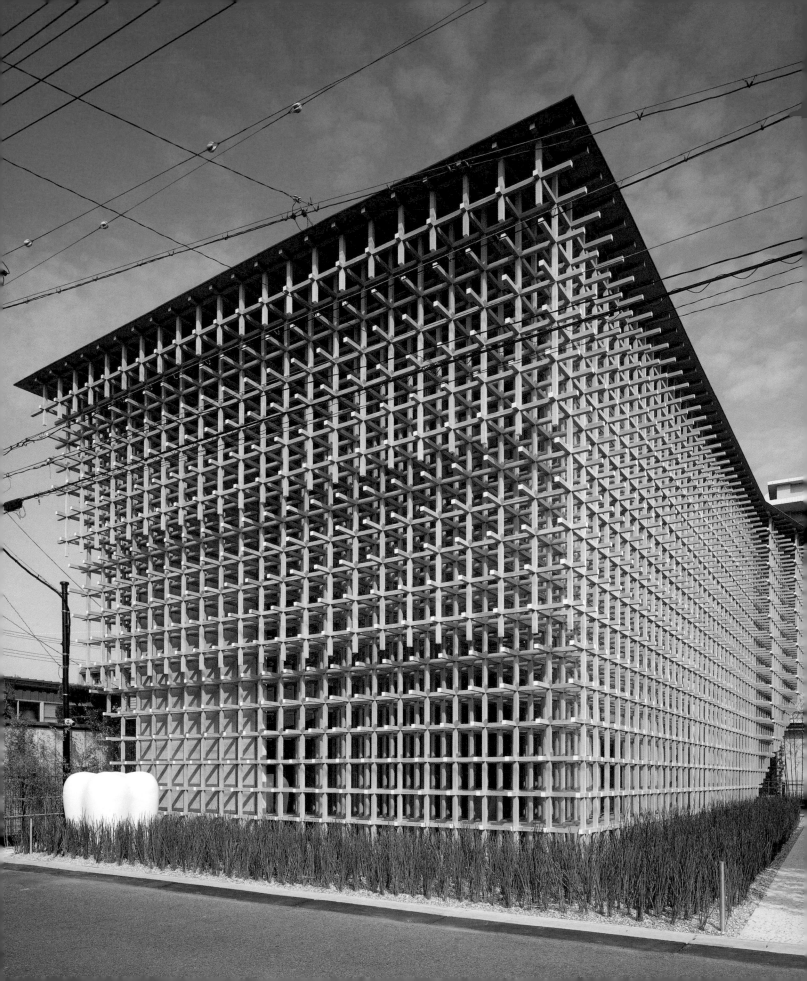

1 (previous spread), 2 (opposite) Kengo Kuma & Associates, GC Prostho Museum Research Center, Aichi Prefecture, Japan (2010).
This showcase for GC, a manufacturer of dental prosthetics, exemplifies Kuma's method of breaking down materials into fragments and then recombining them to dramatic effect. The structural concept is based on the Japanese children's game of cidori, a collection of wooden sticks notched so they can be combined in various ways.

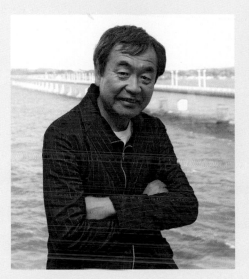

The work of Kengo Kuma (born 1954 in Kanagawa, Japan) builds on the concept of 'weak architecture', developed in part as a reaction to the Kobe earthquake of 1995. This sees architecture as subservient to nature and influences everything from the siting of buildings and framing of the environment to the materials and construction methods employed.

Kuma studied architecture at the University of Tokyo before moving to New York where he was visiting researcher at Columbia University in 1985/86. In 1987 he founded Spatial Design Studio and in 1990 Kengo Kuma & Associates in Tokyo; a Paris office was opened in 2008.

Kuma's international reputation rests on a portfolio covering many building types – houses, city halls, sports centres, museums – as well as on his extensive writings and teaching.

His work is characterised by harmonious, understated spaces that achieve a lot with great economy of means and his buildings embody a sense of vulnerability that humanises institutions which can often overwhelm the individual. Using a limited range of often natural materials in each project, he also experiments with new technologies in construction.

Since 2009 Kuma has been a professor at the Graduate School of Architecture in Tokyo. In addition to his prolific work in Japan, he increasingly undertakes projects across Asia and Europe including the V&A Museum in Dundee and the FRAC in Marseille (2013). He was awarded the French decoration Officier de l'ordre des arts et des lettres in 2009 and is an international fellow of the Royal Institute of British Architects and an honorary fellow of the American Institute of Architects.

3

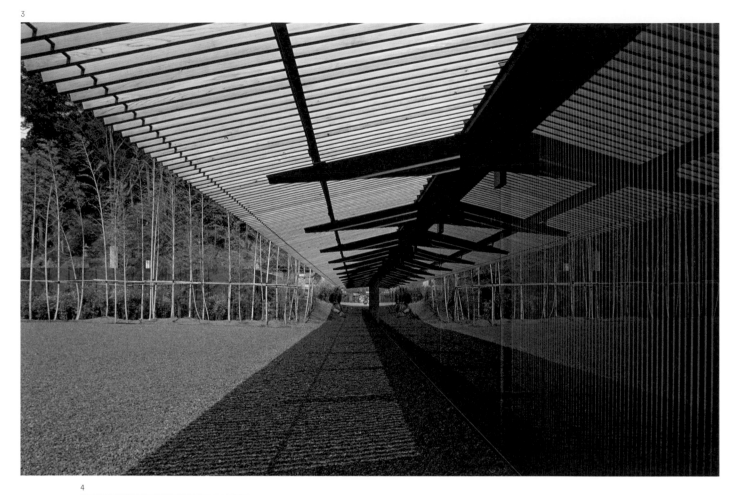

4

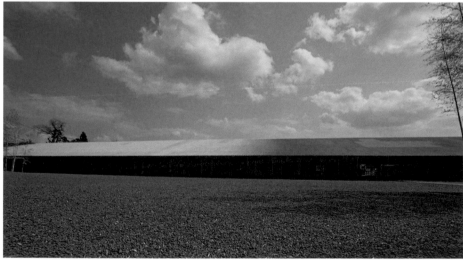

3, 4 Kengo Kuma & Associates, Nakagawa-machi Bato Hiroshige Museum of Art, Nasu-gun, Tochigi Prefecture, Japan (2000).
Kuma's design for a museum for the Edo-period woodblock artist Ando Hiroshige superimposes layers of local cedar to create an equivalent of the spatial world of Ando's work. Some of the detail is inspired by Ando's print 'People on a Bridge Surprised by Rain' – vertical louvres represent falling rain while the roof of the horizontally extruded building suggests cloud over a landscape.

Kate Goodwin: In what ways do you see architecture enhancing human experience beyond shelter and function?
Kengo Kuma: Human beings are tiny, frail creatures, and architecture must offer them comfort as well as protection. For me, the key to achieving this lies in the choice of materials and the scale. I always start with something small, breaking down materials into particles or fragments that can then be recombined into units of the right scale to provide comfort and intimacy. The GC Prostho Museum Research Center, which used some 6,000 uniform pieces of cypress in its construction, is a good example of this process.

Traditional Japanese architecture employs materials that can only be used at a relatively small scale: wood, rice paper, sometimes stone. I believe that if a building is made from a material used on a monolithic scale – for instance, exposed concrete – any sense of intimacy is destroyed. I hope that in my architecture scale and materials do not overpower the beauty of individual elements, so there is a balance between the parts and the totality.

Is this a part of your project to create 'weak architecture'?
The essence of 'weak architecture' is to ensure harmony between a building and its environment. Nature may appear calm and tranquil, but actually it is much more powerful than anything we are capable of making. For many Japanese, the recent tsunamis demonstrated the limits of human progress, with concrete buildings completely destroyed by natural forces. Architecture cannot resist the strength of nature so it needs to find ways of coexisting with it.

My method of design is always site-specific: I don't want to offer a generic response but rather to create something unique with a powerful connection to its surroundings. When it comes to choosing materials, for instance, I talk to local people about the kinds of wood and stone you find in their area. One of my favourite projects is the Hiroshige Museum of Art, which looks as if it has merged with its environment and doesn't trumpet its presence.

'Weak architecture' is also about our relationship with space, and I believe that the human body responds to this kind of weakness. For instance, unlike concrete, the ground is made up of billions of different elements such as leaves or particles of soil. This provides diversity and richness, which is what human beings need to find in architecture. The texture of the floor is very important in traditional Japanese spaces because people don't wear shoes indoors.

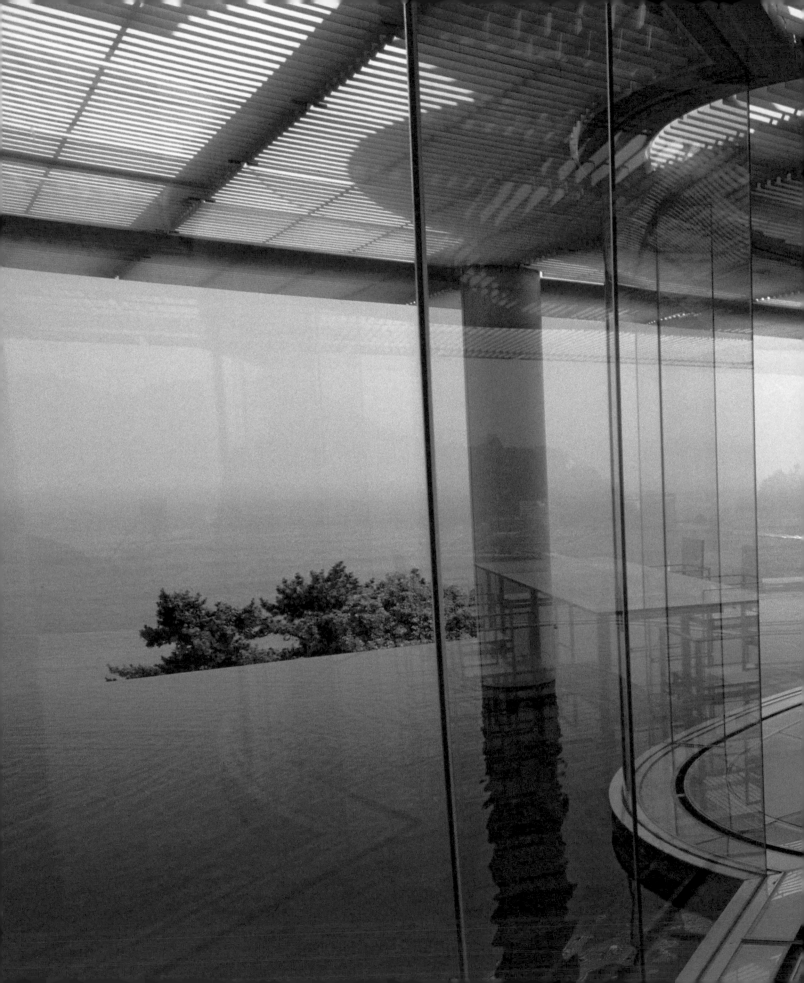

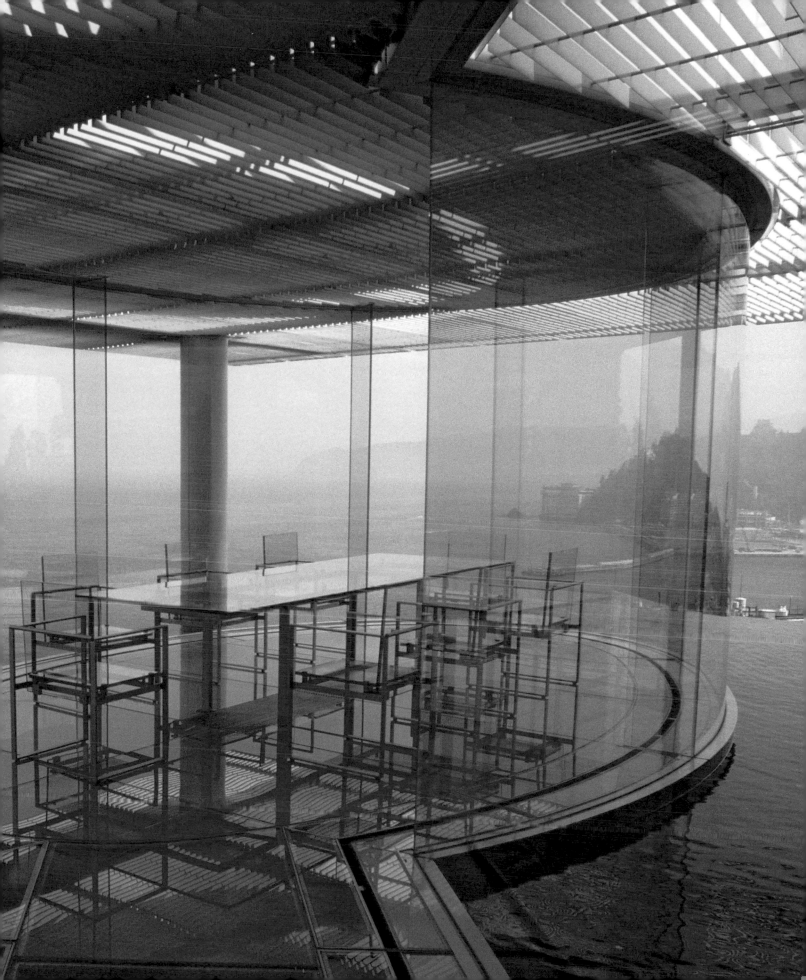

6

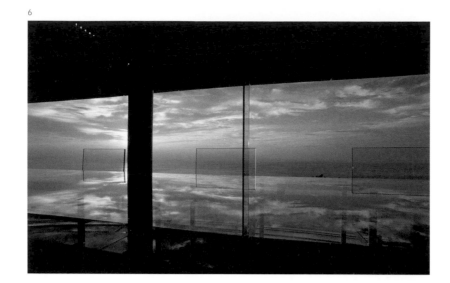

7

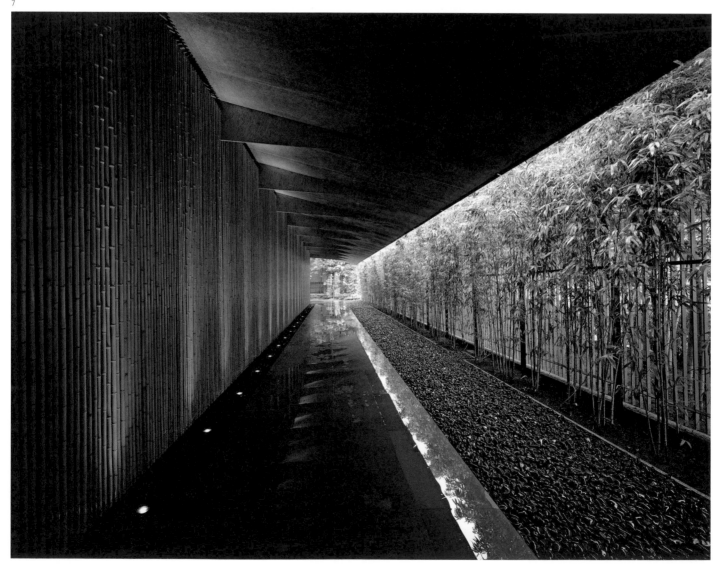

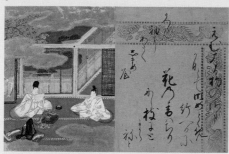

5 (previous spread), 6 Kengo Kuma & Associates, Water/ Glass House, Atami-shi, Shizuoka Prefecture, Japan (1995).
Kuma's villa is inspired by Bruno Taut's Kyu Hyuga Bettei (1936), a synthesis of European formalism and Japanese naturalism. The edges of the glass structure are obscured by water; superimposition, refraction and reflection challenge a simple relationship between the house and the natural world, in which it appears to float.

7, 9 (overleaf) Kengo Kuma & Associates, Nezu Museum, Minato-ku, Tokyo, Japan (2009).
Drawing on vernacular building types, the two-storey pavilion has a massive roof with overhanging eaves which seems to float over walls of glass.

8 Kodo (Way of Incense).
'The Plum Tree Branch, illustration to the 'Tale of Genji' by Tosa Mitunobu, c. 1509–10 (ink, colour and gold on paper, 24.1 x 18 cm).

What other influences have you taken from Japanese tradition and Japanese notions of space?
Architecture and ritual always go together, and this is especially true in Japanese architecture. Without ritual, a tea house is nothing, but when you put the ceremony and the building together you have something very powerful. We repeat rituals on a daily basis – they are an important aspect of human relationships. In Japan taking off your shoes at the entrance is part of the everyday ritual of crossing the threshold.

'Ma', which means space or sense of place in Japanese, is also very important to me. It's more about the experience of space than the building as a physical entity and it's something I always pay attention to. 'Ma' could also be translated as a void or pause – you could describe it as a rich emptiness. It can be created in many ways: through the effect of light, or through attention to details.

'Ma' is something you find in music too – the richness of the silences that enhance our awareness of sound. And in poetry: a Japanese haiku has only seventeen syllables, but people read them slowly to create a silence between the words, so a simple haiku becomes something very resonant.

Within my buildings I hope people feel this same sense of silence, and at the same time are aware of nature – the sound of the wind, or of people walking. I'd like to be able to create both an aural and a visual stillness.

Movement, sequence and progression through space also seem important to you. Is this another key aspect for developing an experiential richness in your architecture?
Certainly. Through movement people discover depth in a simple form. For instance, when you walk past a beautiful screen you experience a changing series of perspectives, or a series of screens offers many different effects and environments. Changing conditions also have a role to play: the evening light can reveal the beauty of paper screens, or on rainy days the richness of the dance of shadows becomes more apparent. With

the Water/Glass House a rainy day makes it seem as if the boundaries between nature and architecture disappear and sea and sky become part of the building.

It's the opposite idea from the building as an object, which to me means the kind of architecture that has been designed to look spectacular in photographs! Photographs can only capture a fixed visual image, whereas for me architecture is about the whole experience of the space. This can include touch or smell – anything that offers a special connection. I remember when American friends visited my office in Tokyo after an interval of five years, they said, 'Ah, your office still smells the same...'

You express an acute awareness of the smell of certain materials used in architecture. Can you say more about the role the senses play in how we perceive and experience space and what this might add to how we engage with architecture?
All the senses are important in our experience of space. It's not about engaging individual senses but more about the whole atmosphere you want to create. Touch is very important too, and each material you introduce has a particular impact. Steel and glass, which are common in modern buildings, are hard and cold, whereas wood, rice paper and fabric are warm and alive.

Smell has been particularly potent in traditional Japanese architecture – the smell of tatami or wood lingers in the memory – and people have chosen particular woods for their aroma rather than their appearance, though this has been lost to some extent today when visual effects are considered more important. The most popular wood was probably hinoki (Japanese cypress) – the smoke from hinoki is very special – but my own favourite is cedar. An authentic tatami mat also has a good smell.

We have a ceremony in Japan, Kodo, which is similar to the tea ceremony, Chado. ('Do' means way or ceremony, so Kodo means 'Way of Incense'.) The ceremony involves bringing in five or six different incenses, each presented in a censer or burner. Then it becomes

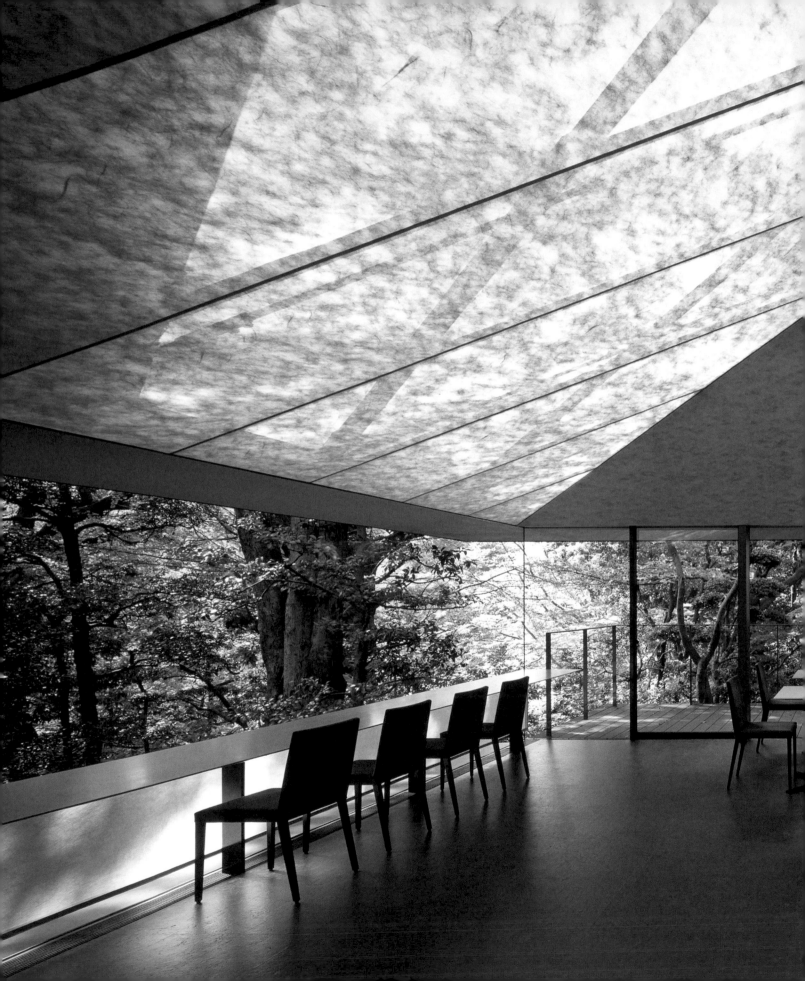

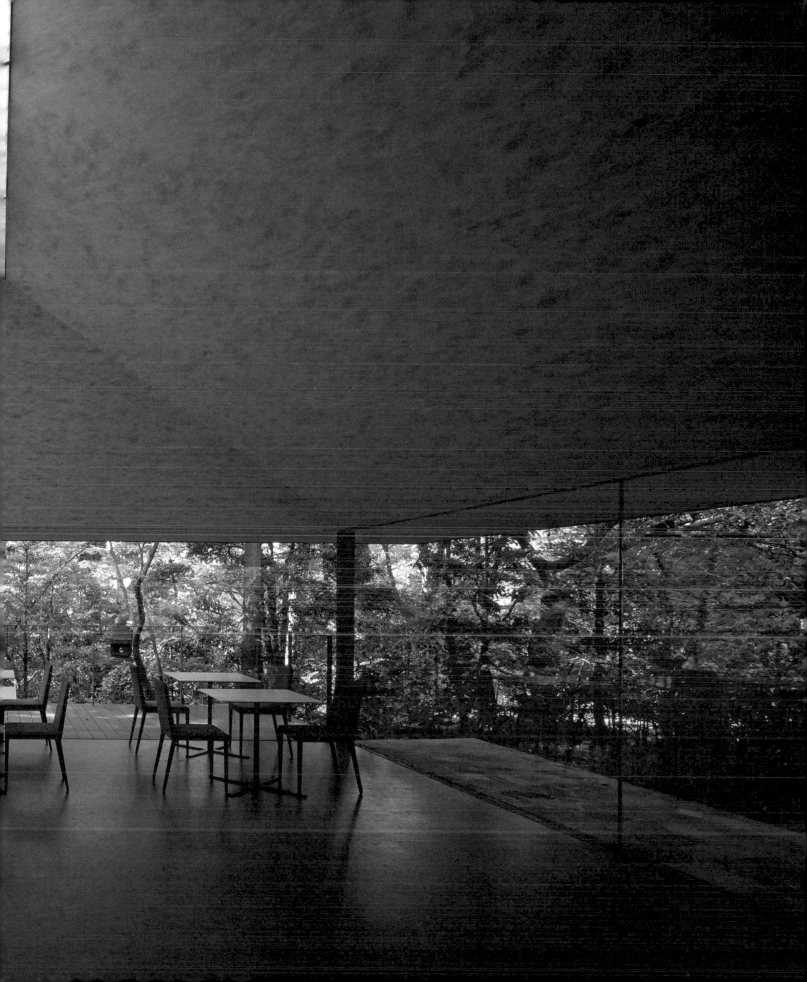

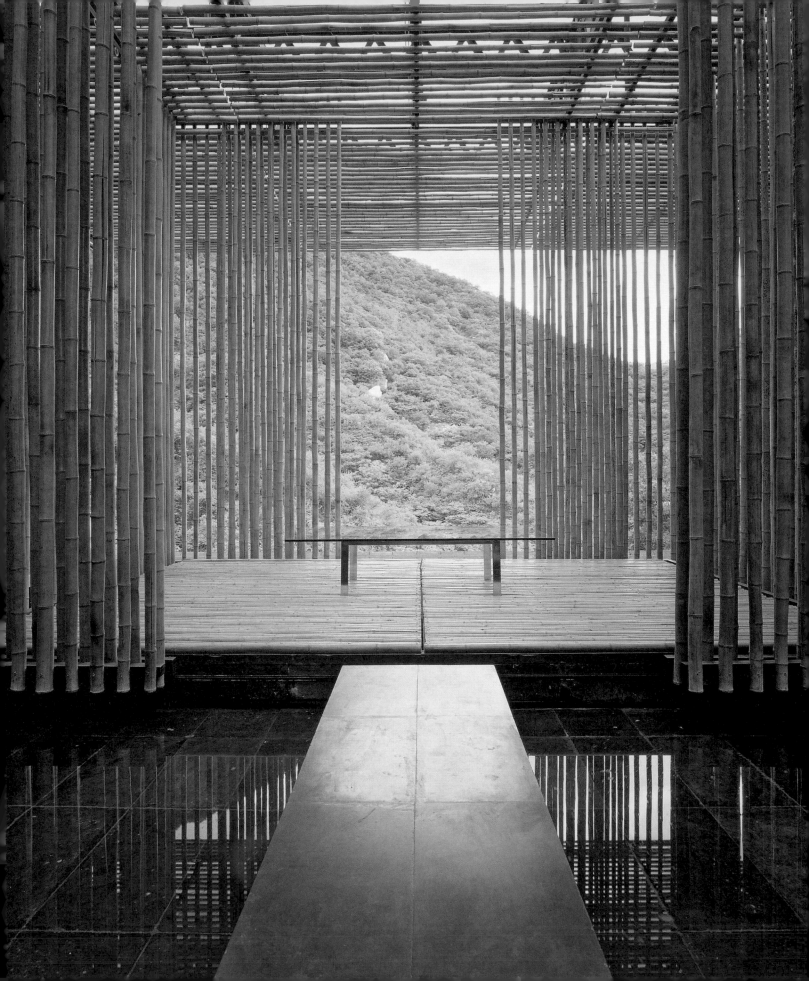

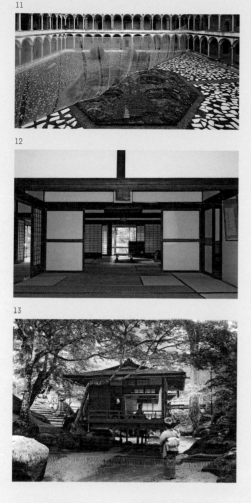

11

12

13

10 (opposite) Kengo Kuma & Associates, Great (Bamboo) Wall, near Beijing, China (2002). This villa for a hotel complex in the Commune By The Great Wall explores the uses of a local material, bamboo, and the formal qualities of the wall as both partition and unifying element.

11 Kengo Kuma & Associates, CCC Wall, University of Milan, Italy (2010). For this temporary installation, a curtain of sheer organza was suspended over the quadrangle with stones and tiles laid underneath.

12 Tatami mats in traditional Japanese domestic architecture. Myosen-ji, Sado Island, Japan (founded 1271), the abbot's quarters.

13 Traditional Japanese tea house, Itsukushima, Hiroshima Prefecture, Japan.

a kind of game, with the participants guessing the names of the incenses. For the master, the selection is related to a story; he creates the story and then chooses the aromas to go with it. The participants' comments are recorded by the master to produce a document of the total experience.

You have to focus to identify different smells, whereas concentration is not so necessary to differentiate between visual effects. The beginning of the Kodo ceremony is always difficult because all the incenses seem to smell the same, but as you concentrate, little by little you make distinctions.

Our spatial imaginations have been developing since we first started exploring the world. Can you recall an early memory of when you became aware of space?
I remember as a boy having a mosquito net that was very beautiful. It had a particular smell and the effect of the light filtering through from the outside was very special. It gave me a feeling of being contained but not enclosed, of being protected but still open to the environment. There was no change to the room itself, but in summer, when the net was up, the space was transformed. I always liked summer very much because of it.

Perhaps as a result I often use fabric in my architecture, especially an organza I discovered some years ago that exploded my definition of what a fabric might be. The first time I saw it, I thought, 'Aha, this is the cloth of angels…'

Can you recall early memories of trying to shape the spaces around you?
I always return to a memory from my childhood, when my family lived in an old wooden house in the suburbs of Tokyo that my grandfather had originally used as a weekend house. My father enjoyed renovating it and extending it, and asked us all for our proposals for the layout: where the toilet and shower would go, how we should plan the spaces. It was like a little competition among the family and I remember my grandmother produced a very good plan; she could

visualise space well. I was flattered when my father adopted one of my ideas.

I also remember in primary school being asked to make a miniature garden using natural materials like sand or twigs. I felt very happy working on this.

Can you identify echoes of these experiences in your own work?
My childhood experience of renovating our wooden house is often reflected in my works, especially when I am choosing materials. A very personal project that reminded me of this was the Masanari Murai Memorial Museum of Art. The concept was derived from the house where the artist had lived, and though the museum was to be newly built, we approached it like a renovation and reused a lot of materials from the old house. Masanari Murai kept everything – every magazine, every sketch, every scrap of paper – so though his house wasn't small, the liveable area seemed minute. He wanted to live surrounded by these things; he didn't want large open spaces. So in the museum I tried to keep as close as possible to the feeling of the spaces he had occupied.

What do you think is distinctive about how you as an architect understand and perceive space?
Architects are said to possess two perspectives: a bird's-eye view and a life-size, ground-based perception of space. They are supposed to be able to move freely between the two. The problem with architects is that too often they design with a god's-eye view, looking down!

Architects are encouraged to believe that physical space and our perception of it are the same, but in fact human beings are not like that. And the idea that our perception and the reality might be different is new territory for architecture and design. For instance, in traditional Japanese architecture, the plan is determined by a standard number of tatami mats, but when you go inside, the experience can be totally unexpected, like magic. This is the wonder of Japanese design!

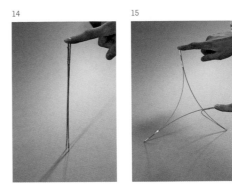

14   15

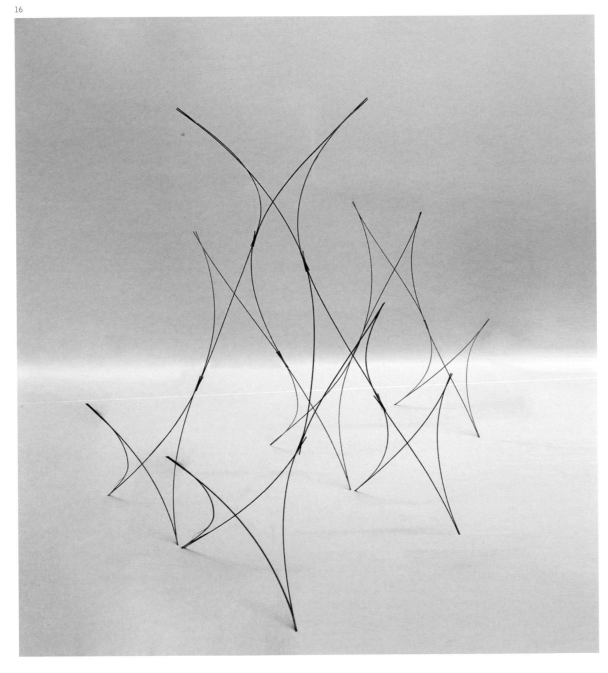

16

The starting point for the installation was an attempt to discover how a minimum of material could induce the maximum effect on the body. Despite being whittled down to 4 millimetres in diameter, the bamboo sticks used to construct the pavilions retain their strength and flexibility (14, 15) and can be combined into structures of great delicacy (16). Tests were made to see how effectively the aromas of hinoki and tatami would rise up the bamboo to fill the gallery spaces (17).

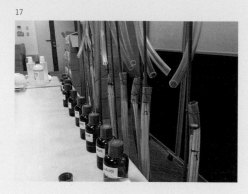
17

What were your initial impressions of the architecture of the Royal Academy?
I liked the high ceilings, and I realised that the contrast between the building and my own, more delicate architecture could be very exciting. If I were creating something similar in Japan, people might think that the Kodo, or materials such as bamboo, were just going back to tradition, but I think they can reveal new possibilities. I am always looking for new ways of using Japanese design principles in other contexts and this is an example that I hope will inform my future work.

Can you describe your installation in more detail?
Our starting point was a question: how can a minimum of material induce a maximum effect on the body? The more the volume of material is reduced, the more sensitive human beings become as they focus on an ever smaller area in order to 'smell out' something from it. The Japanese tea house follows this principle: its frame, pillars and beams are all incredibly slender.

For our installation we designed a 5-metre-high pavilion filled with scent, the 'Pavilion of Incense'. The construction uses whittled bamboo sticks that are only 4 millimetres in diameter, made possible by modern technology. We wanted this delicate structure to deliver maximum effect.

In the end, we decided to build two pavilions in two different spaces. One could be described as the 'architecture of reality' or 'architecture of a father': it stands alone in the space and is filled with the aroma of hinoki. The other is the 'architecture of void' or 'architecture of a mother', a cocoon that envelops your body and is filled with the smell of tatami.

The sequence is important. When the visitors first enter the space, they can't understand it, but step by step as they explore the installation, they begin to grasp what is happening. The experience will start from normal light levels and move towards something darker as the smell deepens, so the lighting conditions and the intensity of the smell change simultaneously.

This is an installation within a room, and I also wanted to design the negative space between the pavilions and the walls. Here in the museum, the space has a very Western rigidity and the in-between space can form a conversation between East and West.

'Sensing Spaces' is not a regular architecture exhibition where people come to see models and drawings, so it is appropriate that the experience will offer a sense of ambiguity – between structure and skin, light and dark, volume and enclosure. We are aiming to create an architecture of experience that dissolves the boundaries between the material and the immaterial.

What opportunities have you found in creating an installation for an exhibition that would not usually be possible in your architectural projects and how have you harnessed these?
Obviously we are given more freedom in installations than in buildings that have to function as shelters so we are able to experiment with new ideas and techniques. If these prove successful, they can then be incorporated into future buildings. So for us, working on an installation is extremely helpful in developing our designs. And we are inspired by the people we meet through exhibitions.

An exhibition can also point to a new direction: in 'Sensing Spaces', for instance, we should be able to show that architecture is no longer just about physical presence and visual effects with other senses as secondary elements. Exhibitions can provide opportunities to hint at the new tide for design and I predict that architecture will soon move into a more sensual mode.

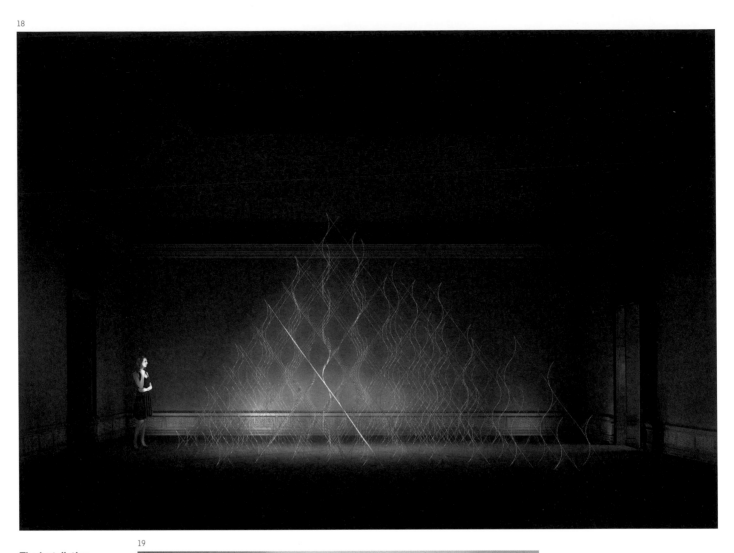

The installation evolved into two different structures occupying two spaces, one large and one small. The 'architecture of reality' or 'architecture of a father' pavilion (18, 19), filled with the aroma of hinoki, stands isolated within the larger gallery so visitors move around it. By contrast, the 'architecture of void' or 'architecture of a mother' pavilion, filled with the aroma of tatami, surrounds and envelops visitors (20, 21).

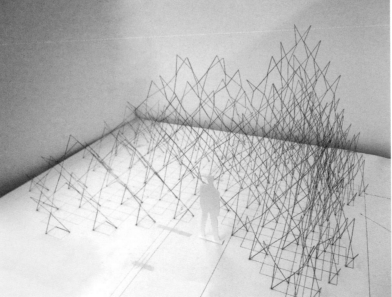

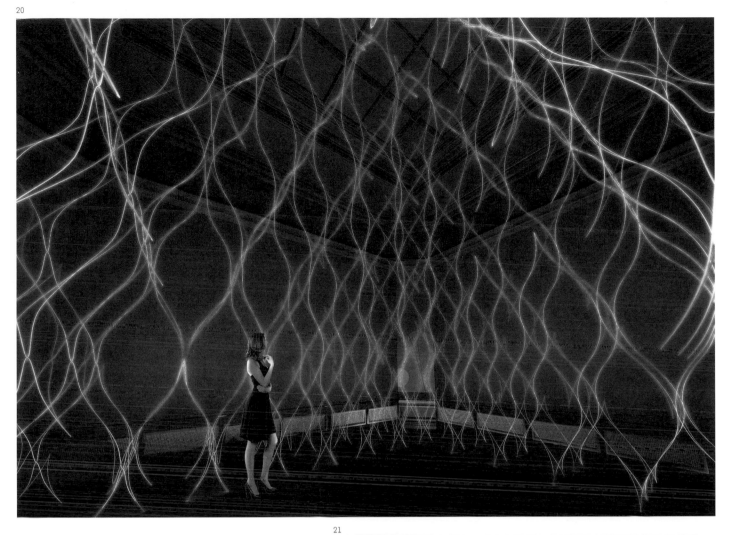

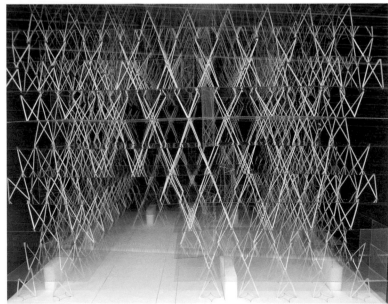

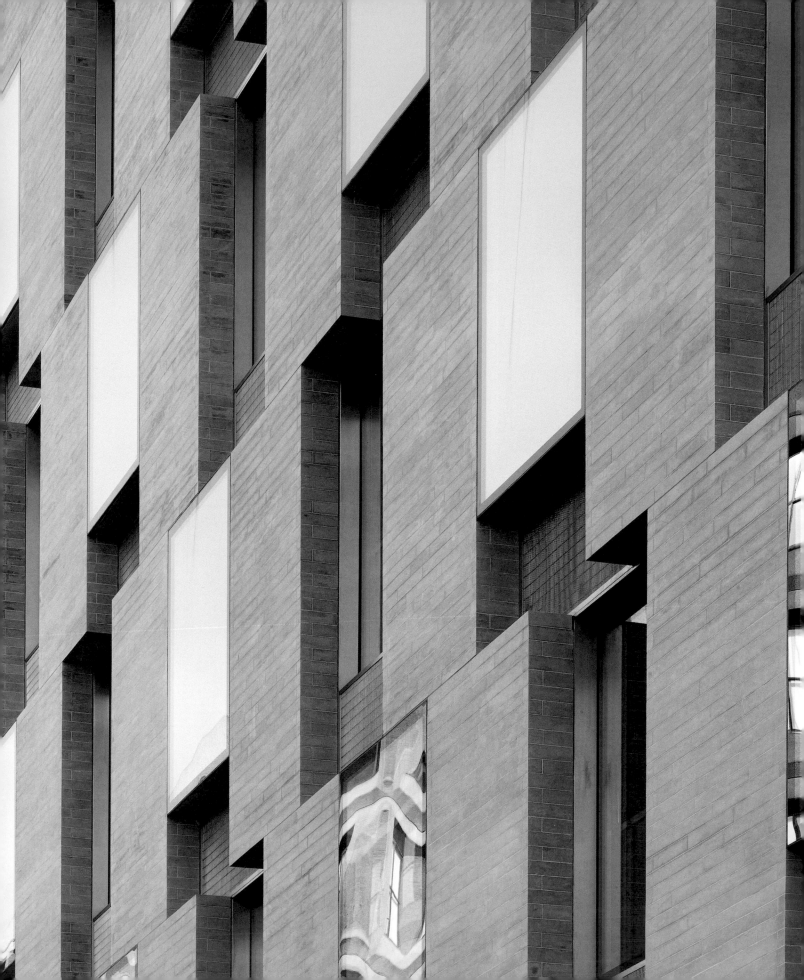

Grafton
Architects

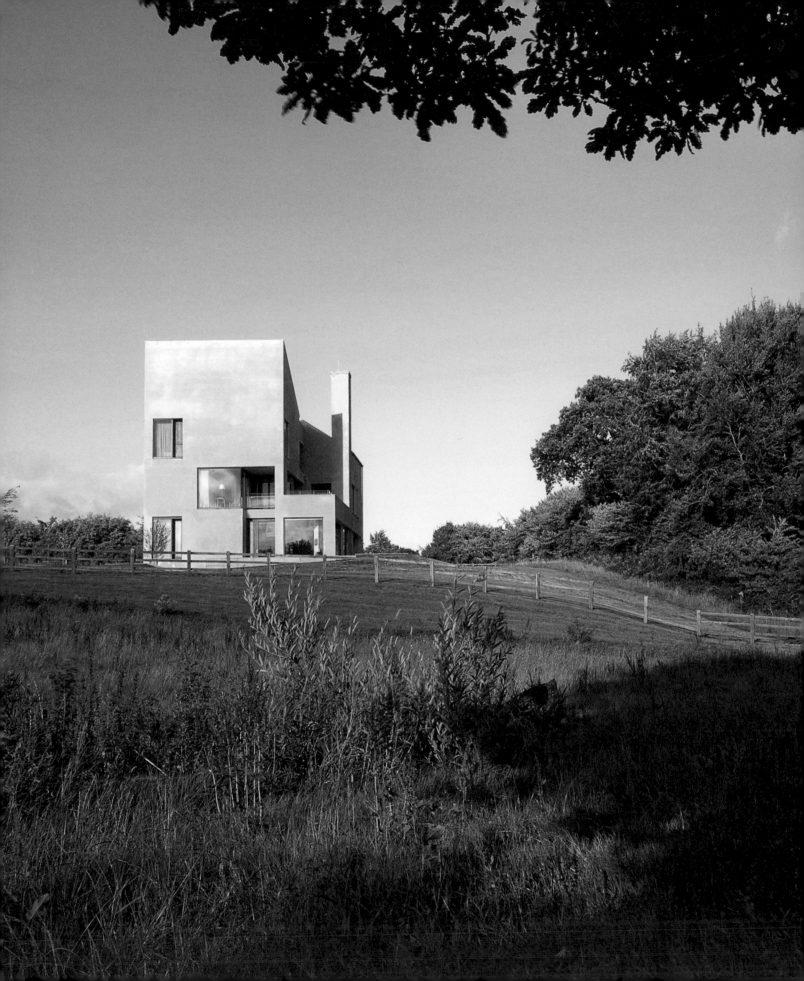

1 (previous spread)
Grafton Architects,
Offices for the
Department of
Finance, Dublin,
Ireland (2007).
Ballinasloe limestone
and glass screen walls
articulate the façade
to create areas of light
and shadow and offer
workers panoramic
views of the city.

2 (opposite)
Grafton Architects,
President's House,
University of Limerick,
Ireland (2010).
A completely modern
house drawing on the
Irish vernacular tradition
in its siting, form,
construction details
and materials,
including lime render
with Wexford sand,
limestone cills and
slate roofs.

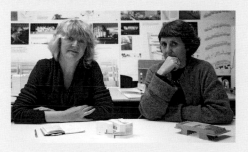

Grafton Architects was set up in 1978 by Yvonne Farrell (born 1951 in Tullamore, Ireland) and Shelley McNamara (born 1952 in Lisdoonvarna, Ireland), then recent graduates of University College Dublin's School of Architecture. The practice takes its name from the Dublin street in which it is located.

Often creating geological analogies for their work, Farrell and McNamara talk about architecture as a 'new geography', seeing buildings not as isolated objects but as part of a wider network that grows out of and contributes to the physical, social and cultural landscape. The aesthetic and structural qualities of materials are a central concern and Grafton Architects are notably skilful in their use of brick and concrete, playing with surface, weight and texture and manipulating light and shadow to convey a sense of gravity or lightness.

While the practice has designed a range of buildings from the domestic to large public complexes, it has become renowned for highly successful university buildings that serve complex institutional programmes with elegant architecture. The Luigi Bocconi University in Milan won the first World Building of the Year Award at the 2008 World Architecture Festival and Grafton's work for the University of Limerick was shortlisted for the 2013 Stirling Prize.

Grafton Architects were founding members of Group '91, the collaborative that won the competition to regenerate Temple Bar, Dublin, in 1991. Farrell and McNamara have held professorships at the Accademia di Architettura, Mendrisio, at the Graduate School of Design, Harvard, and at Yale. They are honorary international fellows of the Royal Institute of British Architects and their exhibition 'Architecture as New Geography' won the Silver Lion at the 2012 Venice Architecture Biennale.

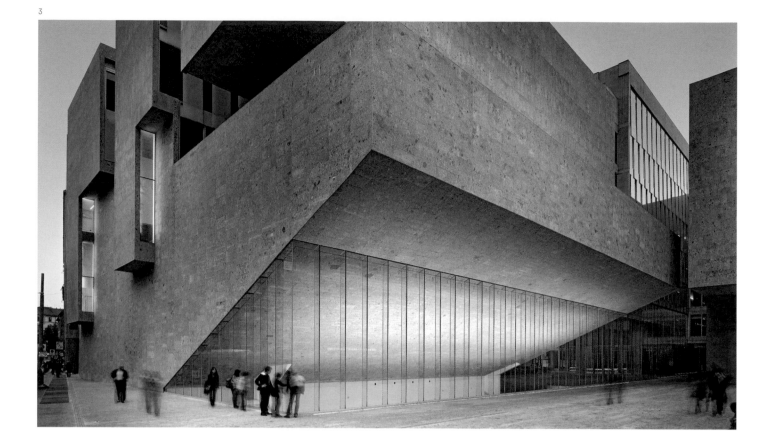

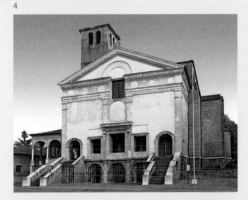

3, 5 (overleaf)
Grafton Architects,
School of Economics,
Luigi Bocconi
University, Milan,
Italy (2008).
The cantilever of the
Aula Magna hovers
over an area of
stone-paved public
space with views down
into the sunken foyer
and meeting space.

4 Leon Battista Alberti
and others, San
Sebastiano, Mantua,
Italy (from 1460).

Kate Goodwin: What do you think
is distinctive about how you as architects
understand and perceive space?
Yvonne Farrell and Shelley McNamara:
As space-makers, we aim to be highly
tuned instruments, with our antennae
alert, in order to absorb our experiences
of space in such a way as to be able to
reproduce or reuse them in our work.

As architects, imagination is our trade.
We imagine… It's humbling that people
come to us with wishes and money and
ask us to translate them into built form.
The result depends on interpretation:
how life is, how life could be.

How do the body and the senses influence
our perception and experience of space?
And what might this add to how we
engage with the architecture around us?
Our whole bodies respond to space,
surface, texture, sound, proportions
and light. Louis Kahn said, 'To hear
a sound is to see its space.'

A term we often use is 'structuring
space' in an effort to describe the central
role structure plays, not just in holding
a building up but in manipulating light,
rhythm and pace of movement, in
giving the feeling of space inhaling and
exhaling, of compression and expansion.

One of the things we try to re-create
within our own work is an ancient
sense of human beings' connection

to the forces of gravity. An example
is the space under the 22-metre cantilever
of the Aula Magna in the Luigi Bocconi
University building in Milan, which
has an 'otherworldly' primal quality
that seems both to anchor and to
liberate the human spirit.

A visitor to the sunken foyer space,
which is 9 metres below ground level,
said to us: 'questo spazio è enorme ma
mi abbraccia' (this space is enormous
but it embraces me). She was a stranger
to us, an inhabitant of one of the
neighbouring streets, and we were very
moved by her response. It confirmed
something to us about the human need
for intimacy within the wider world,
and how architecture might provide this.

There is a definite human enjoyment
of qualities such as tranquility, stillness,
proportions and order. Recently, we
were lucky to be invited to give a lecture
in Alberti's San Sebastiano church in
Mantua and we were completely amazed
by the purity, simplicity and perfection
of the building.

In what other ways do you see architecture
enhancing human experience beyond shelter
and function?
Architecture should offer inspiration,
enjoyment and comfort. A good example
is a group of small houses by J.J.P. Oud.
When you open the entrance gate, there

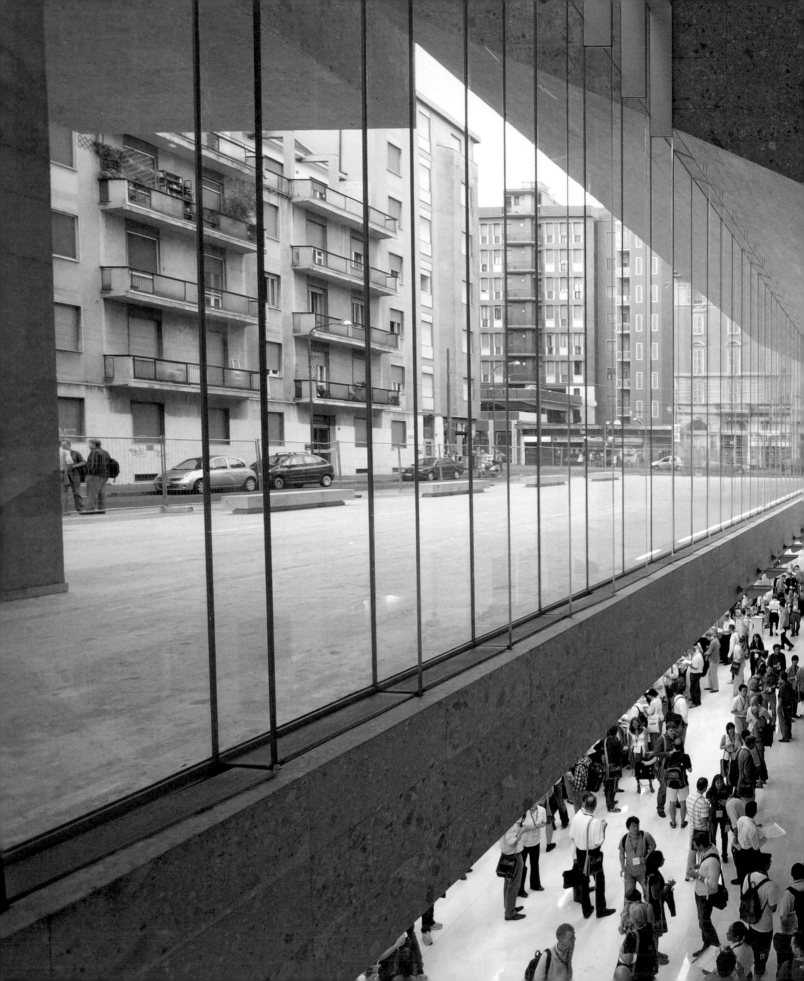

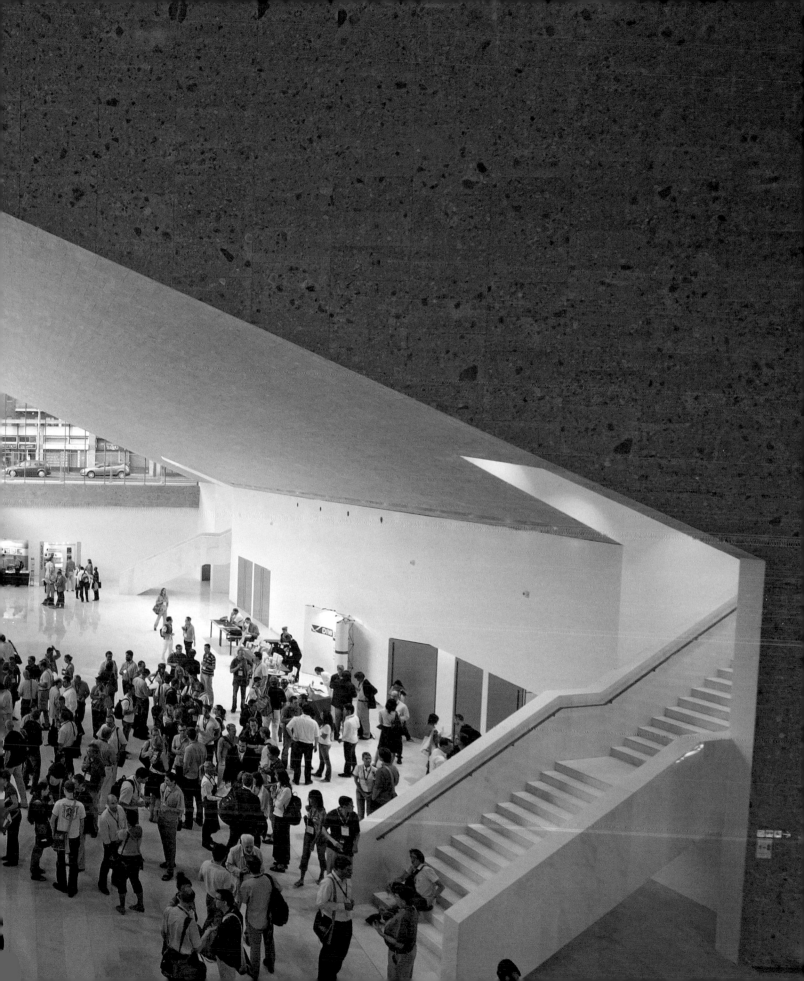

6

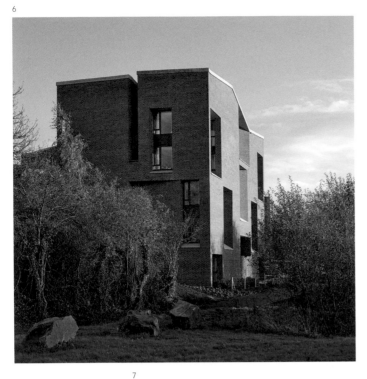

7

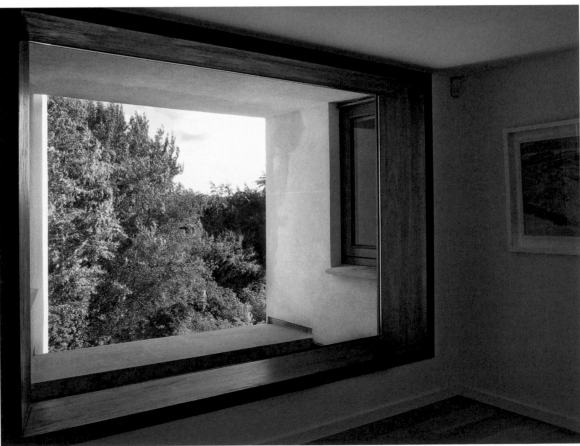

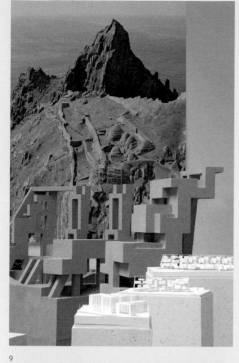

8

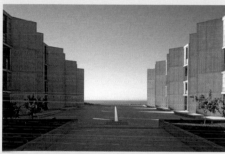

9

6 Grafton Architects, Student Housing, University of Limerick (2013).
A group of three brick buildings for medical students combine with a number of institutions to define a new public space.

7 Grafton Architects, President's House, University of Limerick.
Deep windows create an intermediate space between inside and out and a distinct frame for the landscape.

8 Grafton Architects, 'Architecture as New Geography', Venice Architecture Biennale (2012).
In the foreground are paper models of Toulouse University 1 Capitol and papier-mâché models of the UTEC campus, Lima; in the background is a photograph of Skellig Michael.

9 Louis I. Kahn, Salk Institute for Biological Studies, La Jolla, California, US (1959–66).

is a little seat, then you come through the garden to the front door and you have a strong sense of intimacy, of home and security. We noticed the same feeling of humanity outside Angelo Mangiarotti's apartment building in Milan: again there is a gate, which is small even though the building is big, with steps down to a seat and a shelf, so you can put down your shopping or stop for a chat. You feel the architecture is paced for human exchange rather than being object driven.

It's about thoughtfulness. Someone has thought about how pleasant it would be to sit down while you look for your key. That kind of gesture doesn't just happen: it comes from the architect's capacity for anticipation and practical generosity. There is something beautiful about making architecture that's heroic and at the same time has a sense of humanity.

You have also spoken about how architecture might make connections across place and time.
One of the things we spoke about in exploring the theme of 'Common Ground' for our installation at the 2012 Venice Biennale was a datum linking the geography of Venice with the fifteenth-century Inca site of Machu Picchu in Peru and with Skellig Michael, an island off the south-west coast of Ireland that is home to a monastery built between the sixth and eighth centuries. We were trying to find connections and consistencies. We thought about time and place.

Architecture is a language that conveys feelings and messages, so the places you create have a wide and long-lasting reference. We therefore included images of both Machu Picchu and Skellig Michael in our Venice installation, which we called 'Architecture as New Geography'. What we found so striking when we visited Skellig Michael was that you could almost feel the intimacy experienced by the monk in his garden, with his herbs growing, surrounded by an enormous and threatening ocean. We discovered something similar in the relationship between Machu Picchu and the sky – the human desire for security within that vast landscape. The essential aspect is the contrasting scales: building and geography, window and landscape, the human being and the wider world.

And you also mentioned the dimension of time…
The French architect Laurent Beaudoin wrote about how human time is different from natural time – the time it takes for clouds to cross the sky, for tides to come in and go out. Human time moves quickly, and architecture can be a means of slowing time down, allowing the human to become more in tune with the natural.

To form a relationship with the natural world, you need to make a building that will be like a piece of geography, a building that adapts and grows. In our UTEC campus project in Lima, for instance, we are trying to make a series of gardens that will become bigger and more luscious over time. It's not about preciousness – we imagine architecture as a platform for life rather than a perfect, jewel-like object. Over time some things deteriorate and others get better… a good brick wall improves over time. We often discuss the difficulty of finding components for our buildings with enough muscle to survive.

What makes a powerful and memorable architectural or spatial experience?
We were very moved by something we read by the Spanish architect Alejandro de la Sota in which he encourages architects to make as much nothing as possible. This is a wonderful challenge! We experienced something of this at Louis Kahn's Salk Institute in La Jolla, because the space where the building is not is absolutely charged – the void, the nothing, vibrates as a thing in itself. You are not looking at a building as an object; instead you become aware of the space, of the trapped air between ground surface, blue sky and the ocean visible in the distance, and of yourself held by the containing forces of this space in a way that heightens your sense of being alive in a particular place at a particular moment.

An alleyway, even if it is not pretty, can provide a beautiful experience in the way it catches the light or seems

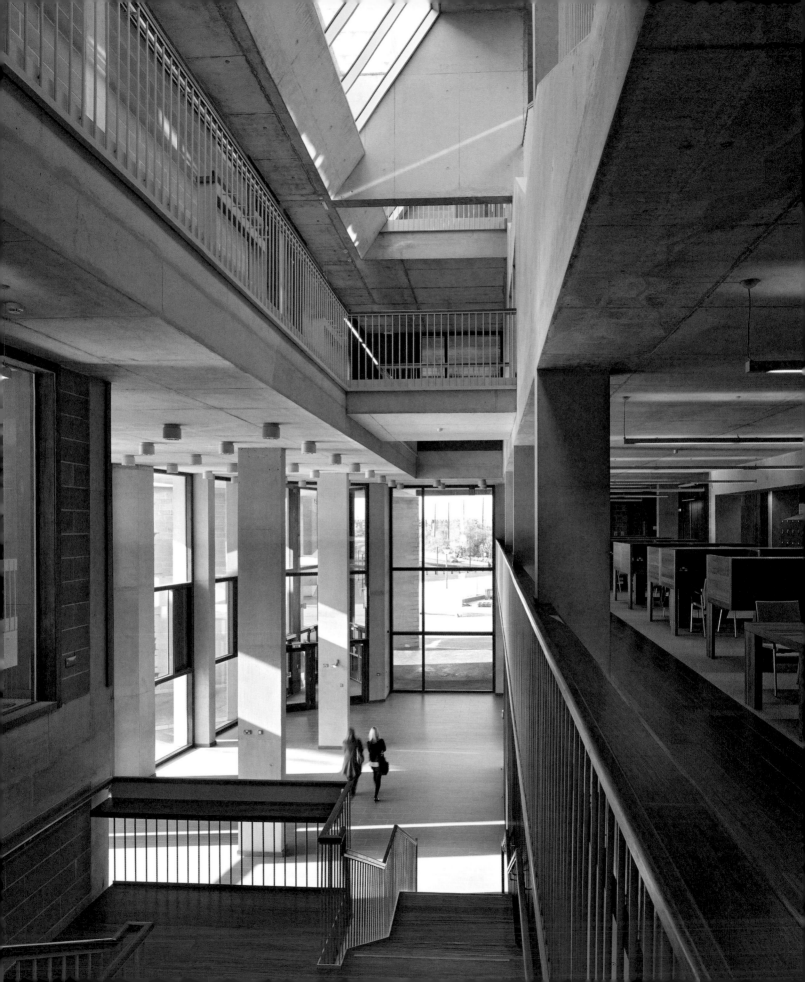

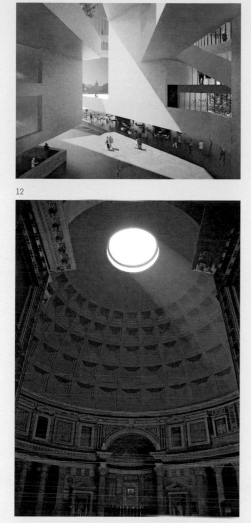

to be carved out of its surroundings. Standing on a cliff overlooking the ocean can be a spatial experience on a grand scale. When we use the term 'architecture as new geography', we are thinking of the architectural experience of being on the edge of something immense. Sometimes the sensation comes from experiencing huge contrasts in scale, as in the architecture of a tiny island in relation to a vast ocean.

Do you see other correlations between 'architectural' experience and the natural world?
David Leatherbrow has written beautifully about architectural phenomenology. He talks about shadow and light, and how the production of shadow was once described as the origin of architecture. Shadow in certain climates promotes certain ways of life: the shadows cast by buildings are the beginnings of the making of public space and the growth of activities – it is about what happens at the edges of buildings. It is very beautiful to go back to basics and talk about light and shade and what it means in different cultures and climates.

The basic building element of the column developed directly from the beauty and elegance of a tree – it's a collective memory, like the enclosure of the cave. After all, the Pantheon in Rome could be described as a crafted cave with a hole in the roof.

We could say that, as architects, we take such experiences of space – the enclosure of the cave, the dappled light of the forest – and try to make them concrete. Recently when we were doing a school competition, for instance, we talked about how a school could be a meadow, a tree house, a forest...

You could also argue that architectural experience is the consciousness of architecture in relation to people and place. In the Toulouse School of Economics (UT1C) and in the Luigi Bocconi University in Milan we are trying to heighten people's awareness of where they are – the buildings don't obliterate and make new, but rather bring out the sense that you are in a particular place.

Our interest is to engage the public: it's about imagination and memory, because if you can touch those chords, you create something very powerful. Architecture can feed people emotionally – it is not just owned by the client, it's not a commodity to be bought. It is shared.

You have spoken about the relationship between people and architecture, but how might architecture influence the relationships between people?
Sociologist Richard Sennett has put forward the idea that people today feel uncomfortable in the public domain because codes of dress and behaviour are no longer formalised and they can't read the signs. These issues of social connection are part of what we deal with in our work. In the Luigi Bocconi University scheme, we tried to connect the spaces for students and professors not in plan but in section, so they could be aware of each other's presence from above and below, separated but connected.

As architects, our job is one of translation – we are consciously engaged in making spaces that bring together different worlds. For instance, at the UTEC campus in Lima, we are saying that socialising outdoors connects students to a place and to each other, encouraging a mix. Our trade encompasses both sociology and construction – it is a complex profession because the spectrum of translation runs from persuading a tree to grow on the ninth floor to understanding how pleasurable it might be for a student to meet a professor en route to a lecture.

When we think about something as seemingly simple as a table, we think about it as a beautiful creation and a social focus. In Zurich, we once had a wonderful meal at a table made from an enormous tree trunk that was incredibly long and extremely narrow. Because it was so narrow, the people facing each other were closer than usual and this table formed a new type of community along its length. When you come to a table, you take off your jacket and sit down, so you are fully present; you have a cup of tea and a conversation, so it's a shared experience.

10 Grafton Architects, Medical School, University of Limerick (2013).
Behind an angled colonnade, a full-height atrium is both a social space and a link to the laboratories and lecture rooms behind.

11 Grafton Architects, UT1C, Toulouse, France.
A twenty-first-century vertical courtyard frames specific views over Toulouse, allowing the presence of the city to enter the university building.

12 The Pantheon, Rome, Italy (126 CE).

13

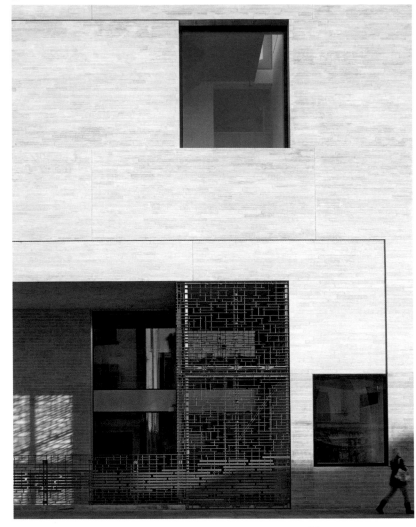

14

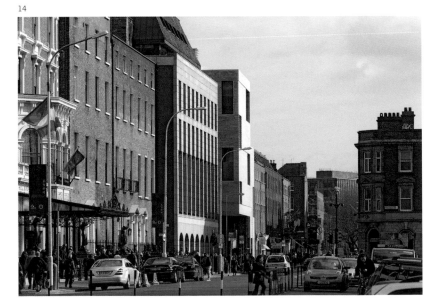

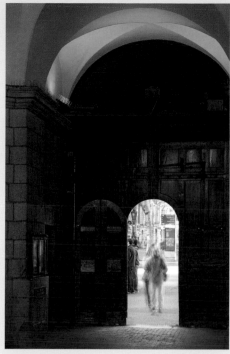

13, 14 Grafton Architects, Offices for the Department of Finance, Dublin.
The building respects and contributes to the street, with the continuity of Merrion Row maintained by a bronze railing and gate and by the 3-metre cantilever of the grand staircase space.

15 Trinity College, Dublin.
The gateway between the university and the city beyond.

We have spoken a lot about the idea of feeling 'present' within a space. What does this mean to you?
Yvonne Farrell: Feeling present is becoming aware that you stand in this space at this time, that you are alive. As a human being, and especially as an architect, it is important to become more aware of our surroundings, to understand the positive and negative effects of different spaces, to notice our own responses and those of others. One technique that highlights this is just to look at the ground as you walk – I do this sometimes, and the variety and patterns I notice are amazing. When we heighten our awareness in this way, it strengthens our sense of being alive and of how we are held and nourished by the spaces around us.

Thresholds are places where we naturally become more aware. For me, this occurs each time I leave the quiet complex of Trinity College in Dublin. Exiting through a small timber door with a metal threshold and entering the heart of the busy city is a moment of contrasts, where you really notice you are leaving one system to become immersed in another. Being present in space is about noticing these moments of change: from one world to another, public to private or vice versa, like the opening of a door, the turn of a key.

One of the places I visit every time I'm in London is the Sir John Soane Museum – its spaces are about intimacy and modernity, expressed in terms of light. Shelley McNamara: Perhaps architecture is when space allows you to be completely within it. It's a vivid sense of being present that you get as much in buildings like the Pantheon as in a snug in a good bar – contemplative places, brown bars with cosy corners, people chatting, a warm bath of humanity.

A memorable experience for me was visiting Le Corbusier's Palace of the Assembly in Chandigarh. The main space is dynamic, with a gracious and easy sense of movement from ledge to ledge within what actually feels like a piece of landscape. When I entered it, it made the hair on the back of my neck stand up! It felt both absolutely ancient and absolutely modern.

I had never realised the impact of the crack of light at the junction of the central space and the perimeter offices. It's a kind of 'light gutter' that casts a strong line of light on the concrete soffit. The light is drawn down into the enormous space by slender columns which become columns of light within what is in fact a dark and moody grand hall. It is one of the spaces we explored as inspiration for our 'Sensing Spaces' installation.

Our spatial imaginations have been developing since we first started exploring the world. Do you think the spaces you experienced in your childhood have influenced your work?
Both of us come from rural towns, and what has probably influenced us is the interwoven presence of street and countryside: there was never a separation between the two because you had the street at the front door and the countryside at the back door. The urban fabric of an Irish rural town is very 'thin', so as you move through it you glimpse the open landscape in the gaps or archways between the buildings.

Maybe that's why in our work we try to have a concurrent sense of city and landscape. For instance, in the school we built in Ballinasloe, we made a dense enclosure, thinking of a school as a small town, as a community, combined with the idea of a conglomerate of courtyards and gardens forming protected landscapes.

What were your initial impressions of the architecture of the Royal Academy?
As with any project, we have been given a site and we want to draw on what is there. We need to think about how we can reinforce the qualities of the existing space and how we can occupy it.

What we find amazing about the Royal Academy is the generosity of the spaces. The volume is like a gift and it would be fantastic to celebrate its grandeur. It is interesting to think about scale – small structures inserted into large spaces – or about how the existing

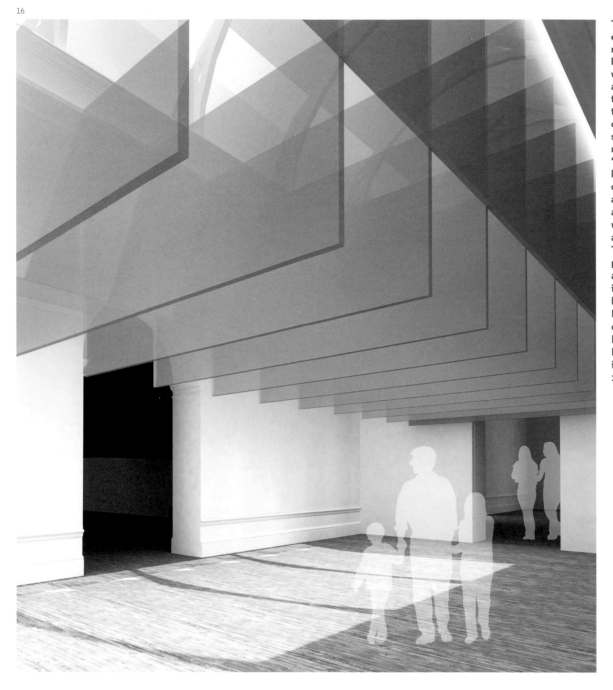

The installation explores the relationship between light and structure within architecture, and specifically the top lighting that is characteristic of the RA gallery spaces. The first room is about 'lightness': here light drawn in from outside is amplified and manipulated, animating the space with the play of light and shadow (16). The project has precedents as diverse as the breakfast room in Sir John Soane's house in Lincoln's Inn Fields, London, c. 1812 (17) and Le Corbusier's Palace of the Assembly in Chandigarh, India, 1955 (18).

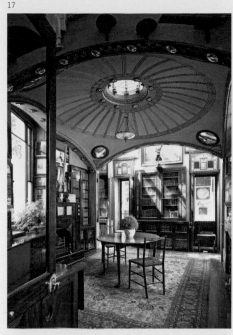

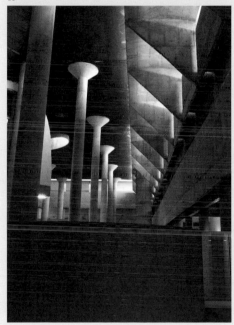

Classical plan and sequence might contrast with the free plans of today. How might you take what is there and encourage people to see it differently?

For us, light is one of the meta-narratives: all the galleries have light from above and we want to use this characteristic, though we will also need to include artificial light to strengthen visitors' awareness of the natural oscillation and qualities of the daylight outdoors. This will make the installation very specific to its time and place.

Can you describe your installation in more detail?
We have drawn on the character and proportions of two adjacent rooms and inserted one main element into each. The first of the two is an exploration of 'lightness'. Lights mounted on the roof are programmed to amplify the fluctuating natural light conditions through the course of the day and the space is animated by the resulting changing shadows on the floor and walls. Blades of light reaching to the sky create a 'waterfall of light'.

The second room is the opposite, exploring weight, containment and carved-out space. Here we are inserting a new element floating 2.4 metres above the floor and extending beyond the rooflight volume on two diagonals. Two cut-away corners funnel light from above, creating a diagonal axis that will draw visitors through the gallery towards the light-filled lantern at its centre.

The open corners and overlapping walls create niches where people will discover intimate views within the larger volume. The walls are made to feel weighty and thick and the 'niche' area is roofed so

it is relatively dark and sombre to contrast with the central lantern of light. As with the other room, roof-mounted lights amplify the changing natural light conditions outdoors.

What opportunities exist within an exhibition that would not normally be possible and how have you harnessed these in 'Sensing Spaces'?
There are beautiful places in the world made by architects, but people don't know what architects do. Often people seem to think that buildings arrive in the world fully formed. Throughout our work we have always had the same agenda – how do you make the general public appreciate how important architecture is? Our aim is to communicate the pleasure and power of architecture, and to make the public aware of its effect.

For 'Sensing Spaces' we took the opportunity to examine core themes in architecture and to find ways of communicating its joys and mysteries. We looked at the actual spaces of the Royal Academy to understand their particular characteristics and thought about essential elements of architecture and how we might emphasise aspects of them. We mined our architectural influences, inspirations and reference points in order to deepen our understanding and awareness. We wanted to rediscover known territory and reveal its wonders so the public could enter into the world of architecture with us, with a shared sense of discovery.

Great poets and writers capture architectural experience and powerfully describe spatial experience. Here we are describing spatial experience using not words but light.

19

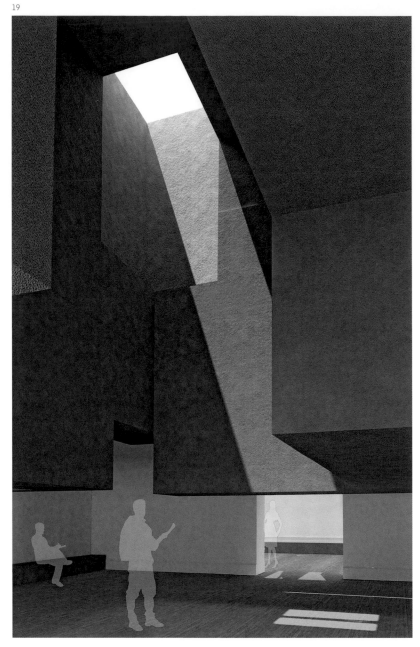

The second room
explores ideas
of weight and
containment.
A new large form
is inserted into
the aperture of the
existing rooflight,
hovering at 2.4
metres above floor
level. Light is brought
in through two voids
in the form located
at opposite corners
to create a diagonal
axis. As in the first
room, natural light
conditions outside
are amplified (20, 21).
The new structure
creates niches in
which people can
sit, observing the
changes in light
and discovering
views into the
larger volume (19).

20

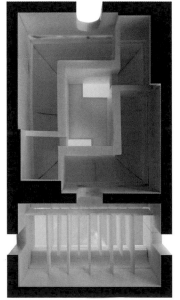

21

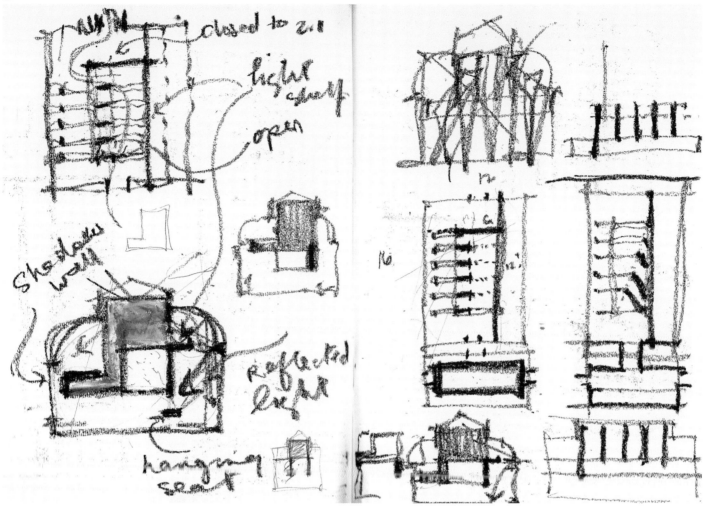

closed to z.11

light shelf

open

Shadow wall

Reflected light

hanging seat

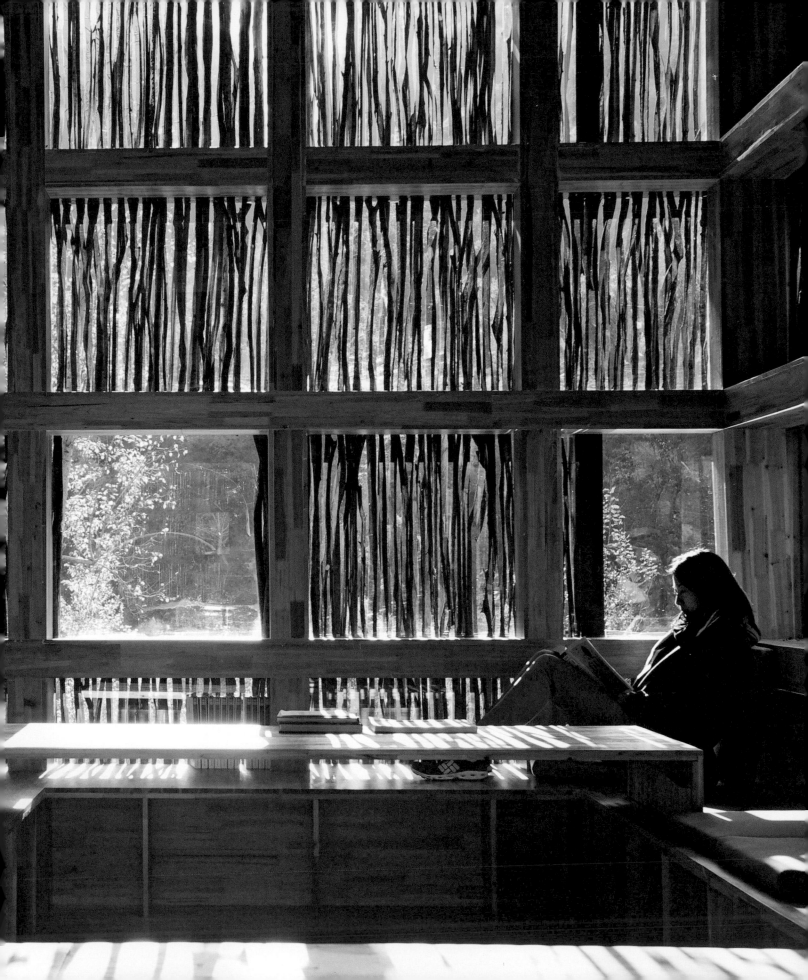

Li Xiaodong

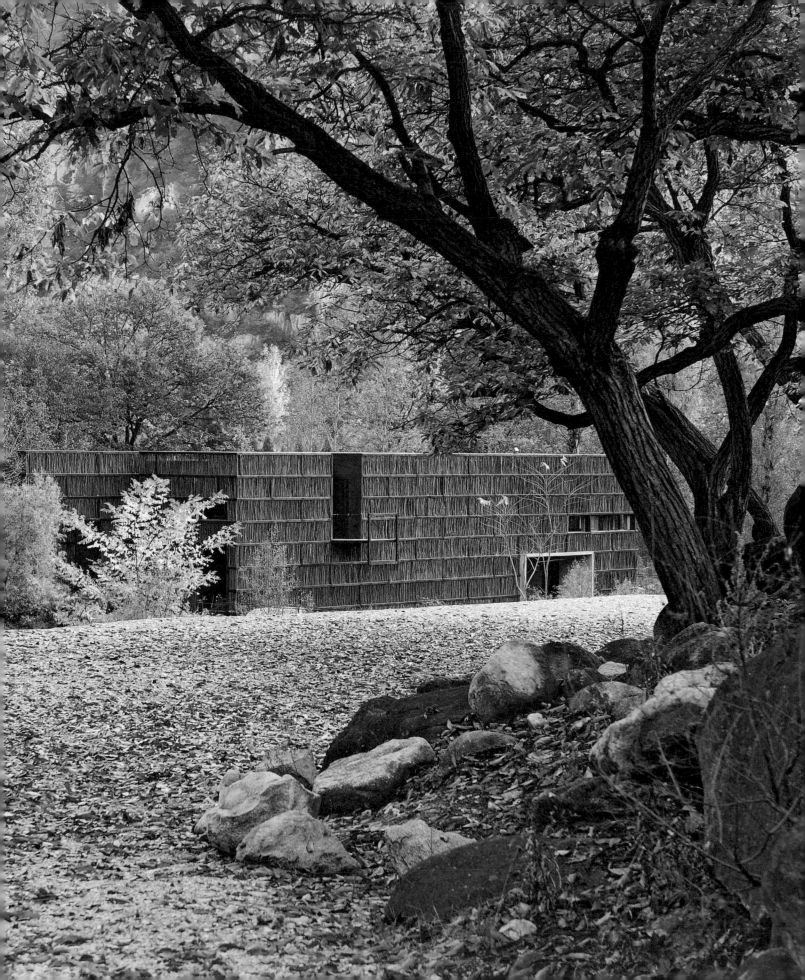

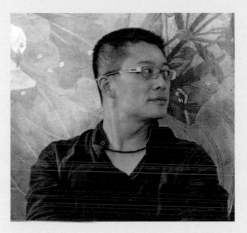

Focused on small, often self-initiated projects, Li Xiaodong (born 1963, China) develops propositions about an appropriate 'Chinese architecture' that brings together traditional and contemporary modes of expression, technical knowledge and artistic judgement. His architecture combines a spiritual exploration of ideas with rational thinking and is based on a continuing enquiry into the underlying concepts of space in the Chinese context first explored in his book *Chinese Conception of Space* (1991).

After studying architecture in Beijing, Li completed a master's degree and a PhD in architecture at the Delft University of Technology in the Netherlands. He now combines his practice with a role as Professor of History and Theory at Tsinghua University School of Architecture in Beijing.

Strikingly modern in form, Li's designs are rooted in the vernacular, often using local construction techniques and responding to the specific features and landscape of each location. He pays close attention to climatic conditions and the changing seasons, so the experience of his architecture is constantly in flux.

Li's work includes the Bridge School, Fujian, China (2009), which won an Aga Khan Award for Architecture in 2010. He was made an honorary fellow of the American Institute of Architects in 2012.

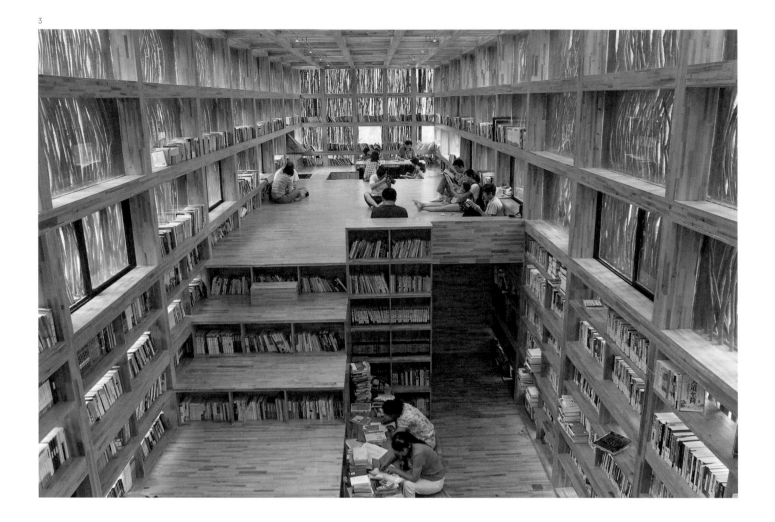

4

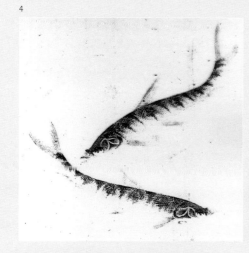

**3, 5 (overleaf)
Li Xiaodong Atelier,
Liyuan Library.**
Interior and exterior
in winter.

**4 Detail after a
thirteenth-century
handscroll.**

*Kate Goodwin: You have written a book
called* Chinese Conception of Space.
*Do you feel there is something very
particular about the ways your culture
understands space?*
Li Xiaodong: The book began as
a research project comparing concepts
of space in China and the West.
I found that there is a clear distinction:
the Western tendency is to look
at the world as a series of objects,
while in China and the East we tend
not to differentiate between subject
and object. So Western architecture
develops from perspective, with
the building as an object to be looked
at from 'without', while Chinese
architecture develops from the
idea that the building is something
to be experienced from 'within'.

Space in Chinese tradition has been
articulated within a defined framework
that allows for reinterpretation
in different contexts through the
use of the imagination rather than
through logic. This possibility of
reinterpretation is what makes the
culture sustainable – it's like the
characters in Chinese writing, which
were created thousands of years ago but
still form part of a living language. The
Chinese tend to focus on the intangible
rather than the tangible – you see this
in Chinese painting, in which the

blank surface is often just as important
as what is inscribed. For instance,
in a handscroll that shows a pair of
swimming fish, the presence of water,
which can be inferred from the blank
background, is a vital part of the image.
Allowing room for the imagination
is essential if a space is to become
a satisfying physical experience.

We can also see the difference
between Chinese and Western ideas
in the way architecture has been
represented within the two traditions.
For the Chinese, an artificially created
space is first of all cosmological and
should be in harmony with the order
of nature. The articulation of space
in Chinese culture has been regarded
as an art form alongside painting,
calligraphy or poetry, as in the history
of private garden design from the
Ming and Qing dynasties.

*In what ways do you think contemporary
architecture can bridge the gap
between traditional Chinese culture
and present-day conditions?*
The technical language of Chinese
architecture was already defined back
in the Han Dynasty, about 2,000 years
ago. There were columns, beams
and then a big roof, with three or four
different roof types. For the next two
millennia, the only changes were to

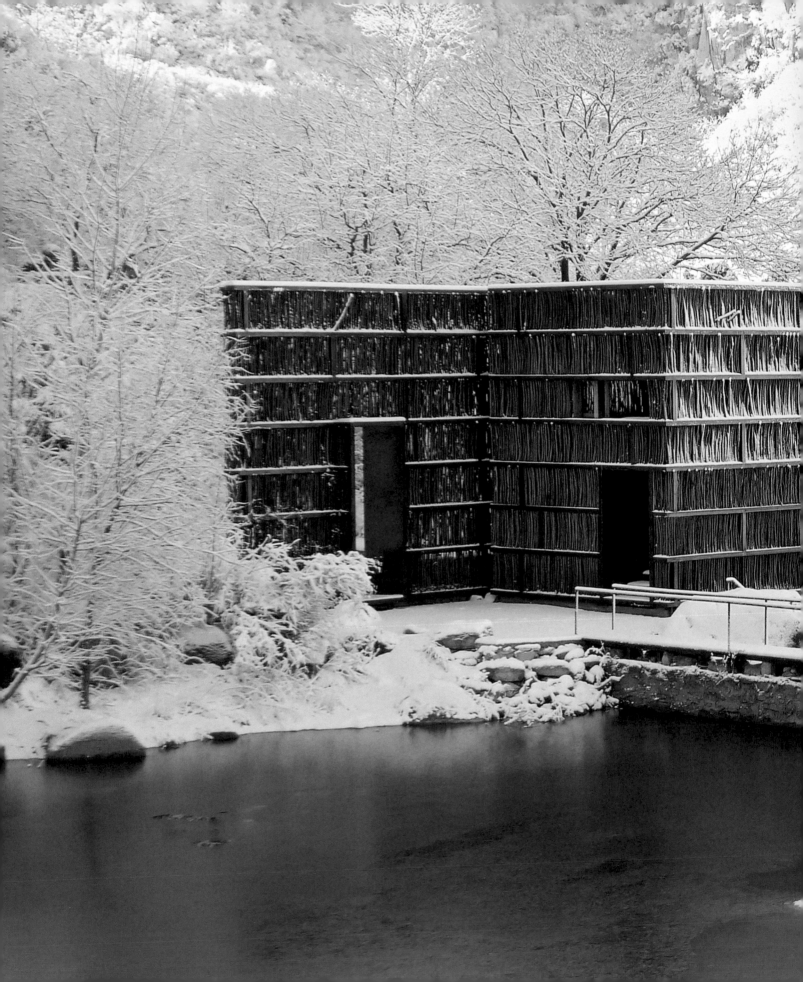

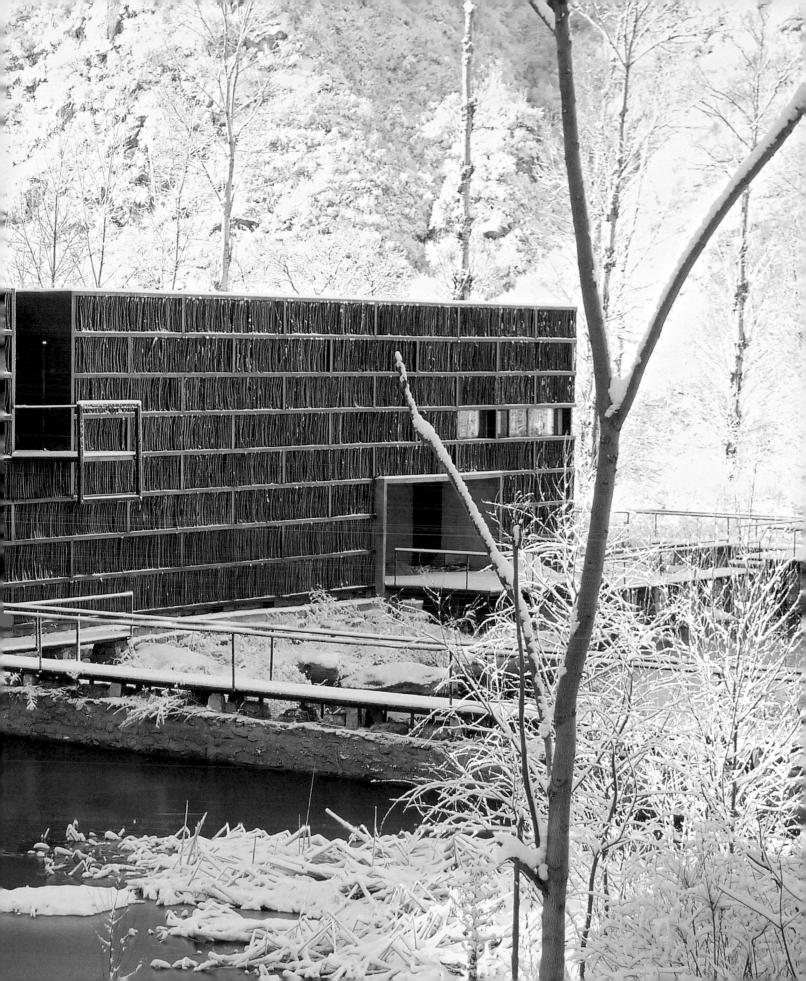

6

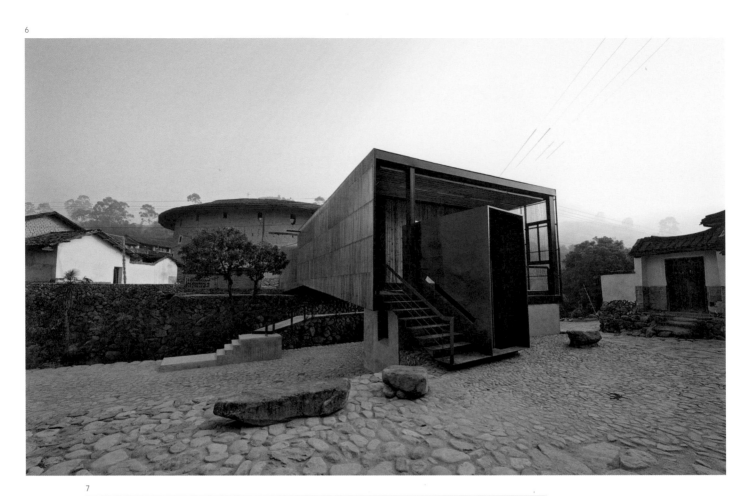

7

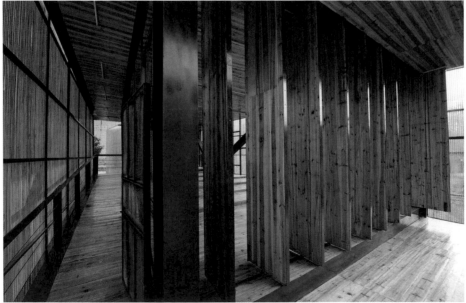

8

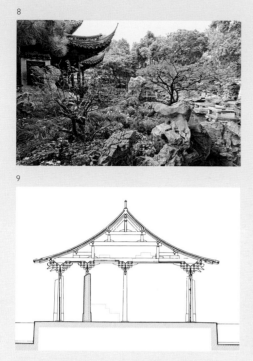

9

do with colour and space. So within Chinese tradition, architecture is less about individual building forms than about how space is defined by the structures that surround it.

The Forbidden City in Beijing, for instance, is about experiencing space after space after space rather than appreciating individual buildings. It's a concept articulated by the ancient Chinese philosopher Lao Zi, who said that what is important is what is contained, not the container. This is also exemplified in the courtyard typology of traditional Chinese housing.

Modern architecture is an invention of the West, and we Chinese have had to adopt this new way of thinking. Liang Sicheng, the 'father' of modern architecture in China and the founder of the Architecture Department at Tsinghua University, where I was trained, based his teaching on ways of combining Chinese tradition and knowledge with modern forms, which, of course, was an important stage for us in discovering relationships between identity and modernity. But the question for me is: can we really modernise a traditional Chinese form if Chinese architecture has never been about form?

Much of my own research and design work has been focused on exploring whether contemporary architectural theory and practice could be enriched through dialogue with our ancient culture, and on how Chinese tradition might be expressed conceptually in modern ways. This is what matters: we need to find ways of developing our architecture without aping Western models or relying on a superficial imitation of traditional Chinese forms and decoration.

How are these ideas manifesting themselves in your own practice?
It seems to me that the last hundred years have been about the development of tectonic languages of architecture – Modernism, Postmodernism, Deconstructivism and so on.

Theory and debate have created a useful working vocabulary, but in the twenty-first century globalisation and cultural conflicts have changed the issues. So I think architecture today should try to reintegrate ideas with real-life conditions.

What I am trying to do in my own practice might be described as reflexive regionalism. It's more about identifying original conditions than inventing original forms.

To take an example, my project for a conference centre in Bali creates a sense of regional identity by mixing modern, functional thinking with traditional materials and culture. In the tropical jungle, order is of primary importance for human settlements and my design grows from that principle. For instance, local buildings use bamboo to filter the light – it's a functional thing – but the repetition in the material also reflects the sense of order you find in Balinese villages. It's about combining technology, local materials, modern thinking and a traditional sense of identity.

You have described how key the relationship of building and environment is to your work. Can you recall a moment when you first became aware of the spatial potential of the environment and your place within it?
A formative experience from the start of my career was my stay from 1984 to 1986 in the Yellow Mountain range while I was supervising the construction of a hotel. The changing seasons and weather, the distances and dimensions, as well as my consciousness of the vast timescale of the mountains' creation, all contributed to a change in my perceptions.

From a distance you think of a mountain range as a series of objects seen in silhouette. But once you are within it, you start to perceive it as a series of spatial relationships that surround you. Your awareness of scale, distance, texture and enclosure all come alive and you become

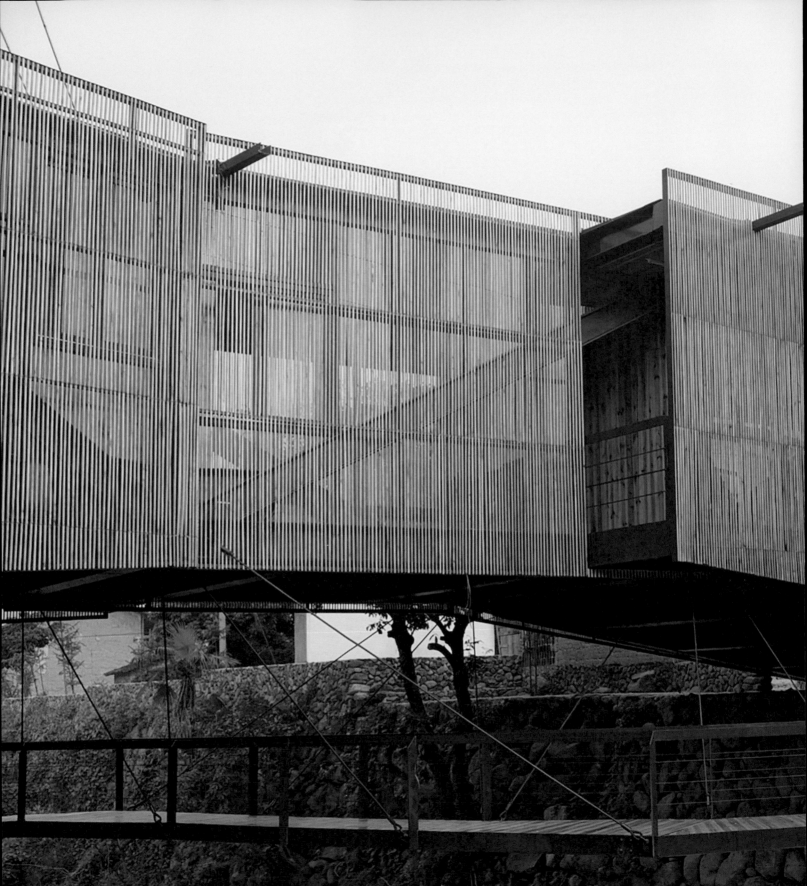

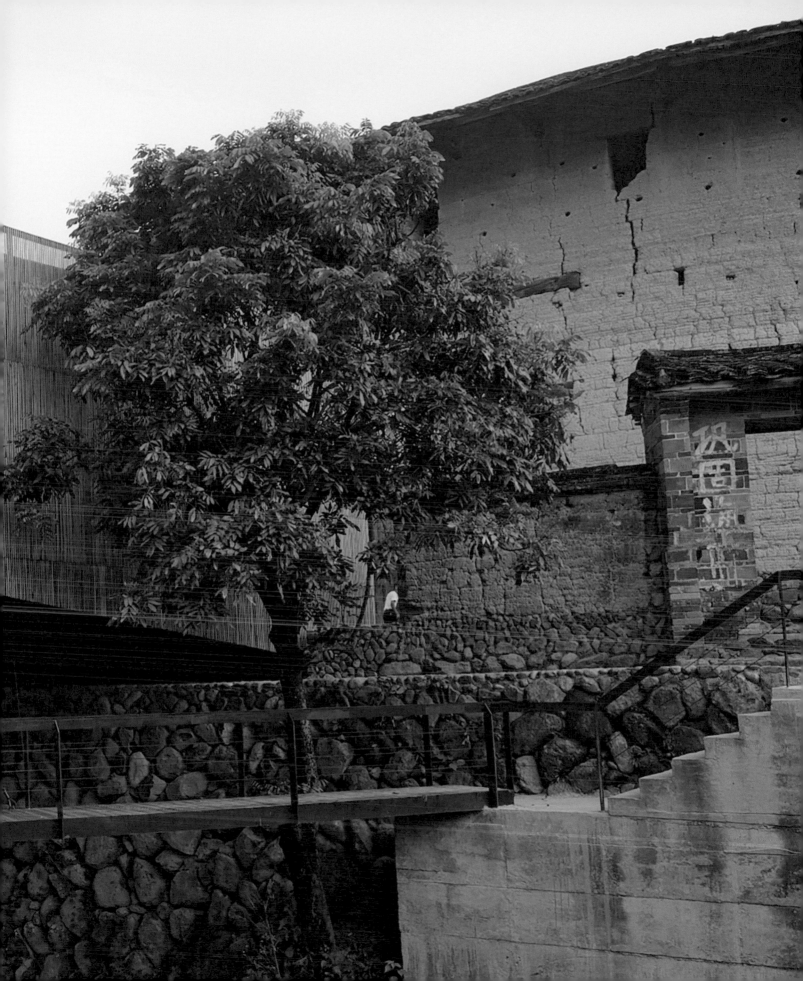

11

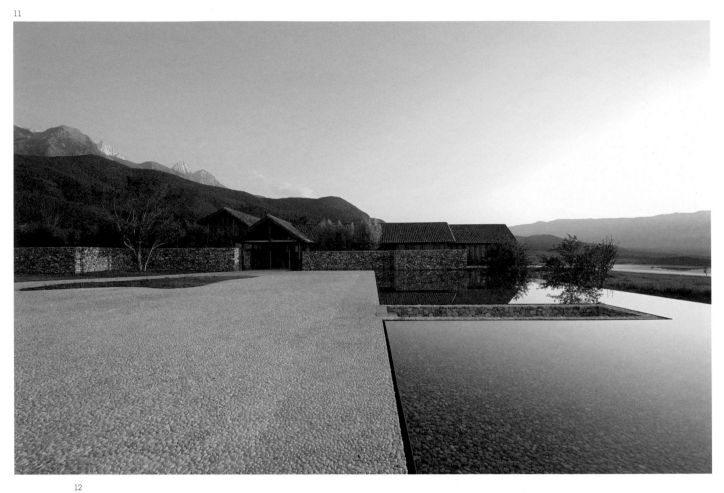

12

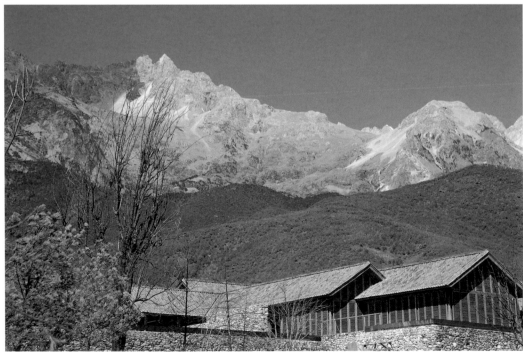

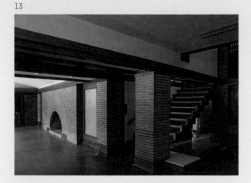

13

11, 12 Li Xiaodong Atelier, Water House, Lijiang, Yunnan, China (2010).
The complex employs traditional forms and construction methods in a series of simple timber and glass pavilions with lightweight slatted walls. Through its materials, form and siting, the building becomes part of the mountain landscape. The town is famous for its network of waterways and bridges and water is threaded through the site.

13 Frank Lloyd Wright, Darwin D. Martin House, Buffalo, NY, US (1903–05).

conscious of your own presence within it. Recognising this was a beautiful moment.

Can you identify any influences of this experience within your own work?
Both the Water House and the Liyuan Library reflect the impact of this experience. They are about the relationship of a building to its surroundings rather than a building as a discrete object.

The architecture of the Water House is integrated into the setting of the Jade Dragon Snow Mountain. House and landscape complement each other so the quality of the whole environment is improved. It's like a system within which the relationships between the parts are more important than the parts themselves, or a kaleidoscope, where the integrity of the system predominates and the significance of the individual elements disappears.

With the Liyuan Library, the intention was to create a framework that would help you to appreciate the natural environment. It is simple because simplicity allows you to appreciate nature more readily.

I have discovered that if a building is too complicated, you risk diluting your intentions. The amount of detail you can generate through computer drawings is wonderful, but you need a consistent and simple way of using those details. When I'm working I need to be clear about the issues before I can generate ideas; solutions emerge from a clear definition of the problem. It's not about the details but about how you create a total environment.

What role do you think the senses play in how we perceive and experience space? And what might this add to how we engage with architecture?
There are millions of sensors all over our bodies, taking in information about our environment and transmitting it to our brains. It's like radar, scanning our surroundings and sending back signals. The information we receive can't be quantified, so how we engage with these

perceptions to create or appreciate architecture is difficult to define.

I've been practising tai chi since I was 21 to strengthen my sensory system. Tai chi is about looking inwards as well as outwards; it's a system of breathing and energy flow that makes you stronger and more powerful. It's not just physical: it's about focusing the mind, through which all your senses become more alert.

Through tai chi I also train myself to be more receptive to what we call *qi* (气场), a flow of energy made possible by the systematic relationship and harmony of physical elements. For the Chinese, this idea of energy forever circulating, flowing through all things and continually transforming the cosmos, is very important. So when I start working on a project, the first thing I do is analyse the site and the flow of energy through it. Then with my training as an architect I hope to translate my findings into designs.

What else do you think is distinctive about how you as an architect understand and perceive space?
Architects work through reasoning, instinct and experience and then put the whole thing together. When a space makes an impression on you, you ask 'why?', and the answer becomes part of your vocabulary. Sometimes it's about a critical analysis of space that you incorporate into your own understanding for future use. Things like, 'this lighting is good, these dimensions work, this material is interesting' are perceptions you store up to explore later. Every place you visit generates pieces and puzzles in your mind and so you develop a palette of possibilities. I find that the more experiences I have, the more open to possibilities I become.

Can you recall a space or a work of architecture that has made you particularly aware of yourself and your surroundings, particularly 'present'?
When I recently gave a lecture in Buffalo, New York, I stayed

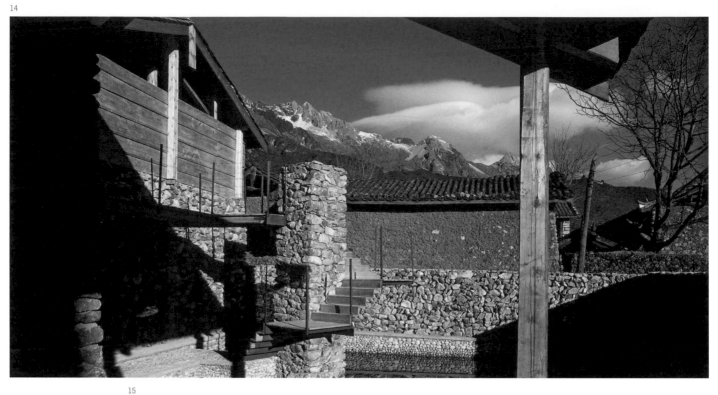

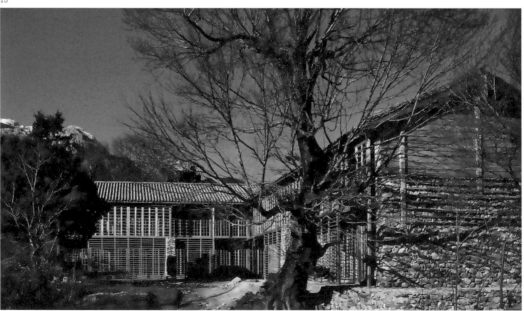

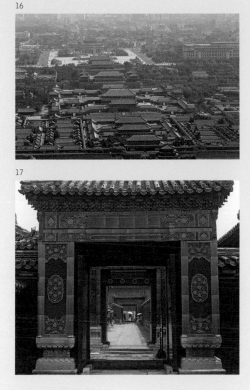

14, 15 Li Xiaodong Atelier, Yuhu Elementary School and Community Centre, Lijiang (2011). Vernacular design elements characteristic of the local Naxi minority population have been reinterpreted to create a modern building providing public gathering spaces in a courtyard and porch, classrooms and a community hall. Construction was undertaken by local farmers untrained in building.

16, 17 Forbidden City, Beijing, China (from early fifteenth century). Aerial view and axial view through portals and courtyards.

in the Darwin D. Martin House by Frank Lloyd Wright. To my mind Wright was the first Western architect whose work focused on space rather than on the building as an object.

To move around inside Wright's houses is to understand his thinking about design. Because he learned about architecture through experimenting with building his home and studio, he was able to establish a clear understanding of what is 'real' and what is 'conceptual'. This is the fundamental difference between 'being present' in a space, where you are absorbed within it, and looking at images of a space, where the mind is detached.

The Kimbell Museum by Louis Kahn is another example of a space where you feel each element contributes to a totality – the architecture, space, lighting, exhibits and yourself within it. It's like yin–yang: without yin, yang could not exist.

In what other ways do you think architecture can enhance or influence human experience?
Space is perceived through a dialogue between imagination and reality. It's like when writers create stories – they use their imaginations to develop and reinterpret the reality of their own experiences.

Chinese literature clearly illustrates the importance of architecture in our lives and the relationship we have to it. Chinese stories often situate their narratives within architectural settings, while Chinese architecture can allude to experiences derived from literary texts. Usually in Chinese poetry, time and space are defined at the outset because without this concrete platform it is difficult for the text to communicate its message. In Chinese literature, every story happens *somewhere*.

Chinese stories often attach a certain meaning to a particular space and this defines how a network of people can associate with each other, so space both determines and describes a social pattern. In Chinese culture,

it is important to be able to grasp one's position in space, time and society, and the establishment of a structure of tangible spatial references facilitates this process. It's like the Forbidden City, again, where you are led through five or six different gates in sequence before you arrive at the palace. The length of each courtyard is different, so the sequence builds a specific momentum, and the thresholds themselves define varying levels of privacy, with regulations to govern how high a threshold can be or how many locks there are on a door, depending on the rank of the individual officer.

The experience of visiting the Royal Academy has a similar sense of sequencing: moving from busy Piccadilly into the Annenberg Courtyard, then entering the eighteenth-century town palace, up the grand staircase and into the nineteenth-century Main Galleries. How does your installation build upon this layering of space and thresholds?
This is already a rich sequence. On the street you have a mix of different textures and noises, different people from different backgrounds. Then in the galleries it's very pure.

Once visitors enter the installation itself, I'd like it to seem like a journey of discovery, with the sense that alternative worlds run alongside their path and intersect with it. Along the way, not everything will be visible and clear; rather the story unfolds like the painted image on a Chinese handscroll, to be appreciated over time. By the end, though, they will have gained a series of impressions that create a new mental landscape.

Can you describe how you envisage the project in more detail?
Metaphorically, you are walking through a forest in the snow at night, which is represented by a maze of slender branches or twigs with the white floor lit from below. As you explore, you discover niches that provide hope and happy surprises. At the end of the maze you arrive

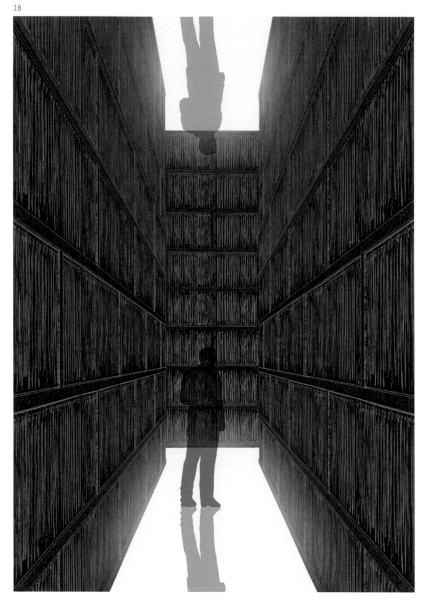

The installation uses a wooden frame (20) to create a labyrinthine route into the more open space of the Zen garden. The armature supports three layers of slender branches, which introduce an unexpected natural material into the galleries (18, 19). An illuminated floor creates the disorienting sense of walking through a forest in the snow at night.

19

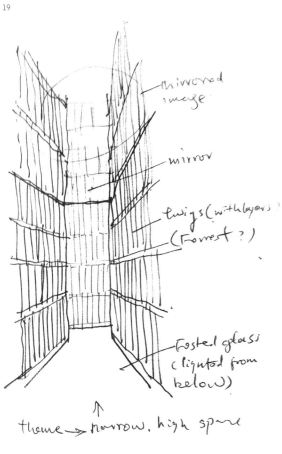

mirrored image

mirror

twigs (with layers) (Forrest?)

Frosted glass (lighted from below)

theme → narrow, high space

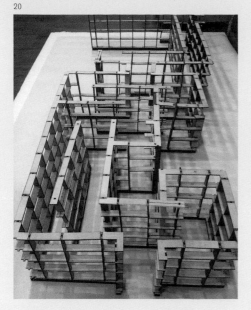

20

at a Zen garden which represents clear-sightedness and inspiration. From an epistemological point of view, this invites you to look and understand, to turn 'blindness' into 'vision'.

I'm using branches because they are a natural material people don't expect to see in architecture, and the unconventional application of a familiar material in an unexpected environment generates an effect. When you want to be creative, it's often not about originality *per se*, but about application and reuse. In the countryside you might try to blend the branches with nature but in London it's about creating a seemingly natural setting within an artificial environment.

I have used a mirror in the Zen garden because mirrors have the power to change the feeling of a space. It becomes not about the physical presence of a wall, but the illusion of something else. The mirror makes the space seem expansive even though it is enclosed. Mirrors are used a lot in feng shui, which is fundamentally about the environment and the flow of energy.

You have spoken about creating a 'pinch of consciousness' for the viewer by way of contrasting spatial conditions. How do you hope to achieve this?
The core concept of the installation

in terms of connection, or rather disconnection, to London is to pinch the consciousness through defamiliarisation.

Much of the effect will come from the changing atmosphere as you move through the space. At first the texture, scale and dimensions are clearly defined and familiar, yet there is also a loss of orientation. Then in the Zen garden you experience a new openness and sense of revelation. This contrast, and the flow of energy through the spaces, invites you to speculate on your experience and heightens your awareness.

In what ways has your approach to creating an installation for an exhibition differed from your usual practice?
In most architectural commissions there is a specified function and programme but with an exhibition it's more about aesthetic experience. On the one hand it's easier, because you don't have to think about the practical issues, but on the other hand it's more difficult because you need to create a space that people will find appealing – they expect something but they don't know what. For me, the main question is how do you arouse their curiosity and generate the kind of impact you want to make?

In contrast to the narrow passageway of the labyrinth, the Zen garden has a sense of openness and expansiveness, enhanced by the inclusion of a mirror (21, 22). The intended effect is to 'pinch the consciousness' of visitors and invite them to reflect on their journey.

21

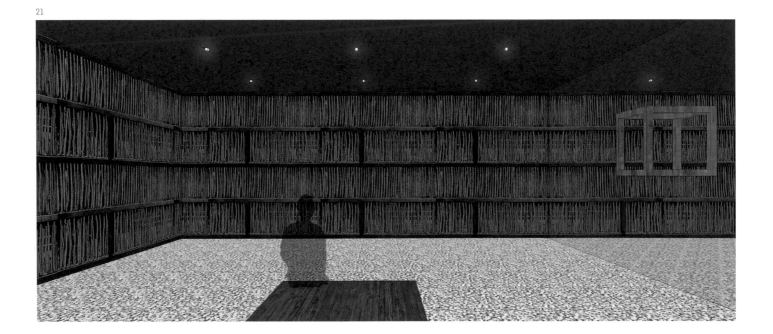

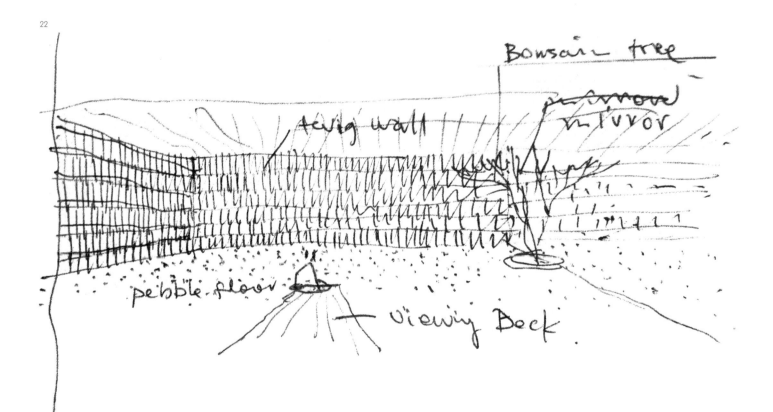

22

Bonsai tree

twig wall

mirror

pebble floor

Viewing Deck

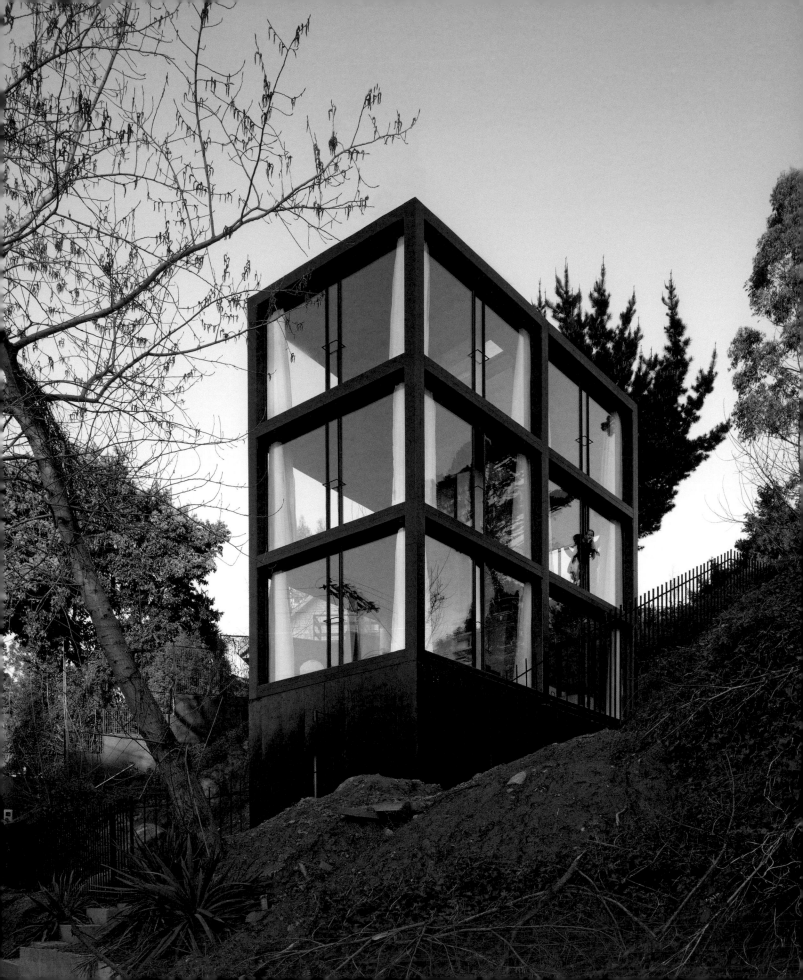

Pezo von Ellrichshausen

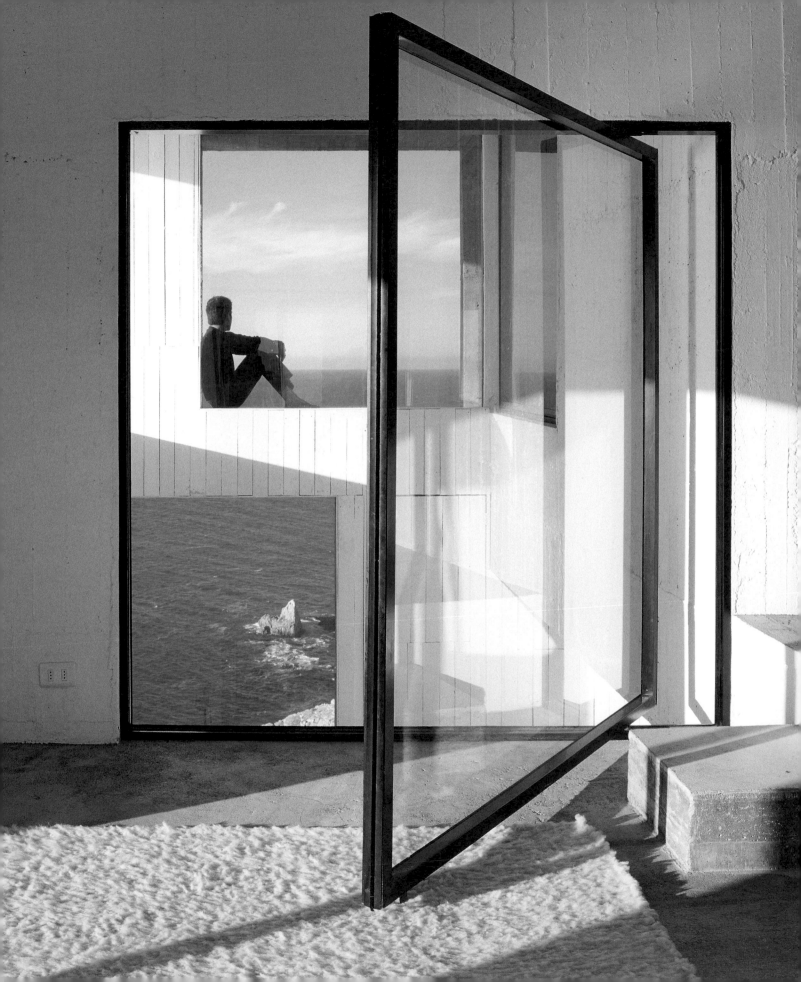

1 (previous spread) Pezo von Ellrichshausen, Arco House, Concepción, Chile (2011). Replacing a house destroyed by earthquake, the Arco House embodies both tension and serenity. The dominating steel structure on its steep hillside frames six glass-walled rooms. At once monolithic and apparently unstable, it is in fact engineered to be earthquake-proof.

2 (opposite), 3 (overleaf) Pezo von Ellrichshausen, Poli House Cultural Center, Coliumo, Chile (2005). Both summer house and cultural centre, the Poli House is a simple intervention in a beautiful natural context.

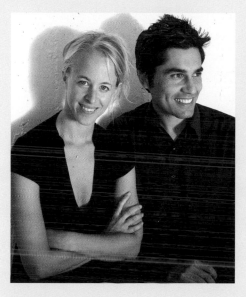

Pezo von Ellrichshausen was established in 2002 in Concepción in Chile by Mauricio Pezo (born 1973 in Angol, Chile) and Sofia von Ellrichshausen (born 1976 in Bariloche, Argentina). The studio's work combines an intense intellectual discipline with an intuitive sense of materiality, light and form, creating spaces of comfort from a limited palette of materials, usually wood and exposed concrete. Occupying a space where architecture and the visual arts intersect, Pezo von Ellrichshausen's buildings and installations challenge traditional perceptions of both.

International recognition was established through a series of houses in Chile, Portugal and Spain, beginning in 2005 with the Poli House Cultural Center in Coliumo, Chile. Though apparently simple, these houses – developed through a rigorous geometric exploration of plan, section and axonometric – are in fact complex, solid, highly organised and humane. Art installations by Pezo von Ellrichshausen, including '120 Doors Pavilion' in Concepción in 2003 and 'Mine Pavilion' in Denver, Colorado, in 2013, show the same focus on developing typologies. They also curated 'I was there', the Chile Pavilion at the 2008 Venice Architecture Biennale and were selected to show their own work there in 2010.

Both partners teach in Chile and have been visiting professors at the University of Texas at Austin and Cornell University in New York. Awards and prizes include the AR Award for Emerging Architecture (2005) and the fourth annual Spotlight Prize presented by the Rice Design Alliance (2012).

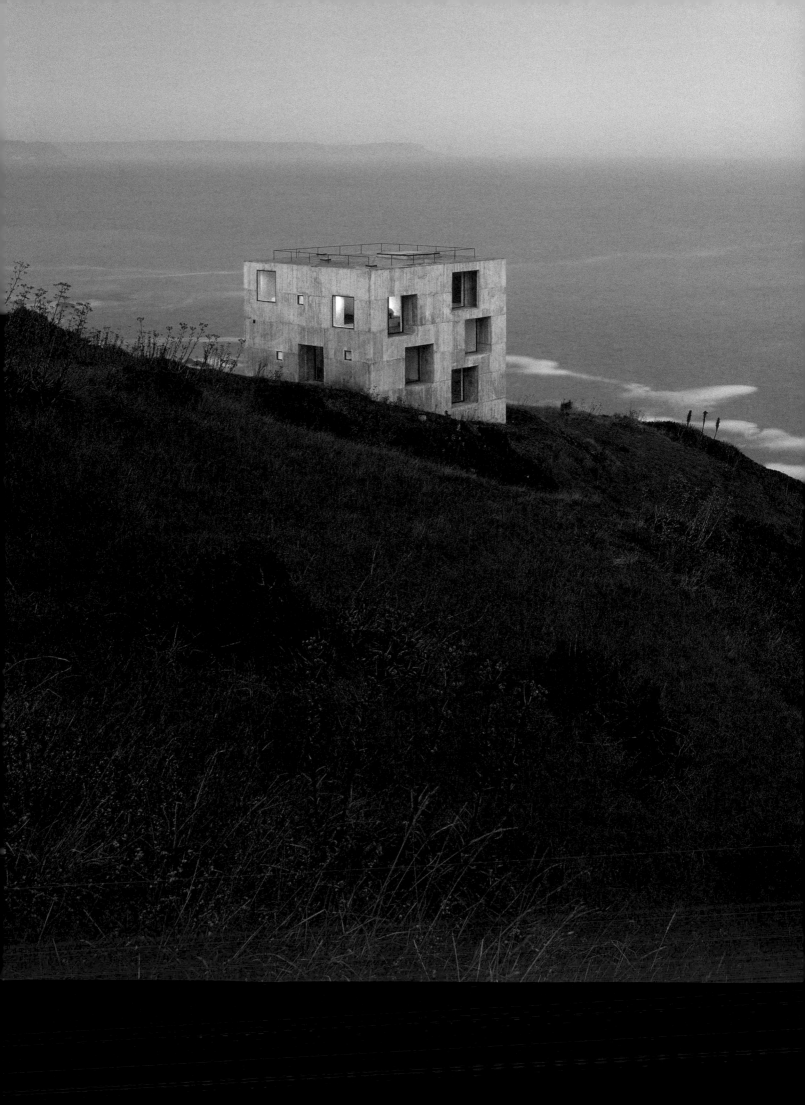

4

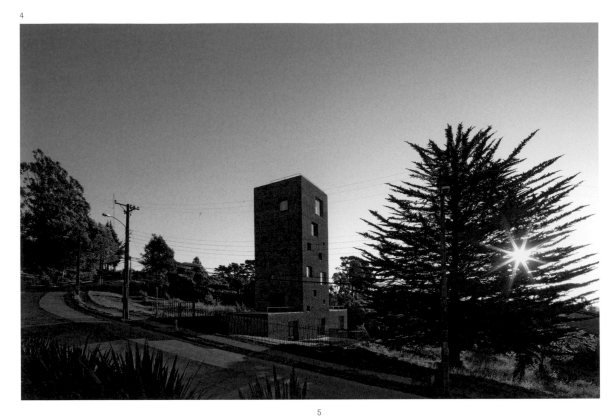

5

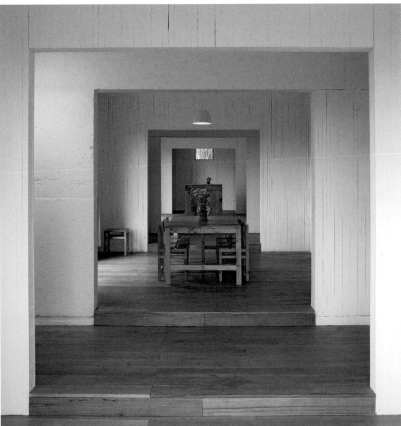

6

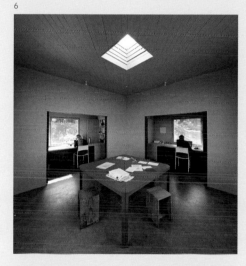

4–6 Pezo von Ellrichshausen, Cien House, Concepción (2011). Five monolithic storeys rise over a two-storey podium to form the architects' own house and studio.

7 (overleaf) Pezo von Ellrichshausen, Solo House, Cretas, Teruel, Spain (2011). On an elevated site, the sculptural structure of the Solo House is raised on a blind podium. The space enclosed by the balcony has no roof and holds a pool of water, a 'soft patio' as deep as the podium itself.

Kate Goodwin: In what ways does architecture enhance human experience beyond its function of providing shelter?
Mauricio Pezo: We are fascinated by the ordinary and familiar and I hope we can contribute to an understanding of this. European architects are working within a defined tradition, but we are talking about something more universal, a tradition of human behaviour. At the same time, there's a degree of inventiveness in what we create just because it's so simple, so basic. You think there must be something more to it – like when you see examples of great vernacular architecture and ask, 'Can something that seems so ordinary have been intentional?'

We try consciously to define the parameters of each project to understand what is essential. For instance, if you take a house, what is the minimum you can do while still providing what is necessary? It's also about understanding how emphasising certain elements produces an architectural statement.

You can see this approach clearly in our choice of materials: we're not trying to innovate for the sake of it, to experiment with new materials or the possibilities of structure. We're not trying to show the effort of a building, its muscles. The emphasis instead is on the proportions of the rooms, their sequence, the way they open – simple things, but which taken together suggest something more complex. Perhaps instead of complexity and contradiction we're trying to produce complexity and integrity, a unitary, coherent artefact.
Sofia von Ellrichshausen: We like the idea that there are basic ways of understanding spatial relationships, a universal language, and so we have been investigating spatial structures in a primitive and topological sense.
Pezo: For instance, in architecture a cross is a spatial relationship you can describe without even making a drawing – it's basically a direction you can understand in any language, at any scale or for any programme. We are interested in this sort of fundamental understanding of architecture.
Sofia: It is also related to a sense of timelessness. People look at our own house, the Cien House, and wonder if it was born old. We do not use the word 'design' because for us design is linked to fashion, an expression of one specific moment within a culture. Our aim is to create structures based on a timeless beauty, which is a consequence of doing things honestly at a given moment.

What are the key factors that have influenced your architectural sensibilities?
Sofia: We started working together twelve years ago, after I moved to Chile

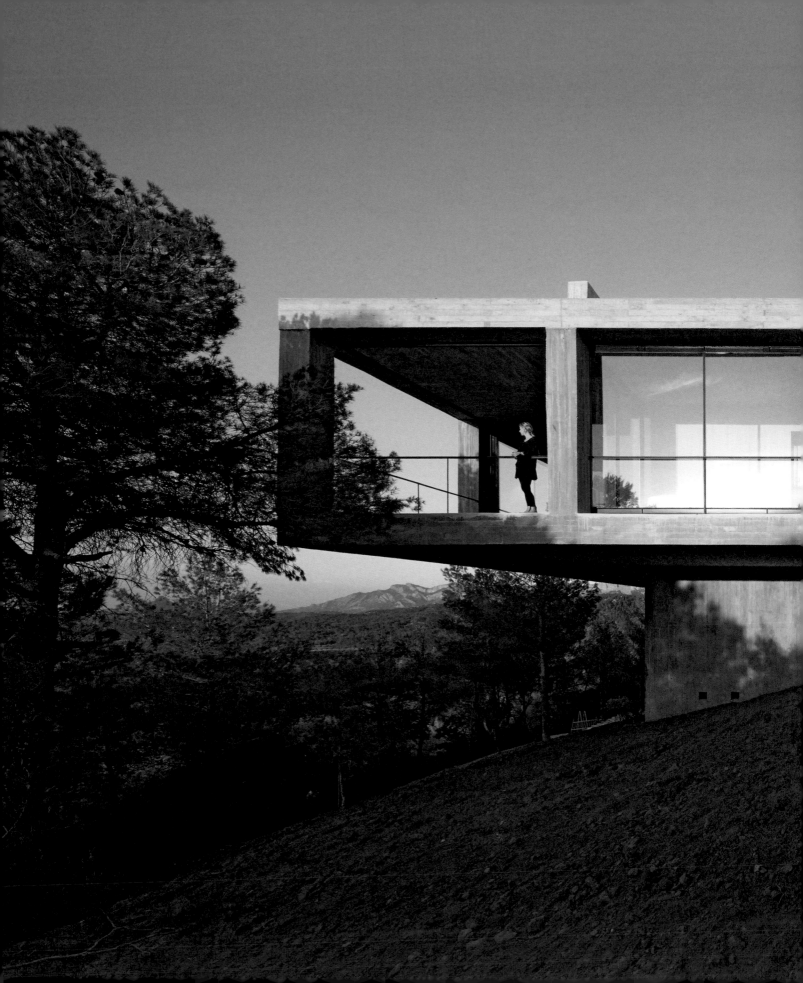

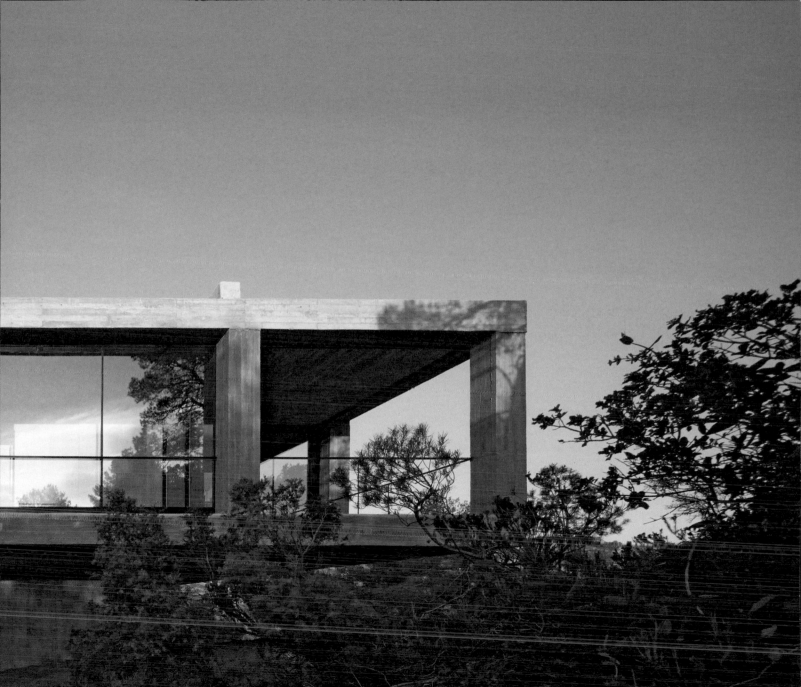

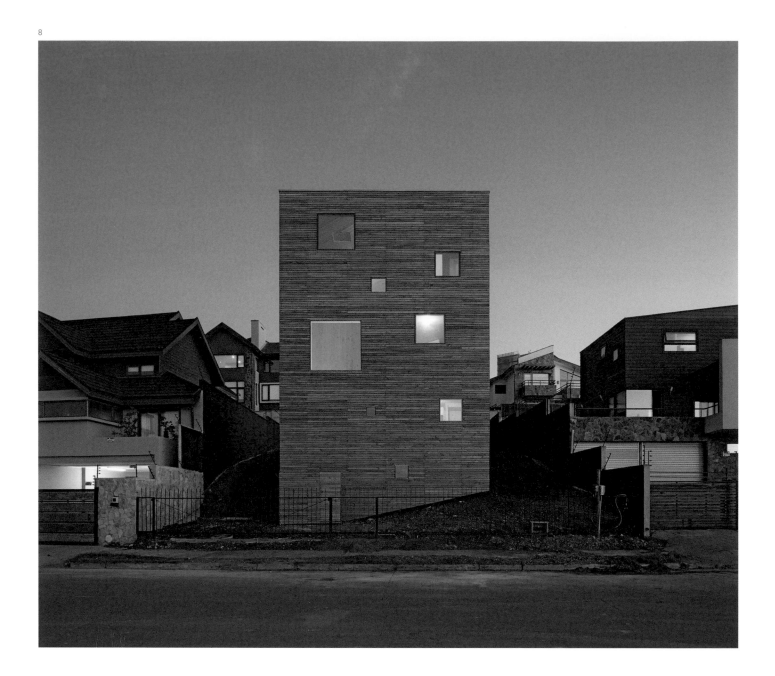

from Buenos Aires. Neither of us had much experience of working for anyone else so we were able to discover our own ways of doing things.

At the beginning we weren't so aware of the way our work was developing, but over the years we started to detect a pattern, to realise we've been insisting on certain ideas. We always ask ourselves, 'Is this really what we are interested in? Is this really what we believe in?'
Pezo: Our priorities are drawn from our physical and cultural place in the world, which has made us very humble and at the same time very ambitious. We have grown up in what has been known historically as the New World, which means we don't carry the burden of a specific architectural heritage, at least not from the modern era. It's a kind of *tabula rasa*: we believe we have the right to start from scratch, to establish our own spatial grammar. But this is also a fragile position because you have to make sure you are not doing something new for the sake of novelty, which is merely a relative term.

When people are operating with limited resources, then producing something spectacular and visually impressive might seem like a way to attract attention. But because Chile provides a beautiful natural context we believe our interventions should be simple and direct. We believe that architecture is a balance between continuity and rupture: for instance, our Poli House and Cien House use ordinary windows, doors and materials but still provide something unexpected. We like the notion of familiar materials within a new spatial logic.

You have talked about the natural setting you operate in as well as your place within the 'New World'. How much of your approach is specific to Chile?
Sofia: In Peru or Mexico the built heritage is a huge influence on the entire culture. But Chile doesn't have that – it's more about geography, a natural inheritance.
Pezo: It's very easy to be romantic or nostalgic or poetic about nature. But for us, this is not about the presence of mountains or water but about a deep understanding of basic coordinates and orientation. The mental image of Chile is an abstraction: a strip of land with forest in the south, desert in the north, mountains to the west and a string of cities in the middle. We think it's important to know how that impacts on our architecture.

Chile's national anthem describes the country as 'the happy copy of Eden': not Eden itself, but a replica. This illustrates that there is no such thing as a pure perception of place but only a construction of the reality we perceive around us. Our feelings about places are influenced by ideas, memories, desires, even prejudices, so when we say we are looking at how architecture can respond to a particular natural environment, we are already making an interpretation of that environment. It is not so much about natural beauty as about the elements we can use to turn that beauty into an architectural experience.
Sofia: Practising in Chile also has a practical impact. Labour conditions are volatile so we know things will have to change in the course of construction. It means we think not of details but of the structure and bones of the piece, the elements that will survive the process.

You often create visual representations of your work – particularly paintings – which present the architecture as an object. How does this relate to how you want people to experience your architecture?
Sofia: We tend to think of architecture in terms of pieces, with each building as a specific piece. We don't have a problem with thinking of a building as an object, but we believe that this is not enough. An object has its own autonomy, as in the Classical notion of sculpture, but architecture, despite the intentions of architects, is never autonomous. There is always a link with a place, a moment, a culture, the natural environment. A piece is a specific object that is articulated within a unique situation.
Pezo: We usually work with axonometrics because they are a synthetic way of depicting the integrity of a piece and representing its formal character.

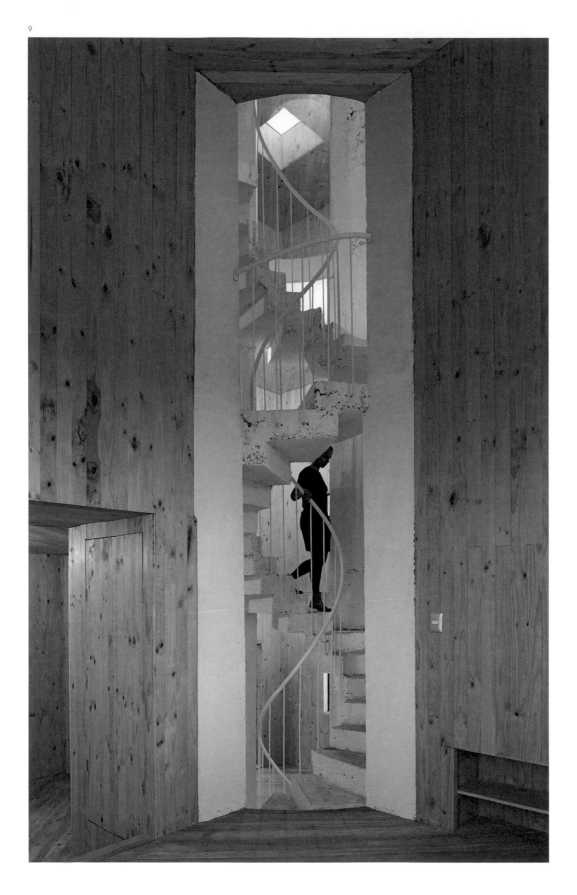

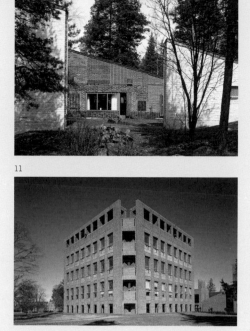

9 Pezo von Ellrichshausen, Gago House.
A spiral stair without landings connects the strata of the house.

10 Alvar Aalto, Muuratsalo Experimental House, Jyväskylä, Finland (1952–54).

11 Louis I. Kahn, Phillips Exeter Academy Library, Exeter, New Hampshire, US (1967–72).

12 (overleaf) Pezo von Ellrichshausen, Fosc House, San Pedro de la Paz, Chile (2009).
The house has three floors of accommodation: bedrooms on the first and third floors are split by space for social activity. The rooms occupy the periphery of the structure with a vertical circulation shaft spiralling through the centre.

The sliced axonometric drawing or painting, which shows both interior and exterior, can be understood as an attempt to highlight the piece's coherence. Every piece can be described as a complete world in itself, with its own character or identity. The experience for the user should be meaningful and unique on both an explicit and implicit level: it is not about the architect's intention, but the capacity of the piece to encourage certain behaviours or evoke a certain idea.

Can you recall a space or work of architecture that has made you particularly aware of yourself and your surroundings, particularly 'present'?
Sofia: In the Muuratsalo Experimental House by Alvar Aalto or the Phillips Exeter Academy Library by Louis Kahn I felt a strong connection with the physical presence of architecture. Most of the places we admire could be described as creating a delicate balance between intimacy and monumentality. There is something simple and schematic in their spatial structure that operates on an intellectual level, but there is also another scale that is very humble, very human.

What role do the senses play in how we perceive and experience space? And what might this add to how we engage with architecture?
Sofia: Good architecture is often invisible, but it allows whatever is happening in that space to be the best experience possible. As we're sitting here in our house, we're not interacting with the architecture but nevertheless the architecture is providing light, a pleasant breeze, allowing us to feel at ease. I think we are coming to a point, more and more, where we don't want to tell people what to do or where to sit but rather to offer them alternatives that allow them to experience different relationships.
Pezo: There is a tendency to think of architecture as a tool to solve problems. But in our view there's also the possibility of considering a piece of architecture as a statement in its own right, something closer to art than to science or technology. The piece in itself can

suggest, evoke, appeal in a sensory way.
Sofia: You have to generate an explicit fitness, a balance, from the essential elements – the site, the programme, the construction. But there is also another variable, which might be called the anti-fitness, some level of discomfort.

Can you describe your initial impressions of the Royal Academy?
Pezo: We find it almost impossible to detach the institution and building from its location. Its position in central London means you feel the weight of history and of the culture it promotes. The building itself is both impressive and puzzling: it has the enigma of being a building within a building, set back from the street, with no presence as an object. Your relation to it is based on a sequence of interiors.

What has shaped your response to the brief?
Sofia: We always felt our proposal had to reflect its position as a temporary installation within the historical space of the institution. Therefore in our approach we were very aware of the morphology and character of the existing building. From the beginning we were fascinated by the size and proportions of the galleries as well as by the clear continuity of the enfilade of rooms. Our project focuses on framing the most permanent yet inaccessible architectural stratum of the gallery: its decorated vaulted ceiling. This is the only part that's in direct contact with the exterior, with the natural light and temperature. It is the silent witness of centuries of temporary art exhibitions but is usually unconnected to the primary experience and is often hidden by artificial lighting and screens.

Can you describe the project in more detail?
Pezo: Our proposal is a small room elevated on four massive columns. The room is square and the columns are circular in plan. This intimate room is contained by low walls but is open to the decorated ceiling of the gallery. The four hollow columns contain spiral staircases that give direct access to this aerial world and there is also another access route: a contained promenade or ramp that

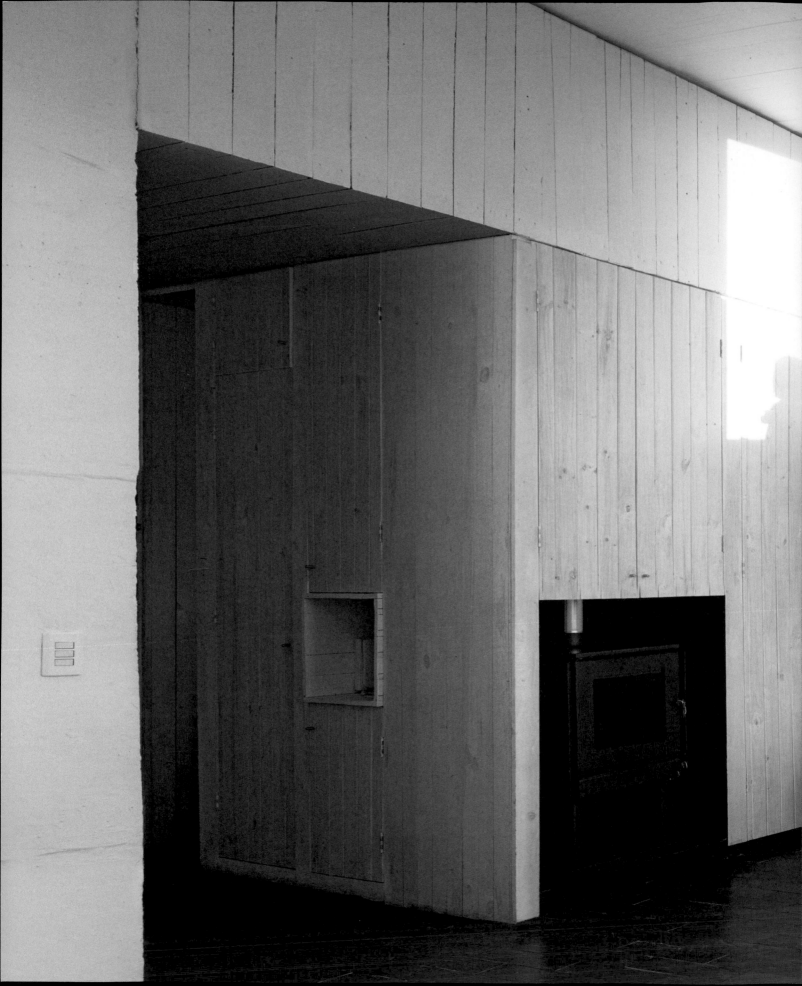

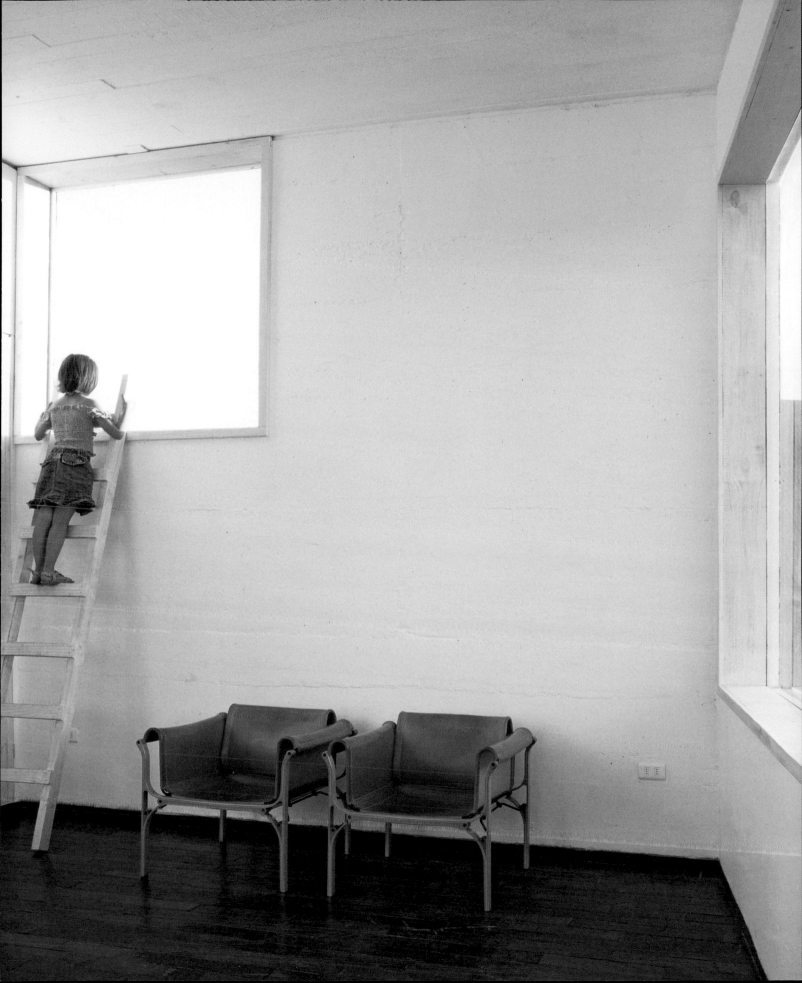

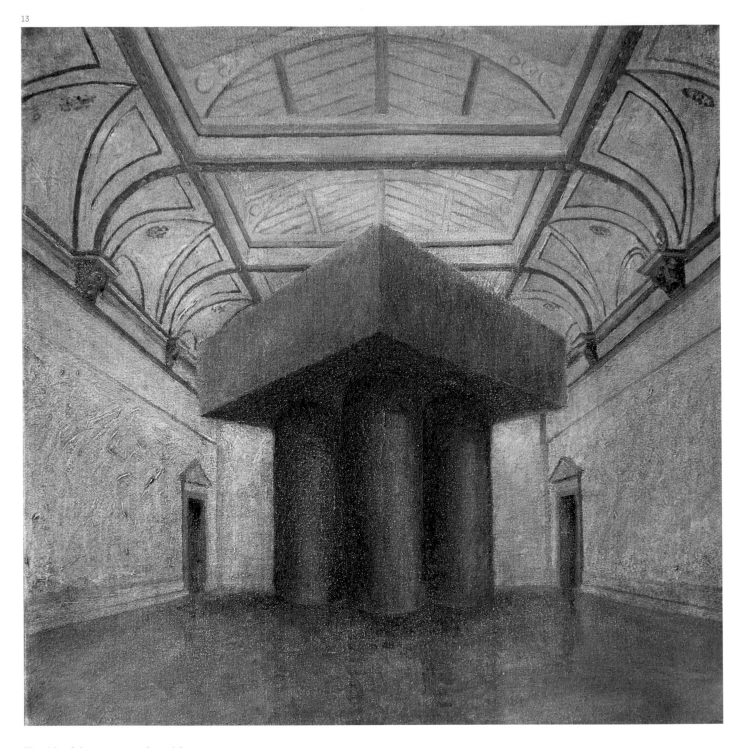

The title of the installation is 'Blue', following Pezo von Ellrichshausen's practice of naming each project with a four-letter word and reflecting the mood they wish to create (13). The installation brings visitors in contact with the most inaccessible level of the gallery spaces – their decorated vaulted ceilings (14).

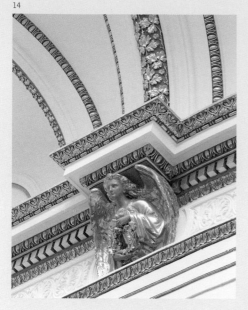

expands the perception of distance and time. As a whole, the structure can be understood as an enigmatic device that invites visitors to abandon the ground plane, the normal strata of the gallery space, and inhabit its upper dimension.
Sofia: This structure provides three different experiences: the collective and open experience under the platform between the massive cylindrical columns; the individual and sensual experience of climbing, or descending, the ramp or staircases; and the surprising collective and intimate experience of being on the platform, almost touching the decorated vaults, steel beams and skylights of the permanent building.

What reactions do you hope this might provoke in the audience?
Sofia: We want people to be aware of the architecture and at the same time to be aware of themselves and of others through the architecture. It's the difference between architecture as the focal point, like a precious object or painting, and architecture as the facilitator for something else.
Pezo: Architecture is often secondary, invisible, but at certain moments, like when you climb a staircase or a ramp, there's a tension between your body and the building. Taking visitors up to this usually unvisited stratum evidences the energy that's necessary when challenging gravity. This is a standard element of architecture, but elevators and escalators meant the physical distance between the ground and upper levels is often forgotten. Our proposal draws attention to gravity as a fact of architecture.
Sofia: We have named the project 'Blue' because of the mood and temperature the word implies. 'Blue' supposes an intimacy and perhaps embodies a sense of quietness, even nostalgia.
Pezo: As with some of our previous projects, 'Blue' is based on a mechanical insistence on a single element and an over-explicit sense of choice offered by the repetition of alternative routes. It is a piece with an undefined scale, perhaps polarising intimacy and monumentality; with a sense of abstraction within a rough

material presence; with a severe and schematic plan but a soft and human construction; with its domestic sounds, colours and hand-crafted details.

You have spoken about timelessness – how does this notion have a resonance in 'Blue'?
Sofia: In 'Blue' the idea is a room within a room. The new room is precisely centred on the openings and roof of the old room. There is a linear transition between the existing and new rooms, by means of a ramp or staircases, which can be translated into a temporal narrative of going from A to B and back to A.
Pezo: We believe a building is both a physical and an intellectual construction. It is what our senses feel about a built space but also what we think about those feelings. We understand time in our buildings not from their character and structure but from their capacity to articulate an experience through an idea. The experience of a courtyard, for instance, is an amalgam of inhabiting that space together with the centrality and enclosure the courtyard produces in the mind of its inhabitant.

You say everything you do feeds into everything else, so can you see correlations between 'Blue' and your other projects?
Sofia: We disagree with architects who say they start from scratch for every project. We find it impossible; each time we finish a building we feel we have executed just one specific variation within a panorama of possibilities for the same idea. We find projects of three or four years too short to exhaust an idea – perhaps the lifespan of personal practice is too ephemeral to develop a wide range of ideas.
Pezo: This is why we don't worry too much about the formal correlation between our projects – their resemblance in terms of materials, character or structure. We find it somehow inevitable. What is more intriguing is the possibility of playing different games with the same set of rules. We tend to see projects as conceptual problems for a specific physical context, so the issue is, to put it in the words of an Argentinian poet, to do the same thing but never in the same way.

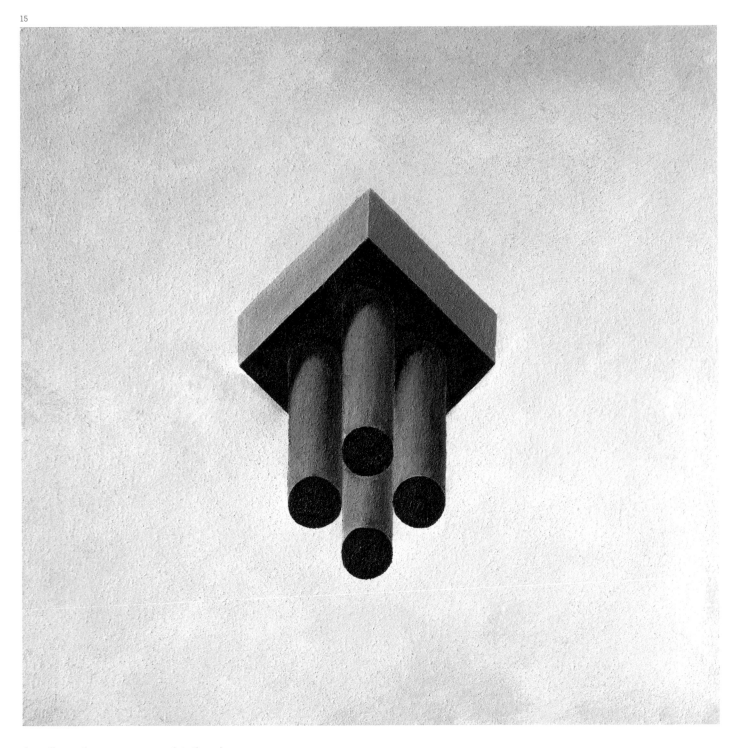

A small room is elevated on four massive columns containing spiral stairs (15). The room is surrounded by a low wall but open to the ceiling so visitors can appreciate the volume of the gallery. As well as access to the room via the stairs, there is also a ramp (16). Both routes emphasise the effort required to move vertically.

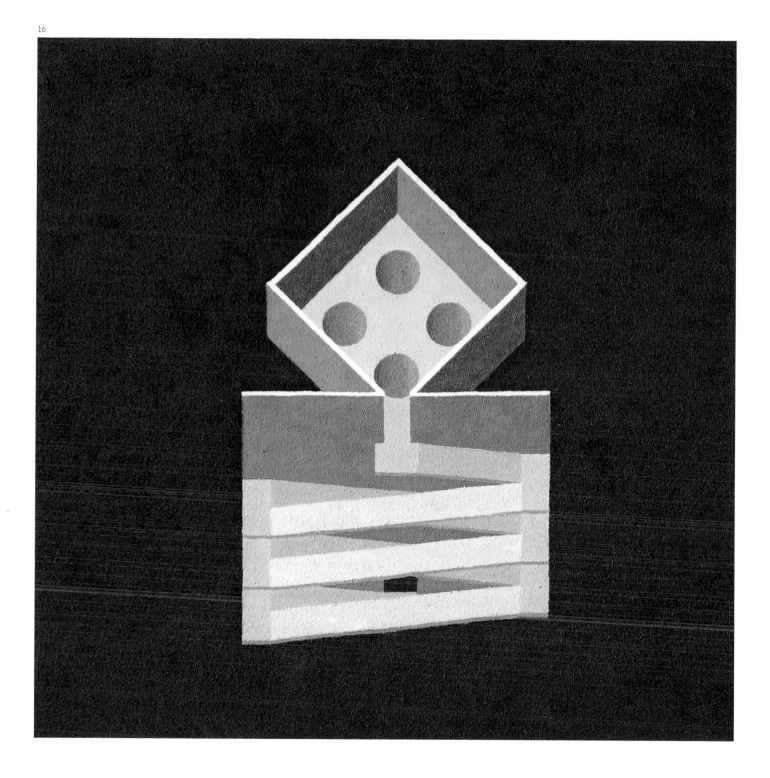

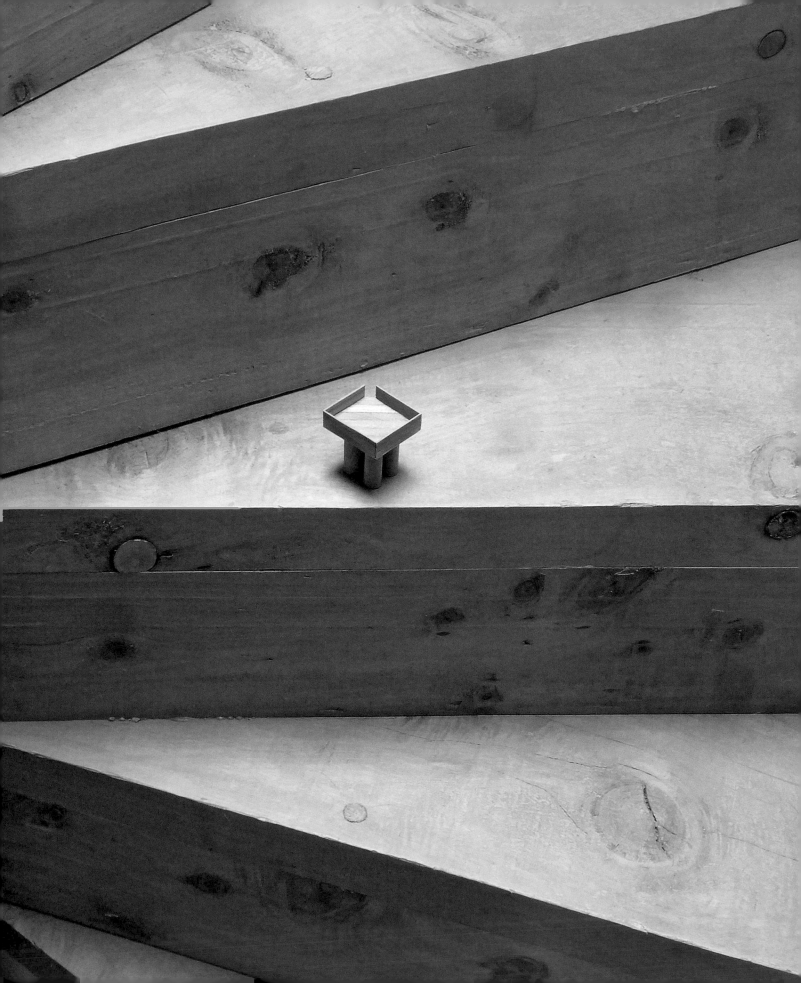

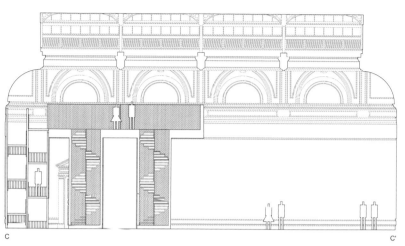

C ⎯⎯⎯ C'

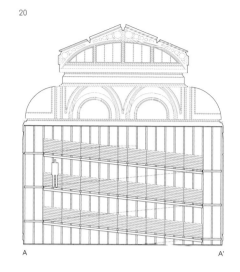

A ⎯⎯⎯ A'

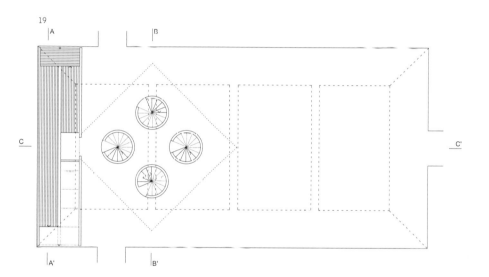

C ⎯⎯⎯ C'

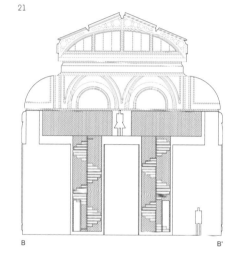

B ⎯⎯⎯ B'

The installation is made entirely of timber (17). It occupies exactly half the gallery space, with the corners of the square room aligned with the ribs of the vaulting. It provides visitors with three distinct experiences of space (18): a collective and open experience between the columns under the platform (19), the individual and controlled experience of climbing or descending the stairs or ramp (20, 21), and the collective experience on the platform close to the vaults and ceiling.

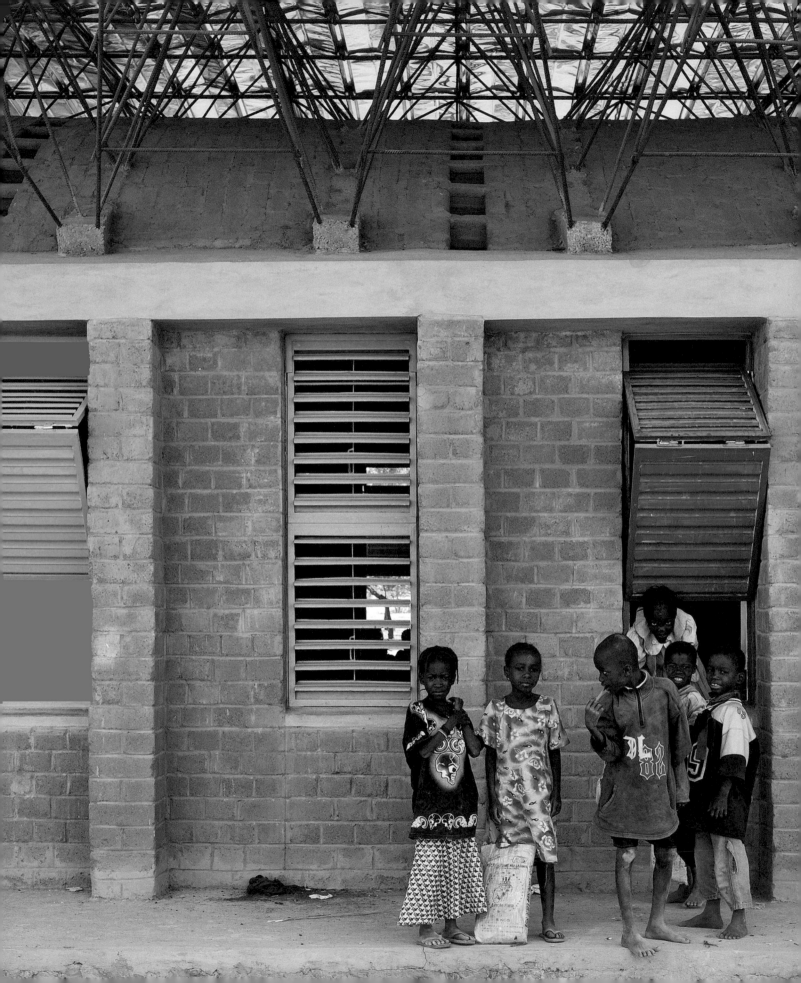

Diébédo
Francis Kéré

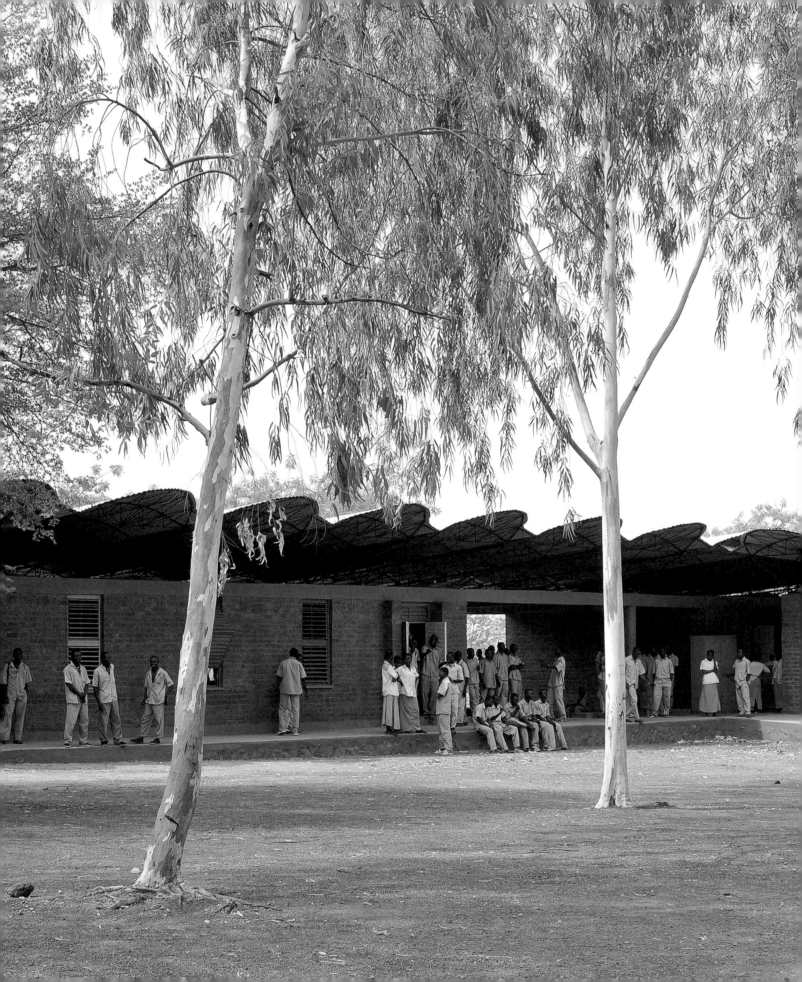

1 (previous spread) Kéré Architecture, Primary School Extension, Gando, Burkina Faso (2009), detail. This project extends Kéré's original school building in his home village with a long single-storey structure using earth-block walls under a lightweight corrugated-steel roof on a spaceframe structure. The oversailing roof gives shade and local people have customised the building by painting the shutters.

2 (opposite) Kéré Architecture, Secondary School, Dano, Burkina Faso (2007), detail. The sheltered but open 'conversation pit' that interrupts the row of classrooms provides a shaded, comfortable space for informal gatherings.

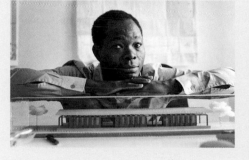

Diébédo Francis Kéré (born 1965 in Gando, Burkina Faso) bridges the worlds of Africa and Europe, promoting a sustainable architecture that uses local materials, labour and building methods enhanced and modified by modern technology. His role as an architect often extends to that of community mentor, fundraiser and builder, and his work places the community at the heart of design, construction and use.

Kéré studied in Germany and established a Berlin-based practice, Kéré Architecture, in 2005. In 1998 he set up the Schulbausteine für Gando, a charity that raises money to improve life for the people of his home village. He has built a number of schools and community spaces in Burkina Faso and across Western Africa: the Gando Primary School (2001) received an Aga Khan Award for Architecture in 2004 and in 2012 the secondary school in the same village received the Global Holcim Award Gold for sustainable construction. Currently on site in Burkina Faso is the Laongo Opera Village, a large and unlikely project initiated by the late German artist and film director Christoph Schlingensief.

Kéré has been an honorary professor at the Technical University of Berlin, guest professor at Milwaukee University, a design critic at Harvard University and a visiting professor at the Accademia di Architettura, Mendrisio. He was made an international fellow of the Royal Institute of British Architects in 2010 and an honorary fellow of the American Institute of Architects in 2012.

3

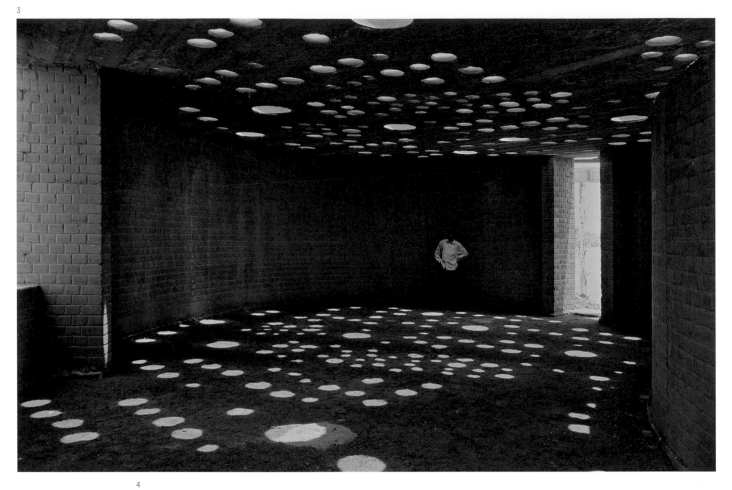

4

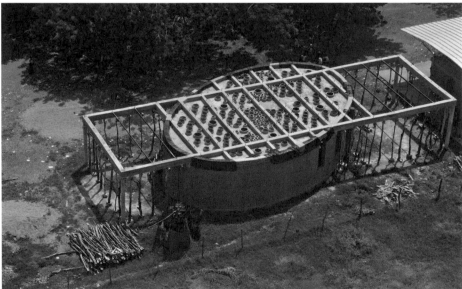

5

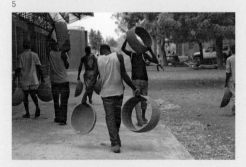

3–5, 6 (overleaf) Kéré Architecture, School Library, Gando (2013). Traditional clay pots cut into sections are set in the ceiling to admit light and promote air circulation. The orthogonal concrete frame was supported by columns of eucalyptus (a material usually used only for firewood) during construction. A corrugated-metal and clear plastic roof sits over the top.

Kate Goodwin: Our spatial imaginations have been developing since we first started exploring the world. Can you recall an early memory of when you became aware of the spaces around you?
Diébédo Francis Kéré: Every night when I was a child my family gathered together. We would sit close to each other in a sort of circle and listen to the adults telling stories; there was no light so we couldn't see each other. It was an intense feeling of being in a safe, protective space that had been created through our presence, along with the lone voice of the storyteller in the darkness. All of us in the circle hung on every word.

I got a similar feeling in the courtyard where we would all eat together, sitting on the ground rather than at tables. So for me, a living space is about intimacy and feeling secure, about having everything you need around you. I think that one of the keys to creating this sense of security is proportion: the right measures of openness and of light and shadow foster feelings of comfort and familiarity.

I remember too that as children we would build shelters using branches and leaves. We wanted to feel enclosed and secure, to define our own territory in the middle of the vast landscape.

What role do you think the senses play in how we perceive and experience space?

And what might this add to how we engage with architecture?
I always like to feel the wind in my buildings; I usually have openings high up so air blows through. This makes me feel absolutely at home. I also like to have natural light, with openings in the roof.

In the school library we created for my home village of Gando in Burkina Faso, for instance, we set sections of clay pots made by the women of the village into the concrete ceiling to create holes for light and ventilation. A corrugated-iron roof sits above this ceiling, extending beyond it to create a shaded area for study or relaxation. As the metal heats up, it draws air from inside the library up and out through the holes in the ceiling to provide a comfortable level of air circulation.

Touch is also very powerful: it offers a sense of substance, the confidence that an object or building will still be there when you wake up next morning. I'm always aware of it in my work – for instance, the contrasting sensations of placing your hand on a wall in the sun and then touching the same wall as you enter the building, where it is pleasantly cool. Touching wood and clay is very different, as is the experience of walking barefoot on a clay floor or over a natural stone floor where you are aware of the form and structure of the stone,

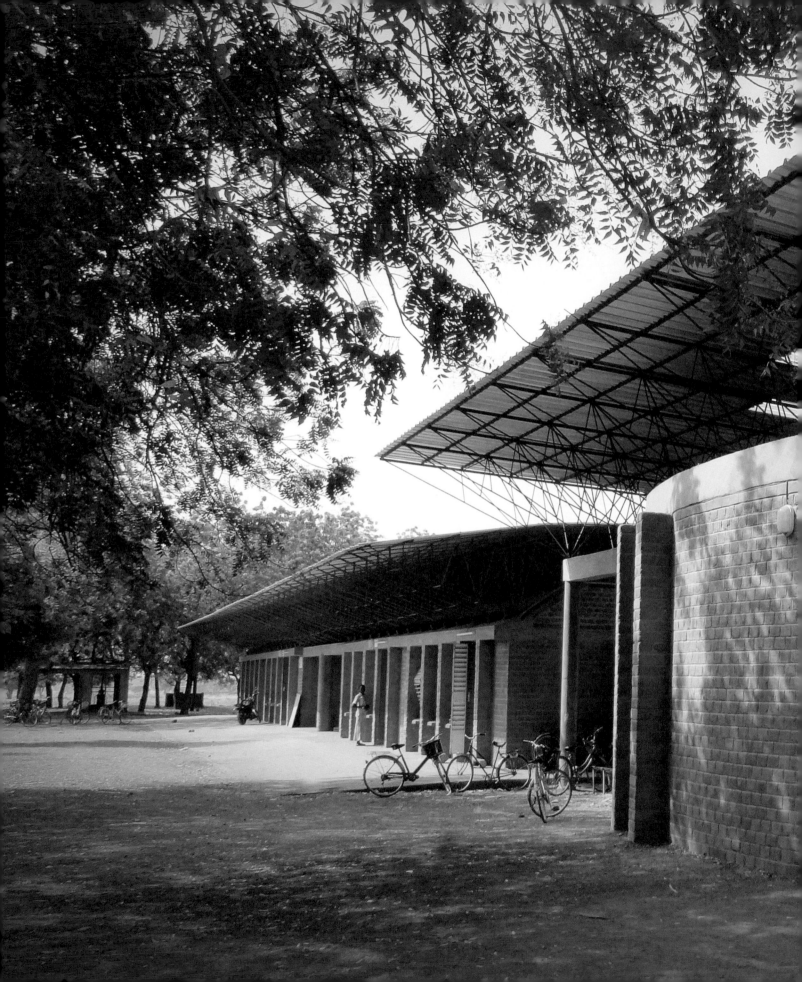

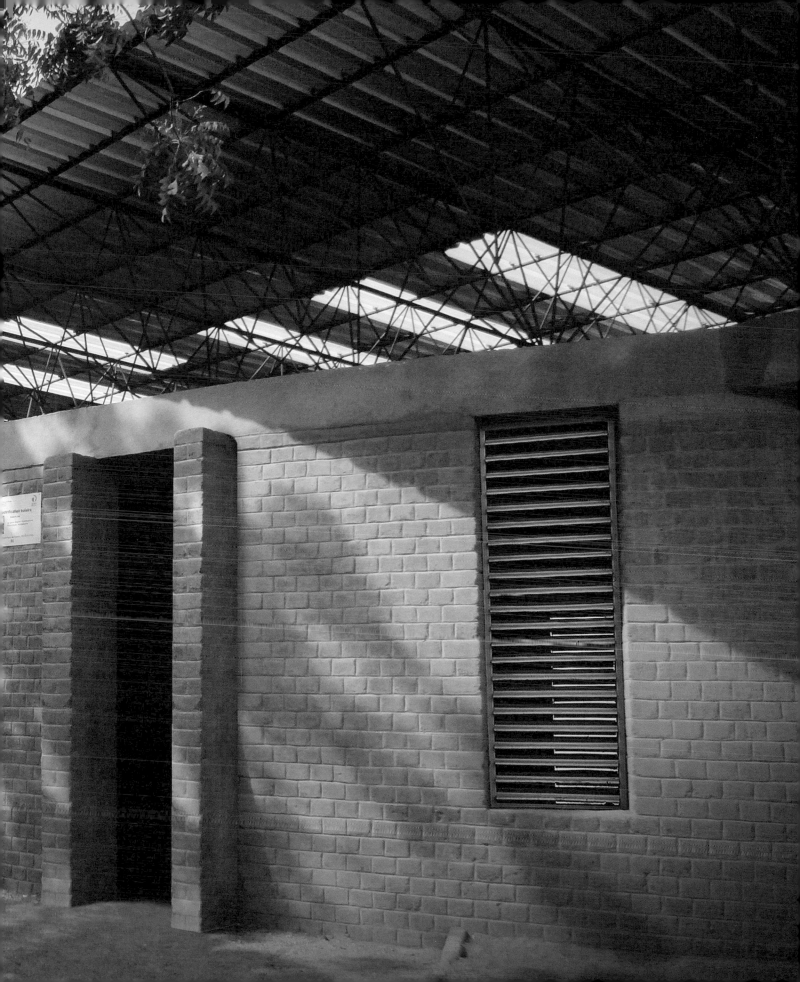

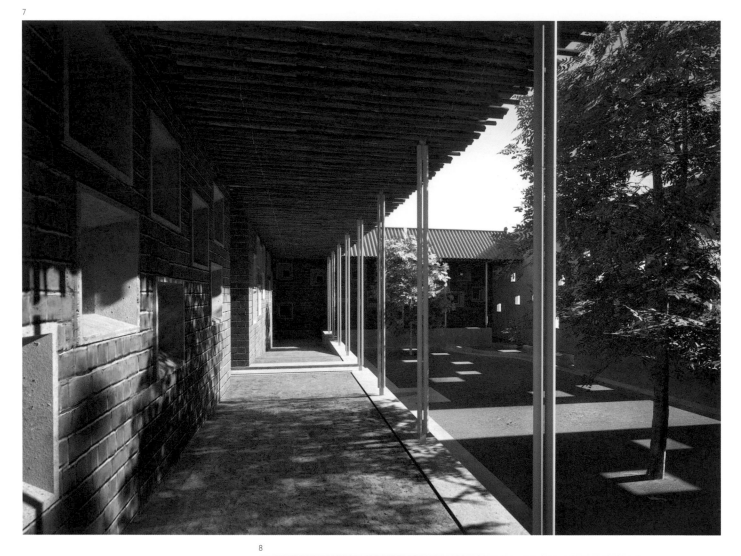

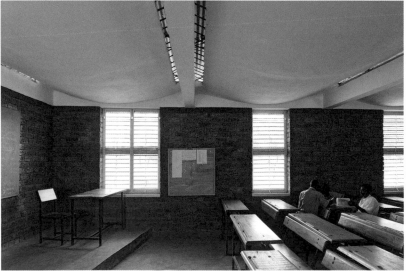

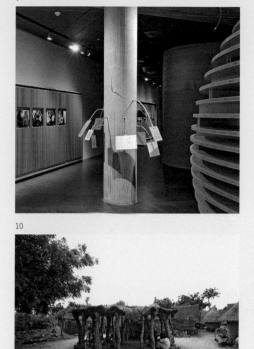

9

10

or sitting on a warm wooden seat rather than a cold steel one. Touch can also evoke emotions, which is something I drew on in the International Red Cross and Red Crescent Museum in Geneva. For instance, the use of cold metal rather than wood to create the 'Tree of Messages' highlights the disjuncture between war and nature.

The part of the museum I designed was devoted to 'Restoring Family Links' and I also used smell to evoke the power of memory and to emphasise the fundamental connections between the family and nature. The walls are made of broken bricks mixed with hemp, which has a very special aroma as well as a natural appearance, so when you look at it you feel grounded. I wanted to make people aware of the wide-reaching human cost of genocides such as Kosovo, but the effect is to encourage them to make connections rather than to deliver messages.

What do you think is distinctive about how you as an architect understand and perceive space?
As an architect I have the ability to consider how a place might be transformed within daily life, to identify elements that could be sources of inspiration for a construction, or to imagine different uses for spaces or materials. But for me, architecture is primarily about people, about asking questions such as 'who is the user?', 'what is going to happen here?' and 'how can I respond to the users' needs?'. If it's a school, I might ask how I can encourage the students to feel comfortable in the space, and then how I can encourage them to learn. And then I try to come up with my own interpretation of what could be done.

Can you recall a space or a specific work of architecture that has made you feel particularly aware of yourself and your surroundings, particularly 'present'?
The seating place for the elders, again in my home village of Gando, is an open area sheltered by a roof supported by columns. It's a light, transparent space

that is completely open to public view. It is made from simple, readily available materials – local wood and straw, connected by cords made of plant fibres – and it is also climatically efficient. It is a temporary structure that is rebuilt every couple of years and has to be completely remade when the head of the elders dies.

As architecture, it is very simple, but as soon as the elders enter it, it changes radically. Then it becomes the most powerful space in the village and the focal point for the entire community.

How have such spaces or structures informed your work?
This simple structure has been a huge influence and I'm always trying to integrate open but shaded public areas into my projects. One of my primary aims is to create comfortable spaces for informal gatherings, like the outdoor 'conversation pit' we made for students at the Dano Secondary School.

For me, architecture is also about process. When we were kids building our shelters we worked without a plan: we'd just look for leaves, or pull down branches and bend them and see what happened. The form of the final object was developed as we went along. And we were not working alone: everyone took part.

Similarly in African tradition, building a house involves the whole community. The women bring water, the men mix it with clay, and the elders who are no longer able to build sit around and give advice. Architecture is defined through the construction process, and I try to take advantage of this collective way of working in my own projects. During construction the building can change shape depending on the availability of labour or materials and the details are worked out as the task progresses. For instance, when we created the Women's Association Centre in Gando, the different sizes or shapes of the pots the women brought determined the form.

There is also a question of sustainability. In Africa, typically, buildings are small, so everyone can help with repairs after the rainy season.

7 Kéré Architecture, Infirmary, Centre de Santé et de Promotion Sociale (CSPS), Laongo Opera Village, Burkina Faso (2013).
A tripartite building arranged around a central waiting room; each of the structures has an inner courtyard with a shaded seating area.

8 Kéré Architecture, Secondary School, Dano, classroom.
Passive techniques are used to keep the classrooms comfortable. Cool air is drawn in through shutters and hot air is drawn up into the roof space through the vaulted ceiling.

9 Kéré Architecture, 'Restoring Family Links', permanent exhibition at the International Red Cross and Red Crescent Museum, Geneva, Switzerland (2013).
Detail showing the 'Tree of Messages'.

10 Seating place for the village elders, Gando.

11 (overleaf) Kéré Architecture, School, Laongo Opera Village (2011).
The first phase of the Opera Village to be completed, the school has a double roof with the corrugated-steel outer skin supported by a steel frame above the massive ceiling, with air circulating freely between them. Outside, a tree provides shade in a traditional circular seating area.

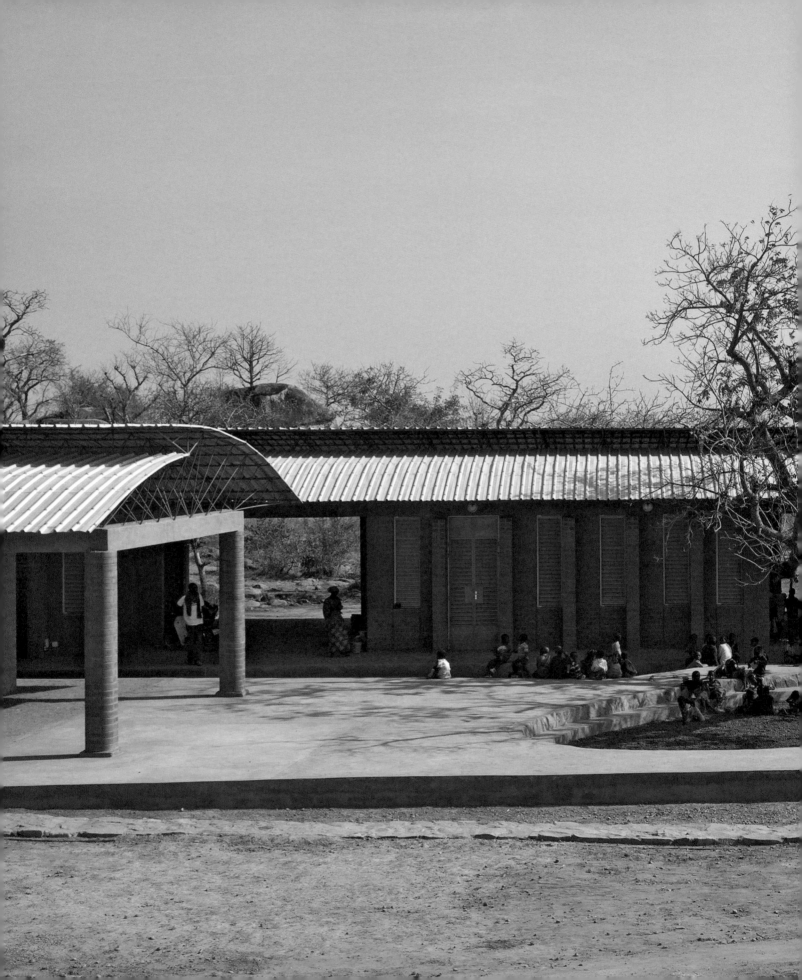

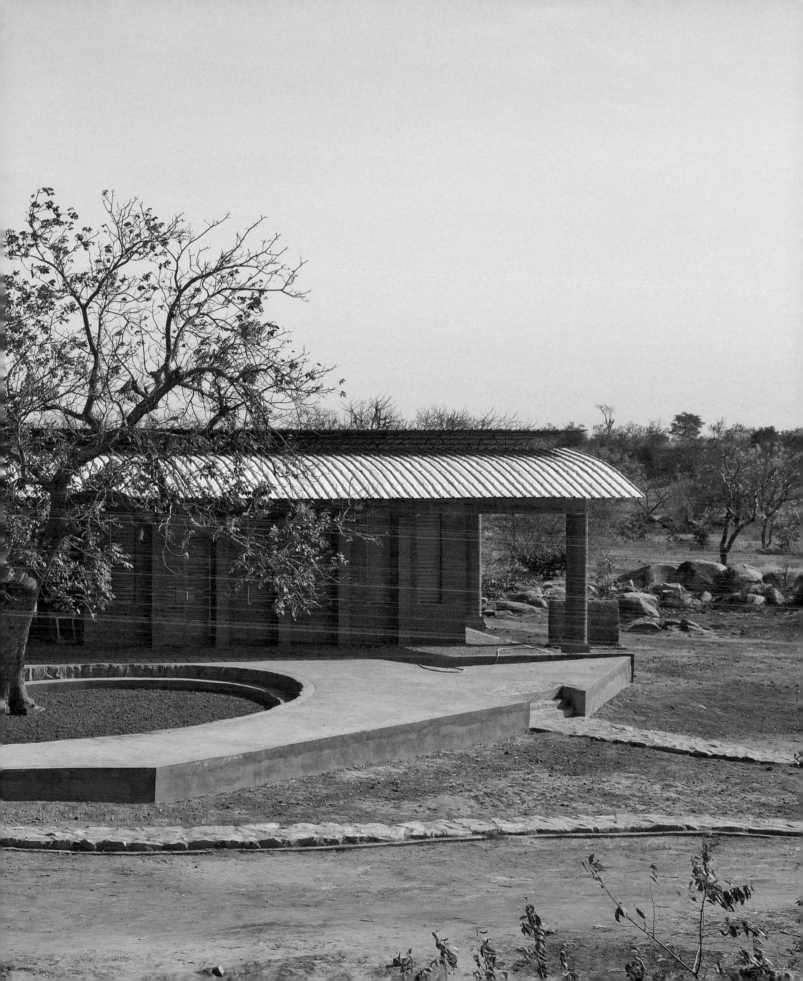

12

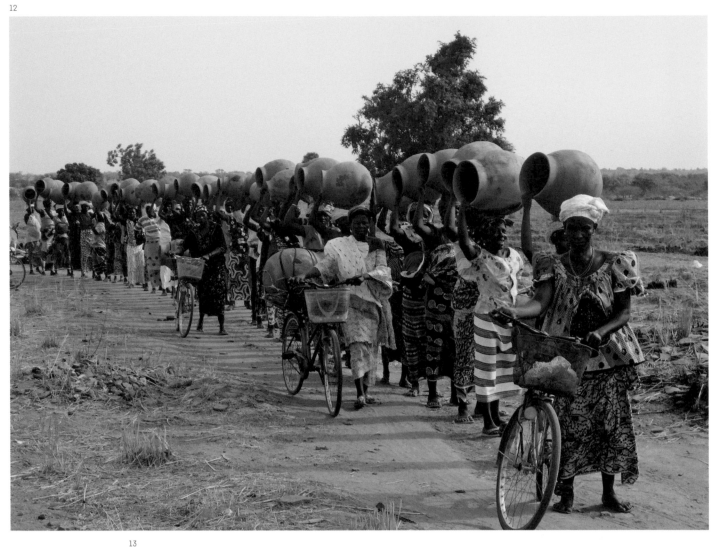

13

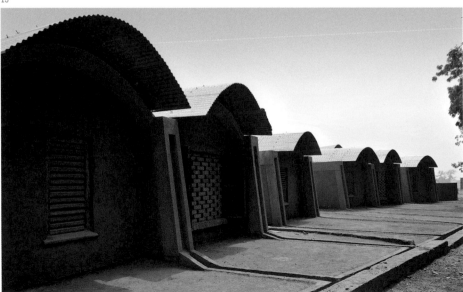

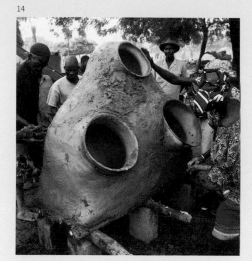

12 Kéré Architecture, School Library, Gando. Women from the community bring pots to be used in the construction.

13 Kéré Architecture, Teachers' Housing, Gando (2004). Each of the six housing units is made of three parallel walls formed of stabilised earth brick supporting compressed earth-block barrel vaults. The exterior walls have become impromptu blackboards.

14 Kéré Architecture, Women's Association Centre, Gando (under construction). Local people work on a prototype for the central storage wall.

As a child, I belonged to a group of kids who would carry materials on site for my uncle, who repaired buildings. Once you increase the scale, however, maintenance becomes more difficult, so I try to ensure that my buildings last longer by experimenting with materials and methods of construction – ways of reinforcing traditional clay, for example, or laying foundations. Each person brings their own contribution, and mine is technological know-how. I try to act as a bridge between tradition and technology.

In what ways do you see architecture enhancing human experience beyond shelter and function?
According to the World Bank, my homeland is one of the poorest countries in the world. But I still want my architecture to go beyond the function of shelter. To move forward, people need to be inspired: they need buildings that enhance their creativity and encourage them to take their future into their own hands. This means building something that is much more than a house or a classroom. I want to build inspiration.

When we worked on the school in Dano, the people had never met an architect before and architecture was a new concept to them. I showed them how they could use familiar materials in new ways and they became enthusiastic and inspired. I asked them new questions, such as 'can you cut this?', 'will it break if you cut it into thin pieces?', 'can you use basic tools to cut it?' and 'how will you work when the rainy season comes?'. I wanted to know about their experience of the materials and to encourage them to test different ways of using them.

What we created was surprising to them, and when they asked how it was possible, we said it was something called 'architecture'. So for the people of Dano, architecture was a wonderful, impressive thing they wanted to be part of. Through the concept of architecture, the whole community came together to share ideas, to learn and to help each other. When I returned to visit, people came from all around because they had heard that the architect was back!

I believe it is important to engage people in the process of building so they have an investment in what is developed; through thinking and working together people find that the built object becomes part of a bonding experience. We are making people responsible, as well as aware of their own potential and capacity to create something. Collective experience is always part of anything you do in Africa.

This collaborative process is central to your work, but to what extent do you want it to continue once the building is finished? Is it important to you that people can change the structures they live in?
Yes, definitely. When you change a building, you become part of its creation. Often I find that people have changed my buildings in unexpected ways, for instance by using a curtain rather than a door or by choosing unexpected colours for different elements. In the Gando Primary School extension they painted the wooden external shutters in bright colours; in the teachers' housing the walls have become blackboards where pupils draw maps or diagrams of the human body. At first I was surprised, but now I am pleased that they have made the buildings their own.

Moving on to your installation at the Royal Academy, can you describe your initial impressions of the site?
As soon as you enter the Annenberg Courtyard you are aware that this is very strong architecture that still has a presence. You feel you want to explore, to go inside. Then the entrance space is full of visitors so it is not until you climb the stairs to the galleries that you become aware once more of the building's substance, the thickness of the walls, the height of the spaces. It is very powerful.

Initially I had the sense that the doors were small but when we came to measure them we found they are almost 2 metres wide; they look small because of the monumentality of the rooms. However, such a seemingly narrow entrance to a vast space has the effect of drawing you in and as you move closer, the door seems

The installation was generated by the idea that the doorways to the RA galleries appear very small in relation to the scale of the rooms and that this has the effect of drawing visitors in. The concept of a tunnel connecting two galleries provides a similar sense of movement through a narrow opening; its form and dimensions were arrived at through computer modelling (15). The pavilion is made of a honeycomb plastic that forms the hidden core of many building materials (16).

15

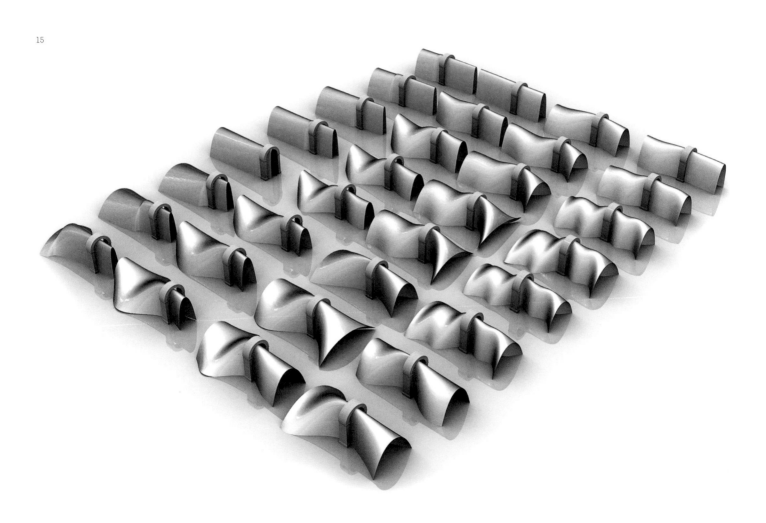

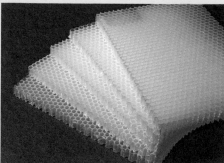

16

to become larger and to absorb you. So I wondered if we could make an installation that people would see as an object before they experience it from the inside, in the same way as you have a strong impression of both the building itself and of the individual rooms before you cross the threshold.

I also wanted people to experience the installation collectively, to have a sense of flowing from a vast space through a narrow opening. And the best way to recreate this sensation of coming together was a tunnel.

Can you describe the thinking behind the project in more detail?
To allow people to experience the space from both outside and within, it is made very clear that this is a room within a room. And you share this room with other people, so even if the visitors don't speak to each other, they are sharing something by being in the same space as well as by being forced closer together as they pass through the opening.

In Africa making a building is an interactive process and I wanted to reproduce something of that interaction here. So visitors are invited to add straws of different colours and lengths to the installation. I envisage parents sitting inside and their children trying to poke straws through the holes at them – you can imagine the shock as the straw touches you or someone else on the neck!

Your architecture usually makes use of local materials, so how are you approaching the choice of materials for an installation in London?
It's not just about sourcing something local but about using a material that is readily available. In Gando the most convenient material is clay, but London is part of an industrial culture and I wanted to reflect that. Plastic is central to Londoners' daily life; it is also economical, transparent and light. So I sourced a plastic honeycomb material that is integral to the city's architecture but is usually hidden – it is used as insulation or as a filler in hotel doors, for instance. I wanted to reveal it within another context, a hive of creativity, a centre for art. So where better than the Royal Academy of Arts? Perhaps it will encourage people to think about other materials and how we use them, or inspire artists to imagine ways to use them differently.

What opportunities have you found in creating an installation for an exhibition that would not usually be possible in your architectural projects and how have you harnessed these?
Exhibitions provide an excellent opportunity to test new materials in an environment free from building regulations, commercial requirements, climatic restrictions and the constraints of the construction industry. It's a chance to be truly creative.

In most exhibitions, the architecture acts as a neutral backdrop or context to facilitate a relationship between the visitor and the display. But when the architecture exhibits itself, as here, it becomes both context and object for the visitor. My pavilion addresses this issue: it is an object in its physical presence, its manipulation of light and its relationship to its surroundings but it also creates its own context by enclosing, by breaking up the space of the gallery, by creating changing perceptions and by its irregularity and transparency. The effect achieved is like a frame that enhances the experience of looking.

My pavilion should be like a living experience in that only through interacting with it can you live it. And likewise the building lives through interaction because only as more straws are inserted can it blossom.

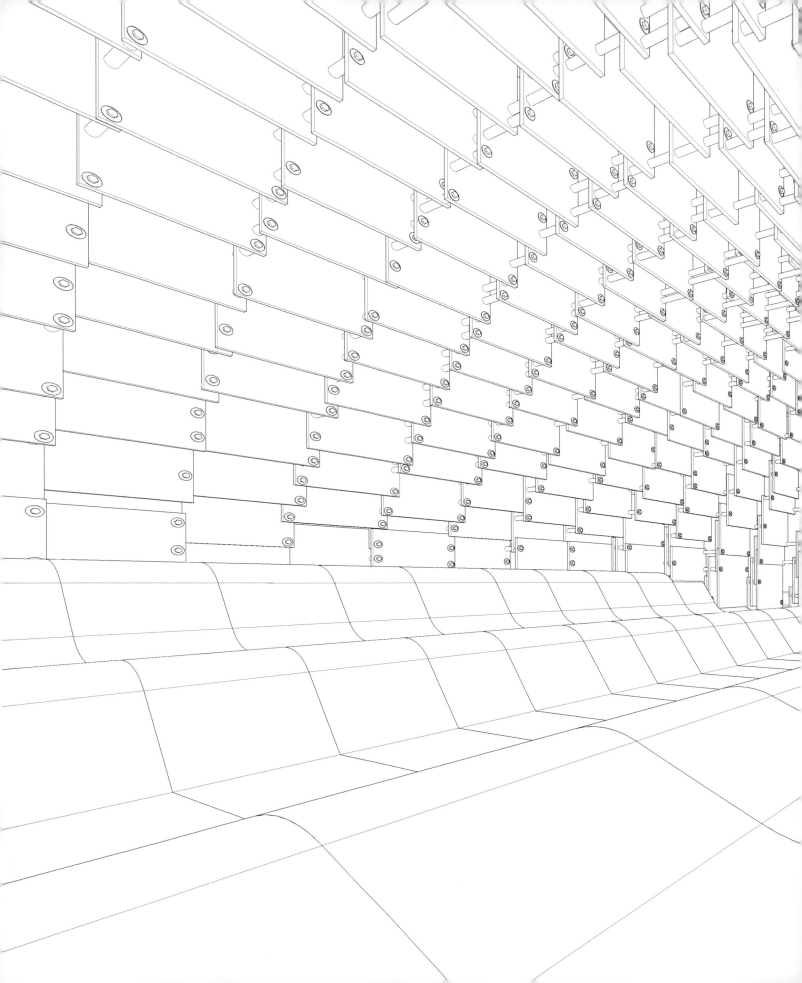

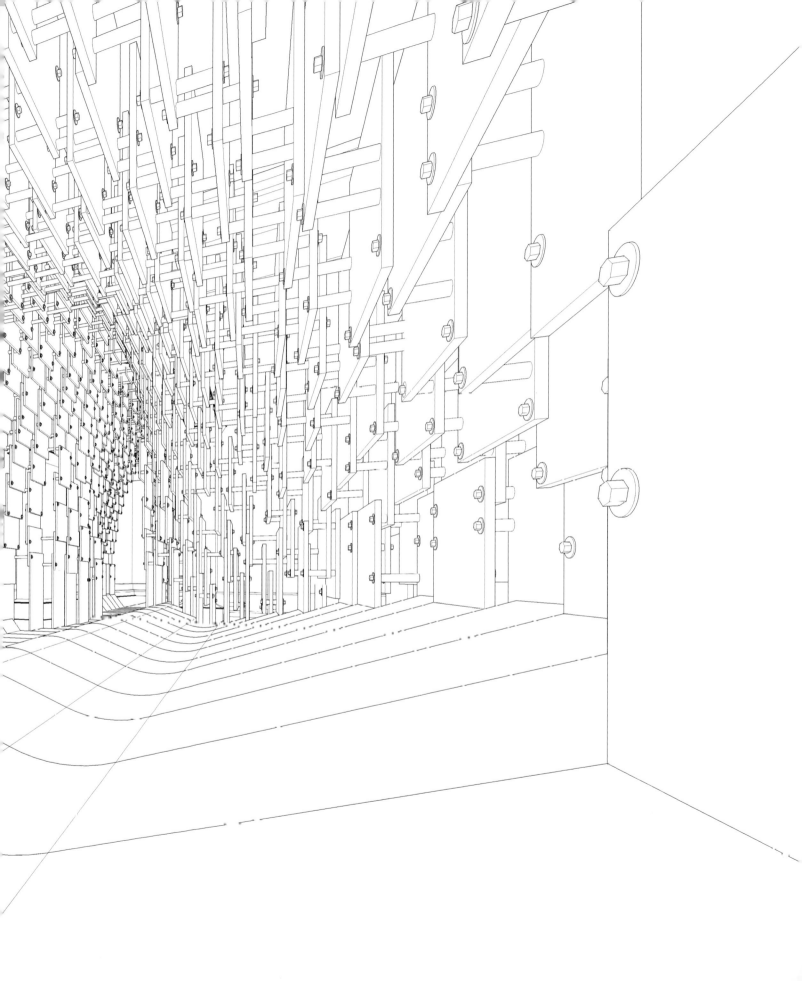

The pavilion is formed by a series of overlapping arches each consisting of rectangular panels of honeycomb plastic connected by spacers (17, previous spread). The structure gives visitors glimpses of the ceiling between the panels and has a degree of transparency when looked at straight on. Visitors are invited to take long multicoloured straws, available at the entrance, and to poke them through the holes in the honeycomb panels (18, 19). The pavilion will become more colourful and clear in form as the number of straws increases (20, 21).

18

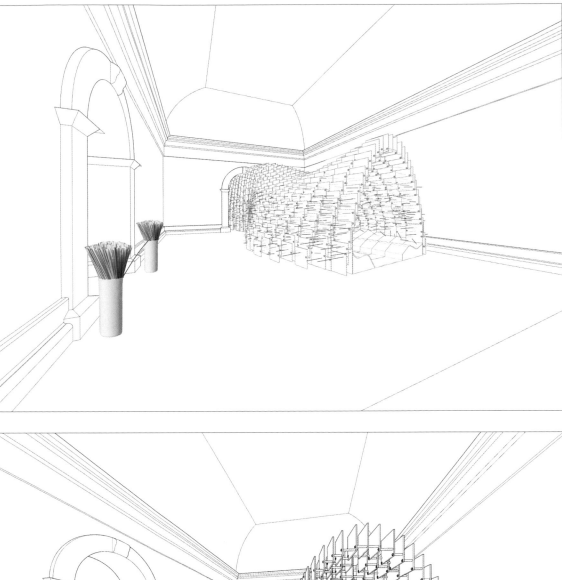

19

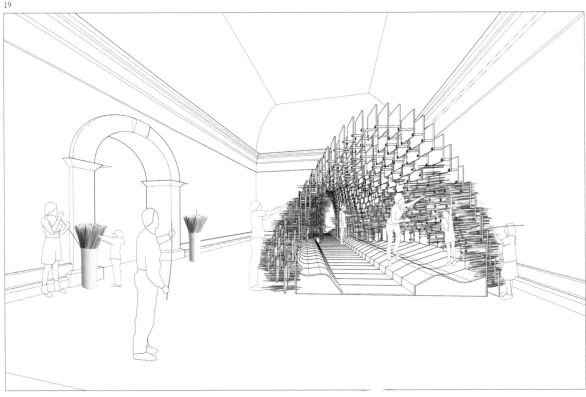

20

21

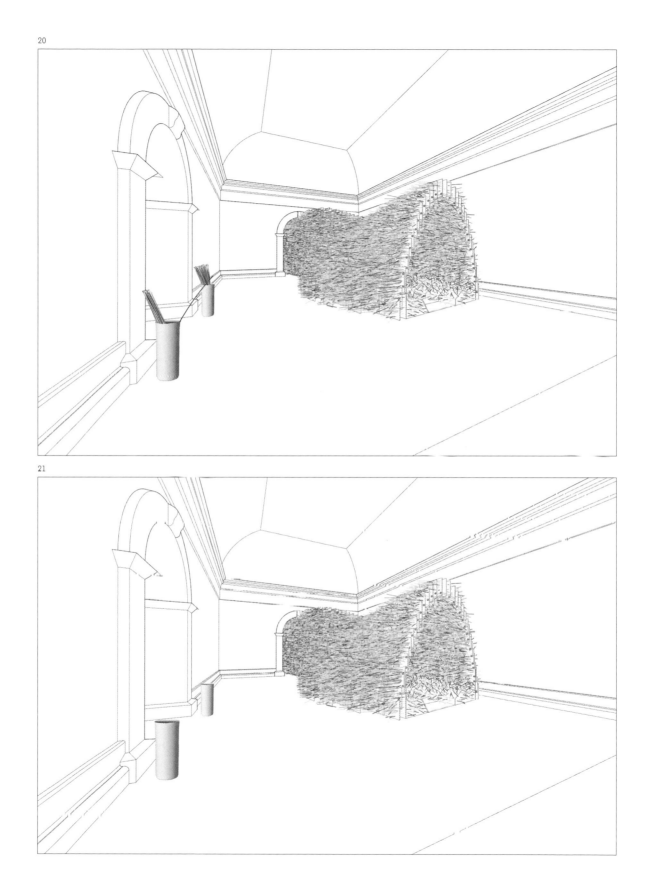

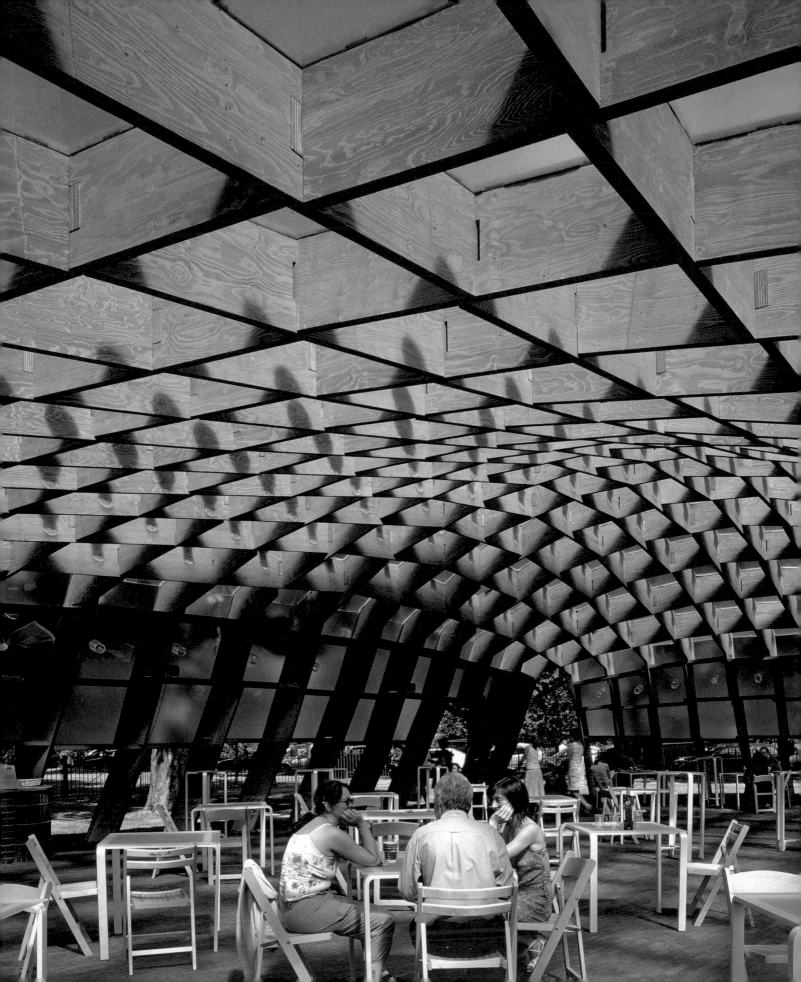

Eduardo Souto de Moura
Álvaro Siza

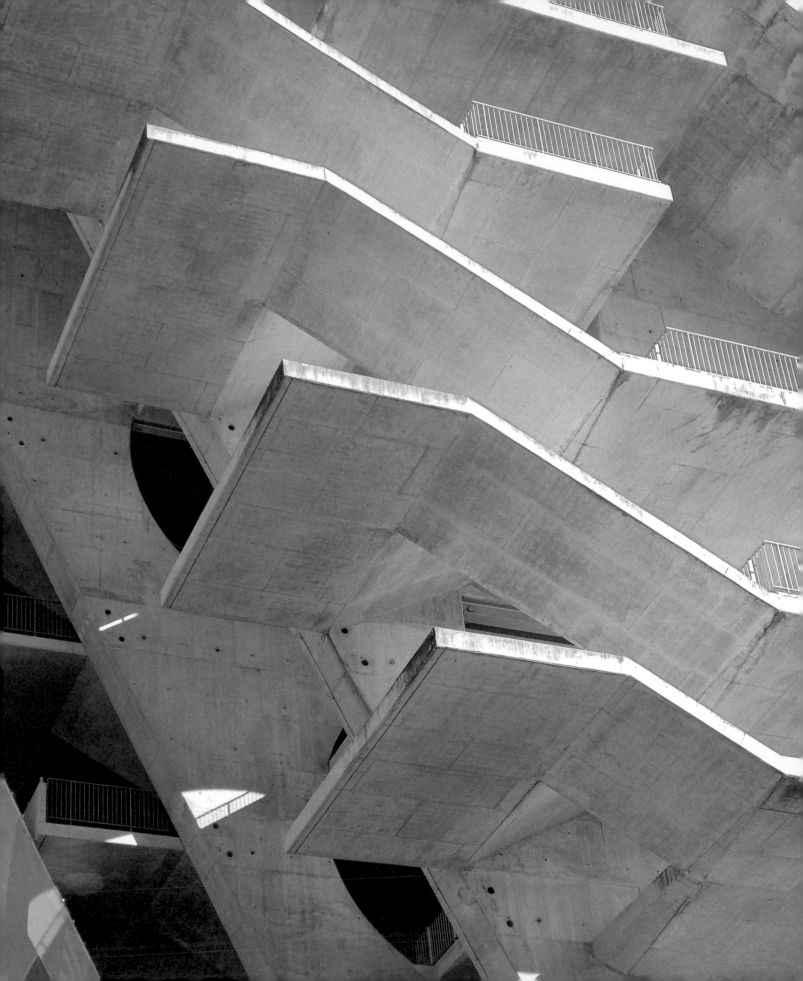

**1 (previous spread)
Álvaro Siza and
Eduardo Souto de
Moura, Serpentine
Gallery Pavilion,
London (2005).**
Working with renowned
structural engineer
Cecil Balmond, Siza
and Souto de Moura
created a temporary
summer pavilion that
employed a totally
different architectural
language to the gallery
itself and gave form
to the space between
the permanent and
temporary buildings.

**2 (opposite)
Eduardo Souto
de Moura, Braga
Municipal Stadium,
Portugal (2003).**
One stand of this
football stadium
is carved into the face
of a former quarry
and the other is sited
independently on the
hillside. The two are
joined by a structure
of steel cables like
tenuous bridges
crossing a ravine.

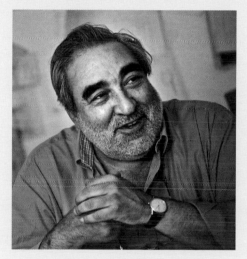

Eduardo Souto de Moura (born 1952 in Porto, Portugal) sees architecture as a continuing story that builds on the past; his contribution is a process of reframing or rethinking earlier models. Nevertheless, his buildings – including houses, office blocks, art galleries and a football stadium – have a striking visual impact, often making dramatic use of geometric shapes or sweeping curves. While these are visually powerful works, they are also human in scale and rewarding in use.

Souto de Moura studied architecture at the School of Fine Arts in Porto. While still a student, he worked with Álvaro Siza before setting up his own practice in Porto in 1980. The minimalist approaches of sculptor Donald Judd and architect Ludwig Mies van der Rohe have been major influences on his work. He aims for purity of form and space combined with free circulation, so his buildings are transformed by the people moving through them. Recent work has been marked by an expressive use of colour and textural materials including wood, marble, brick and steel. His attitude to landscape, which he identifies with Portuguese culture, is one of pragmatism; he seeks not to alter it, but to emphasise its character.

Souto de Moura has taught at the University of Porto and has been a visiting professor at many other institutions including Harvard and ETH Zurich. In 2008 he was awarded Portugal's prestigious Pessoa Prize, in 2011 he was awarded the Pritzker Prize and in 2013 he received the Wolf Prize in Arts.

Álvaro Siza and Eduardo Souto de Moura maintain a close personal and working relationship and have collaborated on a number of projects including the Portuguese pavilion at Expo 2000 in Hanover, Germany, and the Serpentine Gallery annual summer pavilion in 2005 in London.

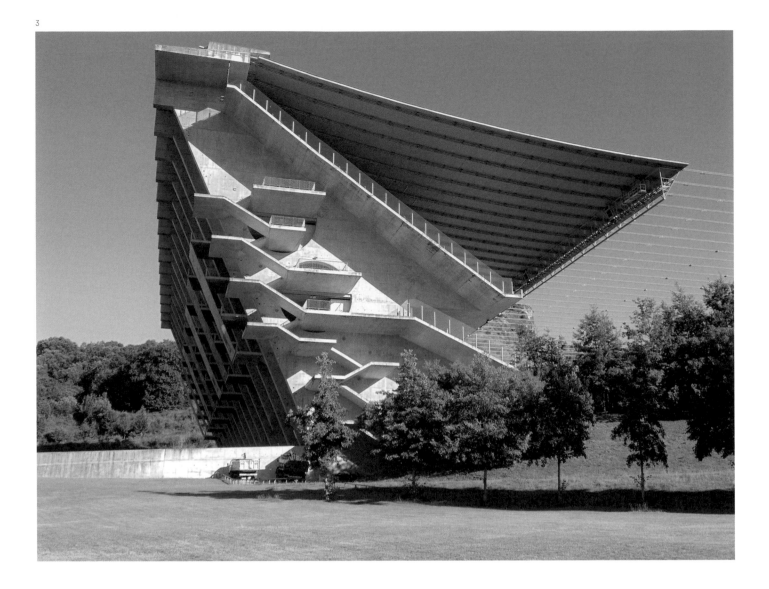

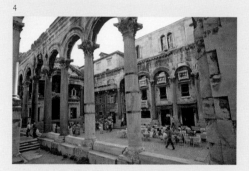

4

3 Eduardo Souto de Moura, Braga Municipal Stadium. The stadium gave Souto de Moura the opportunity to work at several scales, from shaping the surrounding landscape to designing the door handles.

4 Palace of Diocletian, Split, Croatia (early fourth century CE).

5 (overleaf) Eduardo Souto de Moura, Conversion of the Bernardas Convent, Tavira, Portugal (2006–12). Conversion of the former convent into dwellings involved inserting 255 windows into the metre-thick walls; marrying the new and the old required invention.

Kate Goodwin: Which of your buildings have you most enjoyed designing?
Eduardo Souto de Moura: The Braga Municipal Stadium. It allowed me to work on several different scales, which must be every architect's ambition: everything from the interaction of the building with the human body – handles, benches, doors – to redesigning the surrounding landscape by shaping hills or creating forests and roads. It's like the difference between writing a piano sonata and working with a symphony orchestra. This does not mean that some sonatas might not be greater works than entire symphonies, but I do believe that every musician would like to write a symphony.

Álvaro Siza has said that time is a great architect. Do you agree – and if so which building epitomises this process for you?
The Palace of Diocletian in Split is a house, despite being the palace of an emperor. Its architecture is domestic, but because of its large scale it has become part of the city and its interiors have become new outdoor spaces. When you arrive at the palace, you move through streets and squares that were originally interior spaces designed for domestic use. This confusion of interior and exterior can only happen when the quality of design is extremely high, and this is the best example of transmutation

I know of. Le Corbusier said 'Le dehors est toujours un dedans.'

Álvaro Siza and yourself both run your own successful architectural practices but you have also been closely linked and on a couple of occasions you have worked together. How do you work in tandem on projects?
Before starting a project we both think about what we want to do and what we want the project to be. We are not afraid of presenting what we believe to be right or wrong. We have nothing to prove to each other so we put forward our ideas with great openness, which is made possible by mutual intellectual respect. There is also a shared learning, where each of us is keen to bring out the best in the other.

Can you identify a building of Siza's which you find particularly powerful or which has a strong presence?
The public pools at Leça da Palmeira represent a theme I am increasingly interested in – that is, the autonomy of architecture in relation to nature. The pools are one of the best examples of this relationship, where neither the pool nor the surrounding nature outshines the other.
Another aspect of equilibrium in Siza's work is how he has been able to marry specifically Portuguese architecture with

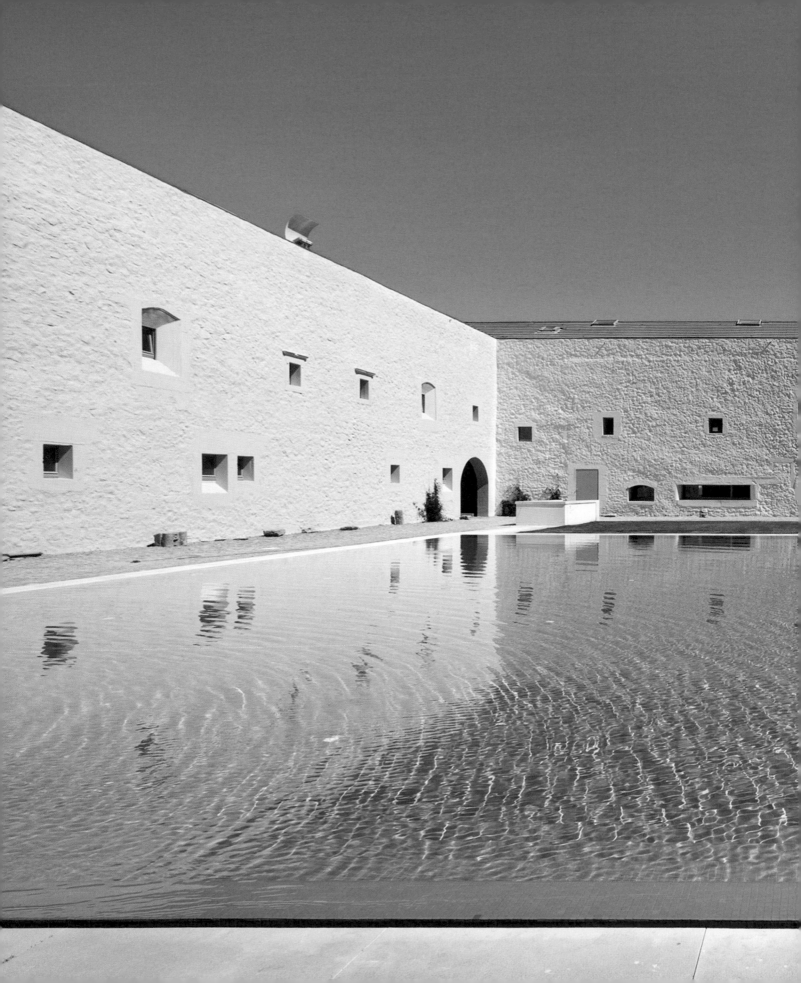

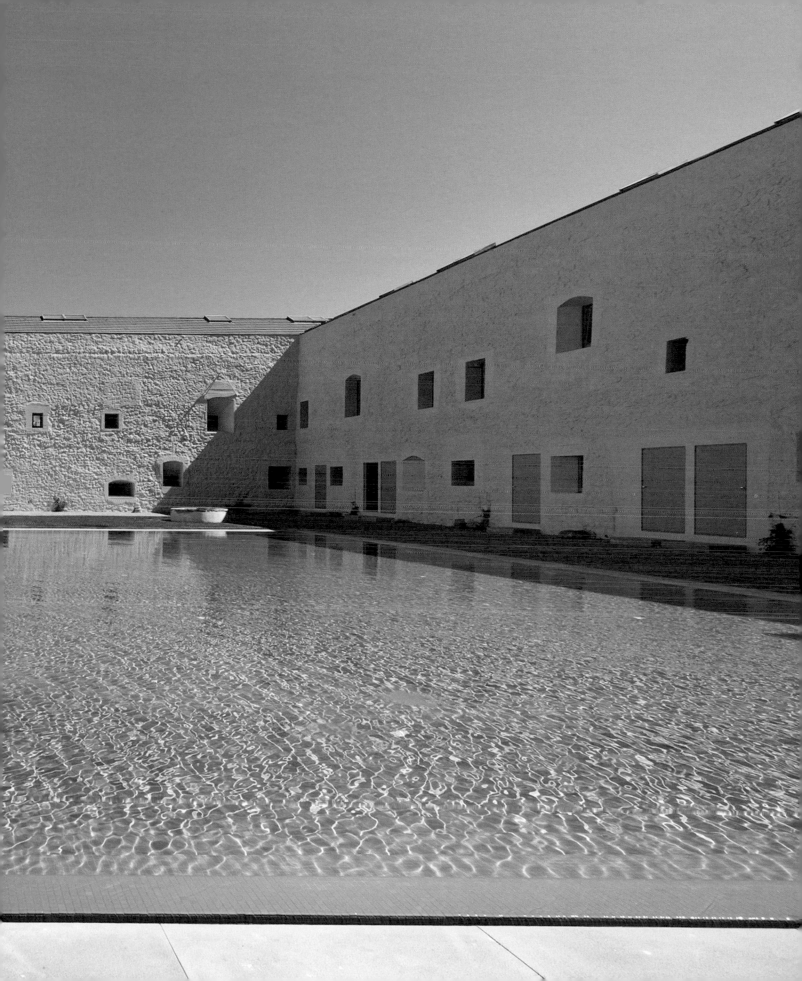

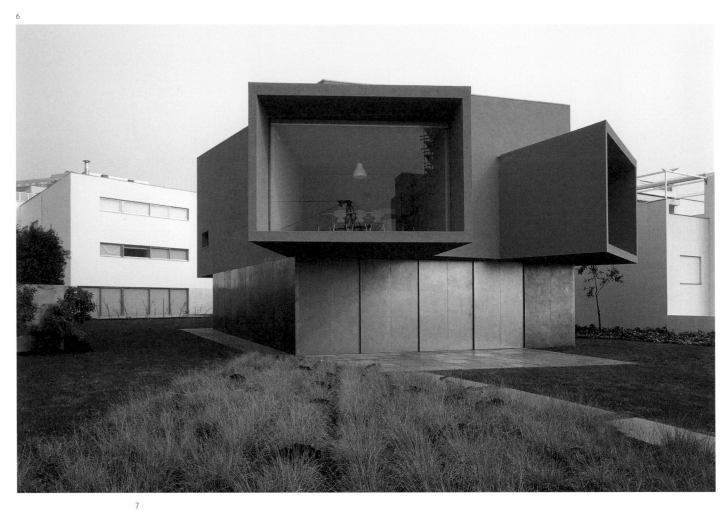

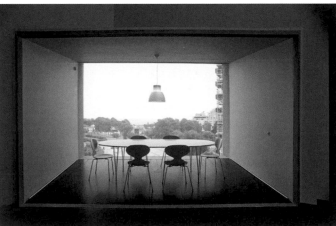

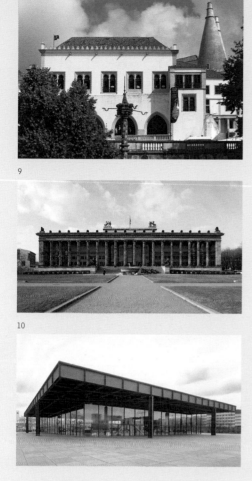

6, 7 Eduardo Souto de Moura, Cinema House Manoel de Oliveira, Porto, Portugal (1998–2003).
An archive for Portugal's veteran film-maker, the building is based on a cube, with the volume put through a series of transformations to reflect the irregular site. Two rectangular extrusions frame the views in a cinematic way.

8 Sintra National Palace, Portugal (from late fourteenth century).

9 Karl Friedrich Schinkel, Altes Museum, Berlin, Germany (1823–30).

10 Ludwig Mies van der Rohe, Neue Nationalgalerie, Berlin (1968).

the universality and abstraction the discipline requires. The church of Santa Maria in Marco de Canavezes is a Portuguese church yet with the proportions of Le Corbusier's Convent of La Tourette. There is a lot of influence from Adolf Loos's Steiner House and from Alvar Aalto, especially the lateral light and slanted wall. What is the twentieth century anyway? It is Le Corbusier, Loos, Mies van der Rohe and Aalto. Siza learns from these masters and gives continuity to the historical and universal. Plus he makes his architecture in Portugal, where it has been embraced by the local community.

What are your impressions of the architecture of the Royal Academy?
I like the fact that it's an axial building, as with all Neoclassical architecture. The Classical language of architecture appeals to me because it is clear, it is organised and it offers a sense of security and continuity. In a building like the Royal Academy, as soon as you arrive at the entrance you know where the exit will be and the doors are just where you expect to find them. It's like a story or a movie that you understand from beginning to end.

Second, I like the fact that the scale is something between a palace and a house. It's big, but it still has a domestic feel. Only English Neo-Palladian architects seem to have achieved this scale. Perhaps because Portugal is small, the cities have a particular scale with no boulevards or axes or large squares. D. João I was one of the most important European monarchs of the 1300s to 1400s but his Sintra National Palace is just a simple pavilion. By contrast, Trafalgar Square was built as a showpiece for the capital of an empire and is monumental in scale.

Can you describe your proposal for 'Sensing Spaces'?
I design by instinct, so I find it difficult to explain my ideas. I think I chose the doors as a site for my intervention because I understand their hierarchy and purpose, which makes me feel secure. But if people ask why I have made two doors, then I can only say that I don't know.

Part of the answer, though, is that for me architecture requires continuity: we have to continue what others have done before us but using different methods of construction and materials. This means that the language too has to change – the same door made in concrete is a different door. The column has been a constant through Egyptian, Greek, Roman, Renaissance, Neoclassical and Modern architecture, even if the vocabulary has changed. For instance, Karl Friedrich Schinkel's Altes Museum in Berlin has twenty stone columns supporting the portico, but the steel portico of Mies van der Rohe's Berlin Neue Nationalgalerie requires only two. The column and its capital have been used in India, China and Latin America, as well as to serve Communist ideology. They form a strong element that can be adapted for different functions: palace, church or state.

You have been looking at two doors with different proportions, one rectangular and one arched.
I think they represent different periods – the arched one is more Classical and the other Neo-Palladian. The Classical door is used along the main axis and it helps to define the hierarchy and orientation of the building. It's an intelligent door, with its shape and construction governed by logic rather than taste or style. It's a door with a function and purpose, designed from science, from history, rather than something Expressionist or Gaudí-esque.

Making architecture is about resolving problems; it is not about communicating your ideas but about your obligation to the requirements of the brief. If you want to express yourself, you should paint a picture or make a piece of sculpture or write a book. I discuss this all the time with Siza: he says that for him architecture is art, but for me it's not art because it has to have a function. I cannot have a car without a road to drive on and in the same way I need architecture in which I can sleep, or eat, or make love. Perhaps you can also engage the emotions, but that is not the purpose of architecture.

The Concorde aeroplane is the most marvellous object of the twentieth

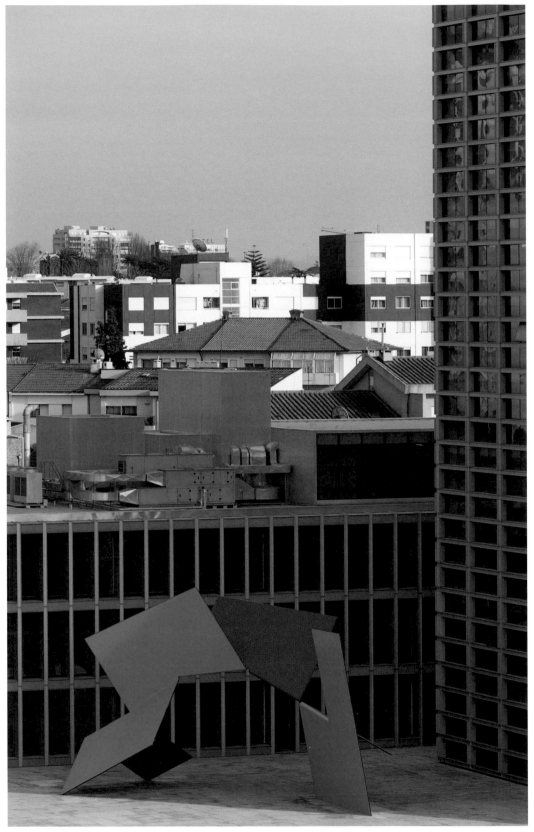

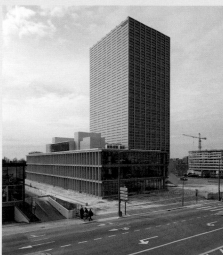

11, 12 Eduardo Souto de Moura, Burgo Tower, Porto (2007). The rhythmic and repetitive treatment of the façades of the two blocks is an exercise in positive and negative, wall and glass. A square partially defined by the buildings is occupied by a massive sculpture by Ângelo de Sousa.

century, and aircraft industrialist Marcel Dassault said, 'For a plane to fly well, it must be beautiful.' In order for architecture to be beautiful, it has to function too.

Within your proposal, do you think that your doors still have a function?
First, they are not architecture, they are sculpture. Second, I think they are elegant. Third, when you cross these thresholds perhaps you experience a sensation, an emotion. Fourth, they are logical.

People will ask why I have made them in concrete, an ordinary material, rather than marble. But concrete is the most efficient form of masonry – it was invented by the Romans, who used it in domes and other structures. Today we can reinforce it with steel or make the same forms using a composite like fibreglass. Perhaps in the future it will all be carbon.

The next question people will ask is why I have repeated what was there, apart from changing the thickness. The answer is perhaps that today we can make everything lighter because of new materials. It's interesting that the first section of Italo Calvino's *Six Memos for the Next Millennium* talks about 'lightness' as a new condition – in planes, buildings, and so on.

Your proposal shifts the positions of the doors from the Classical axis and symmetry to open up a different directionality.
This is because in life there is more than one way to understand things. The axial system seems rigid, but in fact you can open it up to different directions, including the diagonal. I want people to see the work of the other architects and of course I don't know how the way I place something might affect or be affected by their interventions. Cities are created like this, with different interactions and relationships. The city is a collage of time and materials.

Are you interested in the idea of the threshold?
What is interesting in the world are the grey areas. So what I have designed

is a threshold. It's not possible for an architect to design a space – such a concept does not exist. Instead, we design the thresholds and the limits: the walls, windows, doors and so on. And people have feelings about these elements and put them together and create the sensation of a space. I'm interested in designing the elements that give the impression of a space – which is why I like doors.

The dialogue between the container and the contained, the boundaries and the space within them, is an obsession in contemporary culture, where the node is more important than the object. That's why architecture must work at the limits, not invent the shape and language but straddle two worlds, on the knife edge.

A door is usually part of a wall, but you have extracted this element from the wall.
I spent 30 years of my life designing architecture without windows. Instead, I reconstituted the problem as one of positive and negative, glass and wall, as with the Burgo Tower. But I knew I didn't want to die a virgin window-maker – and fortunately in the Bernardas Convent I was obliged to put in 235 windows. When I tried to design them, however, I encountered all kinds of problems.

I could make a copy of a fine old window, but when I came to design my own they seemed ridiculous. I didn't know why at first, but I discovered the reason was because the convent walls are a metre thick and if you design the windows as if they are only 30 centimetres deep then the effect is ludicrous, like a facelift. The Classical language of architecture won't work for the future because we have a new kind of wall. And if architecture is a wall with holes, and the new walls are incompatible with the old openings, then we need to invent new ones.

I believe that avant-garde architecture is a contradiction in terms. Why did all the avant-garde artists, even Mies van der Rohe, live in old houses? I have discussed this a lot with Siza and our conclusion is that they found the avant-garde too disturbing.

13

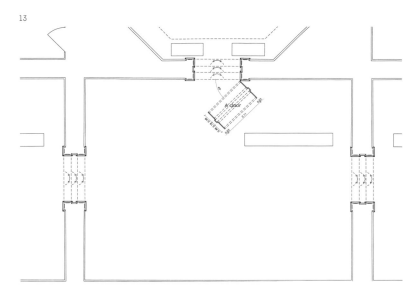

15

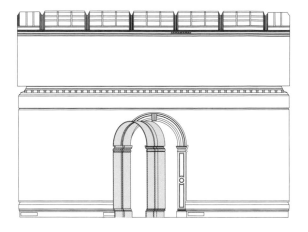

14

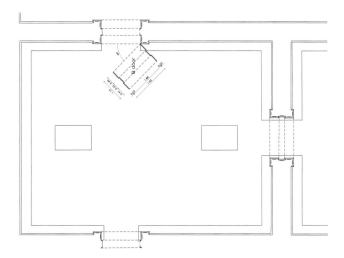

16

The installation takes as its subject one of the fundamental elements of architecture – the door. By inserting a new doorway into two of the RA galleries, leaving the rest of the space untouched, it introduces new diagonal orientations (13, 14, 18) into the building's axial plan (17). The new structures have the same form and depth as the existing doorframes but are made of very thin concrete. They are positioned at 45 degrees from the wall plane (15, 16).

17

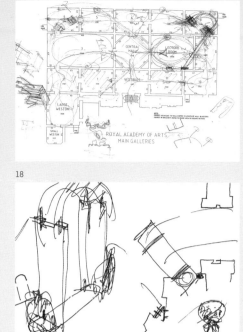

18

Take Picasso – he was so obsessed with painting contemporary woman that he couldn't allow himself to be distracted by a contemporary environment. So he chose to live in houses built in the nineteenth century and then later, as he earned more money, in houses from the sixteenth or seventeenth centuries.

But you and Siza live in a house you designed yourself?
I live in a house designed by me but not for me. It was designed for a client who pulled out and then suggested I should live there myself. And every morning, as I open my window, I ask, 'Why did I do this?'

When I first designed the house it was very minimal, a concrete tube with a living room and bedroom. Then I had to put in a bathroom and it had to have light so I tried inserting a window into the drawing but it looked horrible. I told the builder to start building and to let me know when he got to the level of the windows so I could decide what to do; a few months later I got a phonecall and I went to take a look. In the end I decided to put in the windows with the idea that if I didn't like them I could always brick them up.

When it was finished I liked the house from the inside but not from the outside. Then a year later Siza moved into the floor with the windows. People ask him, 'Álvaro, what's it like living in a house designed by Eduardo?' And he says, 'It's not good, but the bathroom is fantastic because when I take a shower and the sun is shining the room is filled with light.'

After twenty years of working you realise that perhaps you have to forget the seemingly radical, the elegant, and that in fact it is much more radical to propose something natural. It's more difficult to be good than to be original, and often to be good is to be natural.

Discovering what is natural is not a question of ecology or history or philosophy, it's about living with and getting close to the object. When he was in New York, Joseph Beuys lived with a violent coyote, with only blankets and an umbrella to protect him. The first day he kept his distance, the second he got closer, the third day he crept a metre nearer and on the fourth day he and the coyote were touching. To create an empathy with the world, with an object, takes time and energy.

For me the most important thing in architecture now is to have time to think. The quality of architecture today is diminished because architects have no time. Time is money and it's in short supply.

How do you see your work for this exhibition in relation to your architecture?
Most projects take ten or twenty years, so I have enjoyed this very much. But my installation is not architecture, it's a reflection on architecture. I don't yet understand why I have produced these two doors, but with time I will work it out. It's not a question of being minimalist, it's more about stone and concrete, Classical and Modern. Perhaps the Modern is just the Classical without decoration? We will find out once the doors are *in situ*, but meanwhile I will take some time to think about it.

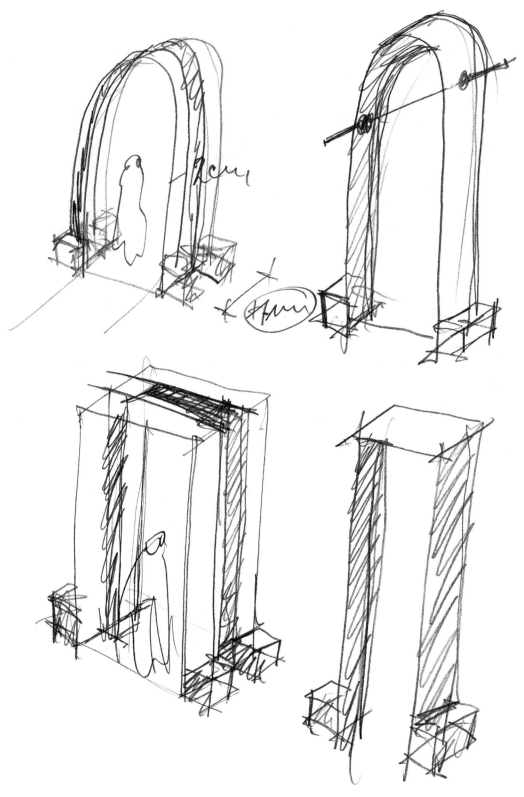

Two kinds of doorways make up the installation: an arched, 'Classical' opening which is used along the building's main axis and a rectilinear 'Neo-Palladian' opening (19). Souto de Moura explored through sketches ways of giving the structure stability (20).

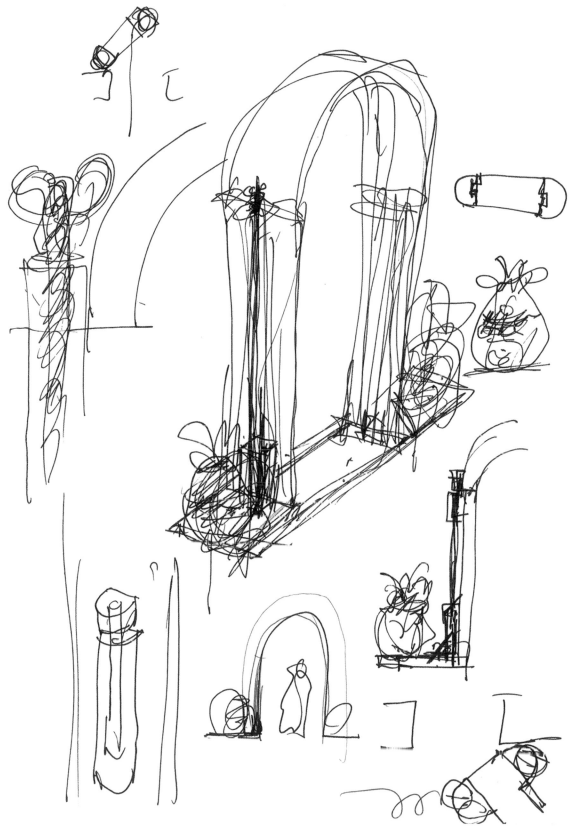

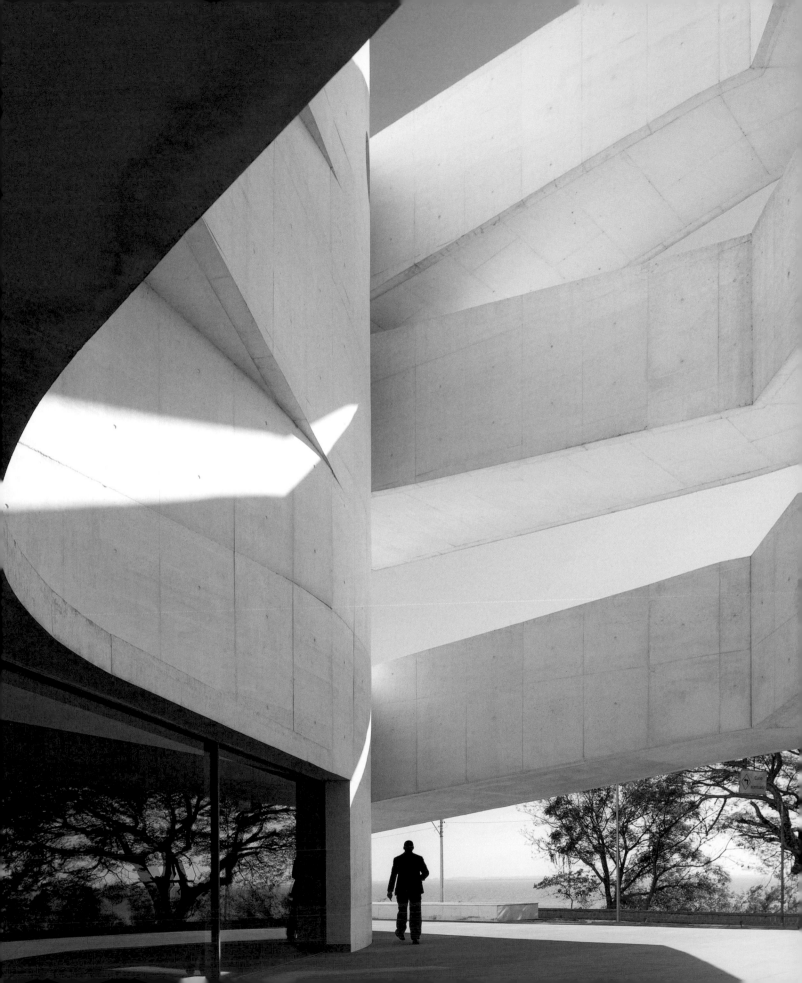

21 (opposite) Álvaro Siza, Iberê Camargo Foundation, Porto Alegre, Brazil (2008). Dedicated to the work of Brazilian painter Iberê Camargo (1914–1994), Siza's first project in Brazil shows the influence of the country's Modernist architects, notably Oscar Niemeyer and Lina Bo Bardi.

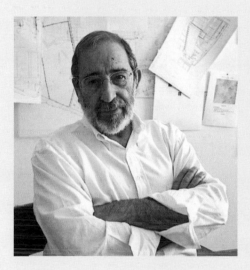

The work of renowned architect Álvaro Siza (born 1933 in Matosinhos, Portugal) is characterised by simplicity and restraint. His architecture treads a delicate line between tradition and modernity, combining craftsmanship with the techniques and materials of the machine age.

Siza believes that architects are not inventors; rather, they transform the reality that surrounds them. Context is all-important, and Siza sets up a dialogue between what he creates and its surroundings, often highlighting the tension between the two. His architecture frames views and captures moments of everyday life using simple, restrained forms with a strong sense of tectonic weight to create coherent spaces.

Siza studied in Porto with Fernando Távora, who introduced him to Modern Movement architects such as Alvar Aalto. He set up his own practice in Porto in 1954. Though he has worked in Germany, the Netherlands, Argentina and Brazil, Siza has made his greatest impact in Portugal, where his work has become associated with the country's rebirth after the 1974 revolution. The low-cost architecture in urban peripheries he designed for SAAL (the national housing association) made an important contribution to social and economic development.

In 1966 Siza began teaching at the University of Porto and he became a professor there in 1976. He has been a visiting professor at the Graduate School of Design at Harvard, the University of Pennsylvania, Los Andes University in Bogotá and the École Polytechnique Fédérale of Lausanne. Among much international recognition, he was awarded the Pritzker Prize in 1992, the Royal Institute of British Architects Royal Gold Medal in 2009, the International Union of Architects Gold Medal in 2011 and the Golden Lion for lifetime achievement at the Venice Architecture Biennale in 2012.

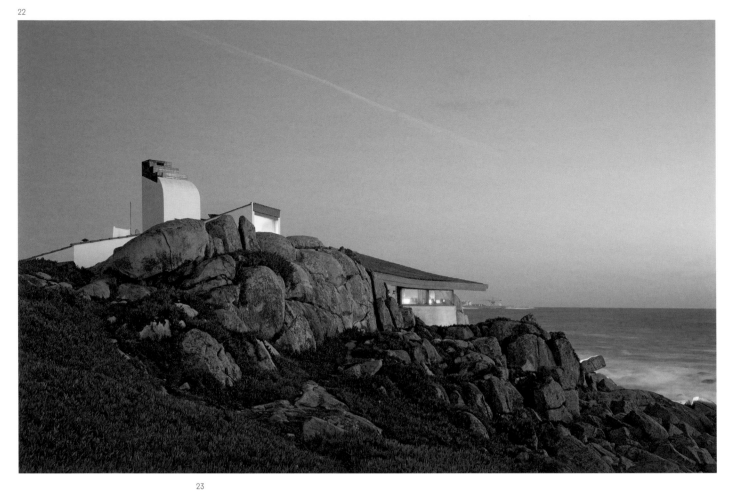

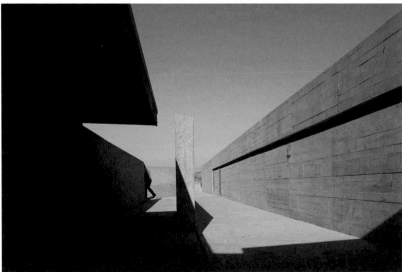

24

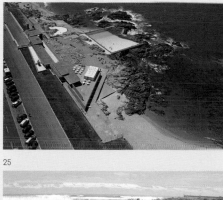
25

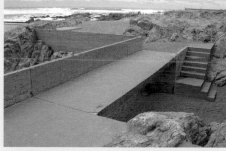

22 Álvaro Siza, Casa de Chá Boa Nova, Matosinhos, Portugal (1958–63).
For this early work on the same stretch of coast as the Leça da Palmeira pools, Siza's aim was to subsume the building to the rocky terrain.

23–25, 26 (overleaf) Álvaro Siza, Leça da Palmeira, Matosinhos (1961–66).
The saltwater pools are an exercise in understanding the site and intervening in subtle but purposeful ways. Siza also tried to imagine the kinds of spaces he would have enjoyed as a child.

Kate Goodwin: Can you describe your relationship with Eduardo Souto de Moura?
Álvaro Siza: Eduardo Souto de Moura began working in my office when he was finishing his degree. He was there for three or four years and he collaborated on designs I did for competitions and so on. Soon I realised he should have his own studio because he is someone with a very strong personality. I could not see him spending years in my office and I wanted a different relationship with his work.

For some time we no longer worked together, but when we resumed our partnership for specific projects it was a very interesting experience. After we finished the Serpentine Gallery Pavilion in London in 2005 a friend of his told him, 'This work doesn't seem yours', and a friend of mine said the same to me. My response was, 'Of course. If the result of a collaboration is something you could have produced on your own, then what's the point of working together?'

We each have our own ideas and our own professional past, and we put them on the table. Step by step we reach a consensus – this doesn't mean that one of us gets his way, but rather that there's a true meeting of ideas.

Can you talk about the dialogue between building and landscape in your work?
Architecture is always set in a particular

place, whether this landscape is natural or urban. As architects, we are always building in relation to something else. What we create is not an isolated object but transforms and is transformed by what already exists.

An example of negotiating this relationship within my own work is the public pools at Leça da Palmeira. When I started the commission I had already built a small restaurant on the cliffs nearby, the Casa de Chá Boa Nova, which was one of my first projects. I remember going to the site in the mornings and making drawings of the shape of the rocks because I wanted the profile of the building to run in parallel with them. The restaurant was very well received, but after it was finished I felt it was too mimetic of the surrounding landscape. It seemed it was simply copying the movement the rock had already made.

By the time it came to designing the pools, I had recognised that we should not try to simulate a scene nature has already created much more beautifully than we can, but should look for points of contact between the two worlds in order to create something new. It was a question of visiting the site, finding that this step should be a little closer to that stone, this line must not be parallel but a little divergent, and so on. What mattered was the connection

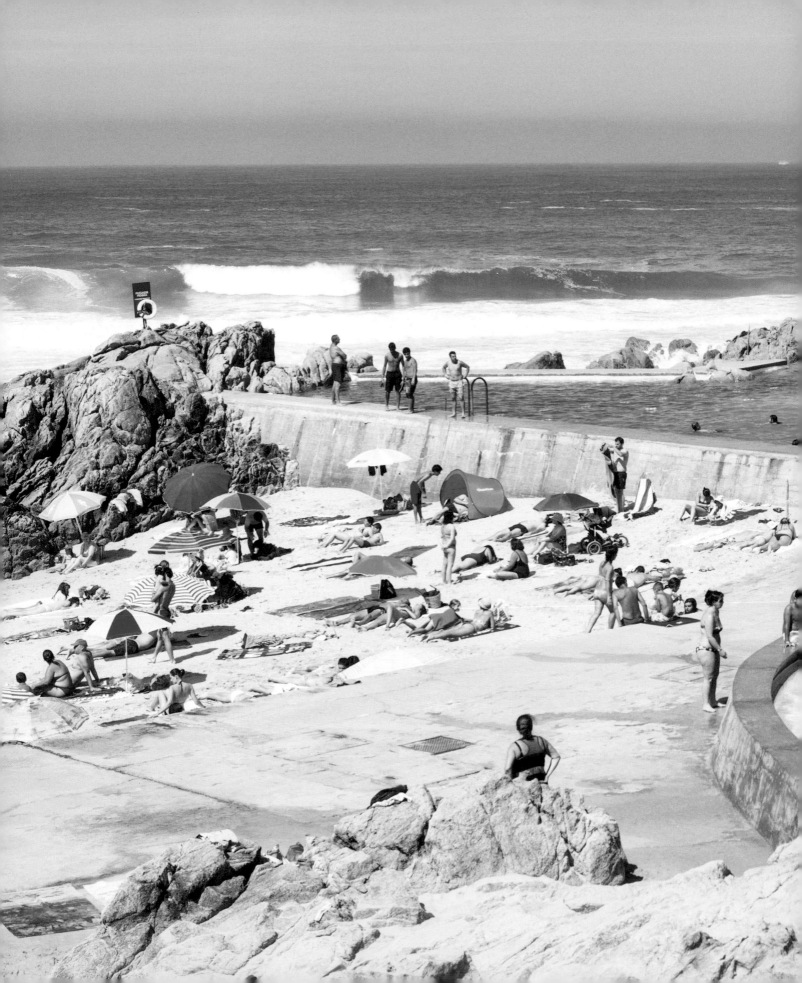

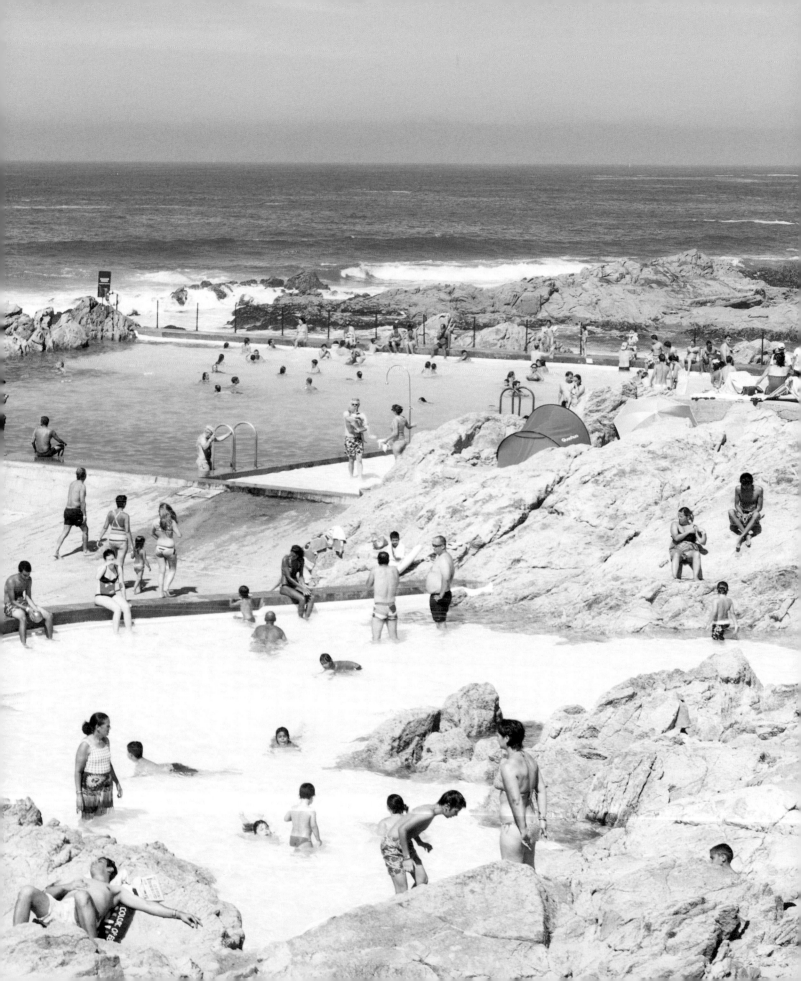

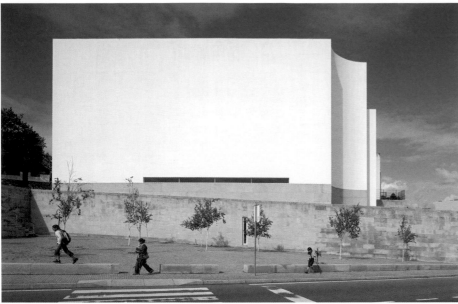

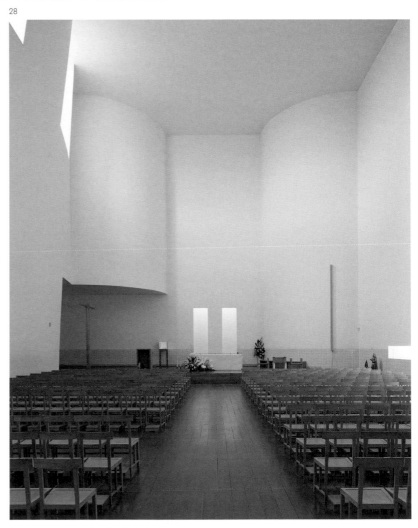

29

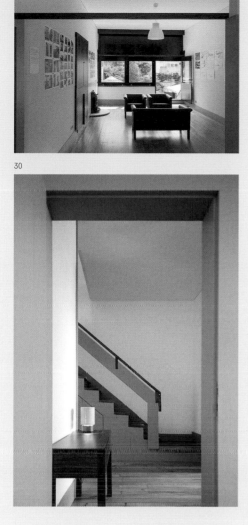

30

between the natural or pre-existent and the few things I could place there. And I tried to place as few as possible.

Your architecture is also about paying attention to the needs and pleasure of the people who use it.
I always try to imagine how people will move around within my architecture and what their needs might be. In the case of the swimming pools, for instance, I was determined not to obscure the views of the sea, even from a car on the road. I wanted to provide as many alternative routes as possible within a journey from the light of the road to the light of the beach, with a zig-zag at the point of access to simulate the sense of a narrow entrance from one space to another, which is reinforced by the change of light. I imagined how the spaces might be organised as open-air rooms for groups to sit in, and what might be fun for children – I thought about what I would have enjoyed as a child, which is how I came to design the curve of the pool and the access passing under the small bridge.

When you design houses are you also thinking about spaces you have spent time in yourself? There seem to be similarities between your early houses in your home village of Matosinhos and your housing project in Bouça near Porto, built some two decades later.
The housing project in Bouça and other similar schemes from the period following the Portuguese revolution of 1974 were very special because we were making homes for people we knew. This meant we could discuss their wishes and put forward our own views – and when there is dialogue, a solution will always be found.

The final scheme is related to the traditional rows of small houses these people lived in, back to back and very crowded. After the industrial migration to Porto at the end of the nineteenth century, half the population lived in houses like these, which had become very uncomfortable. But these people had created true communities. Before the revolution they were often moved out

against their will and their communities destroyed, sometimes for political ends.

The project at Bouça developed after much discussion of the inhabitants' dreams and aspirations, ranging from the internal organisation of the houses to the overall development of the city as there were many similar projects and the different communities came together to talk about them. The people's preferences did not go unchallenged by the architects and because there was honesty on both sides a consensus was always possible. It was a very good moment.

For the house I renovated for my family in Matosinhos, I wanted to keep the spirit and atmosphere but provide more space, a bigger living room, a twentieth-century plan. Almost all my early projects were small houses and my approach was at odds with the radicalism favoured at the time. I wanted to retain elements the Modern Movement had rejected such as wooden doorframes or protective detailing. In Bouça I still used some of the same ideas, though this is less a continuity of language than a continuity of circumstances.

What do you think is distinctive about how you as an architect understand and perceive space?
What we create draws a lot on our past experiences, including our childhoods. For instance, I recognise that parts of my design for the church of Santa Maria in Marco de Canavezes derive from experiences I had as a child – going to church as a family, sitting in the dark space. We notice things and they stick in our memories to help us when we are in trouble with a project! Sometimes we reproduce these things without being conscious of it.

I think that learning for an architect comes from seeing as much as possible. When I began my studies the only reference point was Le Corbusier. Then gradually we discovered Alvar Aalto, Frank Lloyd Wright and the Scandinavians. My teacher Fernando Távora went to England for the Festival of Britain exhibition in 1951. He met members of CIAM and brought back

27, 28 Álvaro Siza, Santa Maria, Marco de Canavezes, Porto (1990–96).
The form of the church on its raised platform is traditional but the building is deeply influenced by the giants of twentieth-century architecture – Loos, Le Corbusier and Aalto.

29, 30 Álvaro Siza, Casa da Arquitectura, Matosinhos.
The house Siza renovated for his parents in the early 1960s, opening up the spaces and expressing the wooden detailing.

31 (overleaf) Álvaro Siza, Bouça Housing Co-operative, Porto (1973–2004).
Initially designed in collaboration with the inhabitants as part of the social housing programme that followed the 1974 revolution, the complex was extended in the early 2000s.

32 (pages 180–181) Álvaro Siza, Iberê Camargo Foundation.
The control of light is a constant in Siza's work – here all the floors can be open to natural light from the atrium.

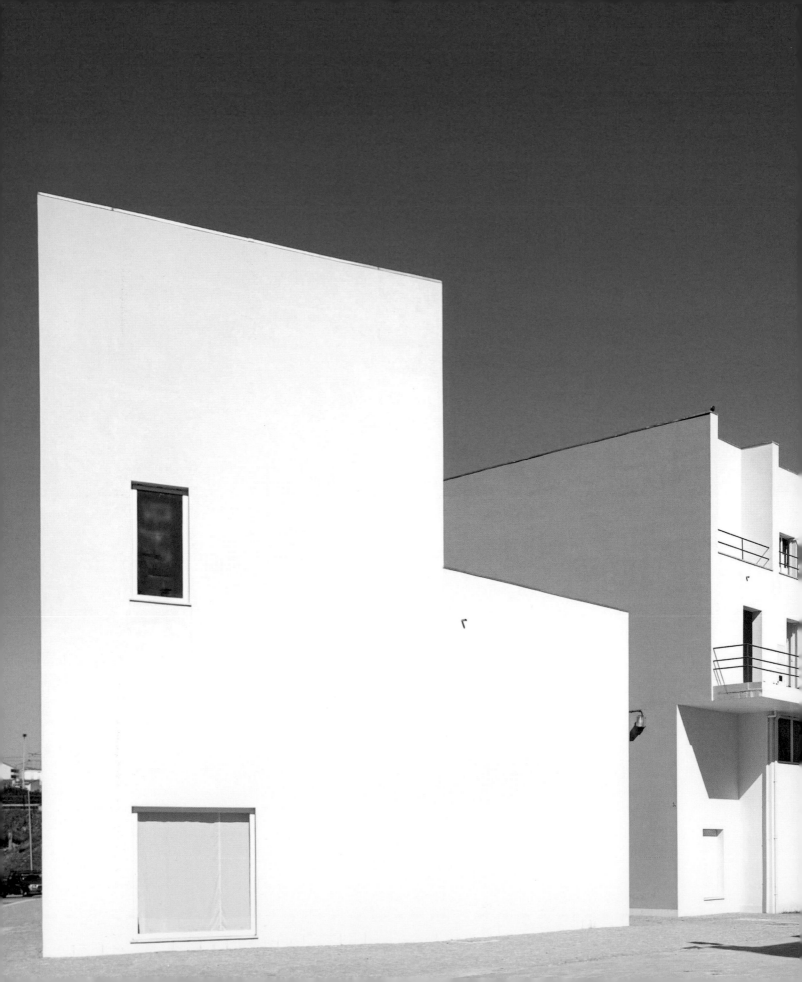

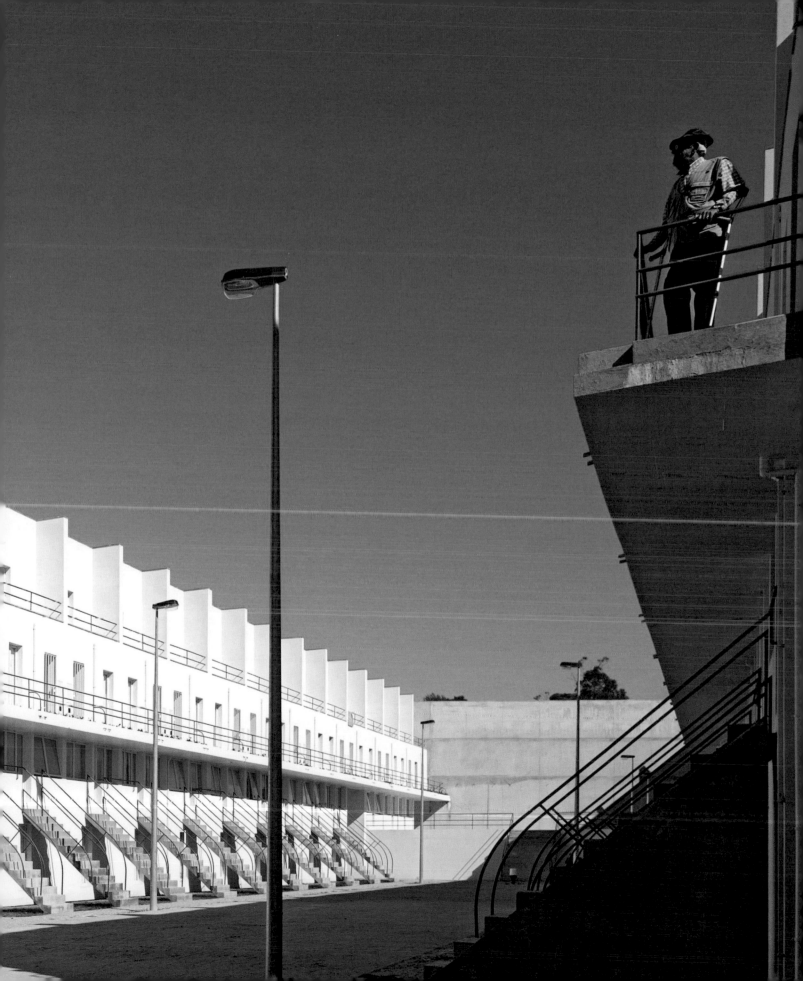

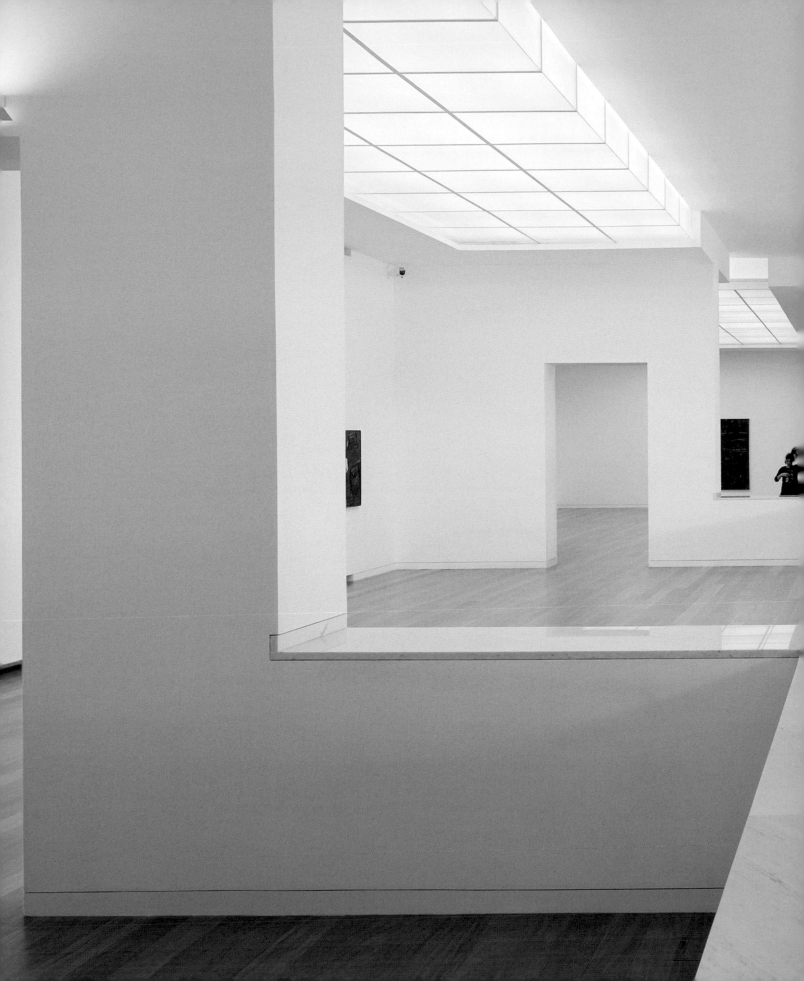

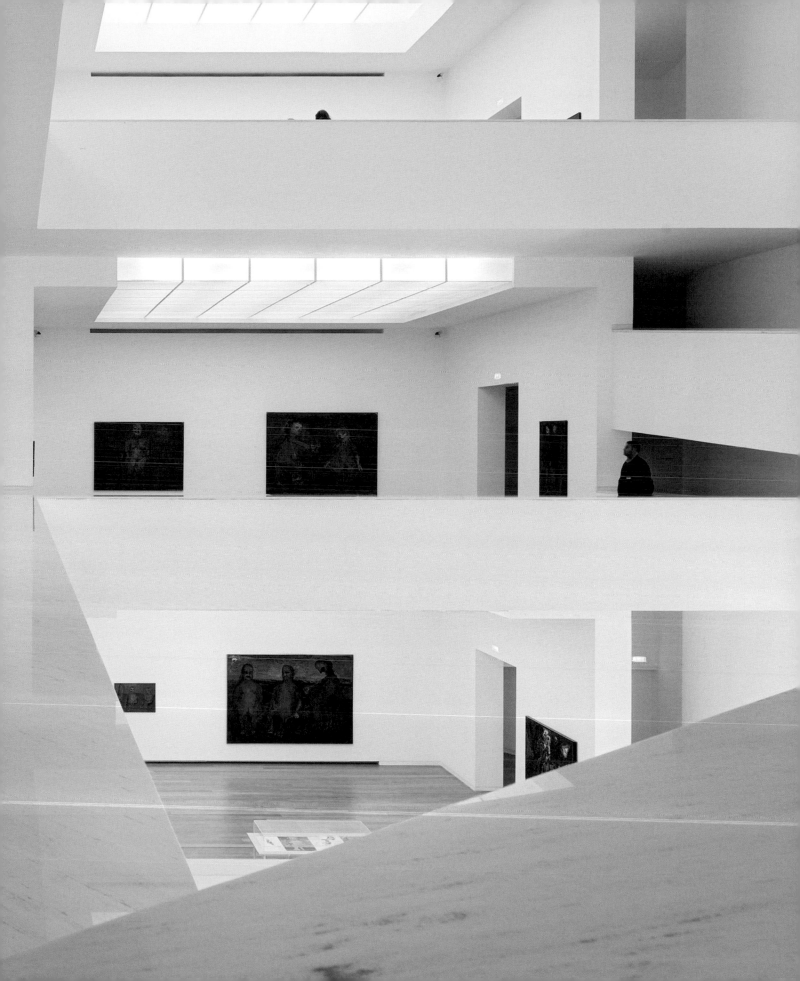

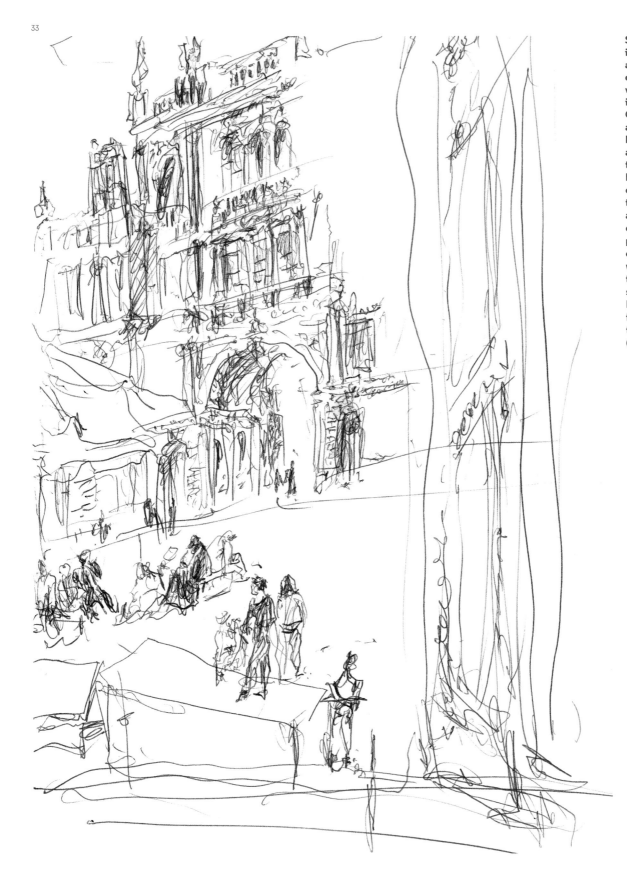

Siza's project is both the first and last installation encountered by visitors; it is located in the Annenberg Courtyard, the anteroom to the RA galleries (35) and a gateway to London (33, 34). His exploration of the birth of the column – an archetypal element of architecture – places the only upright column complete with a capital next to Alfred Drury's statue of Sir Joshua Reynolds (1723–1792), first President of the Royal Academy (36, overleaf).

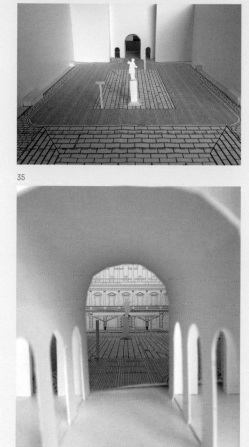

34

35

all the news, which opened our eyes. It is not a question of making copies – these ideas become part of ourselves. Students today, of course, can look on the internet or travel. It is very different.

But can this be a substitute for the sense of presence you get from being in a building?
Today it's more difficult for me to do site visits, so the internet helps a lot. The number of visits you make varies from project to project: if you know the context, then you may not need to go so often – or perhaps you need to go more often so you don't risk slipping into banality and you still have the possibility of making discoveries. An architect is a detective, always trying to discover things.

I remember the stimulus I felt when I first worked in Berlin or Brazil – such experiences provide food for our minds. Local culture is important but it should not be the only thing you draw on.

What were your initial impressions of the architecture of the Royal Academy and of the Annenberg Courtyard?
You walk along the street with all its traffic and find yourself in front of the big archway. Through it you see the courtyard, which comes as a surprise. The scale is domestic rather than monumental, but the building's façade – with its portico and columns, which are whiter than the rest of the stone – has a very strong presence.

My first reaction as I wondered what to do was almost panic. Then the notion of the column emerged and I wondered if I could make an installation that referred to the birth of the column. I have placed one column lying down with its capital beside it, another standing, and a third with the capital in place. I hope that these three elements create an entity which also relates to the courtyard as a whole.

For me, making architecture means starting with what is there. Unless you are building in a desert, there are always lots of things to consider, sometimes too many. Here I am introducing a new element inspired by the sensation I had the first time I entered the courtyard.

Can you talk about how your installation relates to the doors that Eduardo Souto de Moura is making?
From the courtyard, visitors climb the stairs to the beautiful octagonal room, and beyond it they move into the gallery where they find Souto de Moura's installation. The sequence is more intense and richer because you cannot see both his and my installations at the same time. It requires visitors to activate their memories rather than just make visual comparisons.

You both chose to work with fundamental elements of architecture, the column and the door, which suggests a notion of continuity.
In my opinion there is always continuity. Columns and doorways exist everywhere. Sometimes there are periods of seeming rupture but later you understand that what appeared to be completely new was in fact old ideas adapted to new circumstances and conditions.

Yours will be the first installation people come across and also the last. What do you hope they might take away with them?
When you exit the courtyard it is also the entrance to London, so I see my installation as related to the street as well as respecting the architecture of the Royal Academy. For instance, while I was standing in the courtyard I glimpsed a yellow bus through the archway and I had the perhaps crazy idea of painting the columns yellow. I see my installation as a continuity of a lot of movements people visiting the exhibition, but also eating lunch, sitting in the courtyard for a rest, or to smoke a cigarette if it's still allowed!

You connect with the city but also with time, going back to the old and suggesting something of the future.
That is the reality of the city. In a city the atmosphere is all around you and is ever changing. New things will become old things, so the idea of continuity is very real. When you finish a piece of work, it always seems a bit schematic because it's lacking the work of time, the flux of things that builds the city's changing presence. Time is a great architect.

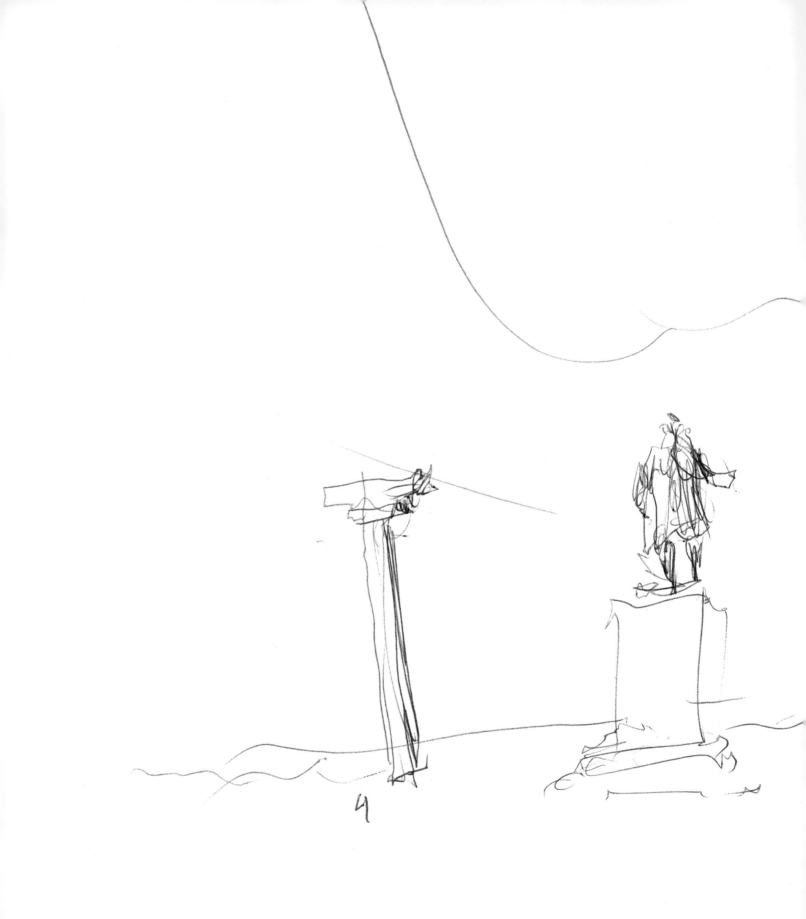

4

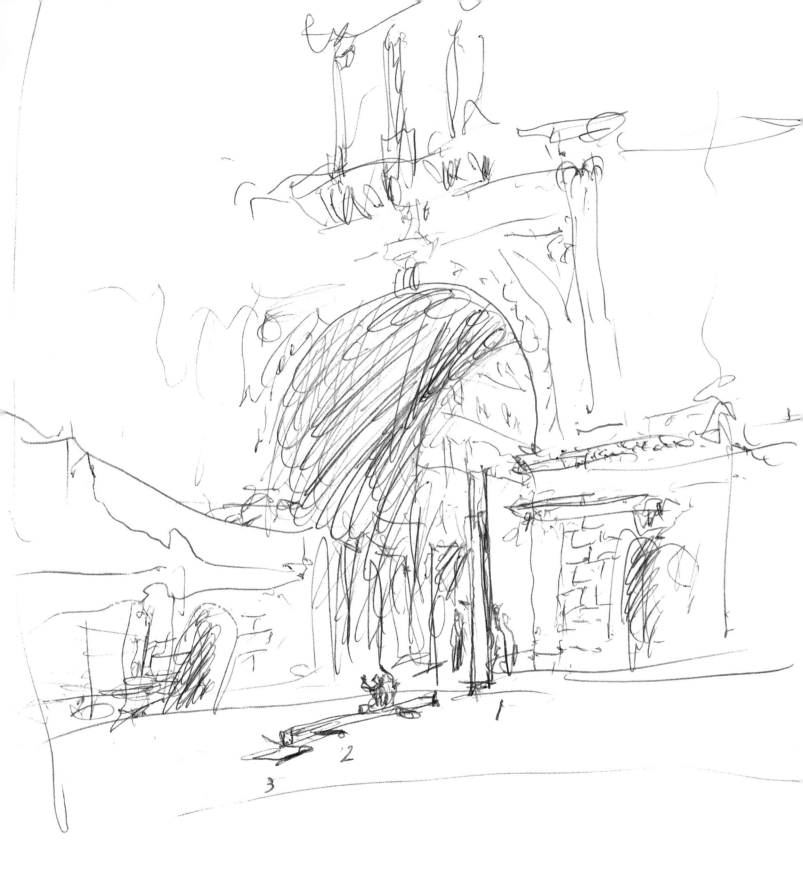

The installation responds to the sensation of entering the Annenberg Courtyard and to the strong presence of the Burlington House façades with their distinctive columns (38). It consists of three elements: one column lying down with its capital beside it, another standing, and a third standing with its capital in place (39). Positioned at the edges of the courtyard's central paved area, the three form an entity that also relates a to the surrounding buildings (37).

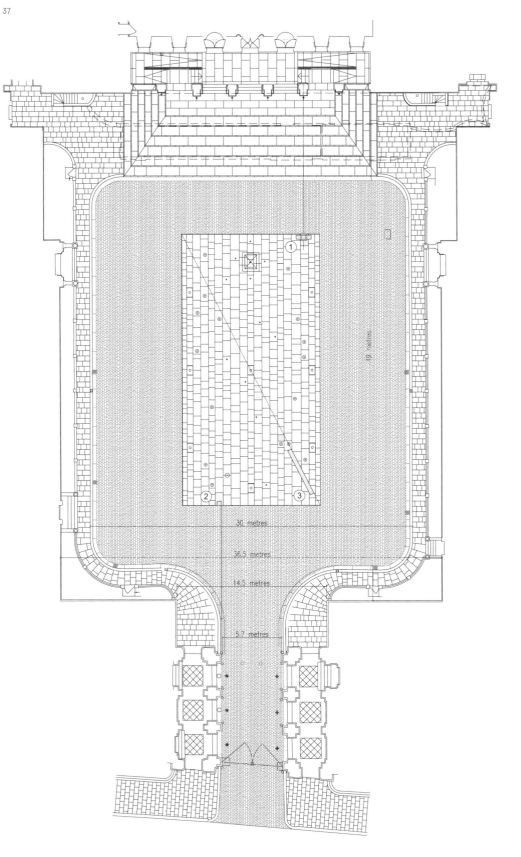

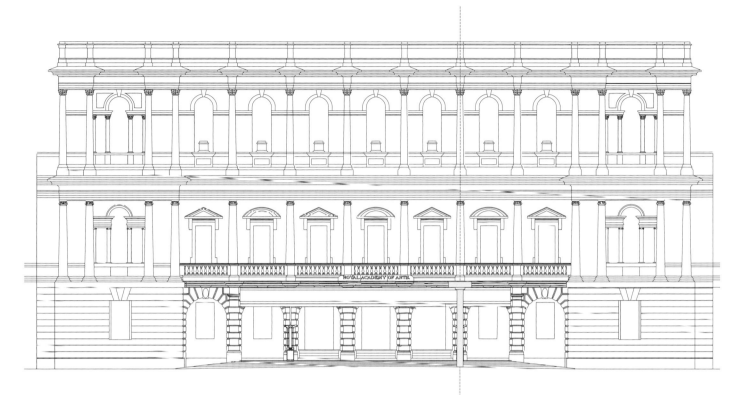

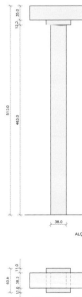

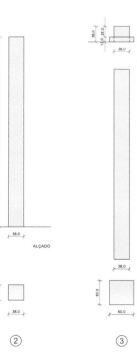

ALÇADO

ALÇADO

ALÇADO

① ② ③

Further Reading

Gaston Bachelard, *The Poetics of Space*, Boston, 1969 (originally published as *La Poétique de l'espace*, Paris, 1958)

Kent C. Bloomer and Charles W. Moore, *Body, Memory and Architecture*, New Haven, 1978

Edmund Burke, *A Philosophical Enquiry into the Origin of Our Ideas of the Sublime and Beautiful*, Oxford, 1990 (originally published 1757)

Italo Calvino, *Invisible Cities*, London, 1997 (originally published as *Le città invisibili*, Turin, 1972)

Adam Caruso, *The Feeling of Things*, Barcelona, 2009

Antonio Esposito and Giovanni Leoni, *Eduardo Souto de Moura*, London, 2012

Adrian Forty, *Words and Buildings: A Vocabulary of Modern Architecture*, London, 2000

Kenneth Frampton, *Kengo Kuma: Complete Works*, London, 2013

Steven Holl, Juhani Pallasmaa and Alberto Pérez-Gómez, *Questions of Perception: Phenomenology of Architecture*, San Francisco, 2006 (originally published as an *a+u* special edition, Tokyo, 1994)

Philip Jodidio, *Álvaro Siza: Complete Works 1954–2012*, Cologne, 2013

Kengo Kuma, *Anti-Object: The Dissolution and Disintegration of Architecture*, London, 2008

Henri Lefebvre, *The Production of Space*, Oxford, 1991 (originally published as *La Production de l'espace*, Paris, 1974)

Li Xiaodong, *Chinese Conception of Space*, Beijing, 2008

Christian Norberg-Schulz, *Existence, Space & Architecture*, New York, 1971

Juhani Pallasmaa, *The Thinking Hand: Existential and Embodied Wisdom in Architecture*, Chichester, 2009

Steen Eiler Rasmussen, *Experiencing Architecture*, second revised edition, Cambridge, MA, 1962

Bernard Rudofsky, *The Prodigious Builders*, Boston, 1977

Leon van Schaik, *Spatial Intelligence: New Futures for Architecture*, Chichester, 2008

Francesca Serrazanetti and Matteo Schubert (eds), *Grafton Architects – Inspiration and Process in Architecture*, Milan, 2014

Francesca Serrazanetti and Matteo Schubert (eds), *Kengo Kuma – Inspiration and Process in Architecture*, Milan, 2014

Junichiro Tanizaki, *In Praise of Shadows*, London, 2001 (originally published as *In'ei Raisan*, Tokyo, 1933)

Nobuyuki Yoshida (ed.), *Pezo von Ellrichshausen*, *a+u*, Tokyo, 2013:06

Peter Zumthor, *Atmospheres: Architectural Environments – Surrounding Objects*, Basel, Boston, Berlin, 2006

Photographic Acknowledgements

Luis Ferreira Alves: pages 160–161, 162 (6 & 7), 164, 165

Daici Ano: pages 56, 58

Arcaid Images: pages 89 (17) (Corbis/photography: Richard Bryant); 125 (11) (photography: Will Pryce/Thames & Hudson); 163 (9) (photography: G Jackson)

Satoshi Asakawa: page 68

bpk/Reinhard Görner: page 163 (10)

British Museum/The Trustees of the British Museum: page 85 (12)

Federico Brunetti: pages 80–81

China Daily: page 96 (Cui Meng)

Alice Clancy: pages 76, 77, 82 (7), 83 (8), 87

Corbis: page 69 (13) (Underwood & Underwood); page 101 (8) (Ocean); page 107 (17) (JAI/Amar Grover); page 159 (Jonathan Blair)

The Courier: page 59

Carlos Coutinho: pages 156, 158

Hans Danuser: page 46

Leonel de Castro: page 157

Luis Díaz Díaz: pages 174–175

Donato Di Bello: page 78

FG + SG Fernando Guerra and Casa Da Arquitectura, 2009: page 177 (29 & 30)

FLC/ADAGP, Paris and DACS, London 2013: page 89 (18)

Mitsumasa Fujitsuka: pages 60 (3 & 4), 62–63, 64 (6 & 7), 66–67

Getty Images: pages 42–43 (Marcello Paternostro/AFP); page 45 (6) (Hutton Archive); page 49 (VIEW Pictures/UIG); page 79 (Mondadori Portfolio); page 109 (16) (Goh Chai Hin/AFP)

Grafton Architects: pages 85 (11), 88, 90 (19 & 20), 91

David Heerde: page 137

International Red Cross and Red Crescent Museum, Geneva: page 143 (9) (photography: Alain Germond)

Dimitrios Kalapodas: page 38

Martti Kapanen, Alvar Aalto Museum, 1979: page 125 (10)

Diébédo Francis Kéré: pages 138 (4), 139, 140–141, 142 (7), 144–145, 146 (12), 147, 148, 149, 150–151, 152 (18 & 19), 153 (20 & 21)

Weneyida Kéré: page 138 (3)

Kengo Kuma: pages 70 (13, 14 & 15), 71, 72 (18 & 19), 73 (20 & 21)

Li Xiaodong: pages 92, 94, 95, 100 (6 & 7), 102–103, 104 (11 & 12), 106 (14 & 15), 108 (18 & 19), 109, 110, 111

Peppe Maisto: page 69 (10)

Maurizio Mucciola: page 173 (25)

Richard Murphy: page 44 (photography: Peter Guthrie)

Maria Manuel Oliveira: page 41

Erik-Jan Ouwerkerk: pages 134, 136, 142 (8), 146 (13)

Cristóbal Palma: pages 112, 114, 118 (3 & 4), 116–117, 119, 120–121, 122, 124, 126–127

Pezo von Ellrichshausen: pages 104, 105 (18, 19, 20 & 21), 115 (photography: Ana Crovetto), 128, 130, 131

Chiara Porcu: page 171

President and Fellows of Harvard College, Imaging Department: page 65

Tian Ren: page 143 (10)

Royal Academy of Arts: page 129 (Paul Highnam)

Phil Sayer: page 34

Álvaro Siza: pages 182, 183 (34 & 35), 184–185, 186, 187 (38 & 39)

Eduardo Souto de Moura: pages 166 (13, 14, 15 & 16), 167 (17 & 18), 168, 169

Swiss Theatre Collection, Berne: page 45

Dr Christopher Tadgell: pages 69 (12), 163 (8)

Markus Tretter: pages 50–51

A. Vieira, Arquivo A. Siza: page 40

VIEW Pictures: pages 74, 82 (6), 84, 86 (13 & 14) (photography: Dennis Gilbert); page 83 (9) (Hans Muenchhalfen/Artur); page 154 (photography: James Brittain); pages 170, 172 (22 & 23), 173 (24), 176 (27 & 28), 178–179, 180–181 (photography: Fernando Guerra)

Alan Weintraub: page 105

Mark Wilson: page 101 (9)

Zhou Limin: pages 98–99

Supporters of the Royal Academy

MAJOR BENEFACTORS

The President and the Trustees of the Royal Academy Trust are grateful to all its donors for their continued loyalty and generosity. They would like to extend their thanks to all those who have made a significant commitment, past and present, to the galleries, the exhibitions, the conservation of the Permanent Collection, the Library collections, the Royal Academy Schools, the Learning programme and other specific appeals.

HM The Queen
Her Majesty's Government
The 29th May 1961 Charitable Trust
The Aldama Foundation
The American Associates of the Royal Academy Trust
The Annenberg Foundation
Barclays Bank
BAT Industries plc
Sir David and Lady Bell
The late Tom Bendhem
The late Brenda M Benwell-Lejeune
John Frye Bourne
British Telecom
The Brown Foundation
John and Susan Burns
Mr Raymond M Burton CBE
Sir Trevor Chinn CVO and Lady Chinn
The Trustees of the Clore Foundation
The John S Cohen Foundation
Sir Harry and Lady Djangoly
The Dulverton Trust
Alfred Dunhill Limited
The John Ellerman Foundation
The Eranda Foundation
Ernst & Young
Esso UK plc
Esmée Fairbairn Charitable Trust
The Fidelity UK Foundation
The Foundation for Sports and the Arts
Friends of the Royal Academy
Jacqueline and Michael Gee
The Getty Grant Programme
Mr Thomas Gibson
Glaxo Holdings plc
Diane and Guilford Glazer
Mr and Mrs Jack Goldhill
Maurice and Laurence Goldman
The Horace W Goldsmith Foundation
HRH Princess Marie-Chantal of Greece
Mr and Mrs Jocelin Harris
The Philip and Pauline Harris Charitable Trust
The Charles Hayward Foundation
Heritage Lottery Fund
IBM United Kingdom Limited
The Idlewild Trust
Lord and Lady Jacobs
The JP Jacobs Charitable Trust
The Japan Foundation
Gabrielle Jungels-Winkler Foundation
Mr and Mrs Donald Kahn
The Lillian Jean Kaplan Foundation
The Kresge Foundation
The Samuel H Kress Foundation
The Kirby Laing Foundation
The Lankelly Foundation
The late Mr John S Latsis
The David Lean Foundation
The Leverhulme Trust
Lex Service plc
The Linbury Trust
Sir Sydney Lipworth QC and Lady Lipworth CBE
John Lyons Charity
Ronald and Rita McAulay
McKinsey and Company Inc
John Madejski OBE DL
The Manifold Trust
Marks and Spencer
The Paul Mellon Estate
The Mercers' Company
The Monument Trust
The Henry Moore Foundation
The Moorgate Trust Fund
The late Mr Minoru Mori HON KBE and Mrs Mori
Museums and Galleries Improvement Fund
National Westminster Bank
Stavros S Niarchos
Simon and Midge Palley
The Peacock Charitable Trust
The Pennycress Trust
PF Charitable Trust
The Pidem Fund
The Pilgrim Trust
The Edith and Ferdinand Porjes Trust
The Porter Foundation
John Porter Charitable Trust
Rio Tinto
John A Roberts FRIBA
Sir Simon and Lady Robertson
The Ronson Foundation
Rothmans International plc
RTZ Corporation plc
Dame Jillian Sackler DBE
Jillian and Arthur M Sackler
Mr Wafic Rida Saïd
Mrs Jean Sainsbury
The Saison Foundation
The Sammermar Trust
The Basil Samuel Charitable Trust
Mrs Coral Samuel CBE
Sea Containers Ltd
Shell UK Limited
Miss Dasha Shenkman
William and Maureen Shenkman
The Archie Sherman Charitable Trust
The late Pauline Sitwell
The Starr Foundation
Sir Hugh Sykes DL
Alfred Taubman
Sir Anthony and Lady Tennant
Ware and Edythe Travelstead
The Trusthouse Charitable Foundation
The Douglas Turner Trust
Unilever plc
The Weldon UK Charitable Trust
The Welton Foundation
The Weston Family
The Malcolm Hewitt Wiener Foundation
The Maurice Wohl Charitable Foundation
The Wolfson Foundation

and others who wish to remain anonymous

PATRONS

The Royal Academy is extremely grateful to all its Patrons, who generously support every aspect of its work.

Chair
Robert Suss

Platinum
Celia and Edward Atkin CBE
Mr and Mrs Christopher Bake
Mr and Mrs Patrick Doherty
Ms Ghizlan El Glaoui
Mr Denis Korotkov-Koganovich
Mr and Mrs Jake Shafran
David and Sophie Shalit

Gold
Christopher and Alex Courage
Mr and Mrs Andrew Higginson
Mrs Elizabeth Hosking
Miss Joanna Kaye
Lady Rayne Lacey
Jacqueline and Marc Leland
The Licensing Company, London
Sir Sydney Lipworth QC and Lady Lipworth CBE
Mr and Mrs Ronald Lubner
Sir Keith and Lady Mills
Jean and Geoffrey Redman-Brown
Mrs Stella Shawzin
Mr Kevin Sneader and Ms Amy Munter
David Stileman
Mr and Mrs Pierre Winkler
Mr Robert John Yerbury

Silver
Lady Agnew
Miss H J C Anstruther
Lord Ashburton
Mr and Mrs Simon Bamber
Jane Barker
Ms Catherine Baxendale
The Duke of Beaufort
Mrs J K M Bentley, Summers Art Gallery
Mr Nigel Boardman
Eleanor E Brass
Mr and Mrs Richard Briggs OBE
Mrs Elie Brihi
Mrs Marcia Brocklebank
Sir Francis Brooke Bt
Mrs Joyce Brotherton
Lady Brown
Jeremy Brown
Lord Browne of Madingley
Mr Martin Burton
Mr F A A Carnwath CBE
Sir Roger Carr
Jean and Eric Cass
Sir Charles and Lady Chadwyck-Healey
Sir Trevor Chinn CVO and Lady Chinn
Mr and Mrs George Coelho
Denise Cohen Charitable Trust
Sir Ronald Cohen
Ms Linda Cooper
Mark and Cathy Corbett
Mr and Mrs Ken Costa
Julian Darley and Helga Sands
The Countess of Dartmouth
Mr Daniel Davies
Peter and Andrea De Haan
The de Laszlo Foundation
Mrs Anita Dinkin
Dr Anne Dornhorst
Lord Douro
Mr and Mrs Jim Downing
Ms Noreen Doyle
Janet and Maurice Dwek
Mrs Sheila Earles
Lord and Lady Egremont
Bryan Ferry
Mr Sam Fogg
Mrs Rosamund Fokschaner
Mrs Jocelyn Fox
Mrs Anthony Foyle
Mr and Mrs Eric Franck
Mr Simon Freakley
Arnold Fulton
The Lord Gavron CBE
Jacqueline and Jonathan Gestetner
Lady Getty
Mr Mark Glatman
Lady Gosling
Mr Stephen Gosztony
Piers Gough CBE RA
Mr Gavin Graham
Mrs Mary Graves
Mrs Margaret Guitar
Sir Ewan and Lady Harper
Mrs Melanie Harris
Richard and Janeen Haythornthwaite
Sir John Hegarty and Miss Philippa Crane
Michael and Morven Heller
Lady Heseltine
Mr and Mrs Alan Hobart
Mr Philip Hudson
Mr and Mrs Jon Hunt
Mrs Deanna Ibrahim
S Isern-Feliu
Mrs Caroline Jackson
Mr Michael Jacobson
Sir Martin and Lady Jacomb
Mrs Raymonde Jay
Fiona Johnstone
Mr Nicholas Jones
Mrs Ghislaine Kane
Dr Elisabeth Kehoe
Mr Duncan Kenworthy OBE
Princess Jeet Khemka
Mr and Mrs Naguib Kheraj
Mr D H Killick
Mr and Mrs James Kirkman
Mrs Aboudi Kosta
Mr and Mrs Herbert Kretzmer
Norman A Kurland and Deborah A David
Joan H Lavender
Mr George Lengvari and Mrs Inez Lengvari
Lady Lever of Manchester
Mr Peter Lloyd
Miss R Lomax-Simpson
The Hon Mrs Virginia Lovell
Mr and Mrs Henry Lumley
Mrs Josephine Lumley
Gillian McIntosh
Andrew and Judith McKinna
Mr Nicholas Maclean
Sir John Mactaggart
Madeline and Donald Main
Mrs Inge Margulies
Mr Charles Martin
Mr and Mrs Richard Martin
Zvi and Ofra Meitar Family Fund
Professor Anthony Mellows OBE TD and Mrs Anthony Mellows
Mrs Joy Moss
Dr Ann Naylor
Mr Stuart C Nelson
Ann Norman-Butler
North Street Trust
Mr Michael Palin
John H Pattisson
Nicholas B Paumgarten
Mr and Mrs D J Peacock
Mr and Mrs A Perloff

Mr Philip Perry
David Pike
Mr Maurice Pinto
Mr and Mrs Anthony
 Pitt-Rivers
Mr Basil Postan
John and Anne Raisman
Mr David Reid Scott
Lady Renwick
Rothschild Foundation
Miss Elaine Rowley
Mr and Mrs K M Rubie
The Lady Henrietta St George
Mr Adrian Sassoon
H M Sassoon Charitable Trust
Mr and Mrs Christopher
 Satterthwaite
Carol Sellars
Mr and Mrs Kevin Senior
Christina Countess of
 Shaftesbury
Mr Robert N Shapiro
Major General and Mrs
 Jonathan Shaw
Richard and Veronica
 Simmons
Alan and Marianna Simpson
The Tavolozza Foundation
Lady Tennant
Anthony Thornton
Mr Anthony J Todd
Miss M L Ultane
John and Carol Wates
Mrs Angela Webb
Edna and Willard Weiss
Anthony and Rachel Williams
Christopher G Williams Esq
Mr William Winters

Patron Donors
Stephen Barry Charitable
 Settlement
Mr and Mrs William Brake
Gerald Fogel
Mr Peter Lloyd
Mrs Bianca Roden
The Michael H Sacher
 Charitable Trust

*and others who wish to remain
anonymous*

BENJAMIN WEST
GROUP PATRONS
Chair
Lady Judge CBE

Platinum
Mr Tony Davis
David Giampaolo
Charles and Kaaren Hale
Ms Dambisa Moyo
Mr and Mrs John R Olsen

Gold
Marco and Francesca Assetto
Lady Judge CBE
Mr Christian Levett
Ms Alessandra Morra
Mr John Peter Williams

Silver
Lady J Lloyd Adamson
Mr Dimitry Afanasiev
Poppy Allonby
Mrs Spindrift Al Swaidi
Ms Ruth Anderson
Ms Sol Anitua
Mr Andy Ash
Mrs Leslie Bacon
Naomi and Ted Berk
Mrs Michal Berkner Jenrick
Jean and John Botts
Mrs Olga But-Gusaim
Mrs Sophie Cahu
Brian and Melinda Carroll
Mr and Mrs Paul Collins
Vanessa Colomar de Enserro

Ms Karla Dorsch
Mr and Mrs Jeff Eldredge
Mr David Fawkes
Mrs Stroma Finston
Cyril and Christine Freedman
Mrs Mina Gerowin Herrmann
Ms Moya Greene
Mr David Greenwald
Mr and Mrs Timothy Hart
Mr Andrew Hawkins
Ms Alexandra Hess
Mr Rashid Hoosenally
Katie Jackson
Suzanne and Michael Johnson
Syrie Johnson
Lord and Lady Leitch
Mrs Stephanie Léouzon
Charles G Lubar
Ted and Patricia Madara
Cornelius Medvei
Mrs Victoria Mills
Scott and Christine Morrissey
Neil Osborn and Holly Smith
Lady Purves
Mr James B Sherwood
Mr Stuart Southall
Sir Hugh and Lady Sykes
Mr Ian Taylor
Miss Lori Tedesco
Mr and Mrs Julian Treger
Frederick and Kathryn Uhde
Mr Craig D Weaver
Prof Peter Whiteman QC
Mr and Mrs John Winter
Ms Regina Wyles

*and others who wish to remain
anonymous*

SCHOOLS PATRONS
Chair
Clare Flanagan

Platinum
Mrs Sarah Chenevix-Trench
Matthew and Sian Westerman

Gold
Sam and Rosie Berwick
Christopher Kneale
Mr William Loschert
Mr Keir McGuinness

Silver
Lord and Lady Aldington
Mrs Elizabeth Alston
Mr Nicholas Andrew
Dr Anne Ashmore-Hudson
Mr Jonathan and Mrs Sarah
 Bayliss
Mrs Gemma Billington
Tatiana Cherkasova
Rosalind Clayton
Mr Richard Clothier
Ms Davina Dickson
Mrs Dominic Dowley
John Entwistle OBE
Mrs Catherine Farquharson
Ian and Catherine Ferguson
Ms Clare Flanagan
Mr Mark Garthwaite
Mrs Michael Green
Mr Lindsay Hamilton
Mrs Lesley Haynes
Rosalyn Henderson
Prof Ken Howard OBE RA
 and Mrs Howard
Mark and Fiona Hutchinson
Mrs Susan Johns
Ms Karen Jones
Mrs Marcelle Joseph
Mr and Mrs S Kahan
Mr Paul Kempe
Ms Nicolette Kwok
Mrs Anna Lee
Mr and Mrs Mark Loveday
Mrs Nicola Manby
Philip and Val Marsden

The Mulberry Trust
Lord and Lady Myners
Peter Rice Esq
Anthony and Sally Salz
Brian D Smith
Mr Simon Thorley QC
Mr Ray Treen
Mrs Carol Wates
Mrs Diana Wilkinson
Mr and Mrs Maurice
 Wolridge

*and others who wish to remain
anonymous*

CONTEMPORARY CIRCLE
PATRONS
Chair
Susie Allen-Huxley

Platinum
Robert and Simone Suss

Gold
Mrs and Mrs Thomas Berger
Mr Jeremy Coller
Helen and Colin David
Mrs Alison Deighton
Matthew and Monika
 McLennan
Mr and Mrs Scott Mead
Ms Miel de Botton
Mr and Mrs Simon Oliver
Mr and Mrs Paul Phillips
Richard Sharp

Silver
Joan and Robin Alvarez
Mrs Charlotte Artus
Mr David Baty
Ms Sara Berman
Viscountess Bridgeman
Dr Elaine C Buck
Ms Debra Burt
Nadia Crandall
Mrs Georgina David
Mrs Elizabeth Davydova
Mr Patrick De Nonneville
Mollie Dent-Brocklehurst
Mrs Sophie Diedrichs-Cox
Mr and Mrs Gerard Dodd
Chris and Angie Drake
Mrs Jennifer Duke
Mr Timothy Ellis
Lady Polly Feversham
Mr Stephen Garrett
Simon Gillespie
Mrs Susan Hayden
Margaret A Jackson
Mr Gerald Kidd
Mrs Fiona King
Anna Lapshina
Mrs Sarah Macken
Mr Penelope Mather
Dr Carolina Minio Paluello
Victoria Miro
Mr and Mrs Jeremy
 Nicholson
Mrs Tessa Nicholson
Mrs Yelena Oosting
Veronique Parke
Mr Tremayne Carew Pole
Mrs Tineke Pugh
Mrs Catherine Rees
Mrs Karen Santi
Edwina Sassoon
Omar Shah
Richard and Susan
 Shoylekov
Mr Ana Stanic
Jeffery C Sugarman and Alan
 D H Newham
Anna Watkins
Cathy Wills
Manuela and Iwan Wirth
Mr and Mrs Maurice
 Wolridge
Ms Cynthia Wu

Patron Donor
Mrs Karen Santi

*and others who wish to remain
anonymous*

LIBRARY AND
COLLECTIONS CIRCLE
Patron Donors
Mr Mark W Friend
Mr Loyd Grossman
Miss Jo Hannah Hoehn
Mr and Mrs Robert Hoehn
Lowell Libson
Pam and Scott Schafler
Mr and Mrs Bart Tiernan
Jonny Yarker

*and others who wish to remain
anonymous*

YOUNG PATRONS
Kalita al Swaidi
Miss Maria Allen
Miss Joy Asfar
Rosanna Bossom
May Calil
Mr and Mrs Tom Davies
Mr Stefano Donati
Mr Rollo Gabb
Miss Fernanda Gilligan
Laura Graham
Soliana Habte
The Hon Alexandra
 Knatchbull
Marc C Koch
Julie Lawson
Lilly Le Brun
Mr Lin Lei
Mr Mandeep Singh
Mr Stephen Sobey
Miss Annabelle Wills
Miss Burcu Yuksel

Patron Donor
Mr Haakon Lorentzen

*and others who wish to remain
anonymous*

TRUSTS AND FOUNDATIONS

Artists Collecting Society
The Atlas Fund
The Albert Van den Bergh
 Charitable Trust
The Bomonty Charitable
 Trust
The Charlotte Bonham-
 Carter Charitable Trust
William Brake Charitable
 Trust
R M Burton 1998 Charitable
 Trust
C H K Charities Limited
P H G Cadbury Charitable
 Trust
The Carew Pole Charitable
 Trust
The Clore Duffield
 Foundation
John S Cohen Foundation
The Evan Cornish Foundation
The Sidney and Elizabeth
 Corob Charitable Trust
The Dovehouse Trust
The Gilbert and Eileen Edgar
 Foundation
The John Ellerman
 Foundation
Lucy Mary Ewing Charitable
 Trust
The Margery Fish Charity
The Flow Foundation
The Garfield Weston
 Foundation
Gatsby Charitable Foundation

The Golden Bottle Trust
The Gordon Foundation
Sue Hammerson Charitable
 Trust
The Charles Hayward
 Foundation
Heritage Lottery Fund
Hiscox
Holbeck Charitable Trust
The Harold Hyam Wingate
 Foundation
The Ironmongers' Company
The Emmanuel Kaye
 Foundation
The Kindersley Foundation
The de Laszlo Foundation
The Leche Trust
The Maccabaeans
The McCorquodale
 Charitable Trust
The Machin Foundation
The Paul Mellon Centre
The Paul Mellon Estate
The Mercers' Company
Margaret and Richard Merrell
 Foundation
The Millichope Foundation
The Mondriaan Foundation
The Monument Trust
The Henry Moore Foundation
The Mulberry Trust
The J Y Nelson Charitable
 Trust
The Old Broad Street Charity
 Trust
The Peacock Charitable Trust
The Pennycress Trust
PF Charitable Trust
The Stanley Picker Charitable
 Trust
The Pidem Fund
The Edith and Ferdinand
 Porjes Charitable Trust
Mr and Mrs J A Pye's
 Charitable Settlement
Rayne Foundation
The Reed Foundation
T Rippon & Sons (Holdings)
 Ltd
Rootstein Hopkins
 Foundation
The Rose Foundation
Schroder Charity Trust
The Sellars Charitable Trust
The Archie Sherman
 Charitable Trust
Paul Smith and Pauline
 Denyer-Smith
The South Square Trust
Spencer Charitable Trust
Oliver Stanley Charitable
 Trust
Peter Storrs Trust
Strand Parishes Trust
The Joseph Strong Frazer
 Trust
The Swan Trust
Thaw Charitable Trust
Sir Jules Thorn Charitable
 Trust
The Bruce Wake Charity
Celia Walker Art Foundation
Warburg Pincus International
 LLC
Weinstock Fund
Wilkinson Eyre Architects
The Spencer Wills Trust
The Maurice Wohl Charitable
 Foundation
The Wolfson Foundation
The Worshipful Company of
 Painter-Stainers

AMERICAN ASSOCIATES OF
THE ROYAL ACADEMY TRUST

Burlington House Trust
Mrs James C Slaughter

Benjamin West Society
Mrs Deborah Loeb Brice
Mrs Nancy B Negley

Benefactors
Mr Michael Moritz and Ms
 Harriet Heyman
Mrs Edmond J Safra
The Hon John C Whitehead

Sponsors
Mrs Drue Heinz HON DBE
David Hockney OM CH RA
Mr Arthur L Loeb
Mr and Mrs Hamish Maxwell
Mr and Mrs Richard J Miller Jr
Diane A Nixon
Ms Joan Stern
Dr and Mrs Robert D
 Wickham

Patrons
Mr and Mrs Steven Ausnit
Mr and Mrs E William
 Aylward
Mr Donald A Best
Mrs Mildred C Brinn
Mr Benjamin Coates
Lois M Collier
Mr and Mrs Stanley De Forest
 Scott
Mr and Mrs Lawrence S
 Friedland
Mr and Mrs Leslie Garfield
Ms Helen Harting Abell
Dr Bruce C Horten
Mr William W Karatz
The Hon Eugene A Ludwig
 and Dr Carol Ludwig
Miss Lucy F McGrath
Mr and Mrs Wilson Nolen
Mrs Mary Sharp Cronson
Ms Louisa Stude Sarofim
Martin J Sullivan OBE
Mr Robert W Wilson

Donors
Mr James C Armstrong
Ms Naja Armstrong
Laura Blanco
Mr Constantin R Boden
Dr and Mrs Robert Bookchin
Laura Christman and William
 Rothacker
Ms Alyce Faye Cleese
Mr Richard C Colyear
Mr and Mrs Howard Davis
Ms Zita Davisson
Mr Gerry Dolezar
Ms Maria Garvey Dowd
Ms Beverley C Duer
Mrs June Dyson
Mr Robert H Enslow
Mrs Katherine D Findlay
Mr and Mrs Gordon P Getty
Mr and Mrs Ellis Goodman
Mr Oliver R Grace
Sir Jeremy and Lady
 Greenstock
Mr and Mrs Gustave M
 Hauser
Mrs Judith Heath
Ms Elaine Kend
Mr and Mrs Nicholas L S
 Kirkbride
Ms Joanna M Lawrence
The Hon Samuel K Lessey Jr
Mr Henry S Lynn Jr
Ms Clare E McKeon
Ms Christine Mainwaring-
 Samwell
Ms Barbara T Missett

The Hon and Mrs William A Nitze
Mrs Charles W Olson III
Ms Jennifer Pellegrino
Cynthia Hazen Polsky and Leon B Polsky
Ms Wendy Reilly
Donna Rich
Mr and Mrs Daniel Rose
Mrs Nanette Ross
Mrs Martin Slifka
Mr Albert H Small
Mr and Mrs Morton I Sosland
Mrs Frederick M Stafford
Mr and Mrs Alfred Taubman
Ms Evelyn Tompkins
Mr Peter Trippi
Mrs Judith Villard
Ms Lucy Waring

Corporate and Foundation Support
American Express Foundation
The Blackstone Charitable Foundation
British Airways PLC
The Brown Foundation
Crankstart Foundation
Fortnum & Mason
Gibson, Dunn & Crutcher
The Horace W Goldsmith Foundation
Hauser Foundation
Kress Foundation
Leon Levy Foundation
Loeb Foundation
Henry Luce Foundation
Lynberg & Watkins
Edmond J Safra Philanthropic Foundation
Siezen Foundation
Sony Corporation of America
Starr Foundation
Thaw Charitable Trust

CORPORATE MEMBERS OF THE ROYAL ACADEMY

Launched in 1988, the Royal Academy's Corporate Membership Scheme has proved highly successful. Corporate membership offers benefits for staff, clients and community partners and access to the Academy's facilities and resources. The outstanding support we receive from companies via the scheme is vital to the continuing success of the Academy and we thank all members for their valuable support and continued enthusiasm.

Premier Level Members
American Express®
Barclays plc
Bird & Bird LLP
BNY Mellon
Catlin Group Limited
CBRE
Christie's
Deutsche Bank AG
FTI Consulting
GlaxoSmithKline plc
Insight Investment
JM Finn & Co.
Jones Lang LaSalle
JTI
KPMG
Linklaters
Neptune Investment Management
Schroders Private Banking

Smith & Williamson
Sotheby's

Corporate Members
The Boston Consulting Group UK LLP
British American Tobacco
Brunswick
Capital International Limited
Chesterton Humberts
F & C Asset Management plc
GAM
Lazard
Lindsell Train
Marie Curie
Moelis & Company
Oracle Capital Group
The Royal Society of Chemistry
Tanya Baxter Contemporary
Tiffany & Co.
Trowers & Hamlins
UBS
Weil, Gotshal & Manges

Associate
Bank of America Merrill Lynch
Bloomberg LP
BNP Paribas
Bonhams 1793 Ltd
Clifford Chance LLP
Credit Agricole CIB
DONG Energy
EY
Generation Investment Management LLP
Heidrick & Struggles
John Lewis Partnership
Lubbock Fine
Morgan Stanley
Pentland Group plc
Rio Tinto
Sykes & Son Limited
Timothy Sammons Fine Art Agents

Supporters of Past Exhibitions
The President and Council of the Royal Academy would like to thank the following supporters and benefactors for their generous contributions towards major exhibitions in the last ten years:

2013
Bill Woodrow RA
2009–2013 Season supported by JTI
The Henry Moore Foundation
Daumier
2009–2013 Season supported by JTI
Australia
National Gallery of Australia
Qantas Airways
The Woolmark Company
Richard Rogers RA: Inside Out
Ferrovial Agroman
Heathrow
Laing O'Rourke
Mexico: A Revolution in Art, 1910–1940
2009–2013 Season supported by JTI
Art Mentor Foundation Lucerne
Conaculta
James and Clare Kirkman
Mexican Agency for International Development Cooperation
Catherine and Franck Petitgas
Sectur
Visit Mexico
Mercedes Zobel

245th Summer Exhibition
Insight Investment
George Bellows
2009–2013 Season supported by JTI
Edwards Wildman
Premiums 2013, RA Schools Annual Dinner and Auction and RA Schools Show 2013
Newton Investment Management
Manet: Portraying Life
BNY Mellon, Partner of the Royal Academy of Arts

2012
Mariko Mori
JTI
RA Now
JTI
Bronze
Christian Levett and Mougins Museum of Classical Art
Daniel Katz Gallery
Baron Lorne Thyssen-Bornemisza
John and Fausta Eskenazi
The Ruddock Foundation for the Arts
Tomasso Brothers Fine Art
Jon and Barbara Landau
Janine and J. Tomlison Hill
Embassy of the Kingdom of the Netherlands
Eskenazi Limited
Lisson Gallery
Alexis Gregory
Alan and Mary Hobart
Richard de Unger and Adeela Qureshi
Rossi & Rossi Ltd
Embassy of Israel
244th Summer Exhibition
Insight Investment
From Paris: A Taste for Impressionism – Paintings from the Clark
2009–2013 Season supported by JTI
Edwards Wildman
The Annenberg Foundation
Premiums, RA Schools Annual Dinner and Auction and RA Schools Show 2012
Newton Investment Management
Johan Zoffany RA: Society Observed
2009–2013 Season supported by JTI
Cox & Kings
Building the Revolution: Soviet Art and Architecture 1915–1935
2009–2013 Season supported by JTI
The Ove Arup Foundation
The Norman Foster Foundation
Richard and Ruth Rogers
David Hockney RA: A Bigger Picture
BNP Paribas
Welcome to Yorkshire: Tourism Partner
Visit Hull & East Yorkshire: Supporting Tourism Partner
NEC

2011
Degas and the Ballet: Picturing Movement
BNY Mellon
Region Holdings
Blavatnik Family Foundation
Eyewitness: Hungarian Photography in the Twentieth Century. Brassaï, Capa,

Kertész, Moholy-Nagy, Munkácsi
2009–2013 Season supported by JTI
Hungarofest
OTP Bank
243rd Summer Exhibition
Insight Investment
Premiums, RA Schools Annual Dinner and Auction and RA Schools Show 2011
Newton Investment Management
Watteau: The Drawings
2009–2013 Season supported by JTI
Region Holdings
Modern British Sculpture
American Express Foundation
The Henry Moore Foundation
Hauser & Wirth
Art Mentor Foundation Lucerne
Sotheby's
Blain Southern
Welcome to Yorkshire: Tourism Partner

2010
GSK Contemporary – Aware: Art Fashion Identity
GlaxoSmithKline
Pioneering Painters: The Glasgow Boys 1880–1900
2009–2013 Season supported by JTI
Glasgow Museums
Treasures from Budapest: European Masterpieces from Leonardo to Schiele
OTP Bank
Villa Budapest
Daniel Katz Gallery, London
Cox & Kings: Travel Partner
Sargent and the Sea
2009–2013 Season supported by JTI
242nd Summer Exhibition
Insight Investment
Paul Sandby RA: Picturing Britain, A Bicentenary Exhibition
2009–2013 Season supported by JTI
The Real Van Gogh: The Artist and His Letters
BNY Mellon
Hiscox
Heath Lambert
Cox & Kings: Travel Partner
RA Outreach Programme
Deutsche Bank AG

2009
GSK Contemporary
GlaxoSmithKline
Wild Thing: Epstein, Gaudier-Brzeska, Gill
2009–2013 Season supported by JTI
BNP Paribas
The Henry Moore Foundation
Anish Kapoor
JTI
Richard Chang
Richard and Victoria Sharp
Louis Vuitton
The Henry Moore Foundation
J W Waterhouse: The Modern Pre-Raphaelite
2009–2013 Season supported by JTI
Champagne Perrier-Jouët
GasTerra
Gasunie
241st Summer Exhibition
Insight Investment

Kuniyoshi. From the Arthur R. Miller Collection
2009–2013 Season supported by JTI
Canon
Cox & Kings: Travel Partner
Premiums and RA Schools Show
Mizuho International plc
RA Outreach Programme
Deutsche Bank AG

2008
GSK Contemporary
GlaxoSmithKline
Byzantium 330–1453
J F Costopoulos Foundation
A G Leventis Foundation
Stavros Niarchos Foundation
Cox & Kings: Travel Partner
Miró, Calder, Giacometti, Braque: Aimé Maeght and His Artists
BNP Paribas
Vilhelm Hammershøi: The Poetry of Silence
OAK Foundation Denmark
Novo Nordisk
240th Summer Exhibition
Insight Investment
Premiums and RA Schools Show
Mizuho International plc
RA Outreach Programme
Deutsche Bank AG
From Russia: French and Russian Master Paintings 1870–1925 from Moscow and St Petersburg
E.ON
2008 Season supported by Sotheby's

2007
Paul Mellon's Legacy: A Passion for British Art
The Bank of New York Mellon
Georg Baselitz
Eurohypo AG
239th Summer Exhibition
Insight Investment
Impressionists by the Sea
Farrow & Ball
Premiums and RA Schools Show
Mizuho International plc
RA Outreach Programme
Deutsche Bank AG
The Unknown Monet
Bank of America

2006
238th Summer Exhibition
Insight Investment
Chola: Sacred Bronzes of Southern India
Cox & Kings: Travel Partner
Premiums and RA Schools Show
Mizuho International plc
RA Outreach Programme
Deutsche Bank AG
Rodin
Ernst & Young

2005
China: The Three Emperors, 1662–1795
Goldman Sachs International
Impressionism Abroad: Boston and French Painting
Fidelity Foundation
Matisse, His Art and His Textiles: The Fabric of Dreams
Farrow & Ball
Premiums and RA Schools Show
The Guardian
Mizuho International plc
Turks: A Journey of a Thousand Years, 600–1600

Akkök Group of Companies
Aygaz
Corus
Garanti Bank
Lassa Tyres

2004
236th Summer Exhibition
A T Kearney
Ancient Art to Post-Impressionism: Masterpieces from the Ny Carlsberg Glyptotek, Copenhagen
Carlsberg UK Ltd
Danske Bank
Novo Nordisk
The Art of Philip Guston (1913–1980)
American Associates of the Royal Academy Trust
The Art of William Nicholson
RA Exhibition Patrons Group
Vuillard: From Post-Impressionist to Modern Master
RA Exhibition Patrons Group

Other Supporters
Sponsors of events, publications and other items in the past five years:

Carlisle Group plc
Castello di Reschio
Cecilia Chan
Country Life
Guy Dawson
Derwent Valley Holdings plc
Dresdner Kleinwort Wasserstein
Lucy Flemming McGrath
Foster and Partners
Goldman Sachs International
Gome International
Gucci Group
Hines
IBJ International plc
John Doyle Construction
Harvey and Allison McGrath
Martin Krajewski
Marks & Spencer
Michael Hopkins & Partners
Morgan Stanley Dean Witter
The National Trust
Prada
Radisson Edwardian Hotels
Richard and Ruth Rogers
Rob van Helden
The Wine Studio

Our World

Weather

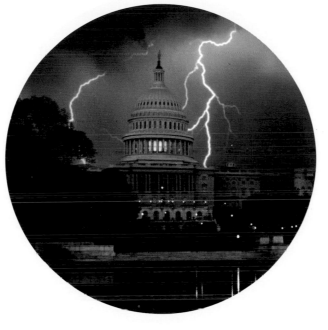

Neil Morris

Thameside Press

Distributed in the United States by
Smart Apple Media
1980 Lookout Drive
North Mankato, MN 56003

Text copyright © Neil Morris 2002

Printed in Hong Kong

ISBN 1-930643-76-4

Library of Congress Control Number 2002 141327

Series editor: Jean Coppendale
Designer: Peter Clayman
Artwork: Chris Forsey
Picture researcher: Terry Forshaw, Jenny Barlow and Ashley Brent
Consultant: Bethan Currenti

Printed in Hong Kong

10 9 8 7 6 5 4 3 2 1

Picture acknowledgments:
(T) = Top, (B) = Bottom, (L) = Left, (R) = Right.

B = Bubbles, C = Corbis, CI = Chrysalis Images, CO = Collections, DV = Digital Vision, E = Ecoscene,
FLPA = Frank Lane Picture Agency, GI = Getty Images, SP = Still Pictures, SPL = Science Photo Library.

Front cover (main) & 19 Jim Zuckerman/C; title page & 24 (B) Craig Aurness/C; 4 Anthony
Dawton/B; 5 Randy Faris/C; 6 (T) Ecoscene/C, (B) Michael Pole/C; 7 (T) Tony Arruza/C, (B) Julie
Habel/C; 8 DV; 9 Jonathan Smith, Cordaiy Photo Library Ltd/C; 10 (L) Bob Witkowski/C, (R) & back
cover (R) Brian A. Vikander/C; 11 Gil Moti/SP; 12 Danny Lehman/C; 13 Gaetan Charbonneau/GI; 14
(L) & 31 (L) Chris Carroll/C, (R) & front cover (inset) Robert Pickett/C; 15 Tom Brakefield/C; 16
Robert Landau/C; 17 (T) & back cover (L) Jean-Pierre Lescouret/C, (B) Morton Beebe S.F/C; 18 (T) &
front cover (inset) Reuters 1999, (B) Stephanie Maze/C; 20 University of Dundee/SPL; 21 & front
cover (inset) Lesley Howling/CO; 22 (T) & 31 (R) Angela Hampton/CO, (B) Anthony T.
Mathews/FLPA; 23 Ecoscene/C; 24 (T) & front cover (inset) Craig Aurness/C; 25 John Tinning/FLPA;
26 Wolfgang Kaehler/C; 27 John Watkins/FLPA.

Contents

All sorts of weather

Weather is made up of sunshine, rain, wind, and **snow**. It plays a big part in our lives. When it is hot and sunny, we wear light clothes to keep cool. But if it is cold and wet, we wrap up warm.

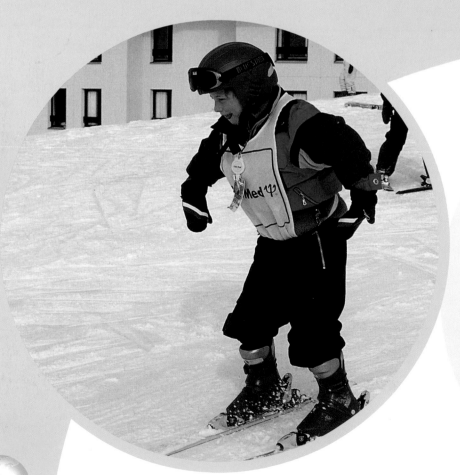

It can be difficult to move around on snow. But learning to ski means you can get about easily

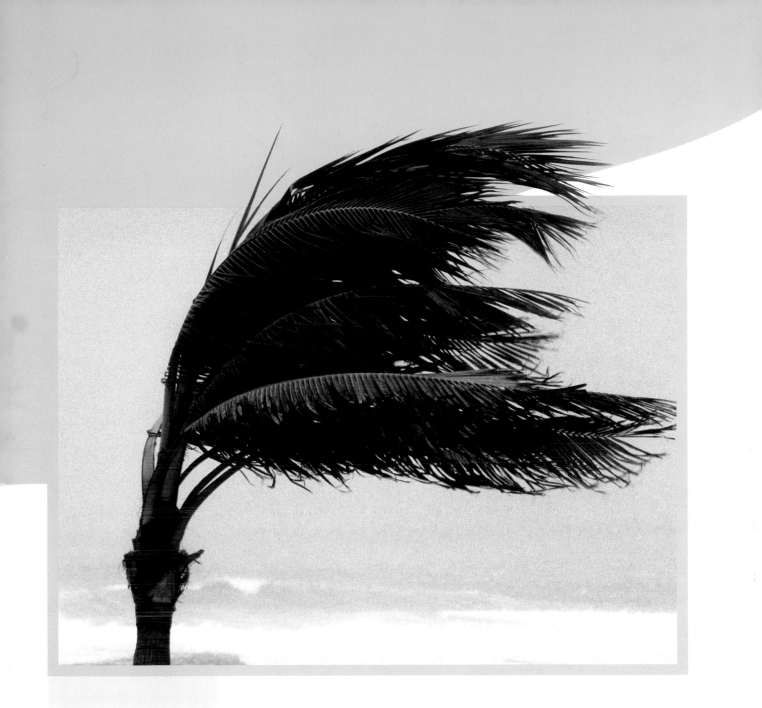

The air around
us moves about
all the time.
We notice it
especially
when it's
very windy.

All the world's weather happens
because of the way air moves
about. Water also changes in the air,
making **clouds**, rain, **fog**, and snow.

Four seasons

Most places in the world have a particular kind of weather at certain times in the year. We call these times seasons. There are four **seasons**—spring, summer, fall, and winter.

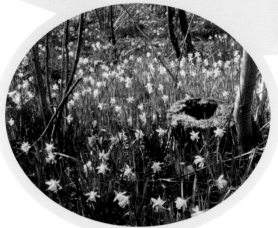

In spring, many plants start to grow as the days become warmer.

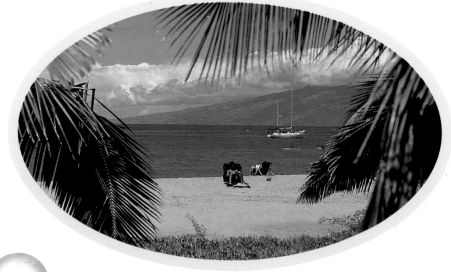

Summer days are long and hot. This is a good time to go to the beach on vacation.

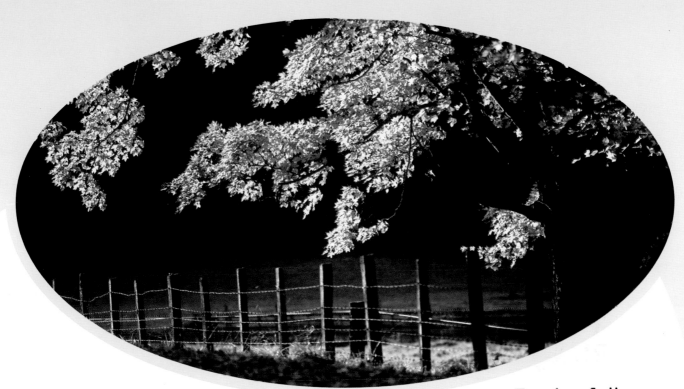

In summer it is usually hot and dry, but in winter it is cold and wet. Spring and fall have weather that is somewhere in between.

In the fall the leaves on many trees change color. Soon the leaves will fall to the ground.

In winter we can have fun playing in the snow.

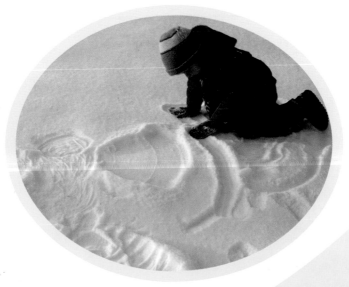

Cloudy days

All clouds are made of billions of tiny water droplets. The water comes from a gas called **water vapor**, which turns into liquid as it rises in the sky and cools down.

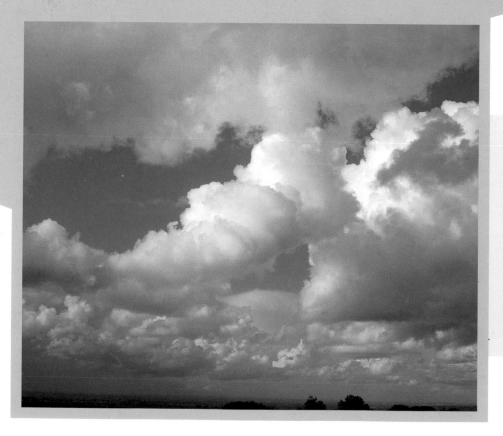

Clouds come in many different shapes and sizes. Some fluffy clouds look like cotton puffs.

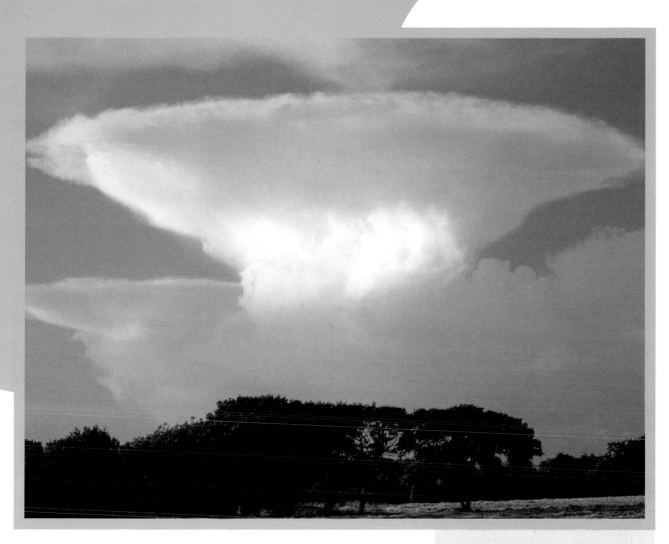

Clouds are so light that they float in the sky and get blown along by the wind. You can watch white, fluffy clouds move across the blue sky on a bright day.

This cloud is called an anvil or thundercloud. Storm clouds like this mean that heavy rain is on the way.

It's raining

If it goes on raining for too long, rivers can overflow and flood the land.

When the sun shines through raindrops, we sometimes see a rainbow.

Sometimes the water droplets in clouds join together. They get so heavy that they cannot go on floating in the sky. Then the droplets fall from the clouds to the ground. That's when we say, "It's raining!"

Some **showers** of rain don't last very long, as clouds are blown along by the wind. But some parts of the world have a wet season. Then it pours with rain every day.

In some countries the wet season can last for weeks or even months. Then floods are common.

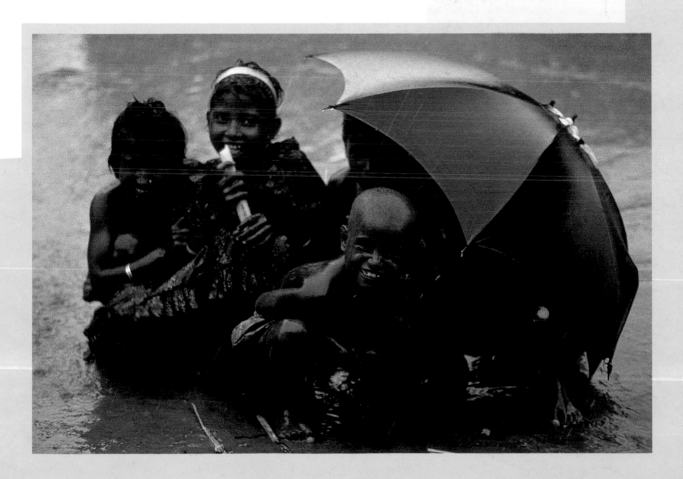

Mist and fog

In the countryside, water vapor rises from wet soil. If the air is cool, the vapor changes back to water droplets and makes fog.

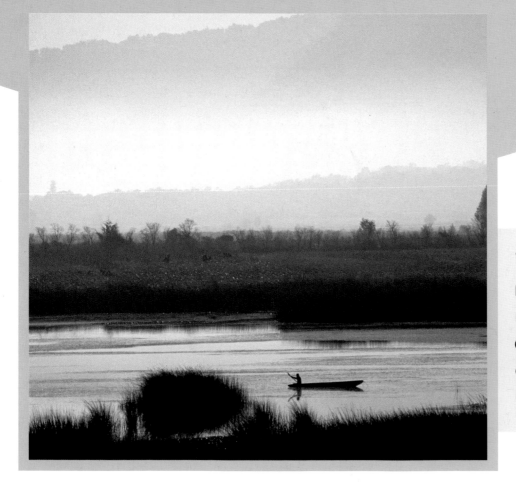

When warm rain falls into cooler air below, it can also turn into fog.

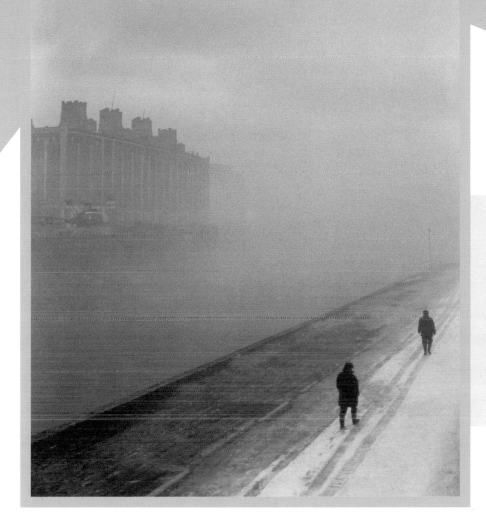

Water droplets gather around tiny specks of dust. This can sometimes cause thick fog in the city.

In a really thick fog you can hardly see your hand in front of your face. **Mist** is a thinner form of fog, with fewer water droplets. It usually clings close to the ground or the surface of the sea.

Snow and ice

High in the sky, the air is freezing cold, and clouds are made of tiny **ice crystals**. Sometimes these fall as snowflakes and cover the ground in a white blanket of snow.

A snowflake seen under a microscope. Snowflakes are all different shapes, but they always have six sides or points.

Everyone loves throwing snowballs. But no one likes being hit!

Swans and ducks have to wait for the ice to melt before they can swim again in their favorite pond. During the freeze, they are short of food.

When it is very cold on the ground, water freezes into solid **ice**. Then ponds and lakes freeze over.

Windy days

Wind is air on the move. When air warms up, it gets lighter and rises up in the sky. Cooler air moves in to take its place, and when that happens, you can feel a breeze.

Gentle breezes and stronger winds can be very useful to us.

It's exciting to watch a kite darting in the wind.

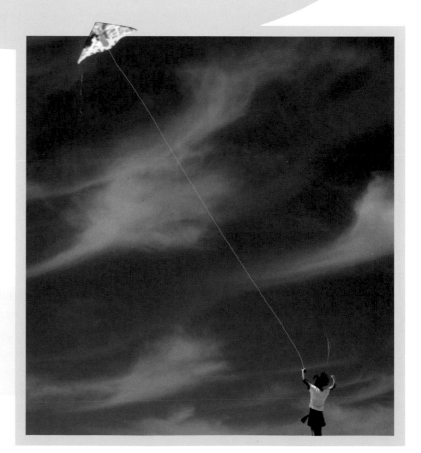

The sails of the windmills are pushed around by the wind. Then they turn wheels inside.

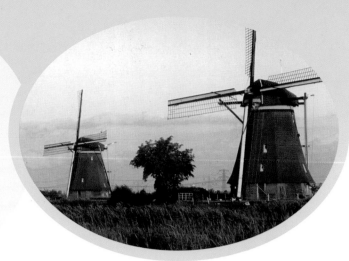

A row of modern windmills form a wind farm. They make electricity to light and heat people's homes.

The turning sails of windmills used to help people grind grain. Today, they are used to make electricity.

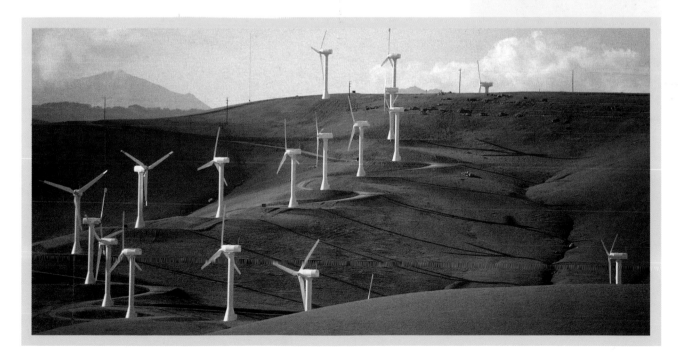

Danger!

Very strong winds can do great damage to people's homes. The most powerful, whirling storms are called **hurricanes**. They start over warm oceans and bring heavy rain and high waves to the coast.

The clouds of a hurricane spin around a small calm area, called the eye.

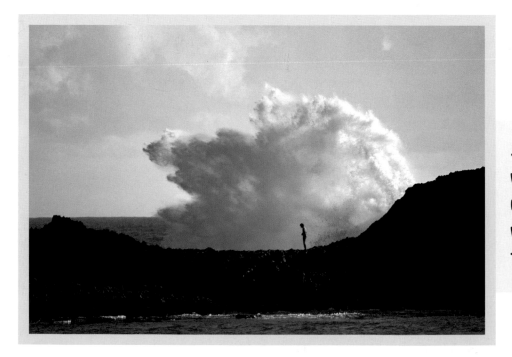

Storm winds whip up ocean waves near the coast.

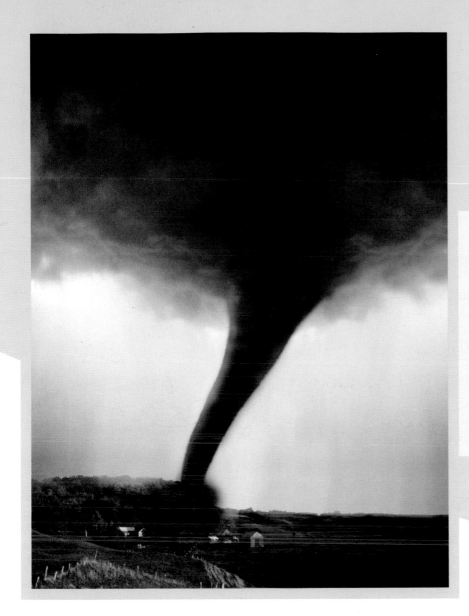

A tornado, or twister, hangs down from a dark thundercloud. It is one of the most frightening and most powerful winds.

Tornadoes are smaller than hurricanes, but their winds can be even stronger. These spinning whirlwinds suck up dust and dirt. They sometimes even pick up and destroy cars and houses.

Highs and lows

The blanket of air that surrounds our planet is called the **atmosphere**. It may not feel like it to us, but air has weight. It presses down on Earth, and this **air pressure** is always changing in different places. This brings changes to the weather.

Weather maps show areas of high and low pressure.

You will often
see a beautiful
red sunset after
a warm, calm day
in summer.

An area of high
pressure usually means
fine and sunny weather.
Low pressure normally
brings clouds and rain.

Sunny and hot

On a cloudy day, we sometimes say that the sun has "gone in." We mean that it is hidden behind the clouds. But the sun is always there, shining on the Earth and giving it heat and energy.

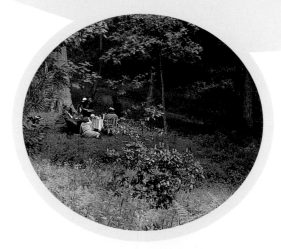

It's best to sit in the shade when it's sunny and hot.

The sun's energy warms up the sea as well as the land.

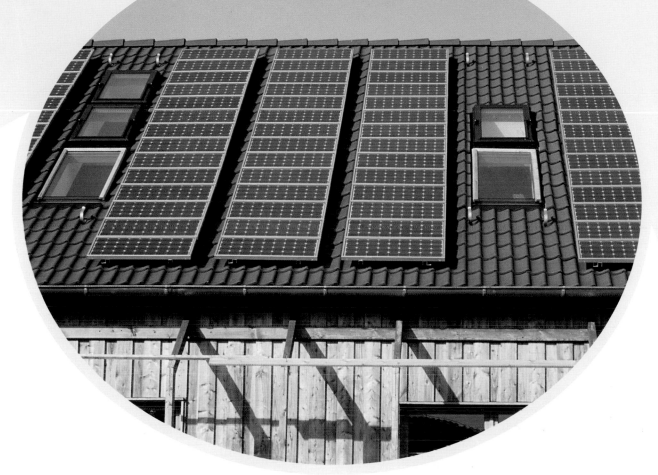

In summer, high pressure brings clear skies and only light breezes. Then the weather is sunny and hot. Places with lots of weather like this are popular for vacations.

We can also use the sun's energy to make electricity. This can heat homes and even run cars.

Thunder and lightning

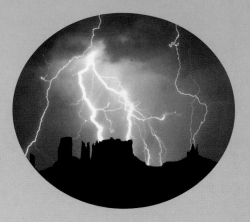

Strong winds can make water droplets and frozen **hailstones** crash into each other. These crashes create electricity, which flashes through the sky as **lightning**.

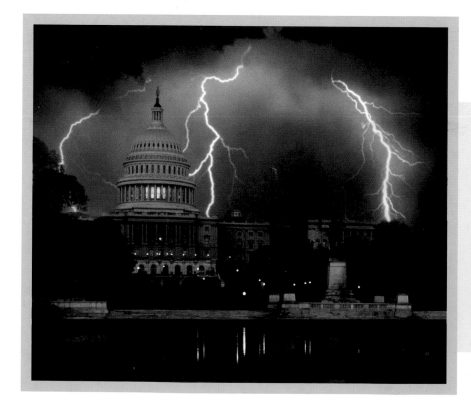

During a thunderstorm sparks jump from cloud to cloud. Some of the lightning flashes right down to the ground.

Lightning heats the surrounding air so quickly that it makes the loud, booming noise of **thunder**. Sound travels much slower than light, so we always hear the thunder after we've seen the lightning.

Metal **lightning rods** are fitted to some tall buildings. They direct lightning harmlessly down to the ground.

Weather forecast

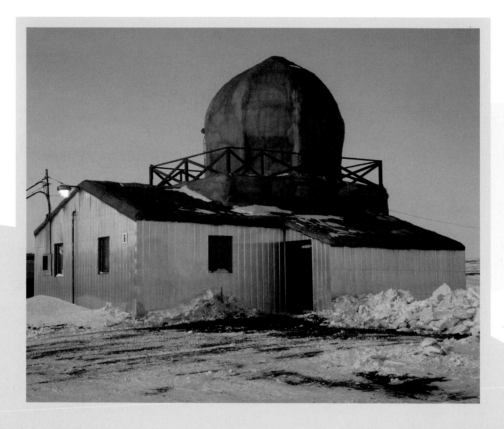

This weather station sends information to a national weather center.

There are thousands of weather stations all over the world. In these stations scientists called **meteorologists** measure rainfall, hours of sunshine, **temperature**, air pressure, wind speed, and other facts about the local weather.

Forecasters use this information and study **satellite photographs** of the Earth. Computers help them to make maps that show what the weather will be like in the next few hours, days, or weeks. But they are not always right!

Weather presenters use maps with simple symbols to show sun, cloud, and rain.

Do it yourself

Make a rain gauge

1 Ask an adult to cut the top off a clear plastic bottle with scissors. Turn the top upside down to make a funnel, and rest it inside the bottle. Seal the two parts with tape.

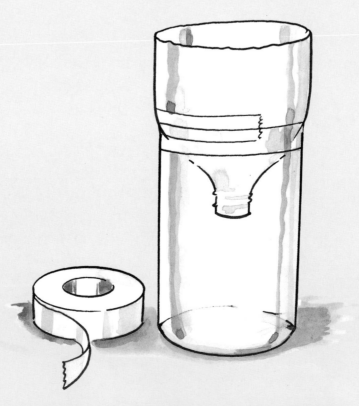

2 Use a ruler to mark off about 2.5 inches on a thin strip of paper. Stick this scale on the side of the bottle.

3 Put your rain gauge outside in a heavy flowerpot, so it won't blow over. You can check the amount of rain that falls every day—or once a week—and make your own rainfall chart.

Remember to empty the gauge after you have taken your reading.

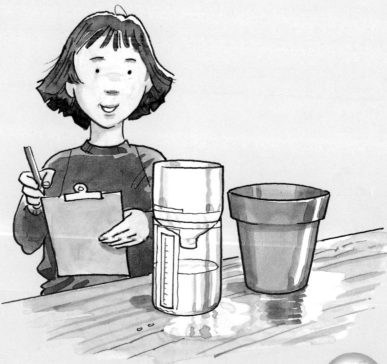

Glossary

air pressure The weight of the atmosphere pressing down on the Earth.

atmosphere The layer of air that surrounds the Earth.

breeze A very light, gentle wind.

clouds Groups of water droplets floating in the sky.

fog A thick cloud of water droplets near the ground.

forecasters People who tell us what the weather is going to be like.

hailstones Pieces of ice that fall from the sky.

hurricanes Violent, whirling storms.

ice Frozen water.

ice crystals Tiny particles of frozen water.

lightning An electrical spark that jumps between clouds or from a cloud to the ground.

lightning rods Metal rods fixed on buildings to stop them from being damaged by lightning.

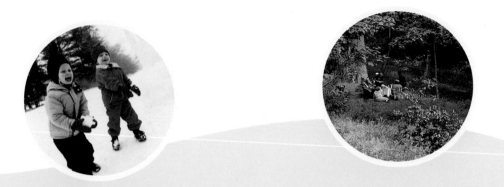

meteorologists Scientists who study the weather.

mist A thin form of fog.

rain Liquid drops of water that fall from the sky.

satellite photographs Photographs taken from satellites traveling in space above the Earth.

seasons The four parts of the year with their own patterns of weather.

showers Light falls of rain that do not last very long.

snow Ice crystals that fall from the sky.

temperature How hot or cold it is.

thunder The booming sound made by a lightning flash.

tornadoes Powerful, twisting whirlwinds.

water vapor Water when it has become a gas that floats in the air.

index

African
Mythology

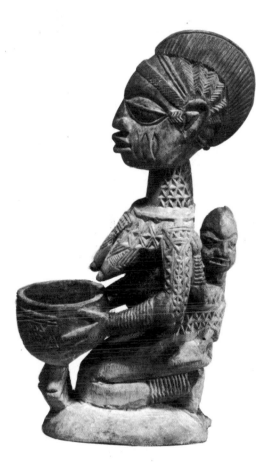

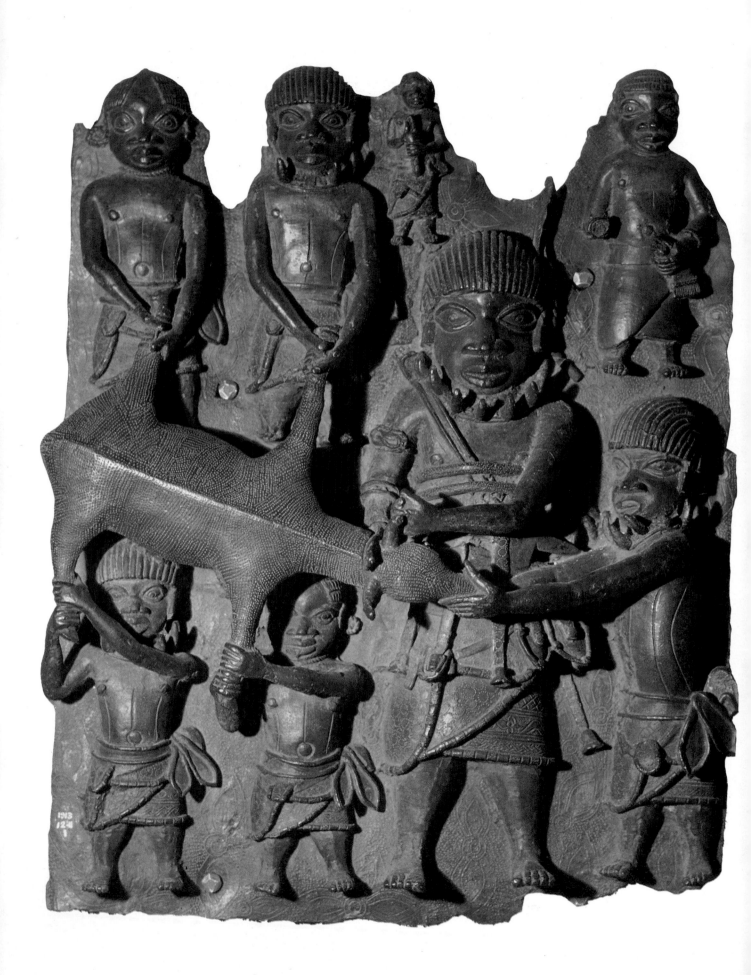

LIBRARY OF THE WORLD'S
MYTHS AND LEGENDS

African
Mythology

Geoffrey Parrinder

HAMLYN

London · New York · Sydney · Toronto

Half-title page. Yoruba vessel for holding
the seeds used in divination ceremonies.

Frontispiece.   Bronze from Benin,
Nigeria, depicting the sacrifice of a cow at
a family altar.

African Mythology first published 1967.
New revised edition published 1982 by
The Hamlyn Publishing Group Limited
London · New York · Sydney · Toronto
Astronaut House, Hounslow Road,
Feltham, Middlesex, England.

ISBN 0 600 34279 4

Printed in Italy

Contents

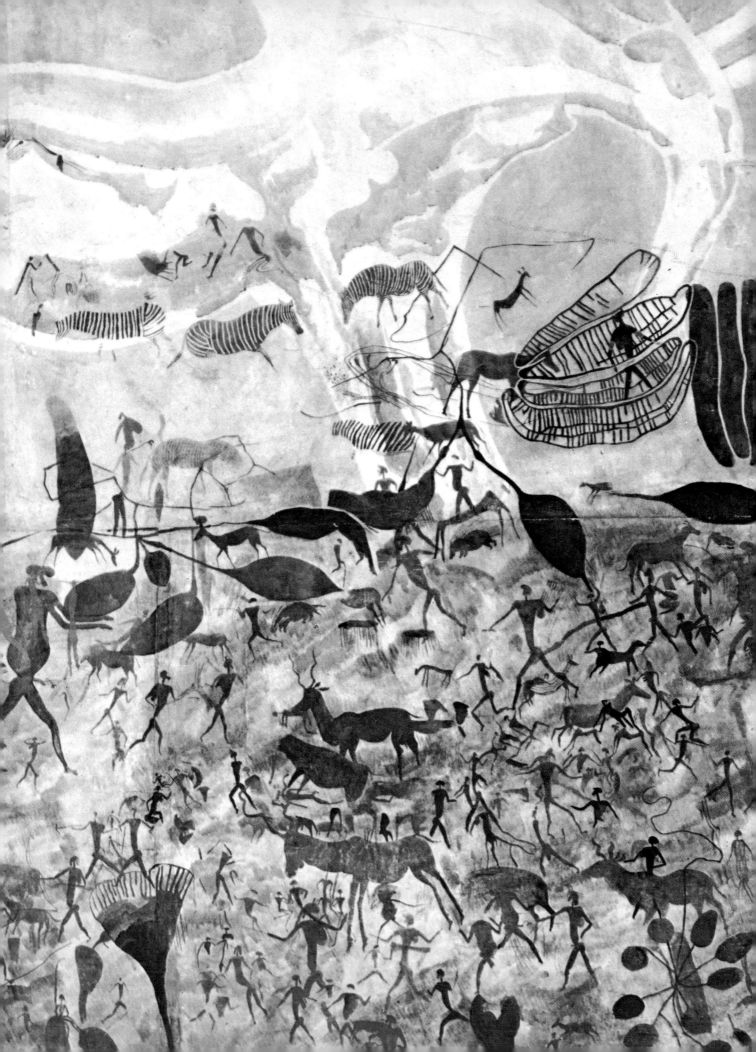

Introduction

New and Old Africa

'There is always something new from Africa,' said the Roman writer Pliny. The emergence of many African nation states in the last few decades brings news of this continent frequently to the front pages of the newspapers. But Africa's traditions are as ancient as any, and some of the oldest forms of human life have recently been discovered in the Great Rift Valley in East Africa. There are still races of Pygmies and Bushmen surviving from ancient times. And behind modern political doctrines there are countless myths and stories which form part of the background to the thinking of African peoples.

Africa is a vast continent, but it divides naturally into two major parts. North Africa, from Egypt to Morocco, and down the river Nile to Ethiopia, belongs mostly to the Mediterranean world, and its dominant religions are Islam and Christianity, with their own thought and story. The Sahara Desert and the tropical forests formed an almost impenetrable barrier to Europeans seeking knowledge of the rest of Africa, until the Portuguese braved the seas and rounded the Cape of Good Hope at the end of the fifteenth century.

Africa south of the Sahara is what Arab geographers called Bilad-as-Sudan, the Land of the Black People. That is what it is from the east and west Sudan, through the tropical and equatorial regions, right down into South Africa. Here black people form the overwhelming majority of the population. It is their mythology that is now to be described.

The Races of Africa

'Black' is a relative term and there is no such thing as a coal black person, any more than there exists a fully white person. There is great variety of shades of colour, height, shape, face and body characteristics, and Africans themselves distinguish between light and dark skinned people in their own communities. The Negro (black) person is roughly described by dark skin, woolly hair, and broad nose. Most Africans are Negroes. The name Bantu is often given to the Negroes of East and South Africa, but it refers to their languages and not to their race.

Small groups of African peoples distinguishable from the great mass of Negroes are Bushmen, Pygmies and Hamites. The Bushmen, including Hottentots, are short in height but not pygmy, with yellowish-brown skin. They travelled down Africa many centuries ago, leaving traces in rock paintings, and were at the Cape when the first Europeans arrived. Now only about fifty thousand of them remain, mostly living by hunting and rearing cattle.

The Pygmies or Negritos of the River Congo forest regions are very short, between 52 to 58 inches (130-140 cm), with broad heads and noses, and they probably come from an early racial type distinct from the

Opposite. Rock paintings are found in many parts of Africa and this lavish example from Mtoko Cave, Zimbabwe, is attributed to the Bushmen who were once here. Large elephants and other animals are easily recognisable but human figures are stylised without clear faces, which suggests that the painters only aimed at helping the chase of animals by magical means. Animals play many roles in African story and this picture is crowded with them, suggesting the flourishing wild life which is chiefly seen in certain reserves and game parks today. Frobenius-Institut, Frankfurt am Main.

Negroes. The Hamites are generally light-skinned, though often mixed with Negro blood, and are related to Europeans. They are found in North Africa and Ethiopia, in the Sahara and parts of the Sudan. Their mythology is strongly influenced by Islamic and Arabic story.

In South Africa there are millions of people of European descent, Coloured people from the mingling of races, and Indians. Their mythology is European or Asian and beyond the scope of this book.

The great island of Malagasy (Madagascar), larger than France and the Low Countries together, is inhabited by a mixed population of which the majority is of Malaysian origin, but other groups are more clearly Negro. The language is Malay-Polynesian, with influences from India, Arabia, and African Bantu and Swahili tongues. A few Malagasy myths are included here which, although different from much African mythology, often deal with similar themes.

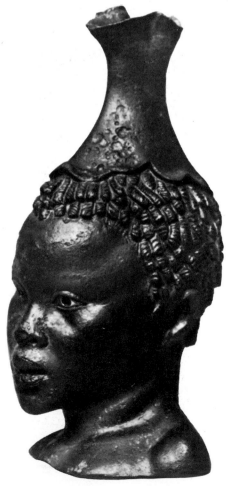

The great majority of all Africans are Negroes, one of the oldest races in the continent. Some of them have been influenced by Hamite blood and culture, and even in the past centuries of isolation there was intermingling in East Africa, a few thin caravan routes across the desert, and some movement round the western coastline. So some African myths resemble stories told in other parts of the world, while there are purely African myths which are found in parts of Africa thousands of miles away from one another.

Myth and Literature

The mythologies of Greece or India are drawn from vast literatures, based on oral stories which were written down and preserved through the centuries in many books. To enjoy the myths one only has to read the books. But in the study of African mythology a great obstacle is met at once. There are no ancient books. There are innumerable stories, for like all races of men Africans loved telling tales. But these were not written down until modern times, and collections are still very incomplete.

The simple reason for this state of affairs is that the art of writing was quite unknown to Africans in the tropical forests and the south. This was due, not to any African inability, but simply to geographical isolation. Desert, forest and sea were effective barriers to the spread of written culture until modern times. The few trade routes took goods or slaves, but little else. From the eleventh century A.D. Moslem missionaries came down the Nile, and round the west coast, and entered the Sudan, taking writing to converts to Islam. But neither the religion nor the writing penetrated the tropical forests, whose people had to wait for written culture till the nineteenth century.

The art of writing is not a common invention. The ancient Britons and Teutonic peoples knew nothing of it, and had to be taught by missionaries from the Mediterranean world. The people of the ancient civilisations of America, Aztecs, Incas and Mayas, built great palaces and temples, but

had no writing. In fact most forms of writing derive from one of two sources: the alphabetic scripts of the Near East, and the syllable writing of China.

Since there are no ancient written collections of African myths, the first modern collections were made by Europeans and Americans, writing down what Africans have told them. Educated Africans also have now started to record the myths of their own people, before it is too late and they disappear or change. The myths given in this book come from recent collections, made by highly qualified writers, who try to present faithfully the stories told to them by old and young Africans.

The Language of Art

Although there was no writing in ancient Africa, there were still means of expression through which Africans themselves recorded their thoughts, their beliefs, and their feelings. These were transmitted in the many and very various forms of African art, though it is not now always easy to understand their meaning.

In this century appreciation of the power of much African art has been given by artists such as Jacob Epstein and Henry Moore, and European art has been influenced by it. African art is not often naturalistic. The famous bronze heads of Ifé in Nigeria, which recall Greek portrait sculpture, are rare. Most African art aims at expressing feeling, not by copying faces and bodies, but by emphasising muscles, power, facial character and mystery.

Since African art was the only 'writing' known in the whole of tropical Africa it was used to interpret life in every aspect. It was employed in religious life, which was not separated from other parts of life, to give spiritual meaning and function to objects used in ceremonies of the individual or the community. It was used to illustrate proverbs and express the wisdom of the people.

So African art provides a sacred literature, giving beauty and solemnity to the face of man. It is deeply expressive yet modest. There were no

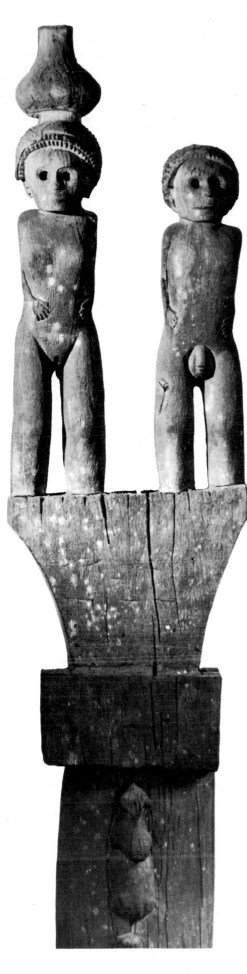

great temples defying the sky, for there was little soft stone, and no explosives to break granite rocks. African art is concerned with human life: with faces and figures showing human nature and human activities. Man and woman together, sometimes as twins, show the nucleus of the African family. Even where polygamy is practised it is the couple that is the basic unit. That man and woman depend upon each other is shown in sculpture and in mythology.

African art shows human beings in every stage of existence: birth, life and death. Motherhood shows the mystery and power of life, portrayed frankly in all parts of the female body. The mystery of death is held to be against nature, and there is a universal belief in survival and triumph over death, demonstrated by the

Opposite. A bronze head in the form of a miniature jug from the Greek culture of Alexandria. Dating from between the third and first centuries B.C., it portrays a remarkably clear representation of a young Negress, one of the race of people who lived beyond the great barriers to the south. Museum of Mankind, London.

Left. There is little sculpture beyond the Niger and the Congo basins, except in Malagasy where these grave posts of ancestors in simple and expressive form show the continuity of life. A Malagasy myth says that God saw his daughter Earth making clay images, and he blew into them to give them life, but when men and women became too numerous he took their breath away again and death came to the world. Musée de l'Homme, Paris.

Centre. Cult figure of the Mende people of Sierra Leone. These idealised and carefully decorated sculptures of women symbolise the guardian spirit of the female secret society, which prepares girls for the life they will lead as adult women. Horniman Museum, London.

Below. Ivory carving is much practised in tropical Africa. This fine example from Benin, Nigeria, may be a goddess or a simple symbol of fertility. Sculptures of African womanhood emphasise the mystery and power of life in the firmly moulded body and the calm, accepting face. Pitt Rivers Museum, Oxford.

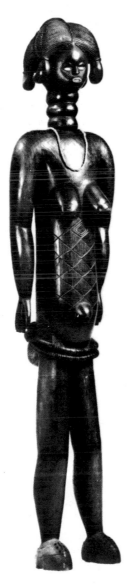

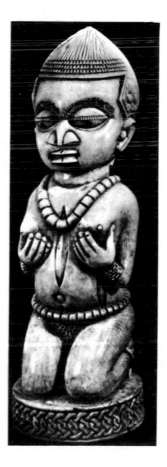

9

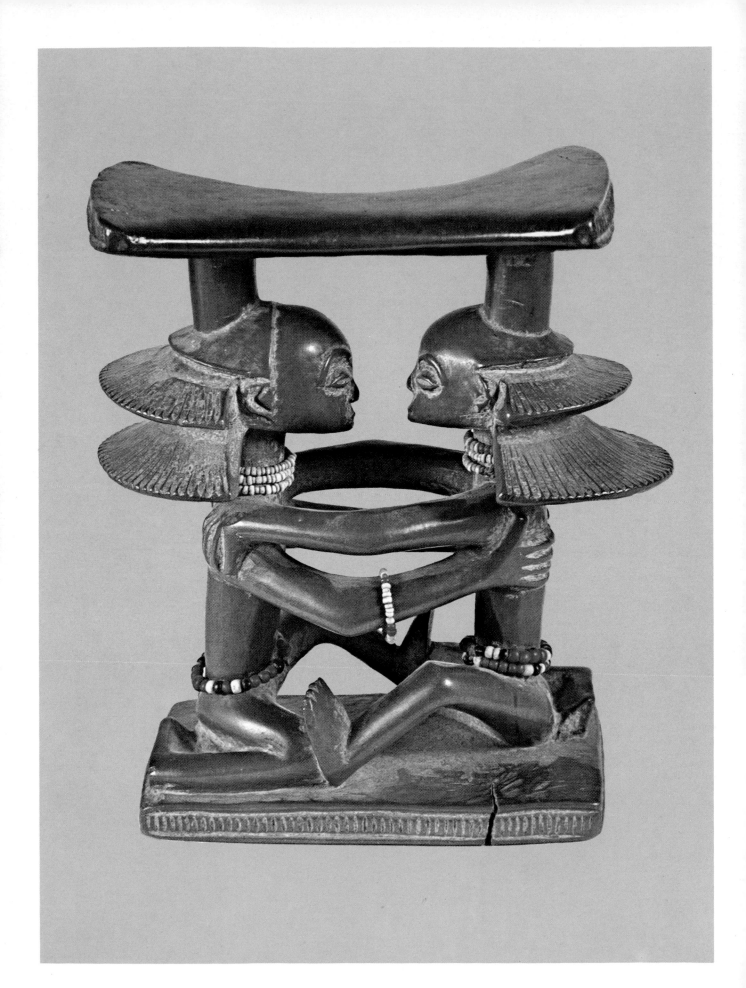

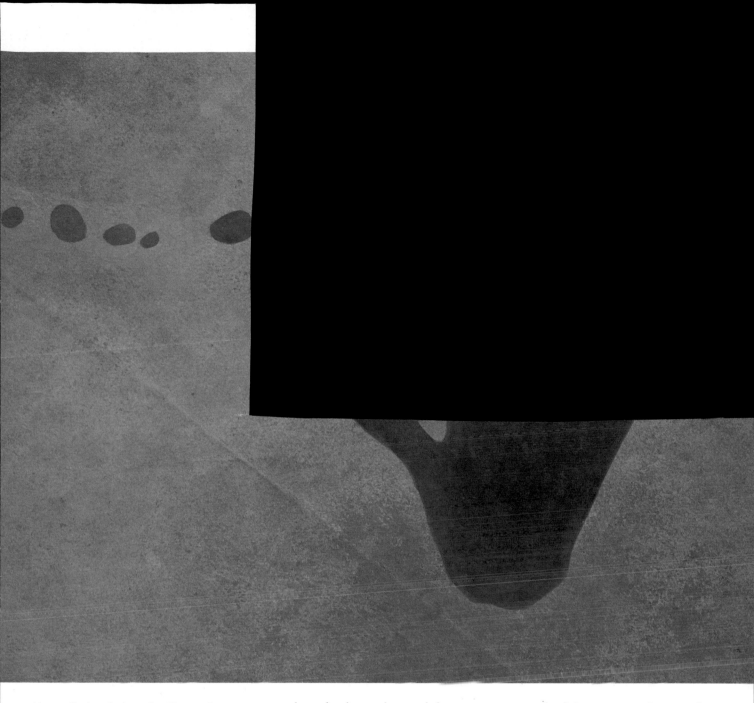

Above. Rock painting of unknown date from Zimbabwe. It resembles cave paintings in many parts of the world: the outline of a hand, dots which may indicate numbering, and a stick-like human figure. The man here is a hunter, with a spear or dart and perhaps a bow.

Opposite. The Luba of the Congo produce fine miniatures like this wooden headrest of a male and female figure facing each other, with fan-like hair styles and bead decorations. Man and woman as the basic unit of human life often appear together in African art and mythology, sometimes as twins, and show their dependence on one another. Museum of Mankind, London

countless death masks, and by societies which represent the living ancestors. The gods, powers of heaven and earth, and the ancestors are all 'clouds of witnesses' to each person's career on earth, and the providence that helps in trouble.

There is great diversity in African art, for there are innumerable racial groups and languages. One survey counted over two thousand languages and dialects in West Africa alone. But there are two extreme points of view to be avoided. One extreme thinks of all African art as the same, whether in east or west, north or south. The other extreme thinks it is all different,

composed of fragments, where each tribe is a separate universe. It is true that there was much division in the past, but there were also great Negro empires, mixture of peoples, and racial migrations. Mythology shows that there are striking similarities between far separated people. But illustrations from different countries also indicate the diversity of art and myth.

Forms of Art

One of the oldest and most widespread forms of African art is painting and engraving on the walls of cave shelters and rocks. These are found in the Sahara, Sudan, East and South

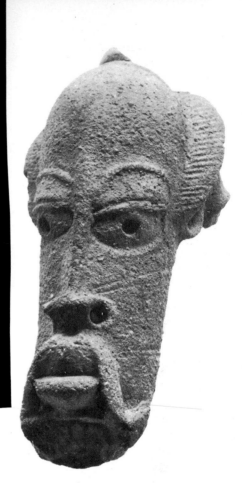

Above. Rock painting from the Brandberg Mountains in Namibia. The Bushmen were great engravers and painters on rock surfaces in red, black, yellow, white and brown. The subjects are usually hunting, fighting or dancing. The practice of the art has almost completely died out, as there are only a few thousand Bushmen left and the survivors rarely know the meaning of the designs. This is clearly a hunting scene and the central figure is called the White Lady, though no more is known about it than the colour. Musée de l'Homme, Paris.

Above right. Terracotta head from Nok, northern Nigeria. The first example was discovered in 1943, and such heads are estimated to be over two thousand years old. They are some of the most naturalistic of tropical African sculptures.

Opposite left. In Sierra Leone and Guinea many ancient soapstone or steatite figures are found. Called 'rice gods' when discovered in fields, they may represent ancestors. They are said to have an 'archaic smile' though the sculptors may not have intended this. The University Museum, Philadelphia, Pennsylvania.

Opposite centre. Portrait head of an ancestor of the Mende, Sierra Leone, made of pink soapstone.

Opposite right. A steatite figure from Sierra Leone, another rice god. Museum of Mankind, London.

Africa, more in the dry than the tropical regions. Many of the East and South African paintings were the work of Bushmen in the past. They are naturalistic, coloured, depicting cattle, wild animals, human beings, and religious figures. Some of these are hundreds, some thousands, of years old, but they are no longer made by Bushmen and so they are not of great value for interpreting mythology narrated today.

Sculpture in the round, in stone, metal or wood, has been practised for a long time in Africa and is still very much alive. It is limited in extent, however, and is found chiefly in West Africa and west Central Africa. This is perhaps partly because the people of the Niger-Congo regions have been settled agriculturalists for centuries, whereas the tribes of the east have been nomads or herdsmen.

The oldest tropical African sculptures are of the Nok culture, found in 1943 in northern Nigeria, and at least two thousand years old. They are made of baked clay, terracotta, and are mostly of human heads, either natural in style or lengthened. Since the people who made them are unknown, so are their myths and religion. But they can be compared with naturalistic terracottas and bronzes that were made over a thousand years later some hundreds of miles farther south in Nigeria. The Ifé bronzes, and related Benin bronzes, gave illustrations of human and royal activities.

There is not a great deal of stone sculpture in Africa, and it is found chiefly in Sierra Leone, Nigeria and the Congo; and some across in Zimbabwe. Soft stone was the chief medium, though quartz and granite were also used. Ivory was carved, often with great delicacy. Clay or mud sculpture is still popular, though as it is highly perishable and cannot be exported; it is not so well known as it deserves.

Of all materials for sculpture wood was and remains the favourite. There are innumerable masks, heads, figures, dolls, head-rests, stools, pipes, bowls, pots, drums, gaming boards, divining trays, screens and doors. And decorative art also appears in rings, bangles, necklaces, girdles, anklets, tattooing and fly-whisks. These form an endless treasury in African art, through which their vitality and dynamic love of life are expressed.

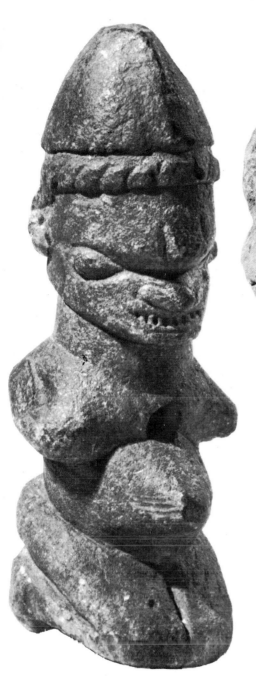

Religion and Philosophy

Like every race of mankind in every age Africans have many religious beliefs. Some of these are philosophical, in that they consider the perennial great questions, such as the origins of all things, the purpose and end of life, death and its conquest. These are often the subject of myths, which are philosophy in parables. The more narrowly religious life is shown in rituals, dances, sacrifices and songs.

Proverbs and myths express joy in life and human activity. It is a 'world-affirming' philosophy, in which life on earth is thought of as good, despite human suffering, sex is to be enjoyed, and children are the gift of God. The family is not only husband and wife and children, but the extended family of grandparents, brothers, sisters and cousins, in which old people are honoured and cared for. Life and health are the objects of prayers, maintained by good magic and medicine, and threatened by bad magic and witchcraft. It has often been said that the chief value of African thought is power, vital energy, or dynamism. The world is a realm of powers; the most fruitful life has the most power and harmony.

God, the Supreme Being, is the greatest power of all, the strong one, who possesses life and strength in himself, and from whom creaturely force is derived. Few if any African peoples have been without belief in the supreme Creator, and even where that belief has been influenced by Islam or Christianity the original idea may still be traced.

The powers of the world act on one another and man tries to keep on good terms with them all. They are not all equal, but are seen to be in a hierarchy of forces. The highest is God, who creates all other powers, and strengthens those who call on him. After God come other great powers, like the chiefs in human society. There are spiritual forces attributed to nature or great human beings, and especially the ancestors who founded the race and who are still interested in it.

It has been suggested that African religion can roughly be depicted as a triangle. At the top, head of all powers, is God. On the two sides of the triangle are the next greatest powers, gods and ancestors. At the base are lower forces, with which magic and medicine are concerned. Humans are in the middle, and must live in harmony with the powers that affect life, family and work. The powers extend into the animal world, for animals have great forces which need to be watched and harnessed if possible. Even supposedly inorganic nature is not dead, but may be the vehicle of power.

A human being is more than body; there is a spiritual element which is the breath of God, sometimes even called God in man. Body and soul are closely interwoven and are often

13

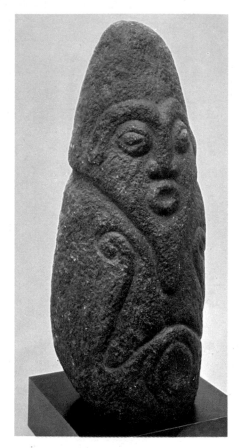

spoken of as if they were one, though it is known that at death the spirit leaves the body. This is not merely the breath, for people distinguish breath, shadow and influence, from personality. Medicine is administered to heal disease, but a spiritual remedy is also needed.

Human morality is behaviour in society, helping or hurting one's neighbour. It is the interaction of forces, but since they are dependent on God so it is God who is the final judge of human deeds. People have the power to kill their neighbours, but no right to abuse that power, for they are God's children, and responsible to him for all their actions. This close relationship and the mutual effects of spiritual and material will become clear as the myths are read.

In modern times new religions have come into every part of Africa. Islam and Christianity bring new doctrines, morality, history, scripture, and universalism. But much of the old remains, many Africans are still untouched by the new religions, and even the millions who have joined them are still influenced by the old outlook and mythology.

Mythology

In the mythologies of every continent there can be distinguished great myths, and others that are of less importance. Some myths dominate and show the character of the religious outlook, while others are less central, repetitive, and fanciful. All kinds of myths need to be taken into account, for altogether they show the values which the society holds dear.

Most myths tell how something came to exist: human beings, the world, animals, social affairs. The myths make a 'sacred history' of the people. But naturally the creation of the world comes first and this myth influences others that follow. There could be no stories of the creation of people or animals if there was not already a world for them to enjoy. So the central myth, telling the origins of

Above. Stone figure from Ekoi on the upper Cross river, Nigeria. Called Akwanshi ('dead person in the ground'), it is a memorial to a head of a clan and may be several centuries old. The shape may be phallic or natural, the figure being engraved rather than sculpted out of hard basalt. Museum of Mankind, London.

Right. In many lands women suffer for the sake of beauty but rarely as much as the Ibo women of eastern Nigeria, who traditionally wore large platelike gold anklets from adolescence. They were fixed and removed by smiths and when walking the legs had to be swung outwards, but a procession of ladies made a fine sight, flashing in the sun. Other women wore copper anklets or spirals of brass which covered most of their legs. Horniman Museum, London.

Opposite. A family group in terracotta. An Ibo (Igbo) husband and his two wives bring a fowl to sacrifice to the spirit of the yams. Museum of Mankind, London.

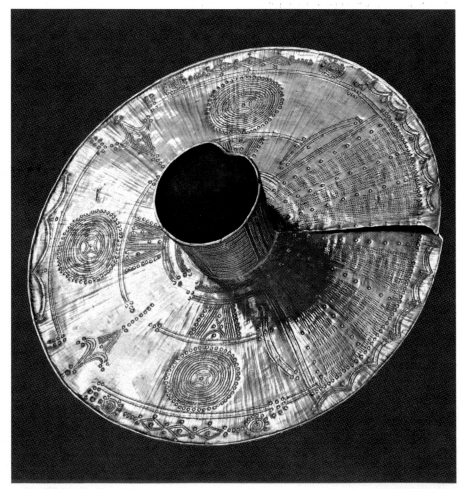

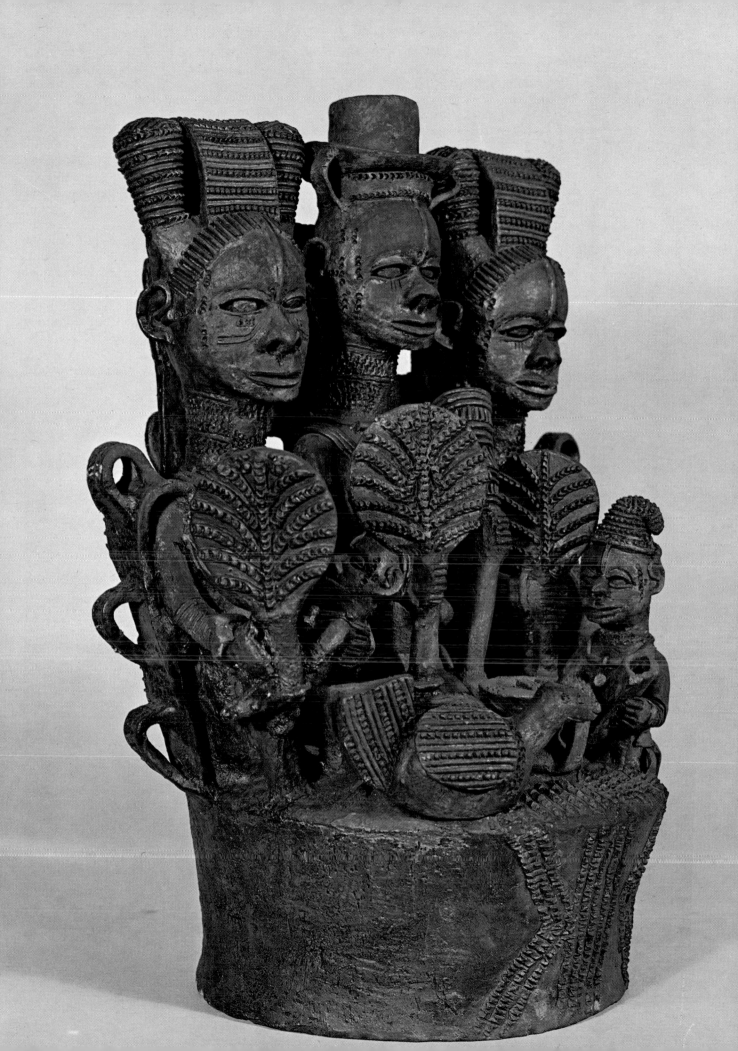

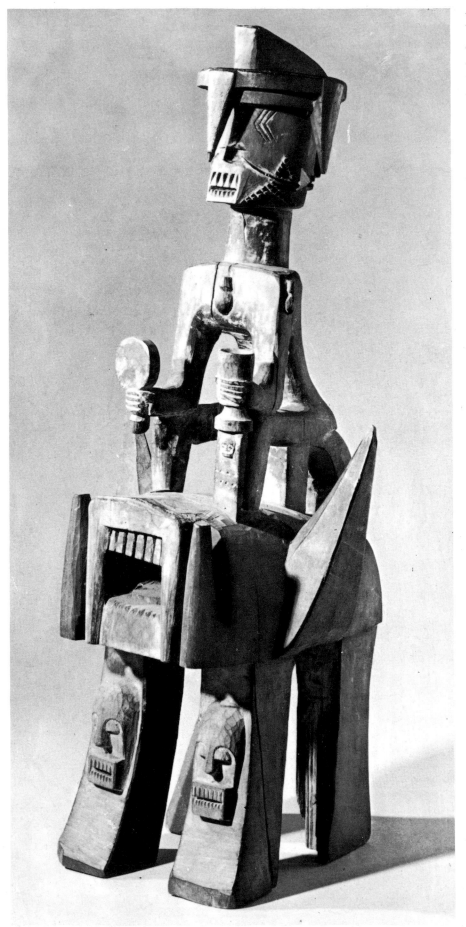

the world, shows that history had a beginning. Legendary events that came later show how the world was changed, and in particular the adventures of human beings, the discovery of sex, the obligation to work, the coming of death.

Myths also tell about supernatural beings, gods and ancestors. The great heroes of the past provided models for human behaviour later. But they show an end as well as a beginning. For although the Supreme Being and other spirits created and lived on earth, they also left it later on or disappeared. Human beings too begin and end their lives on earth.

Myths are stories, the product of fertile imagination, sometimes simple, often containing profound truths. They are not meant to be taken too literally. If details sometimes appear childish, so often do those of classical Greece or Egypt. But most myths express serious beliefs in 'human being, eternity, and God'. Modern psychologists, like Jung, have seen in myths clues to the deepest hopes and fears of mankind, not to be despised as stories, but studied carefully for their revelation of the depths of human nature.

The mythology given in this book has been taken from many parts of Africa, but obviously in such a huge continent many people must be given small space. Some tribes have not been studied at all for their mythology, or very little and inadequately. Others have been favoured by detailed and very careful recording. The available material has been studied as widely as possible, and selections have been made from all over the continent in order to give a picture of some of the major themes in the thought of Africa. Much description of African religion relies upon the external observation of students who do not share the beliefs of the people studied. To record the myths them-

Left. The art of the Ijaw of the Niger Delta is noted for its cubist quality. This figure, called Ejiri, is an impersonal means of controlling life and gaining success. The steed is probably a leopard, with a fierce mouth but with human faces on its legs. Metropolitan Museum of Art, New York.

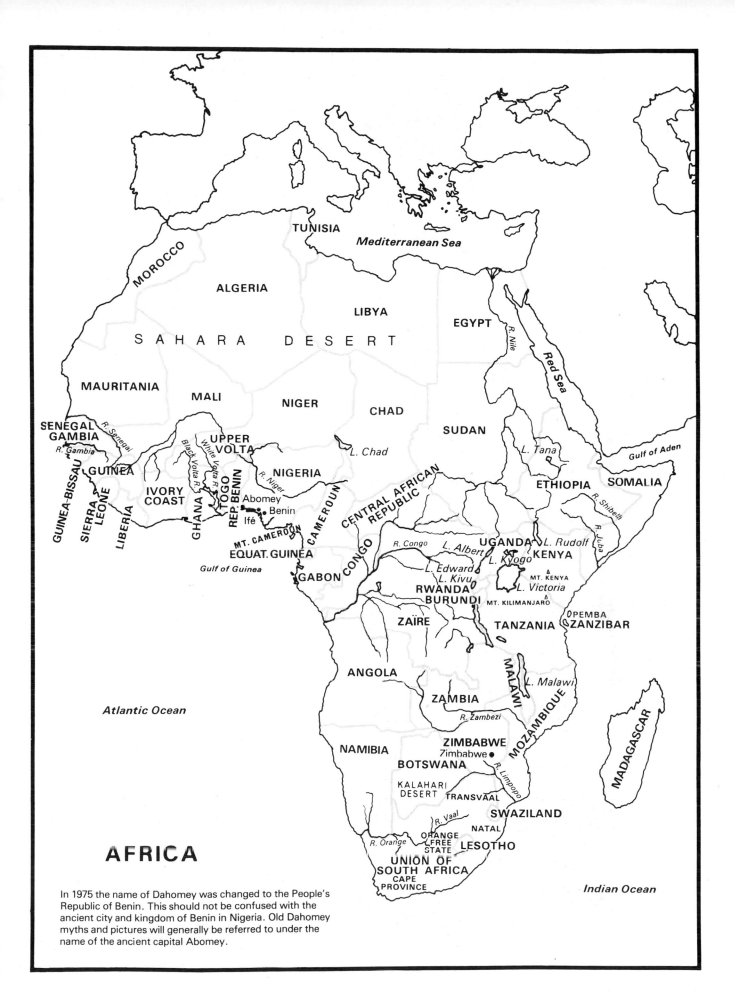

AFRICA

In 1975 the name of Dahomey was changed to the People's Republic of Benin. This should not be confused with the ancient city and kingdom of Benin in Nigeria. Old Dahomey myths and pictures will generally be referred to under the name of the ancient capital Abomey.

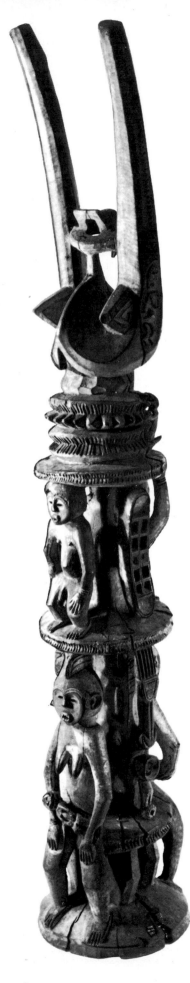

selves helps to reveal the Africans' own thoughts about religion and life and so, with illustrations of art, this begins to provide the basis for a scripture of African religions.

The first and longest part of this book gives what are most properly called myths. That is, stories of supernatural beings and events. Then some traditions of outstanding interest have been selected, from only a few lands, since all peoples have traditions of their origins and rulers, and these are endless. Finally some fables of animal life are included, because these are among the most popular of all African stories. The fables show humans living close to the animal and natural worlds, but they also project human feelings on to animals and reveal attitudes and actions which are both praised and blamed.

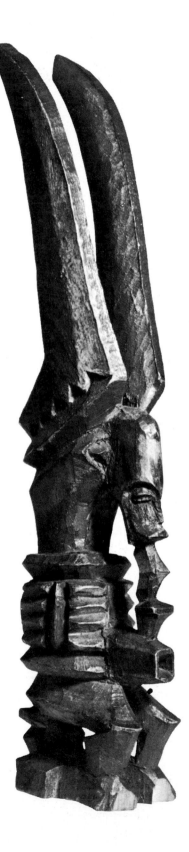

Left. Ikenga (personal shrines) are found in almost every house in Onitsha, Nigeria. As the token of a man's life-force, they are customarily destroyed on the death of the owner. Museum of Mankind, London.

Right. A wooden figure with two horns representing, to the Ibo of Nigeria, fortune and a man's physical strength. It symbolises success in trade, hunting and farming. It is also the personal shrine of a man's 'right hand', or life-force. Horniman Museum, London.

The Creator

There is no doubt that nearly all, if not all, African peoples believe in a Supreme Being, the creator of all things. A supreme god is named in the earliest dictionary of a Bantu language, compiled in 1650, and in Bosman's description of West Africa published in the year 1705. Belief in a supreme being is a thoroughly Negro African conception, current long before there were any established Christian or Moslem missions in the interior regions of tropical or southern Africa.

The names of the Supreme Being vary a great deal, of course, due to the many different languages of Africa. But there are some names which are common over wide areas. The name Mulungu for God is used in East Africa and has been adopted in about thirty translations of the Bible. In central Africa the name Leza is used by a number of different peoples. And in the western tropics, from Botswana to the Congo, variants of the name Nyambé are found. It is possible that the name Nyamé for God in Ghana is related to Nyambé, but West African peoples have many other names: Ngewo, Mawu, Amma, Olorun, Chukwu, and so on to denote the Supreme Being. In this book the English word God will sometimes be used, as the nearest and most convenient equivalent of the quite distinct African conception of the Supreme Being.

God is the creator, and myths told about him seek to explain the origins of the world and human beings. He is transcendent, living in heaven, to which people naturally look up and recognise his greatness. It is often thought that he used to dwell on earth, but he retired to the sky, because of some human misdeed.

Although he is the greatest of all, there are lesser spirits which are often prominent in religious worship. Gods of storm, earth, forest, water, and the like, are popular. In West Africa there are many temples for such deities, though in other parts of the continent they may be only vaguely reverenced and there are relatively few temples for their worship. But the spirits of the dead are important everywhere. Belief in life after death, perhaps the most ancient and tenacious religious belief of all peoples, is found everywhere in Africa. The many secret societies, masked dancers, and ancestral rituals prove this.

It is strange that there are very few temples of the Supreme God, while lesser deities and ancestors have many holy places for their worship. This has led some people to think that he is a distant deity, a necessary creator but now an absentee, often forgotten or only rarely invoked. But the myths to be recorded later will show that he is not only a past creator, but appears very often in the ordinary events of human life. Wise old Africans, when questioned on this point of the absence of worship, say that God is too great to be contained in a house. Solomon in his wisdom said much the same.

Although in myths the Supreme Being is spoken of in a personal manner, as if he were a man with a body, and often with a wife and family, yet many African sayings and proverbs speak of God in an abstract and philosophical fashion. God is the abstract idea, the cause. He is also a personal deity, generally benevolent, who cares for people and does not strike them with terror. Further, he is often an indwelling power, which sustains and animates all. God knows everything, he sees all, he can do whatever he wishes. He is justice, rewarding the good and punishing the wicked. He is the final court of appeal, to which even the poorest and most insignificant can go, when they get no redress from other gods and chiefs. Although people speak of him with a face, and hands and legs, as does the Bible, yet in reality God has no form. He cannot be contained in a temple, the thunder is his voice, yet he is greater than the storm. He is indescribable, the only reality.

These divine attributes appear in proverbs and myths, but of course in stories more tangible human characteristics appear. As Creator he made all things and fixed the customs of every people. He laid out the countryside, arranged the mountains in their places, put in rivers, planted trees and grass. He even fixed the ant-hills that rise up red and hard, great cones which were constructed by the termite white ant.

As Moulder of All he shaped things, like a woman fashioning pots that she makes out of clay. He put things together and constructed them, like a builder making a house of dried clay, layer by layer.

God is father and mother of men and animals. He is not often thought of as having been born, since he is eternal, but there is a story that says he was born of a woman with one breast. His wife is spoken of, and the hard brown rings which form the body of a centipede or millipede are called 'the ivory bracelets of the wife of God'. Yet some peoples think of him as possessing dual natures, male and female, and a famous writer in Ghana used to speak of 'Father-Mother God'. Of course God is beyond sex, though in story he usually appears in human form.

The Supreme Being is in heaven and so he is particularly concerned with rain, upon which men depend entirely for their life. He is rarely associated with the sun, for in the tropics the sun is always present, and there is no need of chants and sacrifices to bring the sun back again, as in ancient Europe and Japan. God rends the sky with lightning and

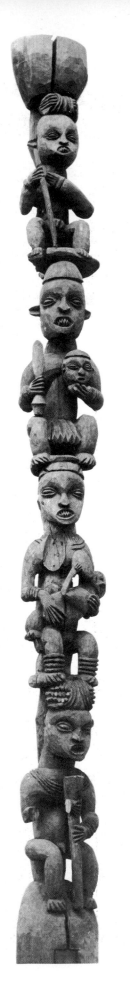

moves the forest so that the trees murmur. Instead of saying 'it', as we do when we say 'it is hot', Africans often say 'God is fiercely hot', 'God is falling as rain', 'God makes the drumming of thunder'. To say 'God is burying eggs' means that as a crocodile hides eggs in the sand and comes back later without mistake, so the thunder will return in time. When rain begins the pleasant freshness is described by saying that 'God has softened the day'. The rainbow is often called 'the bow of God', who is like a hunter.

God is high and over all things; he 'covers' us like the sky. He is powerful and wise, but not easy to understand. There are mysteries about God: he is 'the incomprehensible being'. This comes from the nature of life itself, which has sorrow as well as joy. Like an almighty Fate, he is held responsible for evil and suffering. A man who has lost all his children through sickness or accident may be described as 'one on whom God has looked'. There are moving myths of people who went to God to find out the reason for their sufferings.

Some of the names given to God in African ritual, proverbs and myths show what men think of his character and attributes. He is first of all Creator, Moulder, Giver of Breath and Souls, God of Destiny. His work in nature is shown by titles such as Giver of Rain and Sunshine, One Who Brings the Seasons, the One Who Thunders, the Bow in the Sky, the Fire-lighter. The divine greatness is indicated by the names: Ancient of Days, the Limitless, the First, the One Who Bends Even Kings, He Who Gives and Rots, the One Who Exists of Himself, the One You Meet Everywhere.

The providence of God is shown by names such as Father of Babies, Great Mother, Greatest of Friends, the Kindly One, God of Pity and Comfort, the Providence Who Watches All Like the Sun, the One on Whom Men Lean and Do Not Fall. Finally there are mysterious and enigmatic titles: the Great Ocean Whose Headdress is the Horizon, the Great Pool Contemporary of Everything, the One

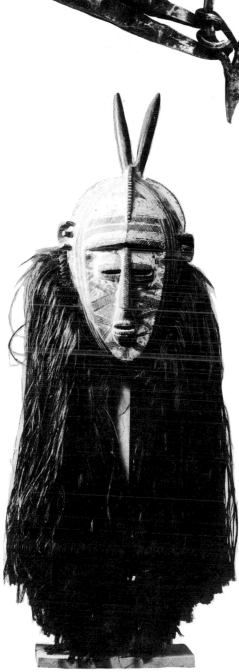

Above. Ceremonial axe from the Songye-Bushongo, Congo. Such axes are carried in many African countries in rites of gods and ancestors. The handle is copper and the wrought iron blade decorated with fifty-eight heads on the two sides. Horniman Museum, London.

Opposite. House post of the Bangwa people of Cameroun. A remarkable piece of carving from a single trunk, it stands ten feet (3 metres) high. The four figures represent ancestors. Staatliches Museum für Völkerkunde, Munich.

Right. Wooden mask of the Bobo, Upper Volta, fringed with hair and raffia. The horns, facial marking, and white face suggest the power and strangeness of the spirit it represents. The body of the human wearer is entirely concealed by the robe. The Brooklyn Museum, New York.

Beyond All Thanks, the Inexplicable, the Angry One, the Great Spider – the clever insect who comes into many stories.

Creating the Earth

The primal myth occurs in many forms, and specimens will now be given from different countries. Shorter references to creating the earth will also be found in stories about the creation of men and traditions of the first ancestors.

The Yoruba of Nigeria say that in the beginning the world was all marshy and watery, a waste place. Above it was the sky where Olorun, the Owner of the Sky, lived with other divinities. The gods came down sometimes to play in the marshy waste, descending spiders' webs which hung across great gaps like fairy bridges. But there were no men yet, for there was no solid ground. One day Olorun – Supreme Being – called the chief of the divinities, Great God (Orisha Nla), into his presence. He told him that he wanted to create firm ground and asked him to set about the task (in some versions it was the Oracle god who did the work, see page 84). Great God was given a snail shell in which there was some loose earth, a

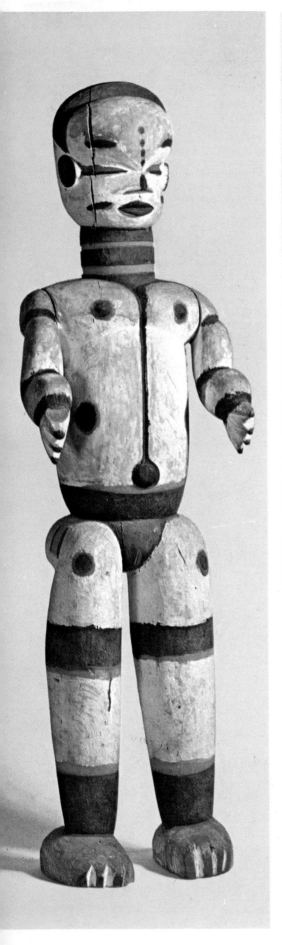

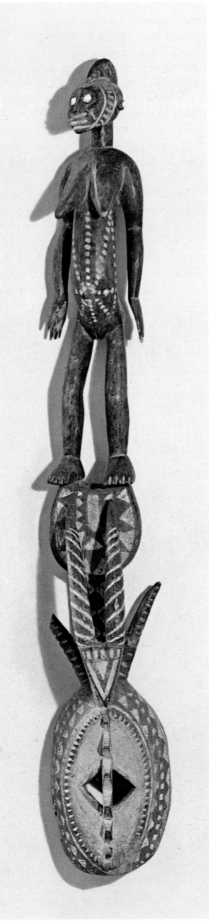

pigeon and a hen with five toes. He came down to the marsh and threw the earth from the snail shell into a small space. Then he put the pigeon and the hen on the earth, and they started to scratch and scatter it about. Before long they had covered much of the marsh and solid ground was formed.

When Great God went back to report to the Supreme Being the latter sent a chameleon to inspect the work. The chameleon is a prominent figure in many African myths, and it is noted for its slow careful walk, its change of colour to suit its environment, and its big rolling eyes. After a first inspection the Chameleon reported that the earth was wide but not dry enough. Then he was sent again, and this time he said it was both wide and dry. The place where creation began was called Ifé, meaning 'wide', and later the word Ilé, 'house', was added, to show that it was the house from which all other earthly dwellings have originated. Ilé-Ifé has been ever since the most sacred city of the Yoruba people, and this story is put out to justify its eminence.

The making of the earth took four days, and the fifth was reserved for the worship of Great God, and ever since a week of four days has been observed, each one of which is sacred to a divinity. Then the Supreme Being-Creator sent Great God back to earth to plant trees, to give food and wealth to humans. He gave the palm nut of the original palm tree, whose nuts give oil and whose juice supplies drink. Three other common trees were planted, and later rain fell to water them.

Meanwhile the first people had been created in heaven and were then sent to earth. Part of the work of making people was entrusted to Great God, and he made human beings from the earth and moulded their physical features. But the task of bringing these dummies to life was reserved for the Creator alone. It is said that Great God was envious of this work of giving life, and he decided to spy on the Creator to see how it was done. So one day when he had finished moulding human forms, he shut himself in with them overnight and hid behind them so that he could watch. But the Creator knew everything and he sent Great God into a deep sleep, and when he woke up the human beings had come to life. Great God still makes only the bodies of men and women, but he leaves distinct marks on them and some bear signs of his displeasure.

Heavenly Twins

Neighbours of the Yoruba are the Fon of Abomey (Rep. Benin), and they have different creation stories. They speak of a supreme god (Mawu) and many other beings related to him. But Mawu is sometimes called male and sometimes female; Mawu has a partner called Lisa, and they may be spoken of as twins. One myth says that these twins were born from a primordial mother, Nana Buluku, who created the world and then retired. Mawu was the moon and female, controlling the night and dwelling in the west. Lisa was male, the sun, and lived in the east. They had no children when they first took up their stations, but eventually they came together in an eclipse. Whenever there is an eclipse of the sun or moon it is said that Mawu and Lisa are making love.

The primeval twins, Mawu-Lisa, became parents of all the other gods. These were all twins too, seven pairs. There is difference of opinion as to which were born first and are senior, but probably the gods of earth, storm and iron are among the first. It is said that one day Mawu-Lisa called all their children together, and gave each of them a domain. The first set of twins was entrusted with the rule of Earth and they were told to take whatever they wished from heaven. The twins of Storm were told to stay in the sky and rule over thunder and lightning. Then the Iron twins were told that since they were the strength of their parents they must clear the forests and make cultivable land; they should also give tools and weapons to humans. Another pair were ordered to live in the sea and all waters and rule the fishes. Yet others were

sent into the bush to rule over birds and beasts and care for trees. The space between the earth and sky was the domain of other deities who were entrusted with the life-span of human beings and they were told to return from time to time to the Supreme Being (Mawu) to tell of all that happened in the world. These Sky gods also prevented other gods from being seen by humans, so people speak of gods as sky or spirit.

To each of the gods the Creator gave a special language and these are the ritual languages spoken by the priests and mediums of the gods in their songs and oracles. One spirit, a divine messenger (Eshu, Legba, see page 86-88), was given knowledge of

Opposite right. The Mossi of Upper Volta use this antelope mask both at funerals and to protect the fruits of the earth. The lower face of the mask is abstract, but on it stands the Earth Goddess with a lively figure and bright painted eyes. Museum Rietberg, Zurich.

Opposite left. The Ekpe or Egbo is one of the principal societies of the Ibibio and neighbouring peoples of eastern Nigeria. It is a club as well as a cult, but the main purpose is the worship of ancestors and the encouragement of fertility. The clubhouse has images and symbols of the spirits, like this figure. Horniman Museum, London.

Below. Ancestral screen with a boat on top from the Kalabari Ijaw of the eastern Niger delta. Such screens were made for the shrines of deceased chiefs in a Dancing People society, and showed them dressed as they might be in plays in honour of the water spirits. Museum of Mankind, London.

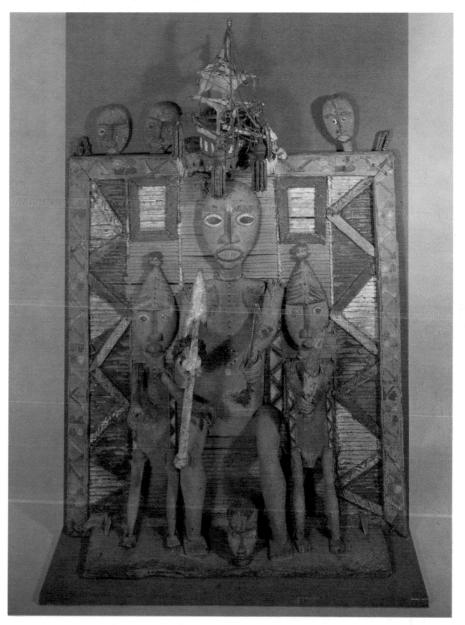

all languages and serves today as intermediary between gods and gods, and between men and all the divinities. It will be noticed that the Supreme Being is often simply called Mawu, and the tendency to unity of thought makes this deity supreme in practice, without mention of male or female nature.

The Universal Calabash

A calabash is a gourd, like a melon or pumpkin, whose hard rind makes it useful to men when the soft inner pulp is cleaned out. It is useful as a waterpot, or with hard seeds in it can be used as a rattle. A round calabash, cut in two horizontally, is put in some temples and contains small offerings or symbolical objects. The calabash is often decorated with carving on upper and lower shells, with a great variety of designs as well as pictures of humans, animals and reptiles.

In Abomey the universe is sometimes said to be a sphere like a round calabash, the horizon being where the upper and lower lips of a divided calabash meet. That is where the sky and sea mingle, in an ideal place inaccessible to man. The earth is thought to be flat, floating inside the larger sphere, as a small calabash may float in a big one. Within the sphere are waters, not only at the horizon but under the earth. This is explained by saying that if one digs into the ground water is always discovered and so water must surround the whole earth. The sun, moon and stars move in the upper part of the calabash. The place of the dead is uncertain: some think that they are above the earth, and others that they are in the invisible part below the inhabited earth.

When God created all things, his first concern was to gather the earth together, fix the bounds of the waters, and join the calabash close. A divine snake coiled itself round the earth to bring it together and keep it firm. He carried God here and there, establishing order and by his essential movement sustaining all things.

Serpent of Eternity

The snake has had a fascination for men in every land; it is mysterious,

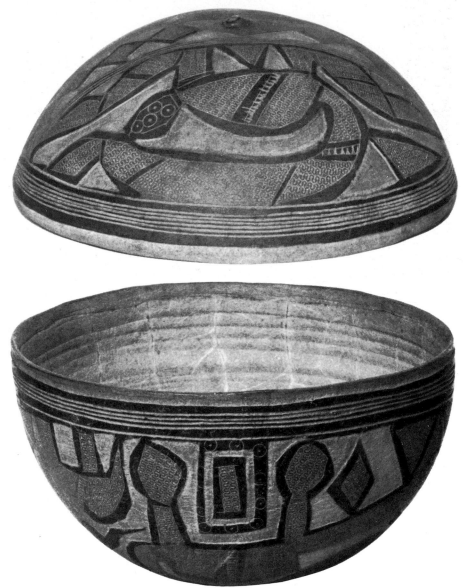

fearful and immortal. Because it goes on its belly without feet, living apart from and dangerous to all living beings, it is feared. Because it sheds its skin yet continues to live, it is regarded as immortal. A snake with its tail in its mouth, apparently swallowing itself yet with no beginning or end, like a circle and sphere, is symbolic of eternity. This is seen in art, depicted on cloth patterns, painted on walls, and worked out in metal. But not all snakes are identical, and the favourite is the python which is not poisonous.

When the world was created, say the Fon, the Snake gathered the earth together with its coils and gave humans a place in which to live. It still sustains the world and its coils must not be loosened lest the whole crea-

tion disintegrates; there are, it is said, 3,500 snake coils above the earth and 3,500 below. In another version of the story the Snake erected four pillars at each of the cardinal points to uphold the heavens, and it twisted itself round the pillars to keep them upright. The three primary colours of black, white and red are the clothes which the Snake puts on at night, day and twilight, and these colours are twined round the heavenly pillars.

The Snake is essentially motion, the symbol of flowing movement, like reeds in water. It is submerged in waters under the earth, dwelling in the ocean and so representing the greatest power in unceasing movement. The coils of the Snake are not still but revolve round the earth and set the heavenly bodies in motion.

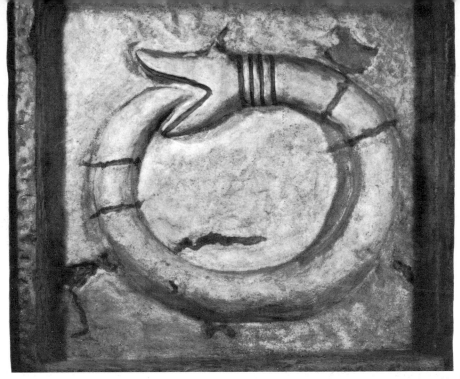

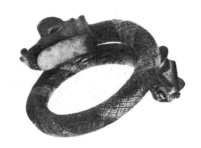

Above. Bronze bracelet from Abomey, representing a two-headed snake. Such rings are worn as lucky charms, and smaller snake rings are put on fingers to protect the wearer against snake bites in the hoeing season, on the theory that snake will not bit snake. Musée de l'Homme, Paris.

Above left. The snake of eternity, with its tail in its mouth. This symbol is common in African art, painted on walls, woven in cloth, and worked in metal and wood. This clay moulding, or bas relief, is from the walls of the palace of King Ghezo in Abomey, now a museum. It is regularly repaired and painted white, with red and blue rings round the neck. Musée de l'Homme, Paris.

Opposite. Calabash from the Hausa of northern Nigeria. This gourd cut in two is used in temples for receiving offerings, and it also symbolises heaven and earth. The top is that inverted bowl we call the sky; the earth is below or floating inside like a small calabash in a large one. The lips where the bowls join represent the horizon. Many calabashes are decorated with patterns of snakes, animals, men or gods. Museum of Mankind, London.

Below. Snakes and tortoises feature in this Yoruba panel from Nigeria. Museum of Mankind, London.

The Snake may still be seen in quiet pools, running rivers, and in the ocean. Or a flash of light may be seen, cleaving the waters, and its voice sounds abroad. In the beginning the Snake found only stagnant water on earth, so he traced out courses for the streams and channels for rivers and thus the world received life. When the Snake carried the Creator through the world, mountains appeared wherever they stopped.

A further version says that the Snake was created first, and it carried the Creator everywhere in its mouth, making the world as it is now. Each night when they stopped great mountains of the Snake's excrement appeared, and so if people dig into mountains they find treasure. When the Creator had finished, he saw that there were too many mountains, trees and large animals for the earth to carry. How could he stop the earth from sinking into the sea that surrounded it? He asked the Snake to coil itself up with its tail in its mouth to support the earth. The Snake became like the circular carrying pad people put on their heads to support

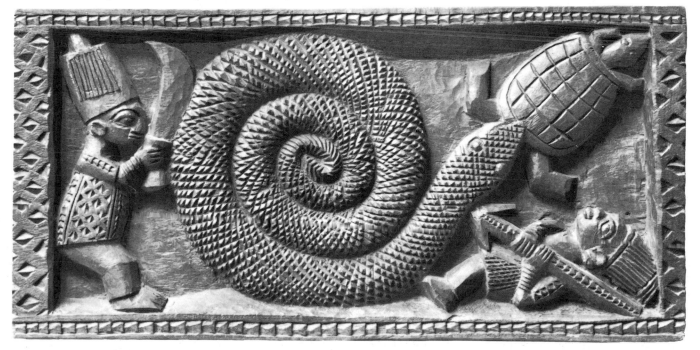

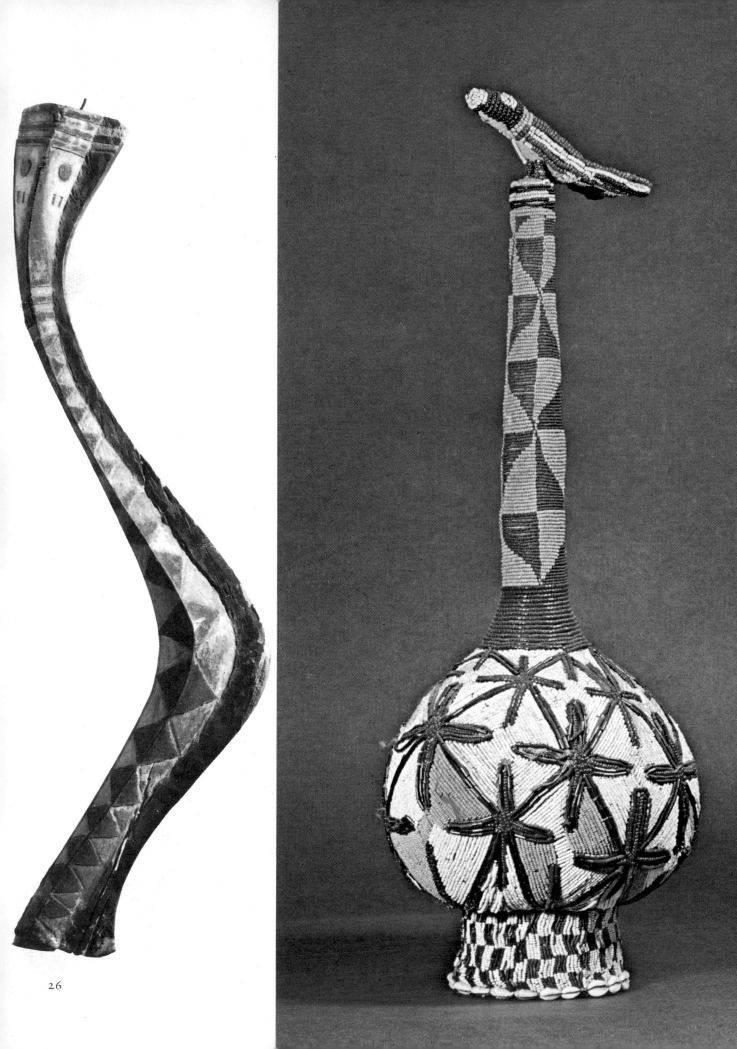

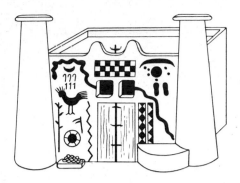

water pots or various other weights. Since the Snake does not like heat, the sea keeps him cool. God told some red monkeys, who live in the sea, to make iron bars for his food whenever he is hungry. Every so often the Snake shifts his position a little and there is an earthquake. If the monkeys fail to feed him with iron the Snake will be obliged to eat its own tail. When this happens the earth, weighed down with even more burdens than at the beginning, with more people and houses, will slide into the ocean, and that will be the end of the world.

God, Earth and Spirits

In Mali, south of Timbuctoo and the bend of the River Niger, live the Dogon people. Remarkable ideas of religion and mythology have been collected among them in recent years that are quite distinct in African studies. It is important to include them, but it must be stressed that it is not known how far other people share similar beliefs, and they cannot be taken as typical. These world views were revealed by a blind old man, Ogotemmêli, who had been chosen to declare the secret mythology of the tribe to his European friends.

In the beginning the one God, Amma, created the sun and moon like pots, his first invention. The sun is white hot and surrounded by eight rings of red copper, and the moon is the same shape with rings of white copper. The stars came from pellets of clay that Amma flung into space. To create the earth he squeezed a lump of clay, as he had done for the stars, and threw it into space. There it spread out flat, with the north at the top, and its members branched out in different directions like a body, lying flat with its face upwards.

Amma was lonely and drew near to the female Earth to unite himself with it. But his passage was barred by a red termite hill. He cut this down and union took place, but the interference made it defective and instead of twins being born, which would have been natural, a jackal was born instead. This jackal was a trouble to him afterwards. The myth justifies female circumcision, which is practised by the Dogon and many other African peoples.

There was further union between God and the Earth and twins were born. They were like water and green in colour. Their top half was human and the bottom half snake-like. They had red eyes and forked tongues, sinuous arms without joints, and their bodies covered with short green hair, shining like water. They had eight members and were born perfect. These two spirits were called Nummo, and they went up to heaven to get instructions from God, since he was their father and they were made from his essence, which is the life-force of the world, from which comes all motion and energy. This force is water and the Nummo are in all water, or seas and rivers and storms,

Opposite left. Stylised representation of a snake from the Baga people of Guinea: a single piece of wood six feet (1.8 metres) tall, carved and painted. One myth says that all water on earth was still, until the serpent came and traced the courses for the rivers; thus the world received life. Metropolitan Museum of Art, New York.

Opposite right. Royal calabash from Cameroun, covered with patterns of coloured beads and sometimes used to hold the bones of ancestors. Other beaded calabashes are used as musical instruments – filled with seeds and shaken to accompany songs and dances. Horniman Museum, London.

Above. Sketch of a Dogon ancestral temple. It is a cube about nine feet high, with towers in front and an iron symbol like lightning above the door. The walls are painted with pictures of snakes, birds and abstract patterns. The platform at the right of the door is for priests to sit on during ceremonies, and to the left are meal-grinding stones. Inside are altars of earth, thunderstones, pots and iron or wooden tools. From Griaule: *Conversations with Ogotemmêli.*

Below. Wooden carving of a warrior and horse from a Dogon ancestral sanctuary in Mali, representing the Guardian of the World. Griaule Collection.

in fact they are water. They are also light and emit it constantly.

When the Nummo spirits looked down from the sky they saw Mother Earth, naked and in disorder. So they came down, bringing quantities of fibres from heavenly plants which they made into two bunches to clothe Earth in front and behind like a woman. The fibres were moist and full of the essence of the Nummo spirits. By means of this clothing Earth obtained a language, elementary but sufficient for the beginning.

The Jackal, deceitful firstborn of God, was jealous of his mother's possession of language. He seized the fibre skirt in which language was embodied. Earth resisted this sinful attack and hid in her own womb, symbolised as an anthill in which she changed into an ant. The Jackal pursued her, and, although Earth dug down deep, she was not able to escape. The Jackal seized his mother's skirt, gained the power of speech, and so is able to reveal the plans of the Supreme Being to diviners.

The result of this unfilial attack was the defilement of Earth, and Amma decided to create live beings without her. But when he had formed their organs the Nummo spirits saw that there was a danger of twin births disappearing. So they drew a male and female outline on the ground, on top of one another. And so it was, and has been ever since, that every human being has two souls at first: people are bi-sexual. But a man's female soul is removed at circumcision, when he becomes a true man; and the corresponding event happens to a woman at excision. The myths continue with the coming of the first people, and, though they still refer back to God, they will be considered later under a separate heading. Meanwhile the gifts of God to humans occur in a number of myths.

God Sends Food

Across the other side of Africa the Ila people of Zambia say that when God sent humans to earth long ago he gave them grain for food and charged them to take care of it. When they got to the land, they sowed the grain and

there was a great harvest. The corn was gathered, put into bins, and then they all sat down to eat. But people were greedy and ate all day, as well as at morning and evening. When they were full they said that since there was so much grain it would never be finished, everybody was satisfied now and the grain could be burnt on the fire. So they set to and burnt all the grain. Then in due course a famine arose and men had no food. They left their village and went to God to say what had come about. God told them they were silly people, eating till they were satiated and then burning the rest. Now he said he would give them fruits, and since they had burnt the grain they would have nothing but roots and fruit to eat. It has been so ever since. Humans act in a foolish way. Grain is wasted; some brew beer from it, others burn it, others eat too much, or at the wrong times, or use the grain improvidently. Then when stores are exhausted they have to turn to roots and fruit. The story refers to the hunger that comes when supplies have run low and before the new harvest is ready, and blames this on human greed and improvidence.

A story told in Malagasy of the origin of rice says that a woman took her child to the river one day and let it play there while she was working. The child saw an insect and asked his mother what it was that jumped so high. She replied that it was a grasshopper, and he asked her to catch it for him. So the mother caught it and gave it to the child as a plaything. But when she was ready to go home the child cried because the grasshopper had jumped away. The mother searched everywhere but could not find it, and the child was so sad that it became ill and died. The mother wept bitterly and her cries went up to God. God took pity on the woman and told her to bury the child in a deep marsh. A month later a plant began to grow from the spot where the child had been buried. It grew up and bore grains, which birds came to eat when they were ripe. Then God told the woman to pound the grains, cook and eat them. This was the beginning of rice, so called after the name of the child.

Another Malagasy story tells of rice and of the work appropriate to every man. There were four men on earth, each with his own work, but they could not agree together. The first was a hunter with a spear, the second a trapper, the third gathered fruit, and the fourth cultivated the soil. As they never agreed they decided to ask God to change their lot, so that they could live together. When they arrived God was pounding rice, and said that he had no time for them that day, but he gave each of them a handful of rice and told them to keep it till he saw them in two or three days time. Then each of the men went his way. The first saw some game, dropped the rice, and went hunting. The second heard a bird screech, put down his rice and went after it, and when he came back the rice was gone. The third reached for some fruit and dropped his rice in a river. The fourth put down his rice and began to dig the ground; when he came back the wind had blown the rice about, but

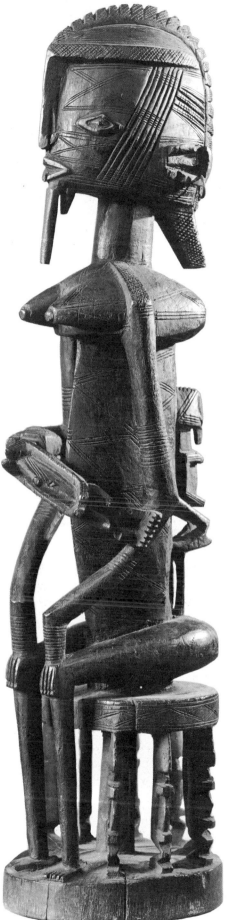

he managed to gather some of it. When God called the men he asked for the rice and each told his story. Then God said that it showed that their fate could not be changed. The hunter remains a hunter, and so on. Thereafter each man stuck to his lot and was content.

God and Fire

The discovery of fire marks a great stage in human life, and there are many stories which agree that at first there was no fire, and it came from God or the celestial regions. A story of the Ila people says that it was brought from heaven by the Mason-wasp. This is one of the commonest insects of Africa, with blue wings, yellow middle and striped legs. It builds mud nests on any object: walls, curtains, sticks and fireplaces; there it lays eggs, puts in grubs to feed them and goes off; in due time the eggs hatch out, break free from the cell, and eventually the new insects lay eggs in the same way, never having met their parents. Because the Mason-wasp likes the fireplace so much the stories see him bringing fire from heaven, like the Greek Prometheus. Originally there was no fire on earth, and all the birds and insects came together to ask how they could keep warm. Someone said that perhaps there was fire with God. The Mason-wasp said he would go and see, if somebody would accompany him. So the vulture, fish-eagle and crow volunteered. They said farewell to the birds and flew high in the sky.

Left. Female ancestral figure of the Dogon of Mali. The aloof face and highly stylised body indicate the power of the ancestors. The University Museum, Philadelphia, Pennsylvania.

Opposite left. The Bambara of Mali are unique in carving double antelope headdresses, highly stylised and used in rites which re-enact myths of the birth of agriculture. Musée de l'Homme, Paris

Opposite right. Hunter carrying an antelope, made in bronze, from southern Nigeria. In his left hand he holds a bow, as well as two legs of the deer, and his dog rubs against his right leg. Found at Benin, but probably Yoruba work. Museum of Mankind, London.

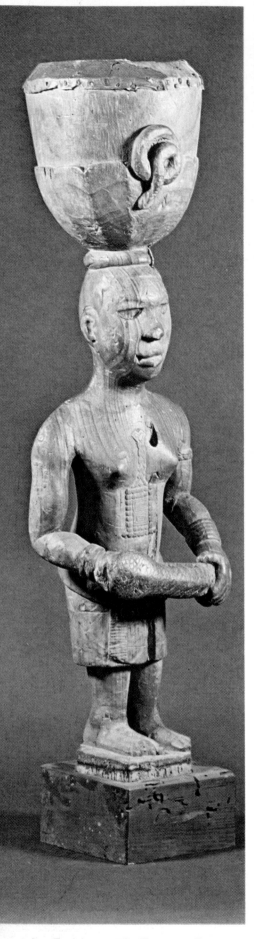

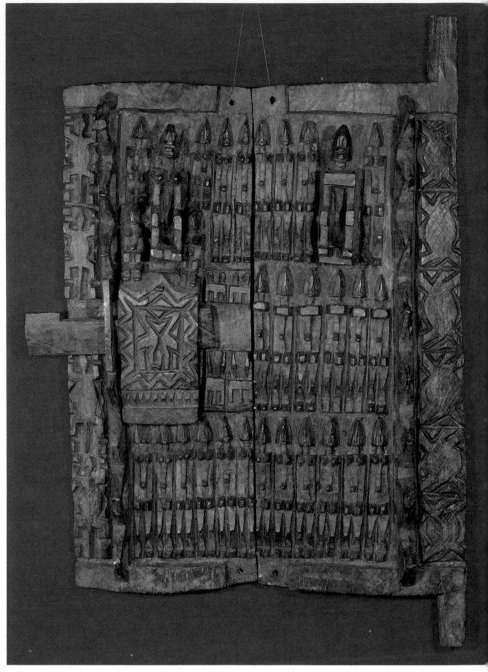

About ten days later some bones fell down to the ground, they were those of the vulture. Next, more bones fell down, from the fish-eagle. Finally other small bones, which were those of the crow. The Mason-wasp went on alone for thirty days, resting on the clouds but never managing to reach the top of the sky. God heard that the Mason-wasp was near and came down to ask where he was going. The Mason-wasp said he had no particular route, his friends had fallen behind, but he had kept on flying to reach the Chief of All to beg for some fire. God took pity on him, and said that since the Mason-wasp alone had reached him he would be head of all birds and insects in future. He told him to build a house for his child near a fireplace, leave the egg there, return after many days, and he would find it had changed into a wasp like himself. So it has been ever since. The Mason-wasp builds his nest near the fireplace because God commanded it to do so. There is some confusion in the tale between the gift of fire and building the nest, perhaps because it combines two stories.

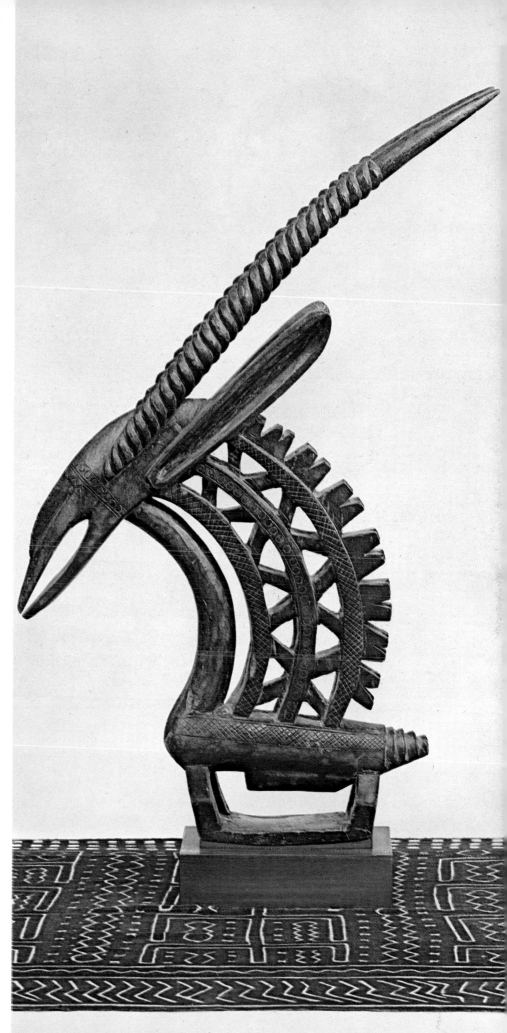

Opposite right. Decorated shutter of a granary from the Dogon of Mali. In Dogon mythology the world was like a granary which contained compartments for the different seeds God gave to mankind. The original granary came down from heaven on a rainbow, crashing to the earth and scattering human beings, animals and vegetables. Old granaries were made of clay, standing free or built into walls, with low doors for entry. Musée National des Arts Africains et Océaniens, Paris.

Opposite left. A kettle drum stands on the head of a wooden cult figure, which comes from the Bakongo, who live near the mouth of the Congo (Zaïre) river, and whose natural style may be partly due to long contact with Europeans. However, the snakes on the drum and in the hand are of African inspiration. Horniman Museum, London.

Right. The mythical buck of the Bambara of Mali was sent by the Creator to teach men how to cultivate corn. The cotton robe is painted with patterns symbolising the universe. Masqueraders dance in pairs in the fields to ensure fertility of crops and families.

The Dogon tale of fire says that when the first ancestors were ready to come to earth they had no fire. The Nummo spirits, children of God and earth, were heavenly blacksmiths and an ancestor stole a piece of the sun from their smithy. The female Nummo threw a flash of lightning at him, but the ancestor protected himself with a leather bellows that he had made to contain the piece of sun, and lightning could not penetrate it. Then the male Nummo cast a thunderbolt, and this also failed, though the ancestor slid down a rainbow to earth with such speed that he broke his arms and legs. Formerly these limbs had been sinuous, like those of the Nummo, but since that time men have had joints at knees and elbows. The story continues with the granary that the ancestor made, and will be told later.

There are several interesting myths of fire told by the Pygmies in the Congo forests. They say that they were the first to obtain fire, and later passed it on to the Negroes who think they are their masters. Once when a Pygmy was chasing an elephant he arrived by chance at the village of God and saw fire burning. He seized a brand and ran off with it, but God caught him and made him give it back. Three times this happened, as Pygmy stories often have three stages. Finally God was tired and made a fence of liana round his village. But the Pygmy jumped over the liana easily and brought the fire safely back to his camp.

A variant Pygmy myth says that originally God had fire, in front of which his old mother sat most of her days trying to keep warm. He also had a swing of lianas on which he flew through the air from one river to another. When God was away on his swing a Pygmy who was lost in the forest came to the place where fire was burning. God's mother was asleep and the Pygmy stole the fire. She awoke with the cold and called her son. God comforted her, jumped on his swing, caught the Pygmy and brought the fire back. The Pygmy told his story to his fellows in their camp and another offered to fetch the fire, but the same misfortune happened to him. Then a third took some feathers off a bird and began to fly. He flew about until he reached the village of God, where he also stole the fire. The mother of God called her son and he chased the Pygmy, but although they jumped over the hills and valleys, up to the sky and down to the depths, the Pygmy escaped, till at last God admitted that he was his equal and brother. But when God arrived back home he found his mother stretched out dead with cold, and then God decreed that henceforth men should die as a punishment. So although men have fire they have death as well.

Another Pygmy story says that originally it was the chimpanzees who possessed fire, and one day a Pygmy found their village and was delighted to sit by the fire. At once he began to plan how to seize it and take it home. One day, wearing a new bark-cloth which hung down to the ground, he came to the village of the chimpanzees. The old chimpanzees were busy in their plantation, and the young ones made fun of the Pygmy in his strange cloth. But they gave him bananas to eat and he sat down so near the fire that his cloth began to

smoulder. The young chimpanzees warned him that he was catching fire, but he told them not to worry because the cloth was plenty long enough. He sat even closer to the fire till the cloth caught light, and then he jumped up and ran away as fast as he could. The young chimpanzees were taken aback, and called their elders, who set off in pursuit. But the Pygmy was too far ahead and when the chimpanzees reached his village there were fires everywhere. The chimpanzees reproached the Pygmy for stealing the fire, instead of buying it honestly, and they went home grumbling. In another version it is said that the chimpanzees then abandoned their village, and ever since they have lived in the forest without fire or bananas and eat only wild fruit.

The Coming of Darkness

A story told by the Kono people of Sierra Leone says that when God first made the world it never became really dark or cold. The sun shone during the day and at night the moon gave a twilight in which everything could be seen clearly. But one day God called the Bat and gave him a basket to carry to the Moon. In the basket was darkness, but God did not say what the Moon should do with it, though he promised to come and explain later on. The Bat flew off with the basket on his back and set out for the Moon. But on the way he got tired and put down the basket for a rest, and went off to get food. During his absence some animals found the basket by the wayside and started to open it, thinking there was food in it. Just as they were taking the cover off the Bat came back, but darkness had already escaped. Ever since then the Bat sleeps all day long, but in the twilight and dark he begins to fly about everywhere, trying to catch the dark, put it back in the basket, and take it to the Moon according to the command of God. But the Bat never succeeds in catching the darkness, although he chases about in every direction, and before long day returns and the Bat has to sleep again. This kind of story, with its resemblance to the Greek myth of Pandora's box, is

very popular in many parts of Africa. As will be seen later, it has parallels in stories of the coming of death.

The Divine Family

God is often credited with a family in heaven, and the Pygmy story of his mother has been told. But generally few details are given and the stories in which this family is mentioned may simply give material for creaturely behaviour. An Ila story says that the Blue Jay was already married, but custom did not forbid him seeking another wife, even from the very

Wooden statue of a chimpanzee from Zaïre. Musée de l'Homme, Paris.

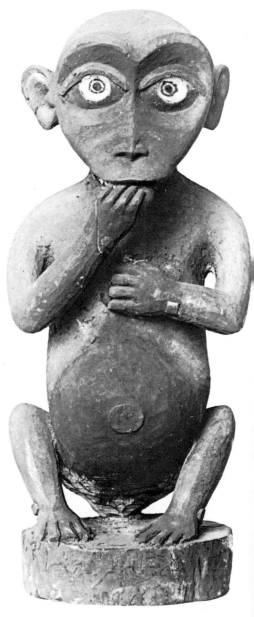

highest quarter. (Later a story will be told about a man who would be satisfied with no other marriage than with the daughter of the sun.) The Blue Jay went to God and asked for the hand of his daughter. God did not refuse, but said that his child must not be given the meat of any large animal to eat. The Blue Jay accepted this condition; he brought the daughter of God to his earthly home, and told his first wife and his mother of the divine law, that his new wife must never eat the flesh of any large animal. His mother agreed but his first wife was jealous. When the Blue Jay next went hunting he killed a zebra and a small duiker deer. He took them home and told his first wife to cook the meat, but not to give the daughter of God any flesh of the zebra. She obeyed, but when the Blue Jay was out again she offered the daughter of God the zebra meat, saying that it was the duiker. God's daughter tasted the meat and fell down dead. When the Blue Jay came in he asked what his new wife had died of, but his first wife replied that she did not know.

So the Blue Jay flew up to heaven to take the news to God. God reproached him for disobeying his command and sent him back to earth. Thirty days later a small cloud arose and God opened his mouth and made thunder. Then he came down and blew open the grave where his daughter was buried and carried her off to the sky. He took the Blue Jay too but did not bear him to heaven – halfway there God hurled him down to earth, and all that arrived on the ground were some very small bones. The story is told to explain the weird cry of the Blue Jay when it flies high in the air. This sounds like a cry of death, and mothers distract children's attention from such a cry lest it become an omen of death for them. The feathers of the Blue Jay are used as a charm against sudden death. The story also shows the danger of neglecting divine commands, the jealousy of a rival wife, and the responsibility of the head of a household for whatever events take place within the bounds of his own dwelling.

Suffering and the Supreme Being

God is the creator of the world, the ordainer of human lives, and the final court of appeal when calls upon other gods and ancestors have failed. So there are some moving stories of men and women who have suffered greatly in their lives and try to get an explanation of their woes from the Great Disposer of All.

An Ila story tells of an old woman who had been much troubled in her life. She came from a big family, but God Leza, 'the One Who Besets', smote them all. While she was still a child her father and mother died and left her an orphan. As she grew up her relatives perished also. The woman managed to get a husband and bear children, yet in undue season her husband passed away. The woman thought that at least she would be spared the children of her womb, and they lived for a time and bore their own children. But then the One Who Besets struck again and both children and grandchildren died, leaving the woman alone as a miserable old crone with nobody to care for her. She thought that at last she would die, and join her family.

But then a strange thing happened. Instead of dying the woman gained energy and became younger. Some people would have attributed this rejuvenation to witchcraft, saying that the woman had eaten her relatives and taken their soul-stuff to strengthen her own. But the woman knew that this was not so, and she determined to put her new powers to a great purpose. She would search out God and demand from him an explanation of all the sorrows of her life. God was in heaven, and she must climb up there somehow, and she tried hard to do it. She cut down some of the tall forest trees, and put them one on top of another, so as to make a ladder up to heaven. She built a great structure, but just when the topmost trees seemed to be getting near the sky the supporting timbers rotted away and the whole pile came crashing down.

The woman was still determined to find God and thought of another way to get at him. If she could find the place where the earth ends and touches the sky, there must be a road to God from there. So she set out to travel from village to village and tribe to tribe. As she passed through each country people asked the purpose of her journey, and she replied that she was searching for God. They asked why she was doing this, and the old woman answered that all her family had died and left her alone, a deserted and friendless old woman. But people retorted that it was not strange to lose friends and relatives. She was no different from every other human being, for all people suffer such bereavements. Leza, the Besetting One, sits on the back of all people; none can ever get free from him. So the old woman was unable to solve her problem and she never found the route to heaven but eventually went the way of all flesh herself.

A similar story, with a happier ending, is told by the Chaga people of Kenya. It concerns a man whose sons had all died and the father was angry with God. Going to a blacksmith he demanded the finest arrows and said that he was going to shoot God. Then he set out for the farthest edge of the world, to the place where the sun rises. There he found many paths, some leading to heaven and some to earth. He stood waiting for the sunrise, and after a time heard the sound of many feet and people shouting that the gate must be opened for the king. The man saw a great host of shining people, and hid himself in fear. The Shining One was in the midst and many others followed after. Suddenly the procession stopped and people in front complained of a horrible smell, as if an earth man had passed that way. They looked around, found the Chaga man, seized him, and took him to God. God asked him what he wanted, and he replied that it was only sorrow that drove him from home, and he wanted to die in the bush. But God replied that he had heard the man wanted to shoot him, so let him shoot now. The man refused, and said that God knew what he wanted without asking. God answered that if he wanted his sons back he could take them: there they

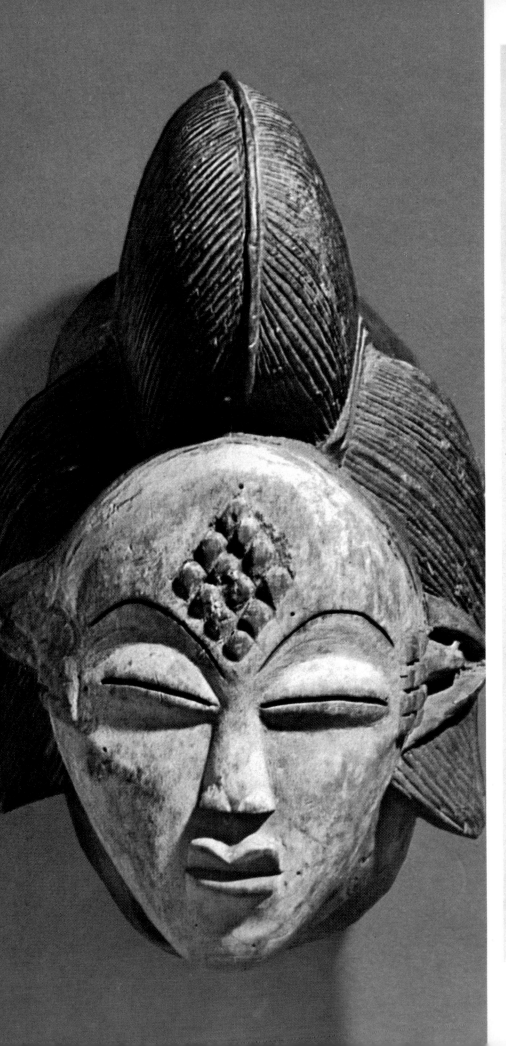
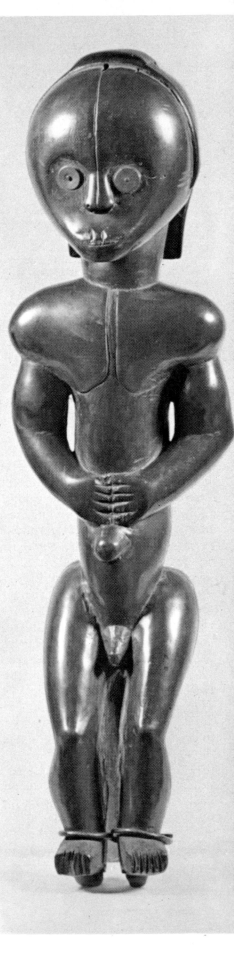

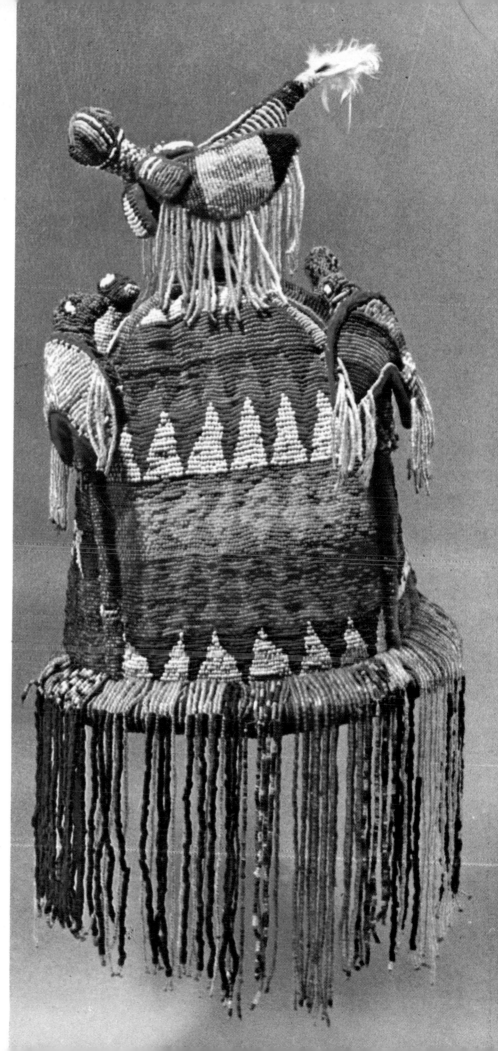

Opposite right. Male ancestor figure of the Fang of Gabon, masters of the sculptured form. Made in carved and polished wood, it was mounted on a cylindrical box which held the bones of the ancestor. Museum of Mankind, London.

Opposite left. Mask of the Mpongwe of the Congo, carved from wood with the face painted white with kaolin. With the impassive features, decorated forehead and elaborate hairstyle it represents a female ancestor. Musée de l'Homme, Paris.

Right. Yoruba king's headdress. Many rulers wore such crowns with beads hanging down in front of the face to add mystery and to emphasise their sacredness. But kings were not absolute, they could be removed from office, and were always subordinate to the spiritual world. A well-known story and proverb declares that there is 'No King as God'. Musée de l'Homme, Paris.

---

were, standing behind him. The man looked and saw his sons, but they were so radiant that he hardly knew them, and he said that now they belonged to God and he must keep them.

Then God told the man to go home, but on the way he must look carefully and he would find something that would please him very much. On the road back he found a great store of elephants' tusks, and was made rich for life. And other sons were born to him and they lived to support their father in his old age. Other stories of visits to the world beyond usually have some promise of good fortune on the way home, if the divine instructions are obeyed.

No King as God

This proverb is one of the most popular in everyday use in West Africa today. It is often painted as a text on the front of motor lorries, to show that God is supreme and the human will must bow to him. The origin of the proverb is given in a Hausa story from Nigeria, but it resembles similar ones in both Europe and the East, as well as other parts of Africa.

When an ordinary man comes before a king he says, 'May the king live for ever.' But once upon a time there was a man who would say each time he came to court, 'There is no king

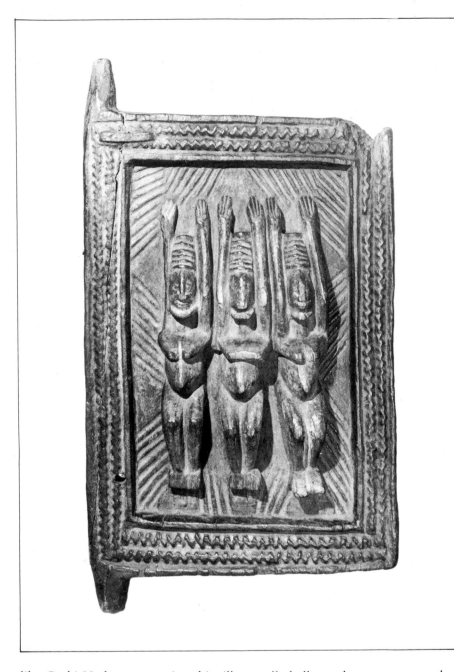

Dogon sculpture on the shutter of a granary. Three female figures make gestures of adoration, while the zig-zag patterns behind the figures and in the border around the panel represent the path followed by the Creator as he passed from east to west and from north to south during the formation of the world. Musée de l'Homme, Paris.

like God.' He kept on saying this till the king got angry and plotted to destroy him. He gave the man two silver rings and told him they were a present to keep, but in reality the king meant to avenge himself through them. The man, whom everybody now called No-King-as-God, took the rings, put them into a dried and empty ram's horn, and gave them to his wife to keep for him. A week later the king called No-King-as-God and sent him to a distant village, to tell the people to come and help build up the city walls. As soon as he had gone the king sent to the man's wife and offered her a million cowries (imported small shells used as currency and ornament), and a hundred head-cloths and body-cloths, if she would give him that which her husband had entrusted to her. Tempted by the splendid presents the wife agreed and brought the ram's horn, and when the king looked inside there were two rings safely stored. He replaced them in the horn, and gave it to his servants with instructions to throw it far into a lake that never dried up. They did so, and as the horn fell into the water a great fish swam by and swallowed it up.

On the day that No-King-as-God was returning home he met some friends who were going fishing. He went with them and caught the great fish. As his son was cleaning it his knife struck something hard and he called his father. The father pulled out the horn, and when he opened it and looked inside he saw the rings which the king had given him for safe keeping. 'Truly,' he said, 'there is no king like God.' They were still bathing when a royal messenger came and told the man he was wanted by the king at once. So he asked his wife where was that precious thing he had entrusted to her. She replied readily that she could not find it and thought a rat had eaten it.

Then the man set off for the royal court. The other councillors all saluted by saying, 'May the king live for ever.' But the man said only, 'There is no king like God.' So the king told the councillors to be quiet, and advancing towards the man he said, 'Is it true that there is no king like God?' The man replied firmly, 'Yes'. Then the king demanded that thing which he had entrusted to the man, and his guards closed round him to kill him. But No-King-as-God put his hand under his robe and pulled out the horn and handed it to the king. The king opened it and took out his two silver rings. 'Indeed, there is no king like God', he said, and all his councillors shouted in approval. Then the king divided his city into two, and gave half of it to No-King-as-God to rule.

God Leaves the World

One of the best known of all African myths, found in many parts of the continent, tells of God leaving the world. It is generally agreed that in the earliest times God lived on earth but, generally due to some human fault, God got angry and went up to heaven. There is some idea of a past Golden Age, when God and the first ancestors were closer together, and some resemblance to the Bible story of the Garden of Eden, though there it is humans who are expelled from paradise. Some ancient Egyptian and classical myths told of the separation of sky and earth by their children, but although in the African stories God is almost identified with the sky, there are important differences in the various accounts.

The Mende people of Sierra Leone say that God made everything, heaven and earth, and animals, and last of all he made men and women. He told them that they could have whatever they wanted if they asked him. So when people were in need they demanded this or that, and God always gave it to them. But they came so often that they thought God's name must be just 'Take it!', which he said when they asked him for anything. And God grew tired of people troubling him so often, and saw that they would wear him out with their demands. So he decided to make himself a dwelling-place far away and out of reach. While the people slept God went away and when they woke they could not find him. But then they looked up and saw God spread out in all directions, and they said that God was great. God said farewell, but warned them not to do evil to one another, for he had made them to live in agreement. Then he went up on high, and men call him 'High'. God also gave man and woman a fowl each, so that they might sacrifice to him if they did wrong to one another. So men still sacrifice and call on God to come down when they offer him a fowl in reparation for wrongdoing.

Along the west coast, in the Ivory Coast, Ghana, Togo, Abomey and Nigeria there are common myths of God retiring from the earth. In olden days God lived very near humans, in the sky, just above their heads. He was so close that people grew familiar with him. Children would wipe their greasy hands on the sky when they finished their meals. Women, in search of an extra ingredient for dinner, would tear a piece off the sky and put it in the cooking pot, and often they would knock against the sky when pounding their meal. This is one of the great female occupations of Africa, where mechanical flour mills have not been introduced. The grain is pounded in a wooden mortar, a scooped out piece of log, and a long wooden pestle is thumped down on the grains of corn. It is said that there was a woman once who had a very long pestle, and whenever she pounded her corn the wooden pole hit against God who lived just above the sky. One day she gave a great bang, hitting God in the eye, and in anger he went away to the place where he has been ever since. This meant that people could no longer approach God so easily. The woman tried to get over this difficulty by telling her children to collect all the wooden mortars that they could find. These were all piled one on top of another and nearly reached up to heaven. Just one more mortar was needed, but they could not find one. So the old woman told her children to take the lowest mortar out from

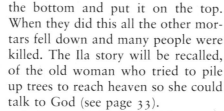

the bottom and put it on the top. When they did this all the other mortars fell down and many people were killed. The Ila story will be recalled, of the old woman who tried to pile up trees to reach heaven so she could talk to God (see page 33).

It is remarkable that right across the other side of Africa similar stories are told. The Nuba people of the Sudan say that in the beginning the sky was low down and close to the earth; in fact it was so near that man could touch it. Women found that it pressed so low that they could not lift up their spoon high enough to stir their millet porridge, and their hands were forced to touch the pots and got burnt. One day a woman got angry at the pressure of the sky and gave her spoon a hard thrust upward. It went right through the sky. Then the sky was angry and retired to the distance it has been ever since. Another version says that the sky was formerly so near that when people were hungry they tore pieces off the clouds to eat. Then the woman stabbed at the clouds with her spoon, and in anger at both these insults the sky moved away; and for this reason also the clouds only give their rain during one short season of the year. It will be noted that women are usually blamed for the disaster, as in the Genesis story, perhaps the most likely reason for this being that the stories were told by men.

The Dinka people, also of the eastern Sudan, say that because the sky at first was so low, men and women had to be careful in hoeing the ground or pounding the grain not to touch God. Death had not yet come into the world, and God had given the first man and woman one grain of millet each day. This was enough for them and they were forbidden to grow or use any more. But one day the woman was greedy and chose to pound more grain than the ration. To do this she had to take a longer pestle, and when she raised it up she hit the sky, and so God went far away. Since that day humans have had to work hard for their food, they are often hungry, they cannot reach God easily, and the two-pronged scourge of illness and death has come to rout them.

Another Dinka story explains the separation of God from humans by saying that a wall in heaven once held human beings in the sky. But eventually people ate part of the wall and God pushed them down to earth. A more elaborate version says that the earth was already created, but it could not be seen because there was no light. So God created a man and pushed him to an opening in the heavenly wall, and then pulled him back. God gave the man eyes so that he could know that he was in the dark, and the man made a rope with which he caught an animal. He gave a leg of the animal to God's wife, who said he should be rewarded. When God asked the man what he wanted, he asked for a chink to see through. God refused this but he did present him with an axe. One day the man struck the earth with his axe and it lit up. God was angry at this and pushed the man down to earth.

A theme that is soon introduced, and often occurs, is that of a rope hanging from the sky, by which some people can get up to and down from heaven. The Dinka say that such a rope hung originally within reach of humans, who could climb up it to God. But when the woman had offended God by hitting the sky, God sent a blue bird to cut the rope so that people could not get to him easily. The Nuer people of the Sudan say that when people grew old they could climb up to the sky by a rope and become young again, and then they could return to earth and take up their life afresh. But one day the Hyena – who often appears in the mythology of death – and a Weaverbird climbed up the rope to heaven. God saw them, and knowing that

Left. Pestle and mortar for pounding grain from Abomey. Horniman Museum, London.

Opposite. Brass weight from Ashanti, showing women pounding fu-fu, cassava, yam or plantain. Used for measuring out gold dust in what used to be called the Gold Coast, many creatures, events and activities are depicted on such weights. Museum of Mankind, London.

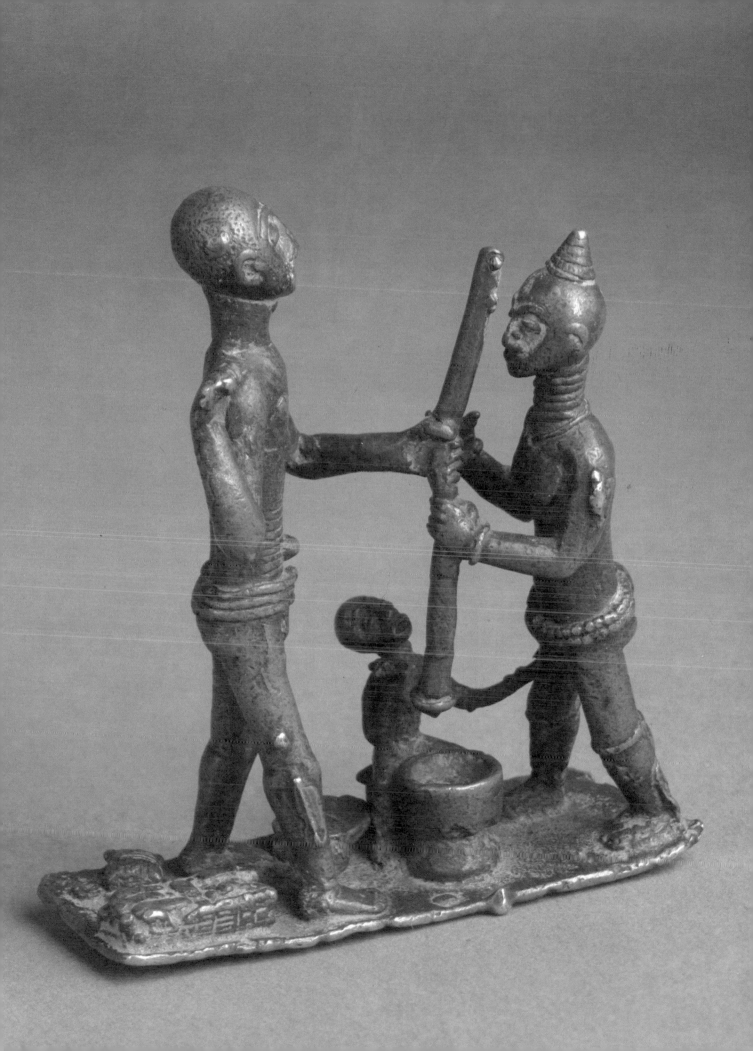

they might cause trouble, he gave orders that these two creatures were not to be allowed to go down to earth again. However the animals managed to escape one night; they climbed down the rope, which the Hyena cut when they got near the earth. The part that was above the cut was then drawn up to heaven, and since then people have never been able to climb up to heaven and death has taken them away.

Many of the central and southern African peoples who speak of God as Mulungu say that he lived on earth at first, but went up to heaven by a spider's thread because men had begun to set fire to the bush and killed his people. Some say that when God was leaving the earth he could not climb a tree, which seems to have been the usual way up to the sky. So he went to the Spider, who could get up and down again easily, and God went up to heaven on a spider's thread. In later stories people sometimes climb up to heaven by a rope or thread hanging from the clouds, like the long spiders' webs that are seen on misty mornings, spun between great trees.

Another kind of story is told in Burundi in central Africa. In olden days God lived among humans, talking with them, going from one to another, and creating the children that were born to them. But one day God created a crippled baby and its parents were angry. They plotted to take God unawares and stab him with a knife. But God, who sees all things, knew about the plot. He decided that if people were going to behave like that he would return to heaven and show himself no more. In that way he could perform his acts of creation as he pleased and not be bothered by complaints from humans. So he departed, and did not reveal himself again. But a few people have caught a glimpse of God, almost by accident and good fortune.

The Lozi (Barotse) people of the upper Zambesi in Zambia say that in the beginning God created the earth and all living creatures. At that time God and his wife lived here below among men. There was a man called Kamonu who was very clever, and

imitated God in all that he did. When God worked in iron so did Kamonu, and when God forged, Kamonu did so too. God began to be rather concerned, and when Kamonu made a spear and killed a large antelope God rebuked him, saying that he was killing his brothers, and drove him out. However Kamonu pleaded to return and God allowed him to cultivate land. Some time later buffaloes broke into Kamonu's plantation and he killed one of them, and when deer came he killed them also. Misfortune then befell his family; he broke a pot, his dog died, and his own child died. Kamonu went to complain about his losses to God and was surprised to see that his pot, dog and child were there with him. He asked for medicine to take them back, but God refused. Then God told his counsellors and his wife that since Kamonu had found his way to their dwelling they must move, and they went to live on an island in a river. But Kamonu made a raft and reached them. Next God made a great mountain and lived on top of it, but still Kamonu followed him.

God could not get away from people and they were multiplying everywhere. He sent out birds to find a place where he could get right away, but they were unsuccessful. He called his diviner, the Wagtail, and asked him to throw the divining bones to find a refuge. The diviner found that they must ask the Spider. So at the order of God the Spider spun a thread which reached right up to the sky, and God and his family climbed up there and have stayed above ever since. But on the advice of the diviner the eyes of the Spider were put out, so that it could not follow them up to the sky. Kamonu continued his efforts to reach God. He and his men cut down many trees and piled them on top of one another, trying to reach the sky. But the weight was too heavy and they all fell down. So every day when the sun rises people still salute God, and when the new moon appears they salute his wife.

There is a Pygmy story, perhaps influenced by Negro myth, that formerly God lived on earth with his

children, two boys and a girl (see page 52). But although he lived among them, they did not see God and were forbidden to try and look at him. He lived in a big house, where they heard him working at a smithy. The daughter was told to bring firewood every day and a pot of water, and leave them at the door of God's house. For a long time she was curious, and then one day she hid herself round the corner of the divine hut. She saw a big arm come out to take the pot, adorned with rich metal bracelets. But God knew that he had been seen and he called all his children together, and said that because of human disobedience he was going to leave them and move far away. He left them arms and tools so that they could look after themselves. The girl he told to marry her brothers and give birth to children. Her first child died two days after its birth and death entered the world.

The First Ancestors

Probably all African peoples have traditions of their first ancestors, and these may also be mentioned in myths of God or legends of history.

The Zulu of South Africa used to say that the first human pair, a man and a woman, came out of a reed or a reed-bed. The Thonga of Mozambique said that one man and one woman came suddenly out of a reed, which exploded and there they were. It was long the custom to put a reed in the ground outside the house in which a baby was born. The Herero of Namibia say that their ancestors came out of a certain tree which is still thought to exist in the veld. Their cattle too came out of this tree, since they used to be great stock-breeders and lived close to the herds. But sheep and goats are said to have emerged from a hole in the ground. They said also that the small Bushmen came out of this hole, though in olden days the Bushmen had no sheep or goats themselves.

One of the versions of the origins of humans current among the Ashanti of Ghana says the first ancestors came to the surface from holes in the ground. Some say that on a Monday night, which is still significant in the seven-day week to certain groups of people, a worm made a passage up through the earth. There came up seven men, some women, a dog and a leopard; the latter is still sacred to some clans. The names of the men and women are still recounted by some old people, on Mondays or Tuesdays only. When the men and women looked around them on the face of the earth, they were very frightened at the strange sights there. Only their leader, Adu Ogyinae, was not afraid. On the Tuesday he calmed the fears of his friends by laying his

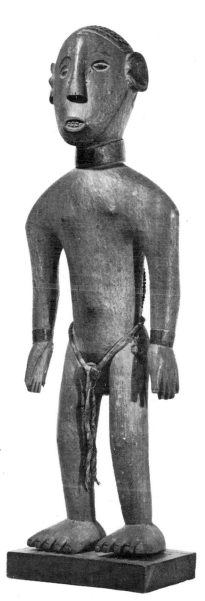

Figure of a woman from the Zulu of South Africa. A Zulu myth says that the first man and woman came out of a reed which suddenly exploded. A similar story is told by the Thonga of Mozambique, and it used to be the custom to put a reed in the ground outside a house in which a baby was born. Musée de l'Homme, Paris.

41

hands on each of them. But when they began to build houses, on Wednesday, the leader was killed by a tree falling on him. Next the dog went out to look for some fire and brought it back to the men. They cooked some food, tried it on the dog first, and then ate it themselves. The God of creation was travelling about the world in his task of making things, and it seems that he met these people who had come up from the ground and took one of them to act as his helper and spokesman. His staff was long treasured by his relatives. There are still pots in the forest which are used for libations at annual ceremonies held in remembrance of these first people.

It has already been told that the Yoruba of Nigeria believe the first people had been made in heaven and sent to earth with the help of Great God. The first man was giver of morality and family order, and he has been respected as ancestor and lawgiver ever since. He imposed taboos and punished anybody who broke them. His tutelary deity was Great God, since he had formed his body. Some of the other gods came down to earth, and of one of them it is said that he did not pay his respects to the first man but acted with disdain towards him. The man took his revenge by poisoning this god's daughter. Every effort was made to heal the girl but without success, and so at last the god came begging to man to heal him. The man was skilled in medicine, and demanded respect and repentance from the god before healing his daughter. The god yielded and gave him this, thus recognising also

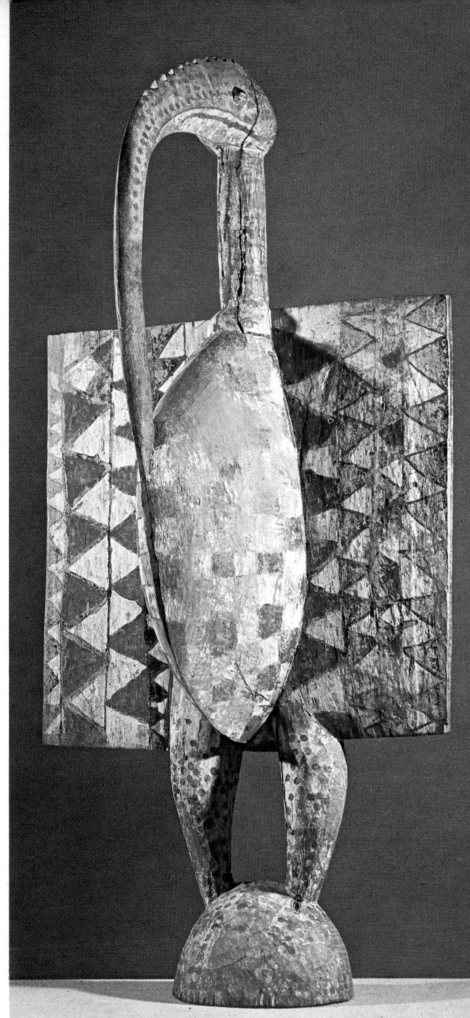

Right. The Senufo of the Ivory Coast make many masks, half-human and half-animal. This figure of a standing bird has abstract patterns on the stylised wings, and genealogical figures on the back which suggest it was originally an ancestor-cult figure. Staatliches Museum für Völkerkunde, Munich.

Opposite. Mask of the Yoruba used in ancestor-cult societies and surmounted by a circular snake being attacked by a bird. Musée de l'Homme, Paris.

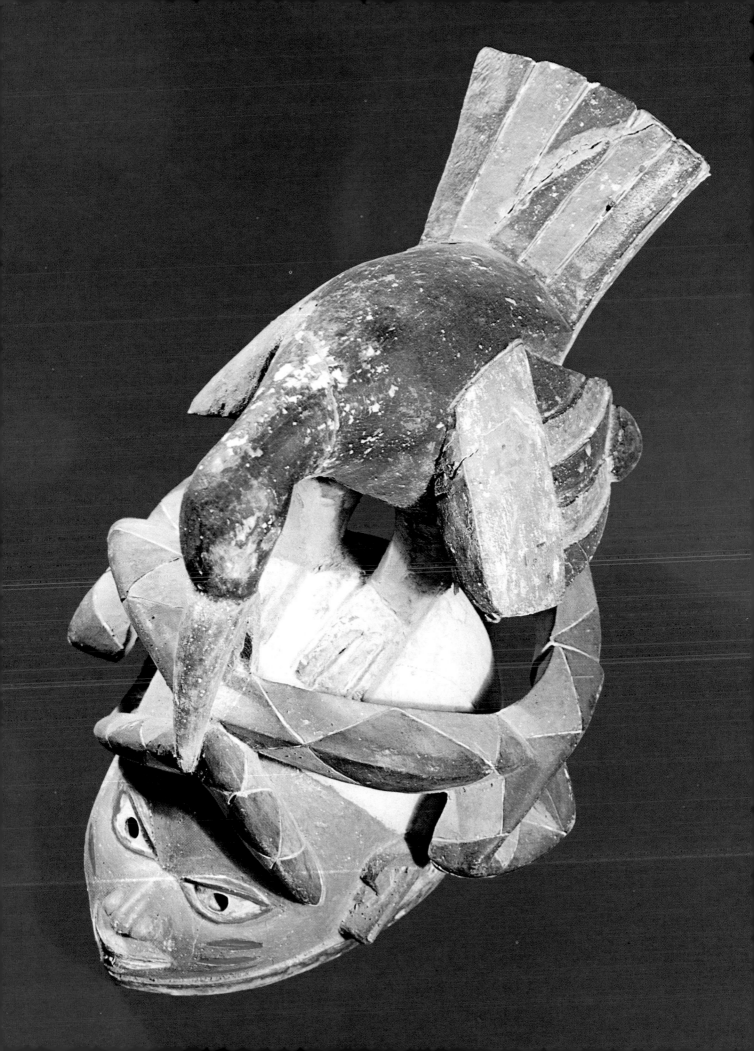

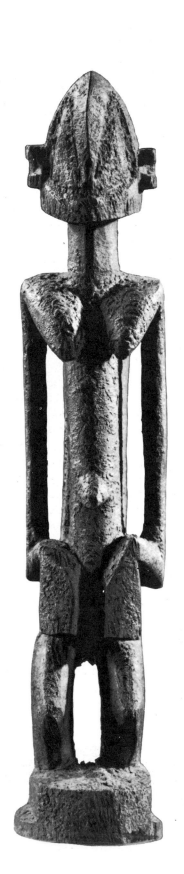

the primacy of Great God, who protected man.

The Shilluk of the upper Nile regions of the Sudan say in the beginning people lived in the land of God, but they ate fruit which made them sick and so God sent them away. This may suggest the Bible story, but it is found among tribes that seem to have had no Christian or Moslem influence. Another story says that in the olden days people used to be able to get to the moon by road, but they became too heavy and could no longer use it. More commonly it is said that humans and animals once lived together and were no different from one another. In those days there was no death, for cattle trampled on people when they were old and they became young again. Then the stories connect the first people with their more historical ancestors, but still with mythological details. The founder of the Shilluk royal house, Nyikang, was the son of a man who came from heaven, or perhaps he was a being specially created in the form of a cow. Anyway he married a woman who was a crocodile, or a river creature who had the attributes of a crocodile, though as the myth develops she appears as a woman. This crocodile-woman represents all the beings of the rivers, and offerings are still made to her at grassy spots on river banks where crocodiles emerge. If any water animal acts in an unusual way it is still looked on as a temporary incarnation of the original woman. She is regarded as the patron of birth and protector of babies.

The Dinka of the Sudan say that the first man and woman, Garang and Abuk, were made very small of clay and put in a pot, but when it was opened they became big. These were the people to whom God gave one grain of corn a day, till Abuk was greedy and pounded more. Garang is also a power, or 'free-divinity', which falls on men from the sky and enters their bodies, becoming their divinity. Such 'men of Garang' often wear leopard-skins, and as they are thought to be powerful doctors their hands are covered with rings and bracelets which mothers give them to

cure their children. Garang is sometimes associated with a snake, of red and white colour, and other animals which have white in association with red or brown are emblems of Garang: such as giraffes and oxen, and there is a tree with yellow-brown fruit. These colours also associate Garang with the sun. Abuk was the primeval woman, whose greed and offence against the sky are viewed indulgently when the story is told. She is connected with the waters and her emblem is a small snake. Abuk is patron of women and their produce, the gardens and the grain used for brewing beer, for which women are responsible.

Many stories are told in Buganda, Uganda, of Kintu, the first man and ancestor. When he came to the country from the gods he dwelt by himself with only one cow and lived on her milk. Then a woman, Nambi, came and fell in love with him, but she had to go back to her father, Gulu, who was king of heaven. Nambi's relatives despised Kintu because he knew of no food but milk and they objected to the marriage. To test him Gulu robbed Kintu of his cow and the man had to live on herbs and leaves. But Nambi saw the cow, and went and told Kintu that it was in heaven and invited him to go up there to fetch it back down to earth again.

When Kintu arrived he was surprised to see many cows, sheep, fowls and houses there. In the meantime Nambi's brothers told their father that Kintu had arrived and a test was arranged for him. A huge meal was cooked, enough for a hundred people, and Kintu was told that unless he ate it all he would be killed. He was shut up in a house with the food, and when he had eaten his fill he did not know what to do with the rest. Then he discovered a hole in the floor so he dropped all the food and beer into it, and called the people to take away the empty baskets. Gulu could hardly believe that Kintu had eaten all the food, and fixed a further test. He sent him a copper axe and told him to cut firewood from the rock, because he did not use ordinary wood. But Kintu found a rock with cracks in it, so he broke pieces off and returned to Gulu. Yet another trial was imposed, and Kintu was told to fetch water which must be only dew. He took the pot into a field and put it down while he thought what to do, but to his surprise when he went to the pot it was full of dew.

Gulu was so impressed that he thought Kintu was a wonderful being, and agreed to let him marry his daughter. He told Kintu to pick out his own cow from the herds, but this was not easy because there were many others just like his own. Just then a large bee flew up and told Kintu to choose the cow on whose horns it alighted. In the morning, when the cows were brought Kintu kept his eye on the bee, which stayed in a tree. He said that his cow was not in the herd. When a second herd was brought he said the same. In the third herd the bee landed on a large cow, and Kintu claimed it as his own. The bee went on to settle on three calves, which Kintu said had been born during the cow's stay in heaven. Gulu was delighted, and declared that since nobody could deceive Kintu he could take his daughter Nambi as wife. The story of Nambi and death is told later.

In Malagasy it is said that in the beginning the Creator made two men and a woman, and all lived on earth, but separately, knowing nothing of each other. The first man carved a woman out of wood, full-size, and was so enamoured of it, like Pygmalion, that he talked to the image all the time and put it in the open so that he could look at it while he worked. One day the second man, walking through the bush, came upon the statue and was struck by its beauty, but its nakedness shocked him and he

covered it with beautiful clothing and jewels. Later the woman came along, lamenting her solitude, and when she saw the image she fell down on her knees and asked the Creator to give it life. He promised to do so if she would take it to her bed.

She clasped the image tightly all night and in the morning it was alive as a beautiful girl. Then the two men came up and claimed the girl as their handiwork. The woman refused to give her up and God had to intervene. He decreed that the first man was father of the girl, since he had made the image from wood. The woman was its mother, since she had given it life. The second man should be the girl's husband, since he had adorned her with so much love. This arrangement was accepted, and of course the first man married the woman, while the second man married the girl. From these two couples descend everybody on earth today. From the first man came the clan of sculptors, and all men must give clothing and ornaments to their wives.

Another Malagasy story says that in the beginning the woman, the cow and the bitch were all children of the same father and lived together. One day God wanted a servant for his throne and sent fever down to earth to get a life from the woman. Her only child became sick and she sent for her relatives to bring all the medicinal plants they could find. But these were no use and the child got worse. During the night God appeared to the woman with a great knife in his hand uplifted to strike. She fell on her knees and begged for mercy. God said he would spare her if she gave him a life in place of that of her child. In the morning the woman went to the bitch, who was the elder, and asked

for help to meet the divine demands. The bitch agreed at first, but when the woman told her dream, and the bitch saw that she wanted one of her litter, she refused, telling the woman to die herself for the child. The woman went to the cow with the same request, and moved with pity the cow gave her the younger and weaker calf of the two that she had. The woman quickly killed it and offered it to God. Her own child opened its eyes and recovered. Then the woman swore that she and her children would always take care of the cow and its young, and look on them as the most faithful companions. But they would not look after dogs, and even though they came from the same parents dogs would always be servants. Thus dogs run in front of humans because they are older, but they have to wait for their masters; they are the lowest of domestic animals and are not allowed to enter houses.

The Luyia of Kenya say that when God had created the sun he wondered for whom it would shine. So he made the first man, called Mwambu. Since the man could talk and see he needed a companion, and God made the first woman, whose name was Sela. They

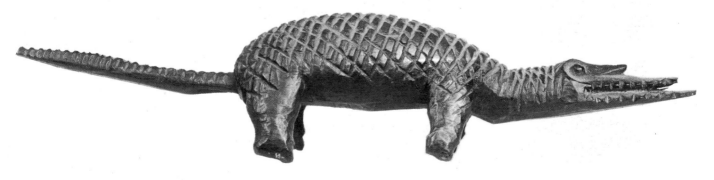

wanted something to drink, so God made water fall from heaven, which filled up the holes and valleys to make lakes and rivers. God instructed Mwambu and Sela in the flesh they could eat: some animals were allowed for food but others were taboo. They were forbidden to eat crawling beasts like snails and lizards, or birds that feed on carrion like hawks and vultures. One day God surprised a buffalo cow with its young, and it ran away leaving the young ones, which were male and female. God took them and gave them to the man and woman. They fed them on an ant-hill, and some people say that originally cattle came from an ant-hill. Mwambu and Sela lived in a house supported by posts, because they were afraid of earthly monsters. Their children came down and lived on the ground, but tree-houses are still used sometimes in forests, and houses on piles stand in the waters at the edge of lakes.

Another Luyia story says that in the olden days people had no idea how to make pots; they simply used calabashes which grew wild, and which many people cultivate now. It was the children who were responsible for finding how to make pots. They saw their mothers with fine calabashes, which they had gathered in the bush, and children tried to make some for themselves, with bits of clay in the shape of calabashes. Somehow their clay pots got in the fire, and they found that if they got hard the water would not leak out as it did when the pots were wet. So children made the first clay pots, and when mothers saw they were good they copied them and made bigger pots for their own use. These large pots were made of damp clay at first and they collapsed. They could not be used till they had been put in the fire and hardened, as the children had done.

Some women are wholly given to special tasks and are freed from the housework that most women do. The Luyia say that this happened first when two sisters lived together. One was so busy making pots all the time that she left all other work to her sister. The sister was so annoyed that she broke all the pots. Then the potmaker was angry and ran away from home. She went for three days on foot till she reached a big lake and saw a tall tree in the middle. The tree noticed the girl at the water's edge and came towards her so that she could climb up into its branches, and then it went back again into the water. The girl's parents had been looking for her everywhere and at last they reached the lake. They saw her sitting in the top of the tree in the middle of the water. They could not get to her and called out, begging her to come home. The girl refused to do this, till at last her lover came and called her too. Then she agreed to return to the shore, on condition that she could do her work without trouble. Her parents agreed, made her some new pots, and excused her all housework so that she never had to do any more.

A Pygmy story of the first humans links up with that character who often appears in fable, the Chameleon. Once upon a time a Chameleon heard some whispering in a tree, like birds chirping or water running. That was surprising since there was no water on earth at that time. The Chameleon took an axe and cut open the trunk of the tree, till at last water came out, in a great flood that spread all over the earth. With this water

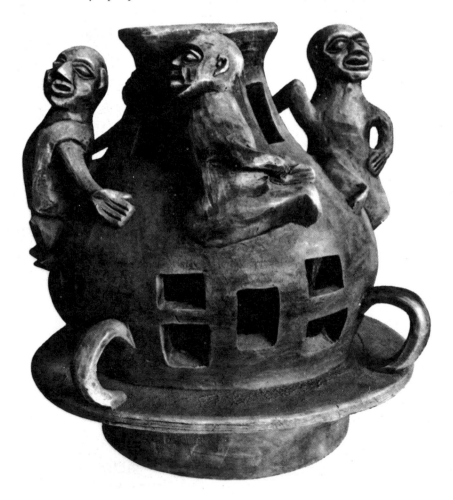

Left. A pottery figure from Abomey represents the Just King. On the left the king stretches out his hand in judgement, the condemned man waits in the middle with his hands tied behind his back, while the executioner on the right lifts his axe.

Opposite left. Two ancestral figures of the Dogon of Mali illustrate the unity of man and woman, the man linking the two with his arm. Twins are also depicted in this manner, as children or adults. Musée National des Arts Africains Océaniens, Paris.

Opposite right. A carved wooden dance mask of the Senufo people of the Ivory Coast, showing a chameleon and a hornbill on a head which combines the horns of an antelope with the features of a warthog. Musée de l'Homme, Paris.

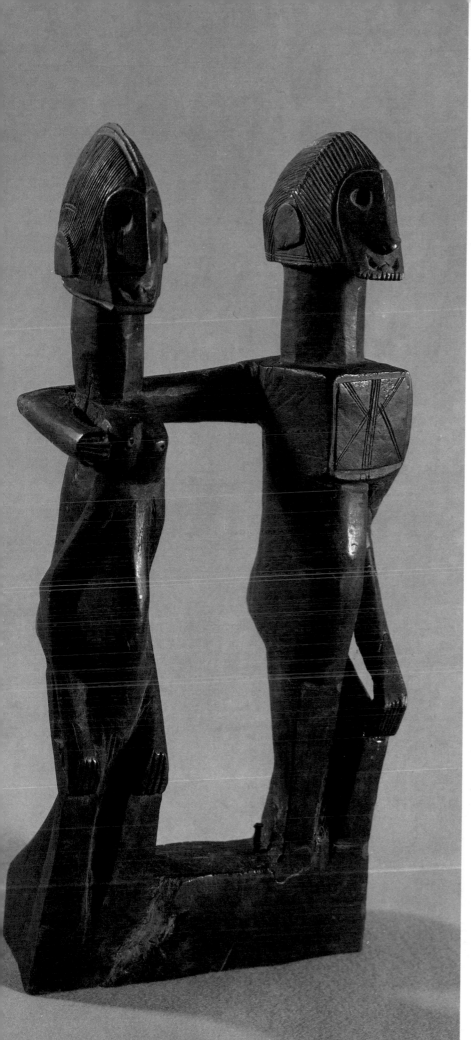

emerged the first human couple, a woman and a man. Both were light-skinned, like the lightest-coloured of the Pygmies. As there were no other people on earth, this couple lived together and gave birth to the first child. Another Pygmy story says that three people were created first (see page 52).

There is a Pygmy story of the first man, called Efé. God had placed him on earth, but after a time he wanted him to come back to heaven as a hunter. He cut a long liana and drew Efé up to heaven by it. He gave him three spears and told him to go hunting. Efé killed an elephant, whose tusks were as big as great trees. All the people of heaven were happy,

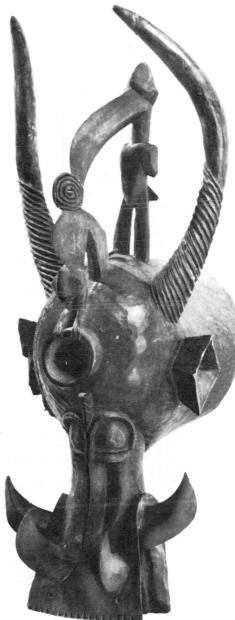

47

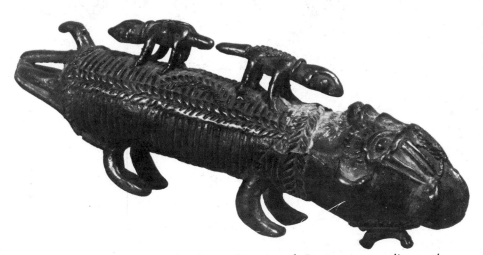

especially the women, who hugged the hunter before cutting up the elephant. Efé stayed for a long time hunting in the sky, but finally he was sent back to earth, taking his three spears and many presents. All the Pygmy camp gathered round for his arrival but nobody recognised him, after his long absence he was a stranger. At last his brother came up and said that even if he should die he would try to find out who the stranger was. Eventually he identified Efé, and asked where he had been for so long. Efé replied that he had been with their father in the sky. 'Is he still alive?' asked the brother. Efé said, 'Yes, and he has sent us these spears and presents.' Then everybody embraced him and rejoiced.

The mythology of the first ancestors told by the Dogon people of Mali is long and complex, following on their creation stories. The first man and woman created bore a series of twins, who were the ancestors of the Dogon tribe. The four eldest ancestors were males, the others females. The oldest ancestor after a time went to the ant-hill or womb of the primeval mother and disappeared into it.

The only trace that remained was a wooden bowl on the ground which he had worn as a hat to protect him from the sun. The ancestor was led by the male Nummo spirit (see page 27) into the depths of the earth, where he shrank to a form like water, which is the seed of God, and finally rose up to heaven. The eight ancestors were transformed in this way and went to heaven where the Nummo reigned. But an extraordinary change occurred with the seventh ancestor. Seven is a perfect number, being the union of four, which is feminine, and three, which is masculine. The seventh ancestor received knowledge of a Word, which brought progress to mankind and enabled it to get ahead of the Jackal, who had taken the first Word. The seventh ancestor revealed his Word by the art of weaving. People also learnt, from the bowl which the ancestors left behind and by studying the ant-hill, how to make better dwellings than the caves in which they had formerly lived.

Up in heaven, however, things were not going well. The eight ancestors were transformed into the same essence as the Nummo pair, but the Nummo were chiefs and they separated the ancestors from one another and forbade them to come together, so as to keep the peace. God had given the ancestors eight different grains each for food; but when all were eaten except the last, the first and second ancestors came together to eat it. So they disobeyed the Nummo orders and became unclean. They then determined to leave heaven and the other ancestors joined them. With the help of God they took with them whatever might be useful on earth.

The first ancestor took a basket and some clay, which was particularly important, as it was a model for the world system. It was moulded with clay on a basket framework, upside down, but when inverted it had a circular base, a square top, and four sides in which were staircases, each of ten steps. The circular base stood for the sun, and the square top the sky; in this roof there was a circle for the moon. The stairs were male and female, and together they denoted the children of the ancestors. They were also associated with men, animals, birds, insects, and stars. This primeval construction was like a granary and was called the Granary of the Master of Pure Earth. It contained compartments, like an earthly granary, for the different seeds which God gave the eight ancestors. They also symbolise the organs of the human body.

The story has been told of the first ancestor stealing fire from the Nummo blacksmith. When the Nummo hurled a thunderbolt the first ancestor loosed the granary and it came down a rainbow to earth, with increasing speed from the blows of thunder and lightning. It landed with a crash and people, animals and vegetables were scattered about. The ancestor came down from the roof of the granary by the steps. He marked out land for fields and distributed it among the descendants of the ancestors. The first ancestor was a smith, and the others began the work and arts of leather-workers, minstrels, and so on. There was trouble with a snake. Some say it was the seventh ancestor, and others that it was the

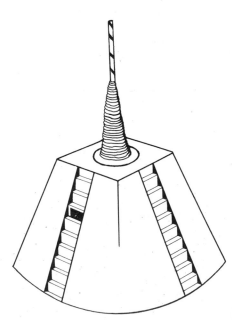

Right. The shape of the Dogon house is symbolical. The floor is like the earth and the flat roof like heaven. The vestibule is a man and the central room a woman, with store rooms at her sides as arms. The hearth at the end is her head. The four posts are the man and woman entwined in union. So the family house represents the unity of man and woman, and God and the Earth. From Griaule: *Conversations with Ogotemmêli.*

Opposite above. A bronze from the Kwale division of the Ibo people of Nigeria, representing an anthropomorphic creature with a man's face. Two chameleons ride on his back. It was possibly used as a weight. Museum of Mankind, London.

Opposite below. Model of the universe in the mythology of the Dogon of Mali. The circular base is the sun and the square top the sky, with a circle for the moon. It is called the Granary of the Master of Pure Earth. The first ancestor came down from the sky by the steps at the side to mark out land for fields for his descendants. From Griaule: *Conversations with Ogotemmêli.*

Below. Dogon symbol of the life-force of their ancestors. This is the outline of every soul which the Nummo spirits make at birth. It is made of different coloured stones, representing the eight ancestors, with an extra stone for the head. The spirits put copper between the legs as the metal which was later used for ritual bracelets. From Griaule: *Conversations with Ogotemmêli.*

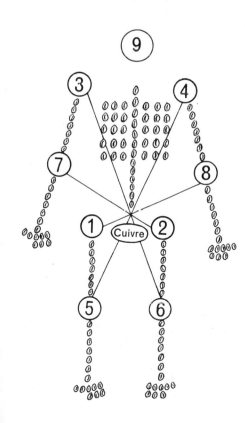

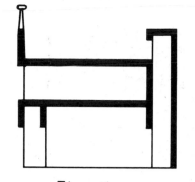

Elevation

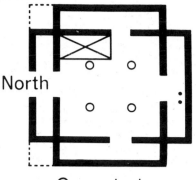

North

Ground plan

granary itself. Anyway the snake was killed and its head buried under a stone in the smithy. It may represent the original granary which was spread far and wide when it came crashing down to the earth.

The Dogon say that for the purposes of God humans had now to be organised. They lived in eight families, descended from the eight ancestors. The eighth family was regarded as superior, since it had speech. The oldest man was called Lebé and he represented the Word. But he had to die, or at least appear to die, though Death had not yet come to earth. He was buried lying on his back, with his head to the north. He was swallowed by the seventh ancestor, who had taken the form of a snake. Then the snake vomited stones in the shape of a body, like the outlines of a human soul. The stones were placed in order, one for the head, eight principal stones for each ancestor marking the joints, and then secondary stones filled in the ribs, spine and other bones. These stones were symbolical of the life-force of the eight ancestors, sent into their descendants and kept later by priests. The arranging of the stones of the joints helped to fix the social system, especially marriages, in which there is alternation of left and right, upper and lower. So the eighth man's body symbolised both human beings and society. He was swallowed so that people should know that his bones had been transformed and that he was present in these covenant-stones. Once Lebé had been swallowed, all that was good from the former Word was put into the stones, and all that was impure was cast away. This was only done in appear-

ance, since Lebé was not really dead or eaten, but it was done for all human beings, to give life-force to the people. There is a great annual sacrifice to Lebé, a victim on behalf of the human race.

The shape of the Dogon house is also explained symbolically. The floor is like the Earth, and Lebé who was restored to life in the earth. If it is placed correctly then the door is open towards the north, and at the opposite end is the hearth, where cooking pots are supported on two stones and the rear wall. The two stones mark east and west, and the wall indicates south. The flat roof of the house is like heaven, in the Granary of the Master of Pure Earth. There may be four small roofs round the central roof, indicating the cardinal points of the compass. The rooms of the house symbolise male and female and their union. The vestibule is the male, while the big central room is the woman, with store-rooms at each side as her arms. The end room with the hearth is her head. The woman lies on her back, and the ceiling above is also the man. Four posts supporting the room are the arms of the man and woman entwined in the act of union. Thus the family house represents the union of man and woman. It also recalls the primeval union of God and Earth.

Like the house the Dogon village also should be orientated north to south, like a prostrate being, human or divine. The smithy should be at the head, like the family hearth. The family houses are in the centre, with women's and men's separate houses like hands on east and west. Mill-stones and a foundation altar are

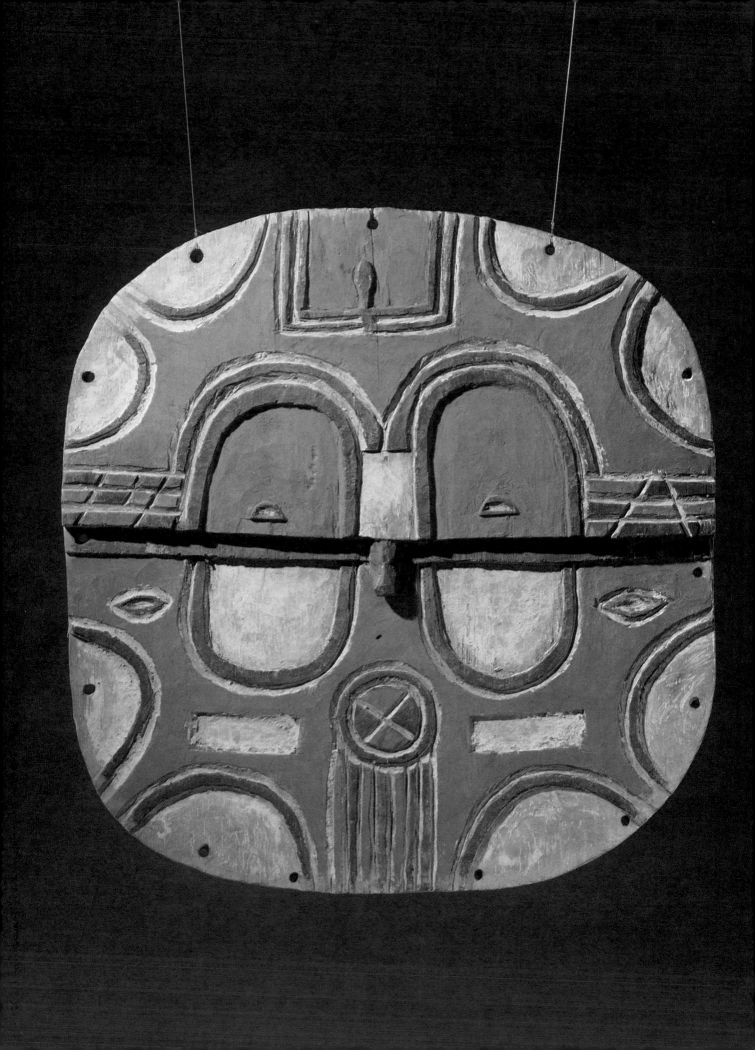

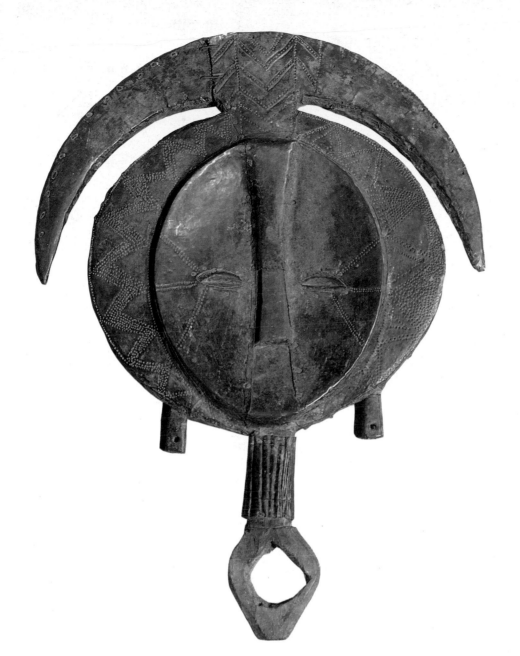

lower down like sexual organs, and other altars are the feet. Villages can only be arranged fully in this manner on the plains, for in hills the contours and rocks force other arrangements. But seen from the air, in the light of mythical explanation, both houses and villages take on a new significance.

Many other Dogon stories, too numerous to relate here, tell of the institution of agriculture, weaving, smithying, trade, dress and love. These are connected with the original myths of God, Earth, Nummo spirits, and the ancestors, and form explanatory patterns and justifications for human activities.

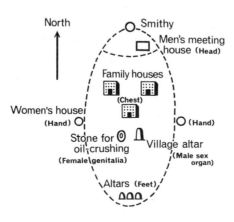

Elevation   Ground plan

North

Smithy

Men's meeting house **(Head)**

Family houses

(Chest)

Women's house
(Hand)   **(Hand)**

Stone for oil-crushing
(Female genitalia)   Village altar
(Male sex organ)

Altars **(Feet)**

Above. Brass and wood reliquary figure, Bakota, Gabon. The face is stylised and the winged headdress semi-circular to make three rounds of mystery and power. Musée National des Arts Africains et Océaniens, Paris.

Left. Like the house, the Dogon village represents human beings. The smithy is at the head like a hearth in a house. The family houses are in the centre and millstones and village altar represent the sexes. Other altars are at the feet. From Griaule: *Conversations with Ogotemmêli.*

Opposite. Mask of the Bateké of Zaïre (Congo). The Bateké live on both sides of the Zaïre (Congo) river. African art is sometimes naturalistic, often stylised, and frequently abstract as here. The lower lids of the mask, representing a dead person, are slightly offset so that the upper part of the head appears to thrust forwards. Musée de l'Homme, Paris.

51

The Mystery of Birth

Another version of the Ashanti story of the origins of humans (page 41) says that long ago a man and a woman came down from heaven, while another man and woman came out of the ground. The Lord of Heaven also sent a python, the non-poisonous snake, which made its home in a river. In the beginning men and women had no children, they had no desire for one another and did not know the process of procreation and birth. It was the Python who taught them. He asked the men and women if they had any children, and on being told that they had none, the Python said he would make the women conceive. He told the couples to stand facing each other, then he went into the river and came out with his mouth full of water. This he sprayed on their bellies, saying 'Kus, kus', words that are still used in clan rituals. Then the Python told the couples to go home and lie together, and the women conceived and bore children. These children took the spirit of the river where the Python lived as their clan spirit. Members of that clan to this day hold the python as taboo; they must never kill it, and if they find a python that has died or been killed by someone else, they put white clay on it and bury it in almost human fashion. The symbolism of the snake is obvious and has been used in mythology at least since the book of Genesis.

A Pygmy story says that at first three people were created, two boys and a girl. One of the boys was a Negro and the other a Pygmy. One day the Negro told the Pygmy that he did not know what to do with his sister, for she was always bleeding despite all the medicines that he put on her wound. The Pygmy had already been told by God the meaning of this physical phenomenon and he laughed at the Negro, saying he would cure the wound. So he took the girl and she bore him children. Then he returned the woman to her brother and explained to him the mystery of procreation as the cure for the female ill. Then the Negro also begat children. Though later this would be regarded as incestuous, in myth it solves the problem of how the first pair had children.

Another Pygmy myth says that the Lightning lived with a woman, as brother and sister, for the way of procreation was not known to them. One day the Moon came to visit the Lightning and, seeing how he lived with the woman, advised him to consummate his marriage. The Lightning refused at first, because he did not know how to proceed. Then the Moon made monthly periods come to the woman. Some say that a young man took the woman first and showed the way. Anyway the Lightning plucked up courage and did the same. The first child was very light-skinned but others were darker, and when at length the woman died the Moon took her up to the heavens where he lived with the Sun.

A Malagasy story says that one day a man was fishing when he felt a strong pull on his line. He drew it in carefully, thinking it to be a big fish. He was very frightened to see a woman emerge from the water, and he threw everything down to run away when the woman called out that he should not be afraid. She said she would marry him, only he must promise never to look at what was underneath her arm. The man agreed, they were married, and had a son and daughter. But when the children were growing up the husband could no

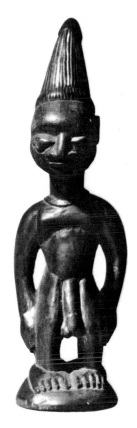

longer resist the temptation to look in his wife's armpit, and he did this while she seemed to be asleep. The woman saw him and said nothing, but next day she suggested that they should go for a bathe. The man went into the water first, while his wife looked after the children on the bank. Then it was her turn, and as she disappeared into the waters she called out that she was leaving him, because he had broken her taboo. Some say that in her armpit she had an extra mouth. Others declare that the taboo was for her husband not to look at her while she was naked – he did this while she undressed and she gave a great cry and disappeared. Both versions may contain veiled allusions to the sex taboo, and the origins of procreation. The woman is claimed as mother of fishing clans.

A story of the Luyia of Kenya says that the first man and woman had no children for a long time. They did not know the secret of procreation and tried to have union in various ways but without success. One day the man saw his wife climbing into the granary and noticed her private parts, and so at night he sought union with her. She refused him at first, saying that he had only seen an ulcer, but later she gave in and suffered great pain. In due course she bore a son, much to the surprise of both parents. Later a girl was born to them.

Further mysteries of birth are children born with some abnormality, and they are usually feared. A baby born with an extra finger may be 'sent back' – neglected or exposed on a river bank – after rites which separate this bad luck from the family. Then there are 'born-to-die' children, from mothers who have had a succession of babies dying at birth; the same child is believed to be born each time. Stories tell of a child whose body is carefully marked at death; the same scar appears on the next child to be born.

Twins, and even more triplets, are regarded with mixed feelings of fear and joy, as abnormal, even animal, births. In eastern Nigeria they used to be exposed in pots in the forest. But in western Nigeria and Abomey they are prized, as the gods themselves, it is believed, were born in pairs. Images of twins, now often sold as curios, were used for rituals, and in front of them offerings were placed in twin pots. If a twin dies, the survivor, or the mother, wears a wooden image of the dead one tucked in the waist cloth. In Buganda twins were said to come from the great god Mukasa, and doctors made ceremonies to ensure health and prosperity. The Thonga of Mozambique called twins 'children of the sky', but thought their birth a great misfortune which needed rituals of purification. They were sent with their mother to live in a special hut outside the village and would not be popular even when grown up. But if storms threatened the village the twins were asked to intercede, since the sky would listen to its children. They stood outside the hut calling on the storm to go away, to thunder farther off and not annoy people. The mother of twins was credited with similar powers, since she had been up to the sky to get her twins and she could speak to it.

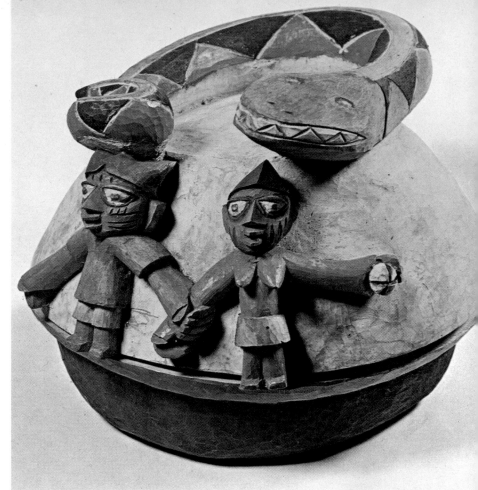

Above right. Man, woman and the snake are common themes in mythology, as shown in this carved and painted wooden bowl of the Yoruba, Nigeria. The snake is the sacred non-poisonous python, the circular symbol of life and eternity, and in some stories it teaches man and woman the mystery of procreation. Museum of Mankind, London.

Right. Wooden twin images from Abomey, joined by seven links, all from one piece of wood without joints. The male twin smokes a pipe. Twin images are used in rituals to ensure the health of the twins, and if they die the mother carries the images in her skirt band. In the possession of the author.

Opposite. Wooden headrest of the Luba of Zaïre (Congo), representing two sisters, possibly twins. In the Zaïre regions headrests are used to protect the elaborate headdresses of their owners from being flattened while sleeping. These figures are naturalistic, but others are stylised because of the heavy weight they have to support. Museum of Mankind, London.

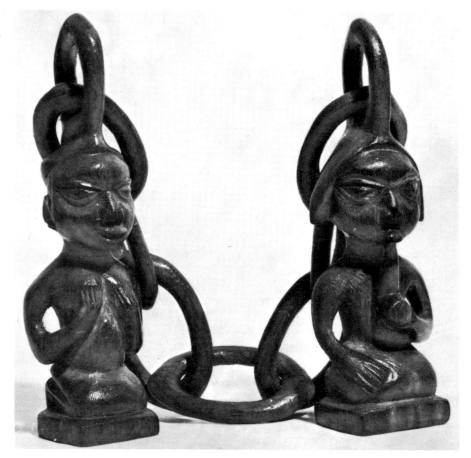

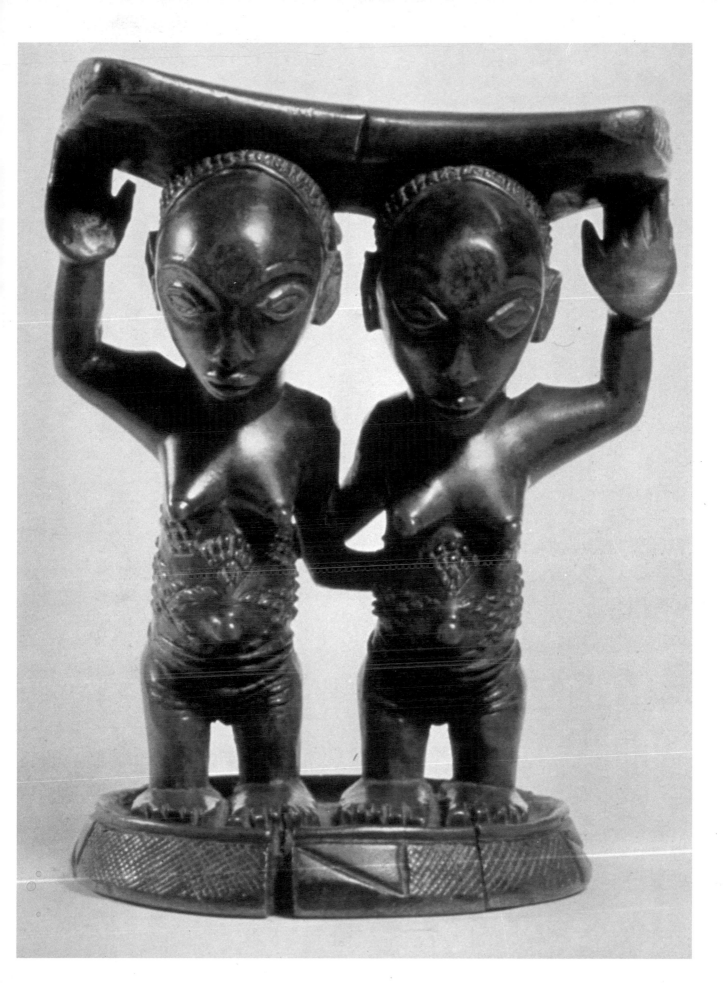

The Origins of Death

Several myths already related have mentioned the coming of death, and all over Africa stories are told which show the belief that death is not natural and was not found among humans at first. Its coming is blamed on some mistake, often the fault of an animal: the dog or the chameleon.

The Messengers
The Kono of Sierra Leone say that in olden times there was the first man and woman and their baby boy. The Supreme Being told them that none of the three would die, but when they got old they would have new skins for their bodies. He put these new skins in a bundle and entrusted it to the Dog to take to man. The Dog went off with the bundle, but on the way he met other animals who were feasting on rice and pumpkins. They invited the Dog to join them and he put down his burden and shared the feast. During the meal he was asked what was in his bundle and he told the story of the new skins that were being sent to the first people. But when the Snake overheard this he slipped out quietly, stole the bundle and shared out the skins with other snakes. The Dog had to confess to man that the skins had been stolen, and they both went to God. But it was too late, the Snake kept the skins, and since then humans have died. The Snake was punished by being driven away from towns to live alone, and if a man finds a snake he tries to kill it.

The Mende of Sierra Leone give a different version, which is also widespread, about two messengers. The Dog and the Toad were sent to take messages to the human race about death; the Dog to say that people would not die, and the Toad to say

they would. The animals set out together, but the Dog stopped on the way. He met a woman who was preparing food for her child, and he waited till he got some for himself.

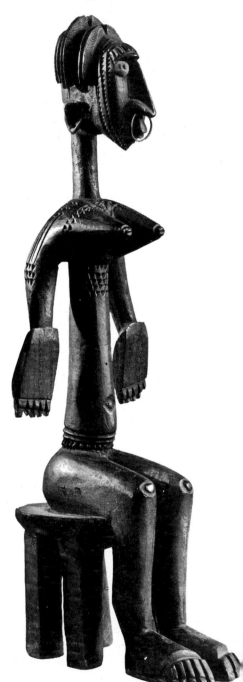

The Toad continued without stopping and arrived at the town, crying out, 'Death has come.' Just then the Dog ran up crying, 'Life has come.' But unfortunately it was too late.

The Nuba of the eastern Sudan say that, at first, when a man died, God told his relatives that he was only asleep; so they put him aside for the night and next morning he would be found alive again. But one day when a man died, and before God told people what to do, a Hare came and told the relatives to bury the corpse in the ground, else God would be angry and would kill them all. So the relatives buried the man and when God came they told him what had been done. Then God was really angry that they had listened to the Hare instead of to him, and he said that in future people would die and not return.

A Nuer story says that when God created human beings he took a piece of a gourd and cast it into the water, as a sign that as the gourd floated so people would live for ever. Then God sent a barren woman to give the message, but when she illustrated it, instead of throwing a buoyant gourd she cast a piece of earthen pot into the water and it sank. Since then men have died.

A Dinka story gives the different explanation that people die because there is not room for them all. The first man and woman were created in the east, on the bank of a great water, under a tamarind tree. They were very small, half as long as a man's arm, made of clay, and laid in a pot. When the Creator took the top off the pot the man and woman stood up fully grown, with completely developed organs. They had children and he told them that they would die, but would come back after fifteen days. The man did not agree and said that if they came back there would be no room for them, no land to cultivate or build houses.

In Burundi it is said that in olden days Death was not among men and God still lived on earth. If Death happened to appear, God chased him away with his hunting hounds. One day Death was being pursued closely by the divine dogs who forced him into a narrow place. He ran into a woman coming from the other direction and promised that if she hid him he would hide her and her family. The woman opened her mouth and Death jumped inside. Then God came along and demanded where Death had gone. The woman replied that she had not seen him. But God, who is the Seeing One and knows everything, knew what had happened. He told the woman that since she had hidden Death, in future Death would destroy her and all hers. God left the woman in anger and from that day death has spread among humans.

A Luyia story says that in olden days people used to die, but after four days they came back to life. But one day a boy died and when he returned his mother sent him away, saying he was dead and ought to stay that way. The boy did go away, but in going he cursed the people, and said that in future those who died would not return.

A further Luyia story says that Maina, son of the ancestor of their people, was sitting outside his house one evening eating his meal after work. As he sat there the Chameleon came and asked for some food. By the laws of hospitality Maina should have given some at once, but he refused. The Chameleon asked again and again until Maina grew angry and drove the beast away. The Chameleon cursed him and said that he would leave, but Maina and all his people would die. Then the Chameleon went on and met the Snake. He asked for food in the same way and the Snake at once shared his food with him. So the Chameleon blessed the Snake and said he would live for ever. People began to breathe bad air,

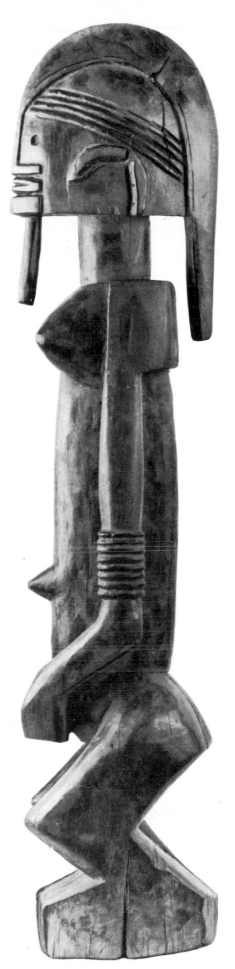

Right. Wooden statuette of the Dogon of Mali, called 'The Figure Which Stands on the Terrace'. Normally kept in a house, it is brought out for the funerals of rich families. Musée de l'Homme, Paris.

Opposite. A seated female figure from the Bambara people of Mali. It is believed to have been an ancestor cult figure, of the kind to which special honour was paid in funerary rites. The University Museum, Philadelphia, Pennsylvania.

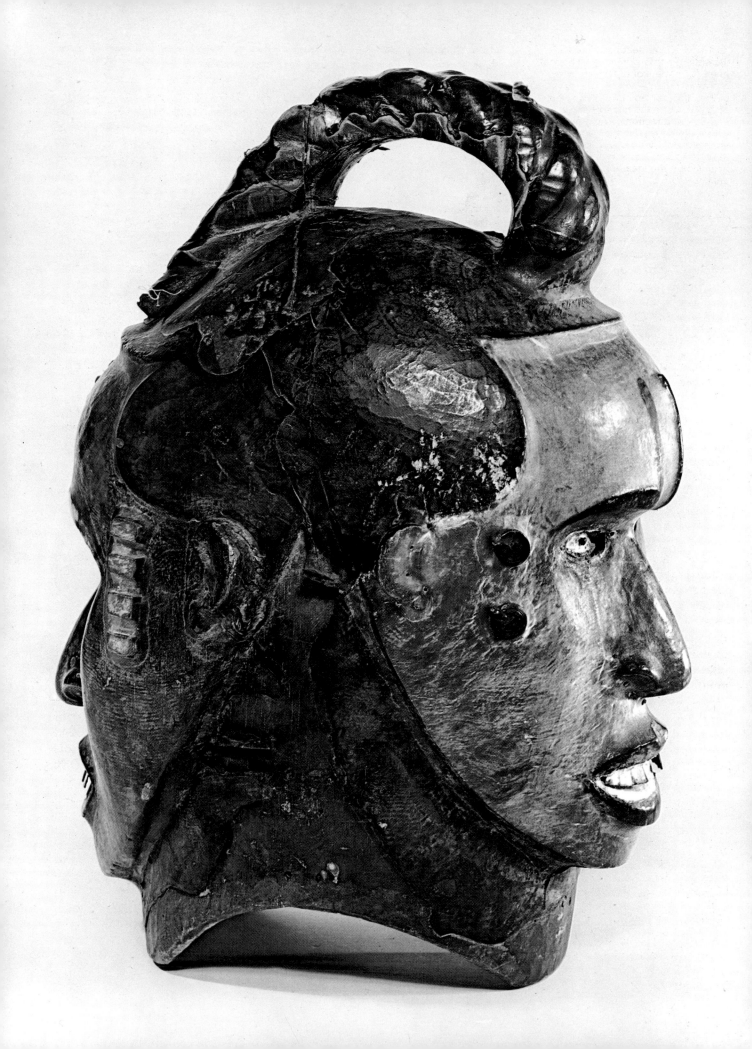

---

sicken and die, while the Snake sheds its skin and goes on living.

Many Bantu peoples have stories in which the Chameleon is associated with death. A Zulu myth says that God sent the Chameleon to humans with the message that they would not die. But the Chameleon walks slowly and it ate fruit on the way. Some time later God sent the Lizard saying that men should die. The Lizard scuttled off, got there first, and gave his message and even returned to God before the Chameleon had reached its destination. People had accepted the word of the Lizard and that could not be changed.

The Pandora's Box theme (see page 32) appears also in a story by the Lamba people of Zambia. The chief used to be a nomad, but finally he wanted to settle down and till the soil. He had no seeds, so he sent to God to ask for some. God gave his messengers little bundles, and one of them in particular they were told not to untie but to give it to their chief intact. The divine insistence on this point aroused the curiosity of the messengers, and when they stopped for the night on the road they began to untie the bundles, to see what God was sending their chief. When they opened the forbidden bundle death came out and spread into the world.

Rather different is a story of the Ila of Zambia. The first man and woman were given by God a choice between two little bags, one containing life and the other death. As one bag shone with a bright light the foolish pair chose this, which of course contained death, and a few days later one of their children died. However God gave the parents another chance, and when they begged him to restore the

child to life he promised to do this, if they would refrain from eating for three days. But their hunger became so great that they could not hold out, they took some food, and ever since then people have died.

In Buganda the coming of death is connected with the myth of the first man Kintu and his heavenly wife Nambi (see page 44). As they were leaving the sky Gulu warned them to hurry because Death would want to go with them, and if they had forgotten anything they must not go back. They set out with cows, a goat, a sheep, a fowl and a plantain tree, a sort of banana. On the way Nambi said she had forgotten grain for the fowl and must go back for it. Kintu tried to dissuade her, but Nambi would not listen and returned to ask Gulu for grain. She tried to steal away, but her brother Death followed her, and Kintu was angry that Death had come. Nambi pacified him by saying they must go on and see what happened. When they got to the earth Nambi planted a garden, and she lived happily with her husband, bearing many children.

One day Death asked Kintu for one of his children to be his cook. Kintu refused, saying that if Gulu came he would be ashamed to say that one of his children was Death's cook. Death asked again, and when Kintu refused again he said he would kill the child. Kintu did not know what 'kill' meant, but the child soon sickened and died. After this other children died at intervals, and Kintu went up to heaven and complained about Death to Gulu. Gulu told him that he had been warned, and if he had not allowed Nambi to return for grain they would have been protected from Death. But after some entreaty Gulu sent Death's brother, Kaizuki, to stop Death killing all the children.

Kaizuki found Death and fought with him but Death managed to escape. Kaizuki told all the people to stay in their houses, with their animals, and he would prepare a last hunt for Death. He also said that if they saw Death they must not call out or make any noise. All went well, and Kaizuki had lured Death from his

hiding place when some children came out with their goats. They saw Death and called out in fear, and at this Death went back into the earth. So Kaizuki told Kintu that he was tired of hunting Death, nothing could be done to catch him, and he himself was returning to heaven. Since then Death has lived on earth; he kills people when he can and then escapes into the ground.

A Malagasy myth says that God had a daughter called Earth, and she played at making little men out of clay. One day God saw the manikins and was interested. He blew into them and the clay images came to life. God told Earth to call them Velo-'living'. The Velo men multiplied and did not die. Soon the Earth prospered, for men worked on the land and produced fine harvests. Another day when God was standing on a high mountain he saw the prosperity of the Earth and was surprised, and perhaps jealous. He called Earth to his palace and demanded that she give him half of the men. But Earth pleaded with him that although everything belonged to God yet she could not be separated from her men, for they made her wealth. God was angry and said he would take away the breath of life that he had given to the Velo. He did this, and Earth wept, crying out, 'O lo Velo', meaning 'Men are decaying.' Since then humans have decayed and died.

Another Malagasy story says that all the animals and birds met one day to see whether a remedy could be found against death, which was always reducing their numbers with unknown maladies. They decided that the kings of all the animals should pray to God to provide a cure for mortal illness. He agreed to, and told the kings to assemble with all their subjects before a great building. They were to appoint the Bull as a guard because the remedy against death would be inside. But God was delayed, and the animals began to drift away. Then the king of the bulls was overcome with hunger and thirst and looked around for something to sustain him. He found it inside the building – and when God arrived he found that the remedy itself had been drunk. Angry, he demanded to know who had done this thing. The Snake, who had not gone far away and had seen what had happened, accused the Bull of the theft. God said he would be punished; he recalled the other animals and told them that if they were ill they must get their remedy from the Bull. That is why men sacrifice a bull when they are very ill.

A Death Giant

A different sort of explanation of death is given by the Krachi of Togo. In the beginning there was a famine on earth, and a young man wandering about the forest looking for food came to a place that was quite new to him. He saw a great lump on the ground, and when he reached it found that it was a giant covered with long silky hair. The hair was so long it would have stretched from one village to another. He tried to creep away but suddenly the giant looked up and asked him what he wanted. The lad said he was hungry and the giant promised to feed him if he became his servant. The youth agreed, and learnt that the giant's name was Death. The food was delicious and the young man was happy to serve Death for a long time. But at last he got homesick and begged leave from the giant, who let him go on the promise that he would send another boy to serve in his place. He brought the giant his brother. The young man went home, but after a time he was hungry again, the famine being still severe, and he longed for the giant's fine food. He returned to the giant and was given as much food as he wanted, under the condition of working for him again. He stayed there a long time, but was surprised that he never saw his brother. When he asked Death about him he was told that the boy was away on some business.

In time the youth was homesick again and asked for another holiday. The giant agreed again, if he would bring him a girl to marry. The lad

Opposite top left. From the north of the Congo an effigy of an ancestor, made of wood covered with brass. The formal design suggests the awesomeness of the dead; the winged head indicates power. The lozenge shape is common in the symbolic art of the peoples of this region. Horniman Museum, London.

Opposite bottom left. Mask of the Mpongwe of Congo, made of wood with the face painted white with kaolin to represent a female ancestor, with impassive features, decorated forehead, and elaborate hair style. The Art Institute of Chicago, Illinois.

Opposite right. Ancestral figure of the Fang of Gabon, some of the greatest African masters of sculptured form. Such figures are attached to gables over doors or put in a bark reliquary containing skulls of ancestors. J. R. Hewitt, Esq.

Below. Wooden figure of a bull from Malagasy. Metropolitan Museum of Art, New York.

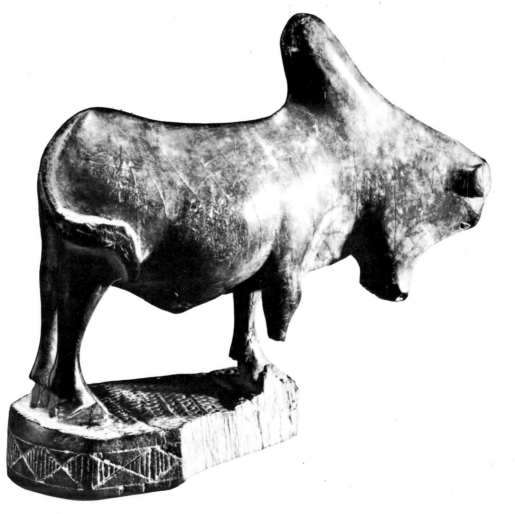

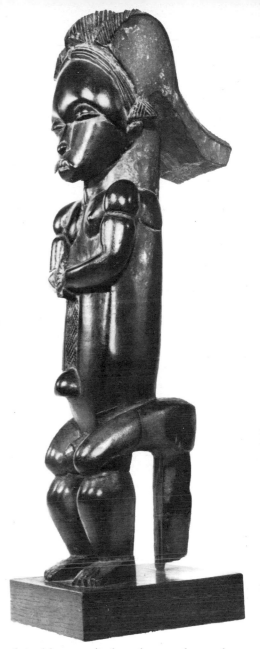

persuaded his sister to marry Death, and she accepted, taking a servant to her new home. Not long after he was hungry again and longed for the giant's sweet meat, so he returned to the forest. Death was not pleased at being bothered so much, but he told the boy to go into an inner room in his house and help himself. The young man was horrified when he picked up a bone and recognised it as belonging to his sister, and when he looked round he saw that all the meat was from his sister and her servant. The village people crept into the forest, and were afraid at the sight of the giant. Then they planned to set light to his long hair, which stretched far all around. They watched from a safe distance and saw the giant tossing and sweating as the flames approached, and at last they reached his head and he lay as dead. When they got near, the young man saw in the roots of the giant's hair a packet of magical medicine. He took it out and showed it to the people. An old man suggested that they might try to sprinkle some of the powder on the bones in the giant's hut. When this was done the missing girls and boy sprang up alive again. The young man suggested putting some of the magical powder on the giant, but the people protested for fear he might come back to life. The boy put just a little powder on the eye of Death. It opened at once, and everybody ran away in fear. It is from that time that Death has come among people. When the giant opens and shuts his eye somebody dies.

Jackal, Snake and Masks

The Dogon stories say that the Jackal who had seized the fibre skirt of his mother Earth had committed incest, and the skirt was reddened with blood. It was put out to dry on the primeval ant-hill, and later was stolen by a woman who put it on and reigned as queen. This spread terror around and eventually men took the skirt from the woman, dressed in it themselves as kings, and forbade women to wear it. But the oldest man had not been told of the theft of the skirt, and this breach of respect to him brought its own penalty. When

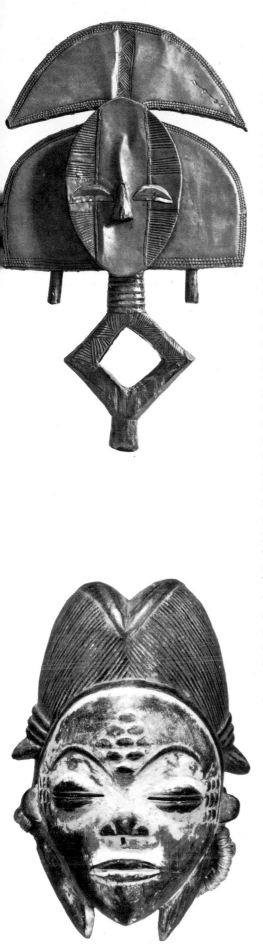

the old man died and was changed into a Nummo spirit, he did not go up to heaven at once, but continued living on earth in the shape of a great snake. One day some young men had put on fibre skirts and were entering the village when the Snake stopped them. He rebuked them furiously, speaking in their own mortal language. But this was a further breach of order: as a spirit he should have used spirit language. Therefore, having cut himself off from the spirit world, he died. So death came to the human race.

The Snake lay dead on the path to the village, and the young men fled in horror to tell their elders. They all came back and resolved to take the corpse to a cave, wrapped in the

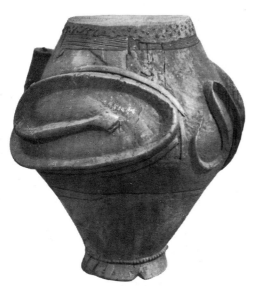

fibres which had caused its death. But the soul of the dead man was looking for somewhere to go, and it entered the womb of a woman in the village. When her child was born he was red like the fibre skirt and spotted like the Snake. He became normal in adolescence, when he was dedicated to the vanished ancestor. In this ceremony a log of wood, in the shape of the Snake, was painted in its colours, and sacrifice was offered to the spiritual principles of the dead reptile. From that time arrangements had to be made to provide places and ceremonies for all who died, and people were chosen for their proper maintenance. From this arose art, particularly the carving of wood. Wooden images represented dead people, and wooden masks represented animals that men killed. Rules and taboos were formed to see that both individuals and groups paid proper respect to the dead.

Struggles with Death

A myth from Togo tells of the river god Tano fighting with Death. Long ago there was a hunter in the forest who for a long time failed to catch anything. After many days he saw and hit an antelope, but it bounded away and a long chase followed. The man went after it but when it went into a cave the creature suddenly turned into the god Tano. The man

was terrified but Tano told him not to fear, for he would protect him in the future. The two set off for the man's home and on their way they met Death. Death challenged them, and Tano replied that he was going to live with a human. Death said he would not allow this, and sang a chant of defiance at Tano. Tano replied, defying Death, and for a whole month the two great beings sang against each other. Death could not force Tano back along his path, but neither could Tano compel Death to let him continue to the man's home. Finally they agreed on a compromise. Whenever someone fell ill, whichever spirit got there first would have power over that person. If Tano arrived first the person would get better, but if Death got to the bed first the person would die. So Tano did get to the human's abode, but Death came too.

A story from the Mbundu of Angola tells of two brothers one of whom, Ngunza, had a dream while he was away from home that his brother had died. When he got back he demanded who had killed his brother, and his mother said it was Death. He vowed to fight Death, and got a blacksmith to make a great iron trap.

He set this in the bush, watched it with great vigilance, and successfully caught Death. Death pleaded with

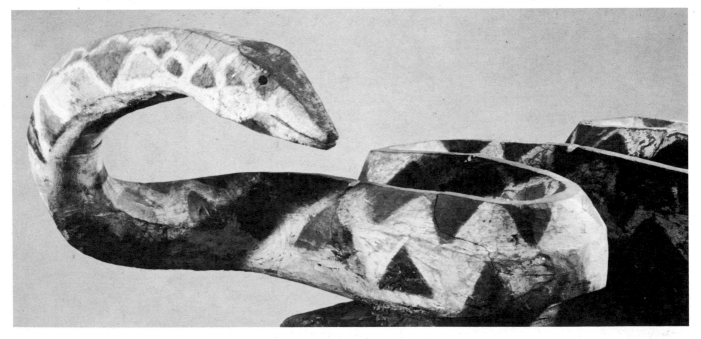

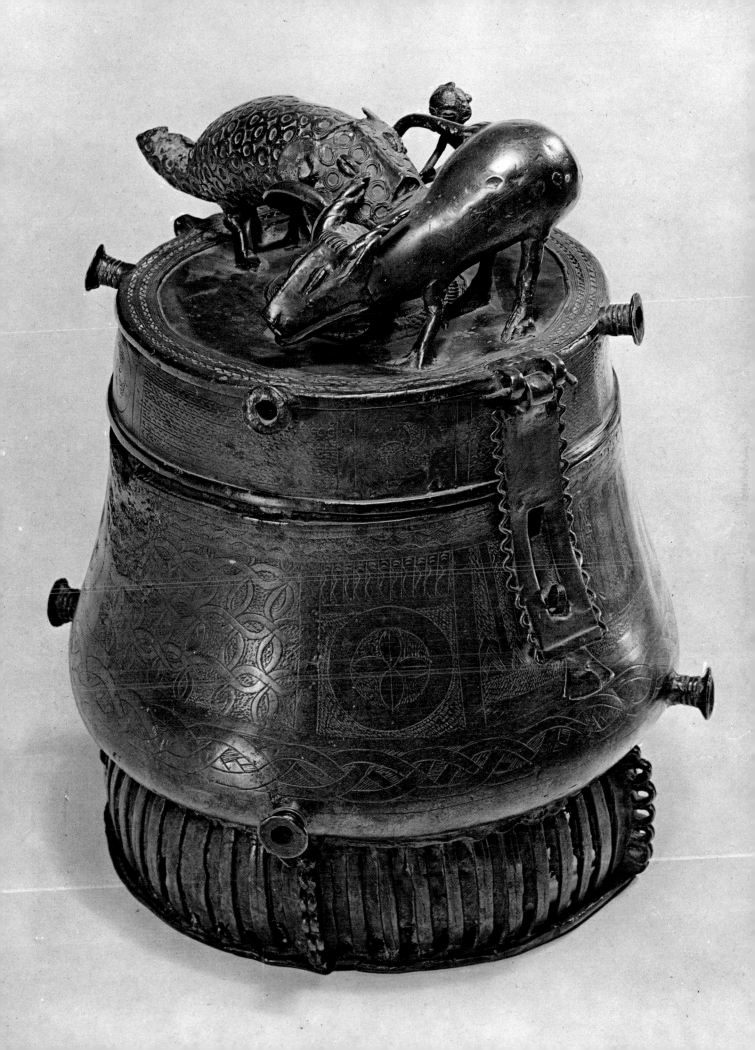

Right. A dance mask of the Epa society of the Yoruba. The dancer's head was enclosed by the hollow 'face' which formed the base and rested on the shoulders. The whole measured three feet (1 metre) in height. Metropolitan Museum of Art, New York.

Centre. An ancestor figure from the Ivory Coast, seated on a stool representing a leopard and with a cockerel – probably used in propitiatory rites – at his feet. Carved wood. P. Verité, Paris.

Below. A wooden cylindrical drum of the Baulé of the Ivory Coast, decorated with copies of masks, figures, lizards, hands, rosettes and abstract patterns, all of which add power to the drum. Musée de l'Homme, Paris.

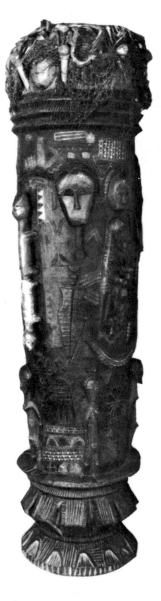

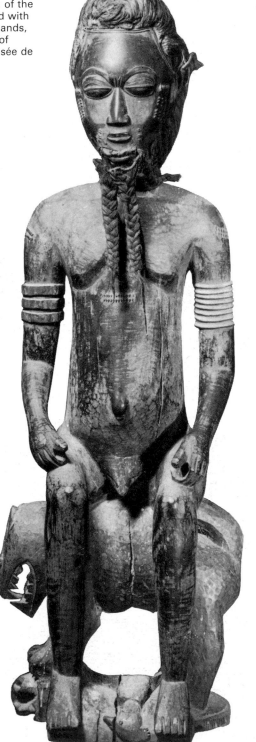

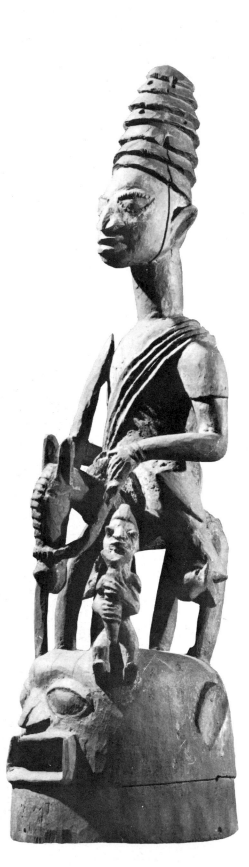

Ngunza to let him go, but he refused, saying that Death was always killing people. Death denied this, alleging that people died by their own fault or that of somebody else, and if Ngunza would release him he could visit his land and see for himself. Ngunza consented and four days later they set off for the family of the dead. Death told him to watch the new arrivals, and of each one he asked what had killed them. Some said it was their own vanity, others jealous husbands, and so on. They had all died through the fault of some human being, and so it was unfair to blame Death.

This fits in with the general belief in Africa that death is never natural, but always due to the malice of some person. Death told Ngunza that he could go and search for his brother, and he was happy to find him living

much as he had done on earth. Ngunza said that they should go back to their earthly home, and he was very surprised that his brother did not want to go, for he was much happier where he was (see the Chaga story of the radiant sons in heaven, page 33). Ngunza had to return home alone, though Death gave him the seeds of all the plants that are cultivated in Angola now; an addition that explains the origin of agriculture.

A further part of the story says that Death came to look for Ngunza himself at his home, and pursued him from place to place. Finally Ngunza protested at this treatment, saying that he had done no harm, and it was Death himself who said that he did not kill anyone. But the only answer of Death was to throw his axe at Ngunza, who turned into a spirit.

A headrest from Mozambique, carved out of a single piece of wood like the better known stools; such headrests were used in ancient Egypt. Antelopes and other deer appear in many African stories. A tale from Togo says that a chief wanted to show his superiority by riding an antelope and sent his hunters to catch one. But he did not know that it was really a ghost, and when he mounted it he was carried off at great speed into the forest and has never been seen since. Musée de l'Homme, Paris.

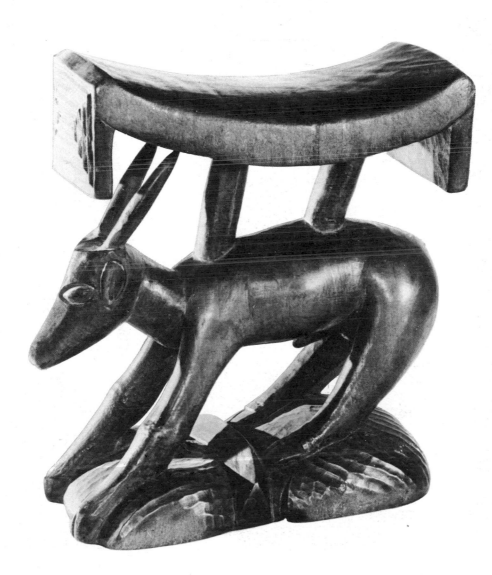

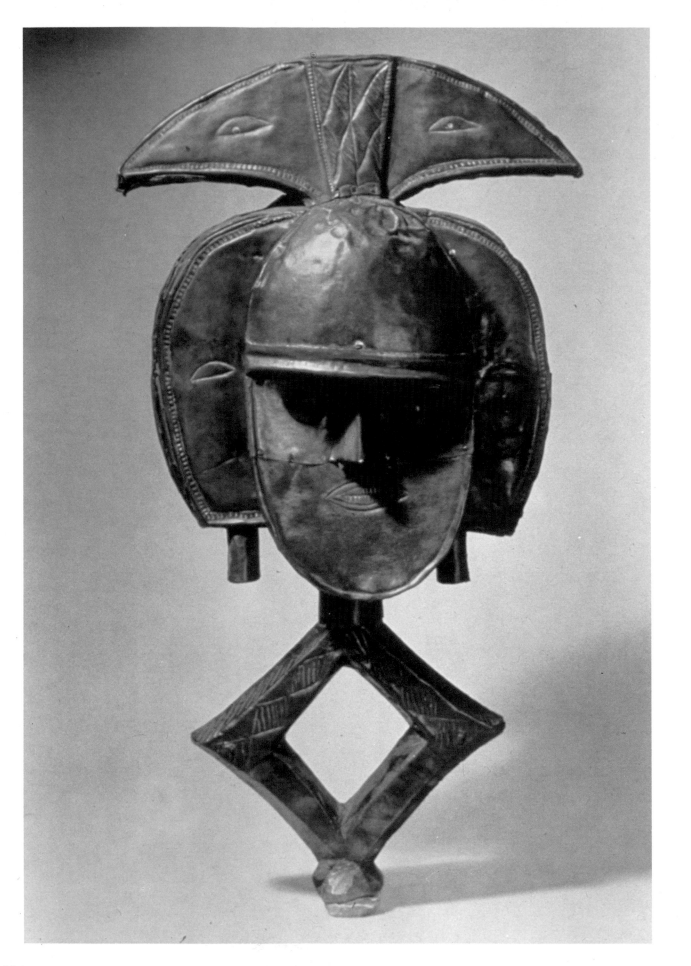

The World Beyond

The last story has told of the land of death, and the myth of Kintu spoke of the heavenly country. Many other myths tell of journeys to the world beyond death, either below ground or up in heaven. The Mbundu of Angola also speak of a king Kitamba whose head wife died. The king was so grieved that he went into perpetual mourning and insisted that all his subjects should do the same. People were forbidden to make noises, or speak in public. The village chiefs protested, but the king refused to change his order unless his wife was restored to him.

The elders in despair consulted a famous doctor and he agreed to help. He had a grave dug in his house and entered it with his little boy. He instructed his wife to dress in mourning but to make sure that the grave was watered every day. The grave was filled in and the doctor and his boy set out for the underworld. They came to a village where they found the dead queen, and she asked them where they came from. The doctor told her of her husband's excessive grief, and the queen pointed to a man nearby and asked if the doctor knew him. When he said he did not, the queen said it was Death, who was consuming them all. Then she pointed to another man, who was chained up, and asked the doctor if he could recognise him. The doctor was surprised to see that the man looked like king Kitamba, and the queen said that in a few years he would die. She affirmed that once a person died he could not return, but she gave the doctor an armlet in proof that he had been to the land of the dead.

Meanwhile the doctor's wife had been pouring water on the grave every day and eventually the earth began to crack. As she looked her husband's head began to appear from the ground, and he came out pulling his son with him. The boy fainted in the sunlight, but with the help of medicines his father restored him. He reported to the village chiefs and received his reward. They gave the news to the king, who recognised the armlet and gave orders for mourning to cease.

In a story told by the Chaga of Kenya a girl, Marwé, and her brother were sent by their parents to watch a field and keep monkeys away from the beans. They sat on guard all day, but in the afternoon they were so hot that they crept off to a distant pool for a drink. When they got back the monkeys had stripped the field bare. The children were so afraid of the anger of their parents that Marwé threw herself into the pool. Her brother rushed off to take the news home and the parents were so distressed that they forgot to be angry. However it was too late, for Marwé had disappeared. She sank down through the water till she came to a hut where an old woman lived with her children. The old woman took care of Marwé, who worked for her and shared the life of the underworld. After a long time she became homesick and asked permission to leave. The old woman did not object, but asked her whether she would like the hot or the cold. The question was mysterious, but a choice of goods is common in such stories.

Marwé chose the cold, which should have been disagreeable, but when she dipped her arms into a cold pot she drew them out covered with rich bangles, and she put in her feet and legs with the same result. The old woman gave her a fine bead petticoat, told her that her husband would be called Sawoyé, and sent her home. Marwé rose up to the surface of the pool and out on the bank. News soon spread that a beautiful and rich girl was there. All the country went out to see her and many wanted to marry her, from the chief down. But Marwé refused all till Sawoyé came along. He had an offensive skin disease and people marvelled at the choice, but it was cured as soon as they were married. With Marwé's bangles they

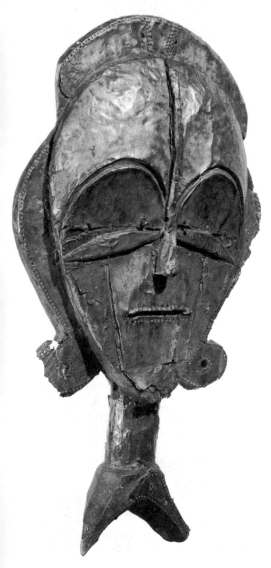

bought many cattle, but this aroused the jealousy of the neighbours and Sawoyé was killed. However Marwé brought him back to life with her magic and hid him inside their house. When the enemies came to divide their spoil Sawoyé came out and killed them. Then the couple lived happily ever after.

Another Chaga story tells of a girl who one day went out with her friends to cut grass. She saw a place where it was growing luxuriantly, but when she put her foot there she sank at once into the mud. Her friends tried to catch hold of her hands but she sanker deeper into the mud and disappeared, singing out that the ghosts had taken her and her parents should be told. The girls ran home and called all the people to the quagmire. Here a diviner advised that a cow and a sheep must be sacrificed. When this was done the girl's voice was heard again, but eventually it faded away and was silent. However on the spot where the girl had gone a tree began to grow, which got taller and taller till it reached the sky. It was a useful tree under which boys would drive their cattle in the heat of the day. One day two boys climbed up the tree, calling to their companions that they were going to the world above. They never returned. The tree was called the Story-tree.

The Ronga of Mozambique tell of a girl who broke her pot on the way to draw water. In great distress she cried out for a rope, and looking up she saw one hanging from a cloud, like the ropes in the stories of God leaving the earth. Climbing up she found a ruined village in the sky and an old woman sitting there asked what she wanted. The girl told her story and the old woman told her to continue walking, and if an ant crawled up into her ear she must leave it alone. The girl did so, and coming to a new village heard the Ant whisper to her to sit down. As she sat at the gate some elders came out in shining clothes and asked what she was doing there. The girl said she had come to look for a baby (a new theme in the story, which is perhaps mixed with another).

The elders took her to a house, gave her a basket, and told her to collect some corn from the garden. The Ant whispered that she should only pull one cob at a time, and arrange them carefully in the basket. The elders were pleased with her work, and with the cooking that she did on the Ant's instructions. Next morning they showed her some babies on the ground, wrapped in red and white clothes. She was going to choose the one in red clothes, when the Ant told her to choose white. This she did, and the old men gave her the baby, and as many cloths and beads as she could carry. Then she found her way back to her family and they were overjoyed at her treasures and her baby. Perhaps she had been barren before; babies are often said to be prepared in heaven and their parents designated for them.

An additional narrative says that the girl's sister was jealous and set off for the heavenly land to seek the same good fortune. She got up to the sky, but she was a very rude and wilful creature, who refused to listen to the old woman or heed the warnings of the Ant. When she saw the babies she chose a red one, there was a great explosion and she fell down dead. Her bones dropped on her home, and people commented that heaven was angry with her because she had a wicked heart.

Left. Bakota head made of wood covered with copper. The eyelids are shown sewn together, presumably as a sign of death. Such heads are placed on top of byeri boxes, or reliquaries for the dead of the family. Byeri boxes play an important part in ritual and in daily life, being a link between men and God and between families and political leaders. Musée de l'Homme, Paris.

Opposite. A spirit figure from the Bayaka of Zaïre. The shape of the nose is characteristic of the region. These spirit figures are much used, enhanced by medicine and spells, to control the forces of nature. Koninklijk Museum voor Midden-Afrika, Tervuren.

God and Spirits

After the Supreme Being there are many other spirits in which people believe. Some of them may be called personifications of natural forces and others glorified heroes of the past; some are both. Groups of gods are worshipped in West Africa, and some other parts of the continent, though often they are vague powers with little mythology. Stories of some of the more important spirits will now be told. But first it may be asked why people pay attention to many spirits, and not one god alone. One answer may be that people cannot afford to neglect any power that can influence their lives, just as they do not pay attention to one person alone but to the many officials with whom they must deal. Another reason is suggested in a story told by the Mende of Sierra Leone.

At first people did not pray, but they came to the Supreme Being with small complaints. God considered how he could make people know his will. He created a mountain and gave it the ability to talk to people, thinking that if people were used to the voice of the mountain, and kept its laws, they would also hear the divine voice and laws. He also gave people the power of dreaming.

One night an old man had a dream in which he saw the mountain coming to him as an old man and calling him friend, saying that he must tell the village chief to get his people to bring food for the mountain to eat. The dreamer asked where the old man had come from and he answered that he came from the mountain. The dreamer looked towards the mountain and saw that it had disappeared, and the old man said that was because he was the mountain. After the old man had gone away the mountain could be

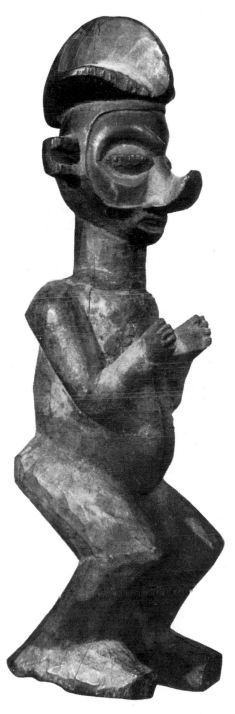

seen again. When the old man awoke he told the chief about his dream. All the people were assembled, the story was told, and it was agreed to give food to the mountain. But they told the old man to ask the mountain for help to catch the animal that would be needed for food. So he went with his sons, picking up twenty stones on the way.

At the foot of the mountain he cleared a space and called out to the mountain that if it really did need food it must arrange the stones so that it could be known how many animals were needed. The dreamer and his sons went home, but next morning they came back and found the stones set out in order. Nine stones faced the mountain, and that

Left. The Ijaw people of the Niger delta carve wooden figures to represent spirit companions, the medium through which they converse with ancestral spirits. The figure is said to tremble when requests for help and guidance are heard. Museum of Mankind, London.

Centre. This male figure holding a bowl was used in making offerings to spirits by the Bafum of Cameroun. Museum für Völkerkunde, Berlin.

Opposite. A door from a royal palace in Abomey, with wooden figures nailed to it. Below is a snake swallowing its tail, and above a chameleon between the sun and moon. A Nigerian myth says that when God created the earth he sent the Chameleon to inspect it, and after walking about slowly it reported that the earth was not yet dry enough. A Zulu myth blames the Chameleon for coming too slowly to the human race with the message from God that they would not die. The Lizard raced ahead and told people that they would die, and so death came. Musée de l'Homme, Paris.

Below. A wooden dish of the Ibo people from the Brass River region of southern Nigeria. Such dishes were used when offerings of food were made to the gods. Horniman Museum, London.

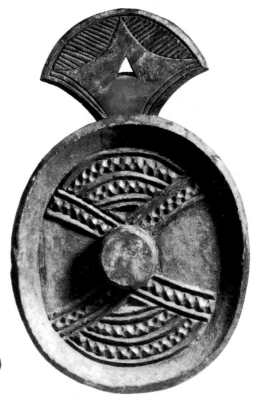

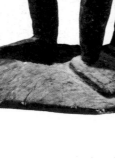

meant that nine animals would escape. Ten stones were facing the man and so ten would be killed. One stone was in the middle and that animal must be kept alive till sacrificed by the dreamer. This was done when the men went hunting. Then the village men collected rice, salt and palm-oil from their women and took them with the meat to the mountain. The women were sent back because there was not enough food for them. The live animal was sacrificed, and meat, rice and oil were put on leaves. The dreamer took a kola nut, which splits into halves and is a sign of friendship. He called on the mountain to show whether the food had been received and appreciated, and tossing the halves of the kola nut into the air he let them fall to the ground. They fell with their white side facing upwards, a sign of acceptance. This was done four times, and the sign of acceptance always appeared.

The dreamer asked the mountain to protect the town against warfare, save women in childbirth, protect children against witchcraft, heal all who were sick, and care for the people as they had cared for the mountain. Every year the mountain was a place of prayer for men, and they brought gifts to it. But God had pity on the women, who were not allowed to share in the sacrifice. He told a woman in a dream to pray at a great rock, and since then men and women have prayed at mountains and rocks, and also at trees and rivers.

Sun and Moon

There is not much mythology of the sun and moon, for in tropical Africa the sun is always present and there is no need to call it back in the winter as men did in the cold countries of northern Europe or Japan. Occasionally some of the gods are connected with sun and moon, like Mawu and Lisa of Abomey (see page 23). Mawu as the moon is more kindly and so beloved of men, while Lisa the sun is fierce and harsh. Mawu is older, woman and mother, gentle and refreshing. During the day men suffer under the sun's heat, but in the cool

moonlight they tell stories and dance. Coolness is a sign of wisdom and age, so Mawu is the wisdom of the world, and Lisa is strength. Sometimes Nyamé, God of the Ashanti, is personified as the moon and represented by the queen mother, whereas another personification of the truly great Nyamé, Nyankopon, is in the sun and the king.

The Bushmen and Hottentots of South Africa tell stories of the sun and moon, which suggest that they paid more attention to these heavenly bodies than the Negroes did. A Hottentot story links the coming of death

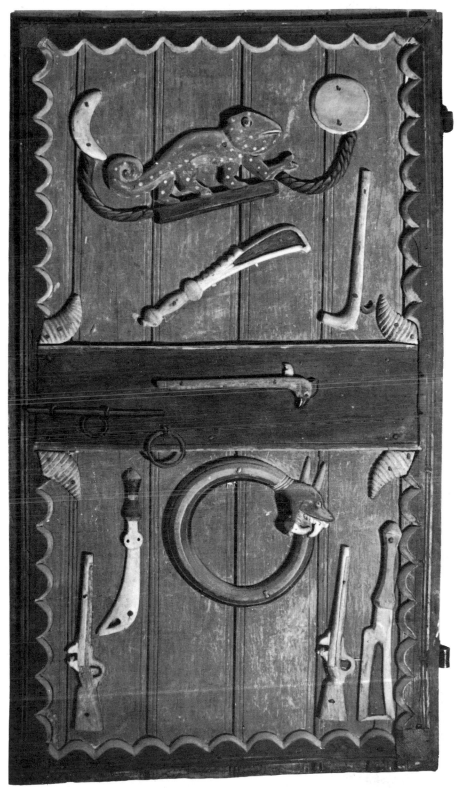

71

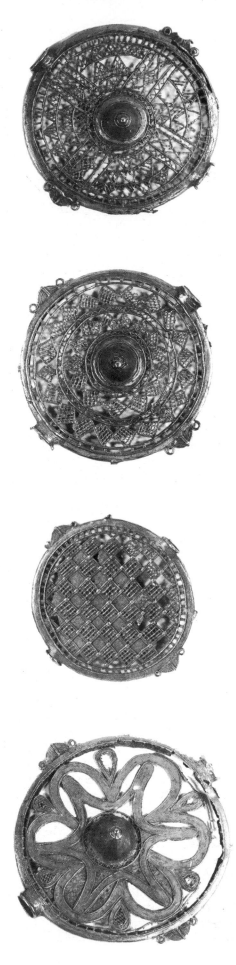

with the rising and waning of the moon, rather than with God as in much Negro story, though the theme of the messengers is the same. The Moon once sent a Louse to assure people that as the Moon died and lived again so would they. On its journey the Louse met the Hare and told his message. The Hare said he could run faster and would take the message. But when he arrived he told people that as the Moon dies and comes to an end so they would die and come to an end. The Hare told the Moon what he had said and the Moon was angry at the distortion of its message to the human race. He seized a piece of wood and hit the Hare on the lip. Ever since then the Hare has had a cleft lip, and its flesh is taboo.

The Cape Bushmen tell a similar story, and also a variant in which a young Hare wept for his mother's death. The Moon appeared and told him not to cry, for his mother was not dead but only asleep and that she would come back alive, just as the moon dies but returns. But the Hare did not believe him and kept on crying, saying that the Moon was deceiving him. The Moon was angry, and cursed the Hare and cleft his lip.

Some of the Pygmies say that it was the Moon who created the first man and put him on earth. His body was moulded, covered with skin, and blood poured inside. Then the Moon whispered to him that he should give birth to children who would live in the forest. The story goes on to say that the Pygmy was told that he could eat of all the trees in the forest, except of a taboo tree; but he broke this commandment and that is why death came to the human race. But, like some other Pygmy stories, this one may have been influenced by Negro or Christian story. However it is told by some Pygmies today. The Pygmy

Gold badges from Ashanti, Ghana, worn by the royal soul-washers or soul-bearers, whose task it was to keep the soul of the king free from danger and contamination by evil. The abstract designs are finely worked in the metal that gave Ghana its old name of the Gold Coast. Museum of Mankind, London.

myth has already been told of the Moon instructing the Lightning in the mysteries of birth.

The Krachi people of Togo say that the Sun married the Moon, and the two gave birth to the many stars. But as time went on the Moon got tired of her husband and took a lover. The Sun was angry and would not have his wife with him in the house any longer. However, he divided his possessions with her, and some of the children stayed with him while others went away with the Moon. But the Moon remains dissatisfied, and she goes into her husband's fields. The children that stayed with the Sun then fight the Moon and her stars, and that is the cause of storms. However the Moon does not like the children to fight too long, and sends a messenger to pacify them by waving a cloth of many colours, the rainbow. Sometimes the Sun himself catches the Moon in his fields, and he tries to seize and eat her. That is why when men see an eclipse beginning they shout and beat drums so as to frighten the Sun so much that it lets the Moon go.

The Dagomba of Togo say that the Sun has a marketplace, which can be seen when a halo appears round the Sun. Here he keeps a ram, and when it stamps its feet that causes thunder, and when it shakes its tail that is the lightning. The rain is the hair falling off the ram's tail and the wind comes from the ram rushing round and round the market. The marks on the face of the Moon are given fanciful explanations. Some say they are an old woman sitting on a stool in the Moon, others that they are an old man beating a drum, and yet others that they are a man on horseback with a spear in his hand.

A story told in Angola says that the son of the first man refused to marry a wife from his own people and declared that he would only have the daughter of Sun and Moon. He tried to find a messenger to take his proposal up to heaven, but animals and birds refused. At last the Frog said he would carry the message. The Frog had found that girls came down from heaven on spiders' webs to draw

72

water, so he hid himself by the well, jumped in one of their jars, and was carried up to the sky. There the Frog gave the message to the Sun, and the Sun said he would agree to the marriage if the youth came himself bringing the first present of the dowry. The Frog went back with the news, the youth asked the price, and the Frog told him it was a sack of money. The young man collected this and sent the Frog up to the sky with it, but he refused to go to heaven himself, for the Frog must bring the girl down. The Frog reached the sky and hid himself in the girl's room that night. While she was asleep he stole both her eyes. In the morning the Sun and Moon discovered this and asked a diviner the cause. The diviner said her suitor had cast a spell on her and if she were not sent to him the girl would die. So the Sun ordered the Spider to weave a cobweb and take his daughter to earth. The Frog went on in advance and told the young man that his bride was coming. When the girl came down the Spider's web, the Frog gave her back her eyes and took her to her husband's house. They were married, and the wife went up to heaven no more. Only the Frog retained this power, and it is said that frogs sometimes fall from the sky in rainstorms.

An unusual story told by the Chaga of Kenya suggests that the Moon-chief and his followers were more backward than people on earth. A boy, Murilé, was being chided by his mother and so he took his father's stool and invested it with magic. He told the stool to go up in the air and it obeyed, carrying him first of all into a tree and then after more incantations right up into the sky. There the boy looked round until he found some people, and asked them the way to the village of the Moon-chief. They made him work for them for a time and then sent him forward with directions. The same thing happened with other groups that he met; he worked for them, and then was sent on, and finally he arrived at the Moon-chief's village. There he was surprised to see people eating raw food, and when he saluted the

Moon-chief he asked why they did not use fire. He was told that they did not know about fire. So he offered to show them, and was promised many cattle and sheep in return. Then with two pieces of wood and dry grass he lit a fire, and was hailed as a great magician.

Murilé became rich, with wives and children, flocks and herds. But after many years he wanted to return home and sent messengers to announce his coming. The Mockingbird went and sang that Murilé was coming back, but the family would not believe it, thinking him dead, and drove the bird away. Murilé too would not believe that the Mockingbird had been to his home, so the bird went again, seized his father's stick in its beak, and brought it back as proof. Murilé then set off, with all his family and herds. But the way was long and tiring; he could not go straight back on his magic stool because he had to take his herds down the slope where heaven joins earth. Murilé was tired, but a great bull in his herd promised to carry him if he would vow never to eat its flesh. Murilé agreed and arrived home in triumph. His family were overjoyed to see him and he settled down in peace. He made his parents promise never to touch the Bull, but when it was very old his father killed it and his mother took some of the fat and put it in Murilé's food. As soon as he tasted it the meat spoke, reproaching him for breaking his promise. Murilé began to sink into the ground, and as he called out to his mother that she had deceived him he disappeared from sight, and that was the end.

Another story of the struggle of the Sun and the Moon, comparable with the Togo myth, is told by the Luyia of Kenya. God created the Moon first and then the Sun. In the beginning the Moon was bigger and brighter, and the envious Sun attacked his elder brother. They wrestled till the Sun was thrown down and pleaded for mercy. Then they wrestled again and the Moon was thrown in the mud and dirt splashed over him so that he was not so bright. God intervened to stop them fighting again, saying that the

Sun would be brighter henceforth and shine during the day for kings and workers. The Moon would only shine at night, for thieves and witches. It is said that the Moon was foolish in showing mercy to the Sun and should have beaten him thoroughly the first time. But it often happens in mythology that the younger brother takes the leading place, as in the story of Jacob and Esau.

When God had made Sun and Moon he made two big stars to shine in the east and west. He made a great red cock who lives in the clouds and sends lightning when it shakes its wings and thunder when it crows.

A Luyia myth tells of another visit to heaven, this time to the Sun. A girl who was being pressed to marry a man she did not like ran away into the bush. After going about twelve miles she came to a rope hanging down from the sky. When she took hold of it she was lifted up to heaven and put down on a rubbish heap outside a village as the day came to an end. As she sat there the mother of the Sun came along and asked who the girl was. She said she was a new arrival, and the Sun's mother said the girl could stay with her, but her son was chief and would want to marry her. The girl agreed to go with her but said she could not marry a chief. The Sun's mother encouraged her and took her home, saying her son was in the garden, and if the girl saw something red and bright she must not cry. When the Sun returned everything looked brilliant as lightning, and the girl laid down to cover her face. The Sun's wives told him that his mother had brought a new wife and he went to salute her. But the girl cast her eyes down and did not answer. Then the Sun sent his chief servant, the Moon, to speak to the girl, but still she did not reply. Six servants were sent in turn, but were all unsuccessful. The servants said they had been wrong in not taking presents to the girl, so the Sun sent her something of all that grew in the land, but still the girl would not speak. Finally the Sun decided to give her his own rays and took them to the girl himself. At last she replied, in a thin voice, and all the

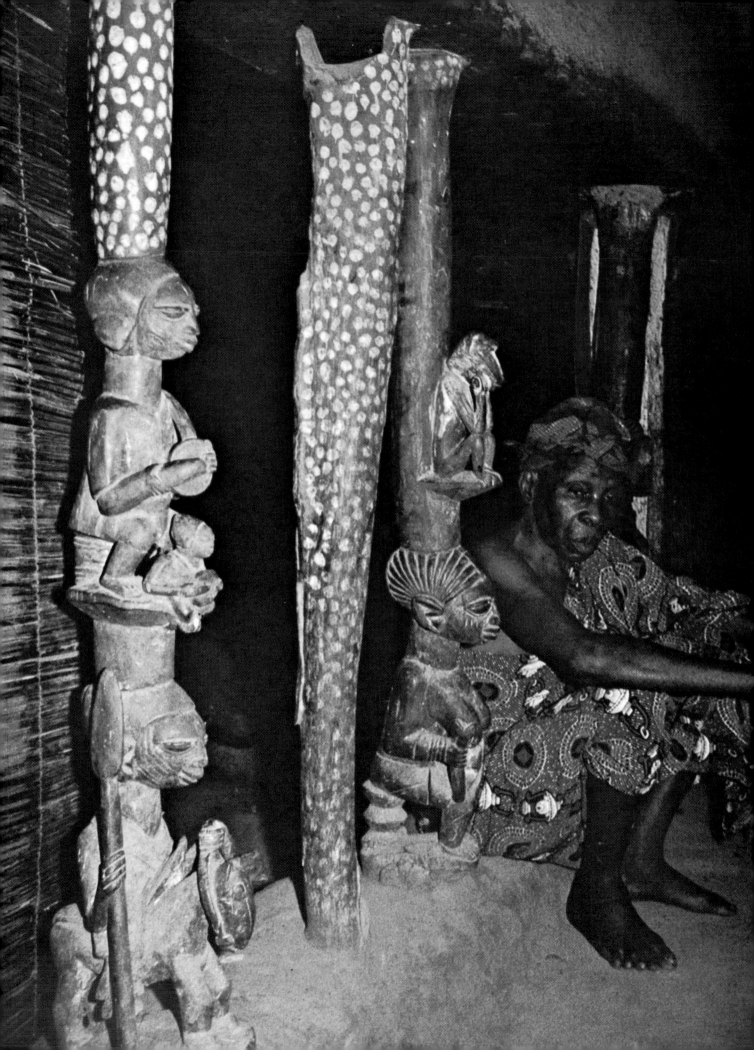

servants brought oil to anoint her as bride. They were married and she bore the Sun three boys.

But all this time the rays of the Sun were in a pot which he had given his wife as a present, and they did not shine on earth. So the wife asked for permission to visit her parents on earth and servants to carry presents to them. The Sun agreed and dropped a rope to earth, down which they all climbed with presents. The girl's parents were astonished to see her, for they thought she was dead or lost in the bush. They brought a black ox to kill for a rite of purification before they could salute her, but she refused it. They brought oxen of other colours, but she shook her head. Only when they brought a white ox did she accept it, and it was sacrificed, and its flesh given to the people who had come from heaven. After three days the girl and her servants set out to go back to heaven, and when they seized hold of the rope they were drawn up so quickly that she had no time to say farewell to her parents. The rays of the Sun had not shone yet, but when they reached the Sun's house his wife opened the pots where the rays were and they began to shine on earth. This brought joy to mankind, and the Sun told his wife that his chief servant, the Moon, would shine at night.

Storm Spirits

More important for ritual in many places are the spirits of the storm, for tropical tornadoes not only bring the expected rains but often cause damage with thunderbolts and flashes of lightning. Remarkable stories are told of Shango, the storm deity of the Yoruba of Nigeria. This divinity was once a man, it is clearly said, and lived as the fourth king of that people, ruling over a kingdom stretching into neighbouring countries. Shango was a strong ruler, and a great doctor, but also tyrannical. He could kill people by breathing fire from his mouth. Eventually his tyranny was challenged by two ministers, and to avoid their attack he set them to fight against each other, hoping that both would be killed. One was slain, but the victor turned on Shango himself, who fled to the forest. He went on horseback, taking his three wives and some loyal followers. But after wandering about for a long time only his favourite wife remained loyal, and finally in despair Shango hanged himself from a tree at a place called Koso.

This shameful end of the terrible king caused a great stir. When travellers brought reports that the monarch had hanged himself, his enemies mocked those who were still faithful to him. So his friends went to a great magician to find out how to bring fire on their enemies' houses. Some say they could make fire descend from heaven, others that they threw small gourds filled with gunpowder on to roofs during storms. Anyway there were many fires, and the followers of Shango said this proved that the king did 'not hang' (ko-so). Shango was showing his anger by sending fire from heaven and sacrifices must be made to appease him. This was done

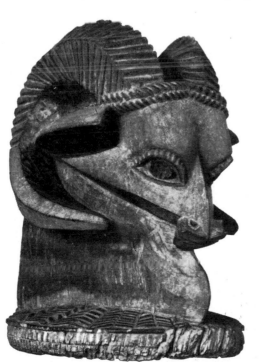

Left. Animals are the source of many African tales, and they also feature in religious rites. This wood carving of a ram's head comes from the Owo of Nigeria and was placed on a family altar to represent an ancestor. The ram is sacred to Shango, the storm god of the Yoruba, and thunder is believed to be his bellowing. Museum of Classical Antiquities, Lagos.

Far left. Wooden carving of a follower of Shango, storm god of the Yoruba of Nigeria. The double-bladed axe on the head is the symbol of Shango, who is said to throw his axe, the thunderbolt, when there is a storm. Museum of Mankind, London.

Opposite. The interior of a famous temple of Shango, god of storms, at Ibadan, Nigeria. The posts are carved with mythical figures of gods and men, and the priest sits among other carvings. Behind him is an altar bearing the thunderstones which are said to fall from the sky during a storm. The spots on the posts are for decoration, though old temples of the smallpox god were also dotted in this way.

75

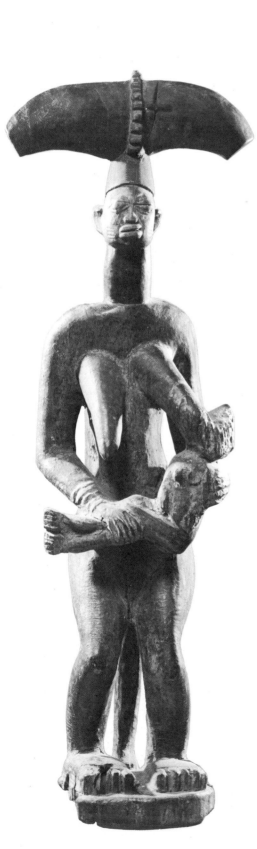

and a temple built at a place still called Koso, to contradict the story that Shango hanged himself. The version of the myth given by priests is that Shango was angry with his discontented subjects, so he disappeared into the forest on a horse. When a search party went after him they only found the horse, and a voice came from the sky saying that Shango did not hang, but ascended to heaven by a chain and would rule from there by thunder.

The Yoruba compare the noise of thunder with the bellowing of a ram, and these animals are sacred to Shango and wander freely about marketplaces. Thunderbolts are called 'thunder axes' and are said to fall to the ground whenever there is a storm. Priests of the storm and their acolytes often carry symbolical 'thunder-axes', with wooden handles and finely decorated thin metal blades. Sometimes these axes are double-headed, like those found in parts of the Mediterranean world.

The Ashanti of Ghana incorporate the activity of the storm with the Supreme God of heaven, Nyamé. Thunderbolts are called 'God's axes' and these, often primitive stone axes, are put in 'God's tree', a forked post standing by doorways containing a pot with simple offerings.

The Fon of Abomey say that when the Creator had made all things, he retired and divided the universe among his children. The Earth was the elder and having quarrelled with the Storm decided to go below, taking all his inheritance. The Creator agreed, and said that the brothers must be like the two halves of a calabash, Storm above and Earth below, and they must not fight. But trouble came when the Storm stopped rain falling. Earth was king below, and people complained that they were dying of thirst under his rule. Finally Earth had recourse to the Oracle to find out why no rain had fallen for

three years. The Oracle said that the Storm was angry because Earth had taken all their father's inheritance. Then Earth remembered that he had stuffed all his property into sacks, but there was no room for fire and water and he had left them behind. On the advice of the Oracle he made a sacrifice of his possessions and sent a bird to report this deed to the Storm. The Storm was appeased, saying that though Earth had taken everything he himself had been able to get all these goods simply by controlling fire and water. As a sign of reconciliation he gave a great clap of thunder and heavy rain began to fall. Since then the brothers have been reconciled and rain falls each year, while the bird that took the message is sacred to priests of Earth.

A story of the Songhay of the upper Niger says that one of the celestial spirits, Dongo, had an axe and flew up to the sky to try it out. He arrived over a village with his companions. One of them made a spark, and Dongo threw his axe. There was a flash of lightning and some men below were killed. Dongo was surprised at this and went off to ask his mother how he could repair the damage. She took him to his grandfather, who gave him an earthenware pot full of water. Dongo plunged his head into the pot and filled his mouth. Then he sprayed it over the dead men, and they all came back to life. Dongo said they had been killed because nobody in the village had sung his praises, but he taught them a prayer-spell which would avert harm from storm.

In southern Africa it is widely held that lightning is a bird, and some people claim to have seen it. It is variously described as a great brown bird, or a fish-eagle with a white neck, or with red legs and shining feathers like a peacock. The bird is said to lay a big egg where it strikes, and some think these bring good fortune while others say they are unlucky and must be destroyed by a doctor. If the Lightning Bird itself can be caught it is of great value for medicine. People who are struck by lightning are said to have been scratched by the claws of the bird.

A standing female figure in painted wood, nursing a child and wearing the double-headed axe insignia of the Shango cult figures. Yoruba work. Metropolitan Museum of Art, New York.

In the Congo region it is said that lightning is a magic dog which gives a sharp bark. A story says that a man found a beautiful dog and took it home. As it was raining he took it into his house and lit a fire to dry the dog. There was a great explosion and man and dog vanished for ever. Sometimes the lightning is called a great chief who goes hunting with twenty-four dogs which are the lightning flashes. Stories are told of men caught up to heaven by the lightning, but allowed by God to return to their earthly families.

One of the most popular spirits worshipped by the Hottentots was a great hero and rain god, Tsui'goab. The myth says that he went to war with a chief called Gaunab, sometimes identified with death, because he killed many people. Gaunab kept overpowering the hero, but the latter grew stronger after each battle, and finally he destroyed Gaunab by smiting him a great blow behind the ear. But as Gaunab was dying he made a last effort and hit his enemy on the knee. Ever since then the conqueror has been called Tsui'goab, meaning 'wounded knee'. He was a great chief and magician. He made the first man and woman, or some say the rocks out of which they emerged. Although he died several times yet he came back and there was great feasting. Tsui'-goab is worshipped as giver of rain, living in the clouds, and invoked with the first rays of dawn. He is called Father of Our Fathers, and implored to send the streaming thunder-cloud and nourish flocks and men. He gives health, and men take oaths in his name, showing that he is regarded as a moral deity. Some writers have taken him to be the Supreme Being, but recent opinion sees him as a hero and rain deity, an ancestor who came from the east, and a father who gives rain and cattle.

Other spirits have the storm as one of their functions. The Dinka of the Sudan believe in Deng, who is an important god but rather difficult to define. Some say he was the ancestor of all the Dinka people. He is closely connected with thunder and lightning and his name is used for the rain. The

lightning is Deng's club, and people struck down by it are not given proper mourning. Both rain and human birth are manifestations of Deng, and in some myths he is the son of heaven and earth.

Kibuka, the Buganda war god, has storm characteristics. He was brother of the great god Mukasa and when a king of Buganda sent to ask for divine help in war, Kibuka was sent to give aid. He was warned to be wary of the enemy and never let them know his battle stations, or have any dealings with their women. Kibuka flew up into a cloud and hovered over the enemy, shooting down arrows and spears on them, while the human army fought successfully below. So Buganda won the first battle and took some women prisoners. One of these took Kibuka's fancy and he carried her off to his hut. But after discovering who Kibuka was and where he posted himself in battle, the woman escaped and told her people all about it. When the battle was resumed Kibuka started hurling down his weapons and the enemy archers sent a volley into the clouds which mortally wounded him. He flew off to a tall tree and died there, and the king of Buganda was killed with many of his people, so that there was no king for some time.

Kibuka's body was found in the tree and taken down for burial. A temple was built for him, enclosing his jawbone, as was done for the kings of Buganda. Priests were appointed to serve him and in time of war some of them accompanied the army to give messages from Kibuka.

Rainmakers and Rainbows
Those who make rain fall and those who make rain cease are found all over Africa. Often they are wise men who observe the signs of the times and the secrets of nature. They are prophets, like Elijah, who can tell whether small clouds in the distance will bring rain. A Luyia story from Kenya says that in the beginning nobody could predict or control the rain, until there was an old woman who had lost her family and wandered about everywhere; she met

many peoples during her travels and gained the knowledge of how to control the rain. She began to show her powers, but when rain fell there came also thunder and lightning, and snakes and crawling things came into houses. So people were afraid and expelled her from their midst. Eventually the woman went to live with a man to whom she revealed the art of making rain fall. As his powers became known people went to ask the man for rain, but he told them that it was not free and they must bring him presents for his work.

An additional story says that the rainmaker was told to demand higher prices after a time, since he was like a chief and spent his time looking at heaven and earth. He should not be content with small gifts of tobacco, but should demand goats and cows. The people brought him goats, but not until there was a long drought did they fear they had not given him enough, so they fattened cows and paid these large fees in time of great need. Since then there have been many people who have known the art of rainmaking. The story of one of the most famous, the rain-queen of the Lovedu, is told later.

The rainbow is regarded not so much as beautiful but as strange and dangerous, though it is also attractive in the sense that it has magic powers. The Luyia say that God created rain and all the water on earth came from it. To stop the rain from falling when it was not needed, God made two rainbows. The male rainbow is narrow and the female is wide. The male cannot prevent rain by itself, but if it appears first and is followed by the female rainbow, then the rain stops.

The double rainbow also appears in Fon mythology in Abomey. It is a symbol of the snake, the red part being the male portion of the snake and the blue the female portion. The snake which supports the earth (see page 24) is often found in double form in art and story, and it is believed that one snake is twined round the lower earth and another appears in the sky. The fantasy of treasure to be found 'where the rainbow ends' is widespread. The treasure may be the bright Aggrey beads which are popular for decoration. Or it is gold which is dug out of mountains and called the snake's riches.

In southern Africa it is said that if someone finds the place where the rainbow ends he or she should run away as fast as possible or be killed. Some people say it is unlucky to point at a rainbow, for if you do your finger will become stiff. But the Ila people of Zambia point at the rainbow with a pestle to drive it away. They think that where the rainbow ends there is a fierce ram which burns like fire.

The Zulu of South Africa call the rainbow the Queen's Arch, one of the frames which form the house of the queen of heaven. Some people call it a sheep, or a being who lives with sheep. But the Kikuyu of Kenya say it is an evil animal which comes out at night to eat men and animals. The Masai of Kenya say there was such a being that lived in Lake Naivasha, where the flamingoes gather, and it swallowed their cattle, till at last the young warriors managed to kill it.

A Chaga story of Kenya tells of a man who was looking for God to ask him for some cattle. He found the end of the rainbow and stood there offering his prayer. He did this many times but no cattle came. So in anger he cut the rainbow in half with his spear. Half the rainbow flew up to the sky, and the other half made a deep hole in the ground. The man disappeared, but some other people came along and found the hole. They climbed down to the underworld and found a rich country, with many cattle, and to prove their words they brought back bowls full of milk. But when other people went down they found lions there and fled back empty-handed. This resembles other stories, of two kinds of people visiting the underworld or heaven.

Other natural phenomena have tales told about them. One day a young man of the Songhay of the upper Niger regions was walking in the scrubland near the bush on his way to market. He saw a whirlwind, a dust-devil, coming straight towards him. In fear he threw his spear at it, and the wind passed him by, but

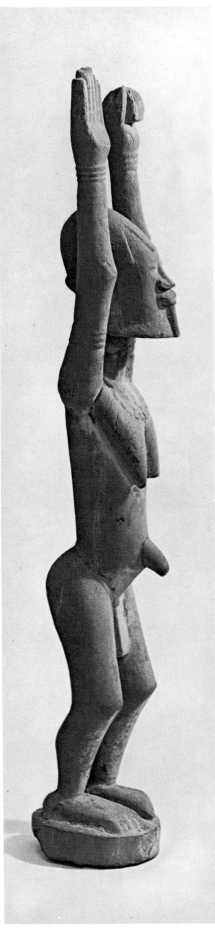

when it had gone he could not find his spear any more. This surprised him, but in time he forgot about it. Then one day as the youth was walking through a market he saw a man who had a spear just like the one he had lost. He went up to him and demanded where he had found the spear. The man smiled at him, for he was the spirit of the whirlwind. He simply asked the youth if he did not remember the whirlwind that had blocked his path one day when he was going to that very market.

Earth Spirits
Belief in a spiritual power animating the earth is almost universal and is found all over Africa. Usually, though not always, the earth is thought of as female, and sometimes as the wife or partner of the heavenly God. Sometimes they are in opposition, or there is conflict between the earth and another celestial deity, and this appears in some of the myths already given.

The Ashanti of Ghana speak of Earth Thursday (Asasé Yaa) because Thursday is sacred to the earth. There is no temple of this deity, but work on the land is taboo on Thursday. In the spring farmers offer a sacrifice of a fowl before digging the soil, praying for permission to dig, protection against accidents, and a fruitful harvest. The earth is also concerned with

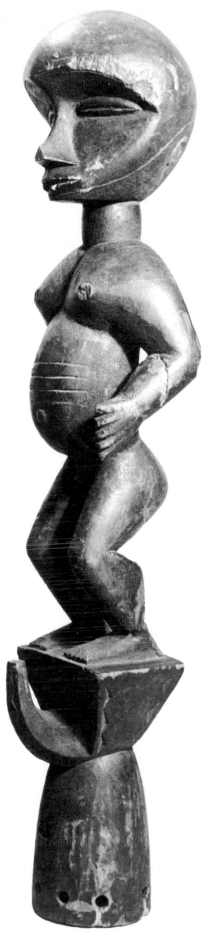

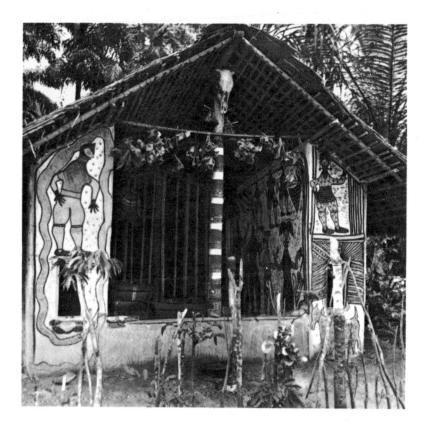

the dead, and before a grave is dug a libation is poured and permission asked. The earth is knocked, a custom that has survived among the descendants of the African slaves in America.

One of the most important earth goddesses in Africa is Ala of the Ibo people of eastern Nigeria. Ala is ruler of men, source of morality, and protector of the harvest. As a mother she gives fertility to the crops, and also to human beings. As queen of the underworld she receives the dead into her pocket or womb. The cult of Ala is shown vividly in sculptures which show the attitude of the people to divinity and to life in general. Shrines to Ala are found all over Ibo country, but in the southern regions of Owerri special houses, called Mbari, are erected. These are only built for particular occasions and are not temples, and once built they are abandoned and new ones erected. The Earth Goddess is always to be seen as the central figure in a group of mud sculpture. Mbari houses are built at the order of priests of Ala, when they say the goddess has sent a sign, such as the appearance of a nest of bees, or a snake, in the priest's garden. Men

and women are chosen to do the work, and they live together in chastity for weeks or months.

The Mbari houses are square, with open verandas round a closed central chamber. They are filled with mud figures, brightly painted. In the middle, facing the road, is Ala, Mother of Earth. She usually has a child on her knees, holds a sword in her hand, and her legs are often painted in spirals like the brass rings that girls used to wear at puberty. Facing Ala is the Storm God, a subordinate counterpart of the goddess. Then there are sculptures of Ala's family, the Water Goddess, and other deities, and with all manner of clay figures of gods, men and animals, and all kinds of occupations, old and new. There are figures of Africans and Europeans, dancing girls and district officers, hunters and policemen, tailors at sewing machines and women giving birth to babies. There are many animals, elephants and snakes, dogs and monkeys, forest creatures and monsters. All the gamut of life is there, without any distinction of sacred and secular. Some of the sculptures are sexual, some tender and pathetic. Ala and her child in some scenes recall the Italian

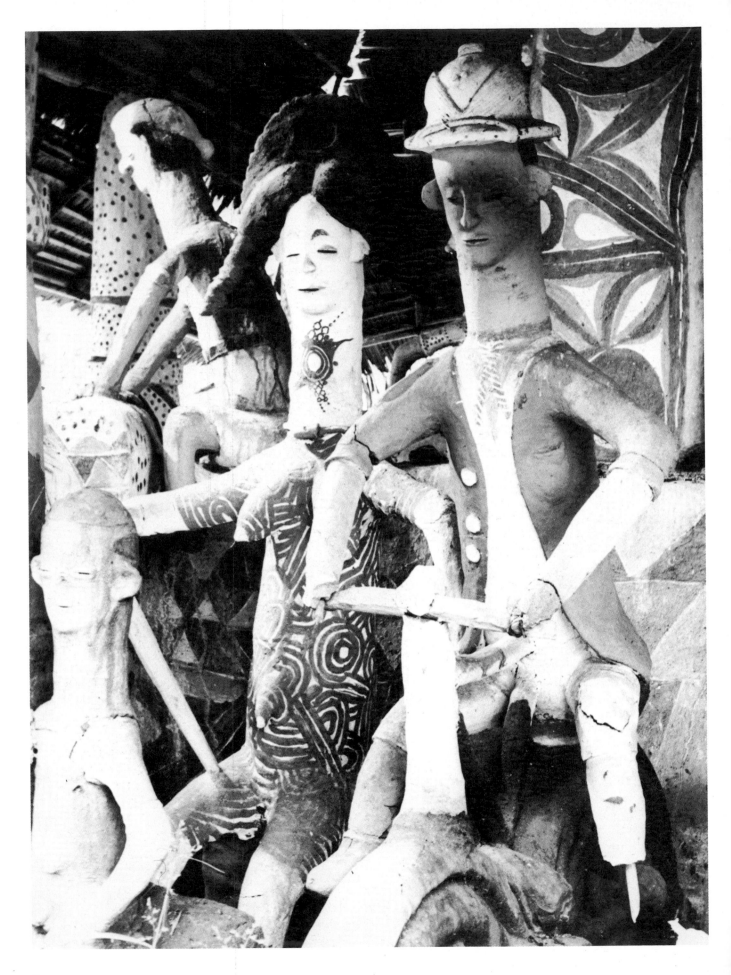

Madonna and Child. Christian symbols are included in the old pantheon.

Earth spirits include those of rocks and hills. Great mountains, like Mount Kenya, Kilimanjaro, and Mount Cameroon are all regarded with reverence and stories are told about their powers and taboos. A king of Buganda who wanted to build on the sacred hill of Boa crossed the stream at the bottom and at once became blind. The blindness remained as long as he stayed on the hill, but left him immediately after. There was a sacred forest there which only a priest could enter, and a temple with a female medium. If the chief of the district allowed the path round the hill to fall into disrepair, or a grass fire caught any of the trees, the medium would threaten him with an illness of burning sores. A story of Mount Kenya will be told later.

Other earth spirits belong to the forest and are patrons of hunters. The Songhay of the upper Niger, though superficially Moslems, believe in a spirit called Musa (perhaps from the Arabic for Moses) who is a great traveller, hunting everywhere, and he surveys the four cardinal points of the compass. Having learnt everything that there was on earth by his travels, he taught humans the secrets of hunting, and of pottery and weaving. Musa had seen his mother take clay and by means of water turn it into pots as hard as iron. He saw the wild tortoise weaving and he told people how to weave strands of cotton together. He knew the ways of the forest, and pointed out the twelve trees whose bark could be crushed into powder and mingled with water, and the resultant mixture would make anyone who washed with it invisible to the animals of the forest.

The gods of iron are often connected with hunting. The Yoruba of Nigeria say that Ogun, the god of iron, used to come down from heaven by a spider's web and hunt in the marshes, in the olden days when the earth was a watery waste. Later, the earth was formed by Great God, who set about arranging everything in order. But he came to thick forest that his tools could not cut, since they

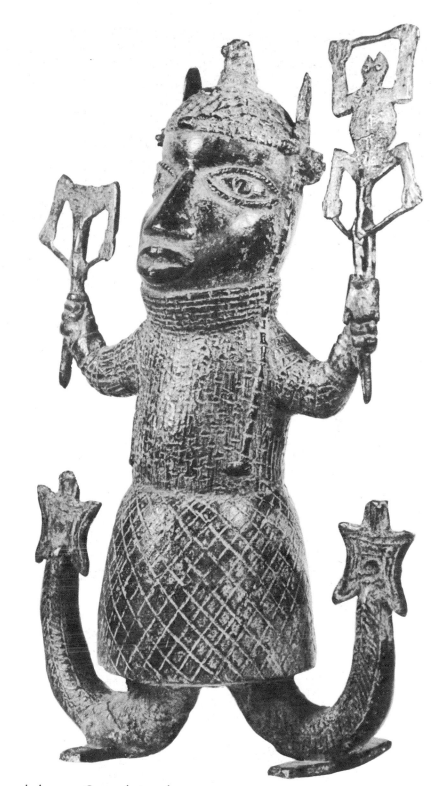

were only bronze. Ogun alone, whose axe was iron, was able to clear a way, and he only did this after the other gods had promised to reward him. So when they built their sacred city of Ilé-Ifé, they gave him a crown. But the Iron God did not want to rule his fellows, since he still enjoyed hunting and battle, and for a long time he lived alone on a hilltop, from whence

Above. A bronze figure of Olokun, sea god of Benin, Nigeria. With a royal coral dress and mudfish legs, he holds lizards in both hands. God of water and wealth, he lives in a palace under the sea with human and fish attendants. Rijksmuseum voor Volkenkunde, Leiden.

Opposite. Painted clay sculptures of the Ibo, Nigeria. The central female figure is the great Earth Mother, Ala. Next to her is a European, wearing a sun helmet and riding a motor cycle.

he could watch over the land and spy out his prey. When finally he came to the gods they did not want to harbour him, for his clothes were stained with blood. So he made clothes from the bark of a palm tree and went to live elsewhere.

A myth told by the Fon of Abomey says that the great deity Mawu sent his child Lisa to earth with a metal sword (in other stories Lisa is the male consort of Mawu, see page 23). Lisa came down to clear the forests and show men the use of metal, so that they could make tools for ploughing the fields and cut down wood for houses. Lisa told men that without metal they could not survive and so he re-created the order of the world, which at first had been without metal. Lisa then returned to heaven and Mawu gave him the sun as his domain. A metal sword is called 'gu' (the Yoruba Ogun) and Gu is the Abomey name for the god of metal to this day. He is protector of warriors, hunters and blacksmiths, oaths are sworn on his symbols, and nowadays he is also claimed as guardian of motor lorries and bicycles, which carry bunches of feathers that have been blessed by his priests.

Water Spirits

All the great waters, and many lesser ones, are believed to be inhabited by powerful beings. The Owner of the Sea, Olokun, is believed by the Yoruba and Benin peoples of Nigeria to live in an underwater palace with a great retinue, the attendants being both human and fishlike. In clay and bronze sculptures the majesty of the Owner of the Sea is illustrated, and stories say that he tried to rival the splendour of the Creator himself. Olokun challenged God to appear in his finest dress and he would do the same, and the winner would be declared by public acclaim.

On the day chosen God sent his messenger, the Chameleon, to fetch Olokun. But when the latter emerged from his ocean palace he was astonished to find that the messenger of God was wearing a splendid dress similar to his own. He turned back quickly, and put on even finer robes

and more coral beads, but when he came out the Chameleon had also changed into the same dress. Seven times Olokun tried to outdo the divine messenger, but each time he was matched by the same costume. Finally he gave up the struggle, thinking that if God's messenger was so glorious God himself must be much greater. Ever since then Olokun has taken second place to the Supreme Deity, even though people pay him more attention in ritual. The myth may reflect ancient stories of the struggle of the sea and the land, or of a primeval flood after which the sea was kept within proper bounds.

In Ghana and the Ivory Coast the River Tano is one of the most important deities and is credited with creation, as son of the Supreme God. A story was told earlier of his struggles with Death, and he was rival also of the River Bia, who was eldest son of God while Tano was the second son. Bia was the obedient child while Tano was often wilful, so when the children came to manhood God decided to give Bia the fertile places and Tano the barren areas. God called the Goat, told him what he proposed, and said he must call the boys so that each could take his lot. But the Goat was a friend of Tano and told him to be sure to get to God's house early in the morning, disguised as Bia, so as to receive the best portion. Then the Goat went on to Bia, gave the message, but said there was no hurry as God was busy. So Tano dressed in his finest clothes and went early to God, deceived him, and received the fertile land. Later Bia came along and God discovered the mistake, but the portion had been given and could not be changed, so Bia had the barren land. The story again resembles that of Jacob and Esau.

Lakes too are believed to be inhabited by spirits and a remarkable example is Lake Bosomtwe in Ghana. Like the Dead Sea this lake has no outlet and the water evaporates in the heat. A story says that long ago there lived an old woman who was a leper and so had no husband or children. One day there came a god out of the lake called Twe. When he tried to

make love to the old woman she protested, saying that she lived by herself and if she bore a child she would not be able to get food and water. Twe said that when she wanted anything she had only to knock on the lake and fish would come. So they were united, and she bore a son called Twe Adodo, son of the lake god, and founder of a clan which claims the lake spirit as protector. Once a week Twe would come out of the lake with his followers, and every year his son would go into the lake and ask his father's help with fishing. Then the lake would 'explode its gunpowder'. This exploding of the lake happens irregularly, when the vegetable matter gathered in the bottom decomposes and the accumulated gases cause loud noises and make horrible smells. The fishermen are forbidden to use iron hooks or nets in fishing, since the lake spirit is thought to dislike them, and they paddle with their hands on logs or rafts.

The Songhay of the upper Niger tell many stories of water spirits called Zin (perhaps from the jinn or genie of Islam). There was a lake belonging to a snake who was a Zin, and one day when the Snake was taking the air it saw a woman and wanted to marry her. The parents agreed but as dowry they demanded ownership of the lake. The Snake gave it to them and went to live with his wife some distance away, where they had a family. From time to time the Snake returned to his house at the bottom of the lake, from where he controlled the fish, crocodiles and hippopotami. When the Snake died his place was taken by his son, who is still guardian of the lake. But he is not pleased with men who have entered the lake with iron weapons, and because of that the hippopotami left the lake.

Another Songhay story says that once a village chief went out fishing by himself at night, and he was astonished to see, in the middle of the river, a sort of round hut. When he drew near he saw a little sheep in the midst of the waters. The chief was afraid and began to recite magic spells. But while he gazed the sheep changed itself into a little baby, and he knew it must be the great snake of the river that had transformed itself. The chief crouched down in the bottom of his canoe and began to shout for help. His brothers in the village heard him and came to his assistance, but when they got there he was dead, for he had seen a Zin, and that is forbidden to mortals.

A favourite story of the Songhay and of many peoples of the Niger bend, tells of a great struggle between a man, Faran, and a river spirit called Zin-kibaru. This spirit had gained great power by magical charms and musical instruments, and ruled over the fishes and animals of the river. Faran had rice fields and every night Zin-kibaru came and played his guitar there and all the fish came and ate Faran's rice. One day Faran went fishing and only caught two hippopotami. He was ashamed to see his mother cook this tiny meal, and calling his assistant he went off in a canoe to fight Zin-kibaru. They met on an island where seven streams crossed, Zin playing his guitar and various drums and violins and dancing. Faran demanded the guitar and Zin-kibaru said they should fight for it, but if he won he would take Faran's canoe. Faran was small and fat, and Zin-kibaru tall and thin. But Faran was winning when his opponent uttered a spell: 'The palm leaf despises the hippo.' Faran fell and lost his canoe. So he went back to his mother in shame and weeping. But his mother said he was stupid, for to fight a spell one must use another and she taught him one. Then Faran took a larger canoe and set off for Zin-kibaru. They met and fought, and the Zin fled. Faran pursued him, they fought again, and the Zin fled once more. A third time they fought, and as Faran was winning, Zin-kibaru said, 'The palm leaf despises the hippo.' But Faran retorted, 'If the sun strikes it, what happens to the palm leaf?' Then Zin-kibaru fell to the ground and his musicians all jumped into the river leaving their instruments behind. Faran seized the guitar, Zin-kibaru's harpoon, and all his slaves, and took them home in triumph. So the human

hero conquered the Zin or dragon, set free other spirits who were subject to him, and gained his musical instruments and weapons.

Most of the Buganda rivers were said to have originated from human or divine beings. Two rivers sprang forth from the son and daughter of King Tembo, who married each other. One of the rivers was said to have been caused by the birth-flood, and later it was worshipped under the form of a leopard because, it was

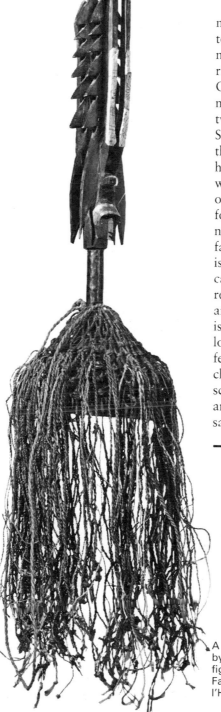

said, a leopard was drowned in it. Another river came from a young woman who was travelling about looking for a lover who had embraced her and then deserted her. On the spot where her child was born a river sprang forth. On each side of the river there was a heap of grass and sticks, and everybody who wanted to cross would throw sticks on the heap as offering to the river spirit, and after a safe transit a thank offering was thrown on the other side.

Some Malagasy clans, whose name means 'son of crocodile', have a myth to explain this. One says that the mother of the clan used to live in a river with a crocodile as husband. One day she was caught in a trap and married a man, but after bearing him two sons she returned to the river. Since that day her descendants hold the crocodiles as taboo and are never hurt by them. Another story says that when a member of the clan dies an old man drives a long nail into the forehead of the corpse so that it cannot move. But when it is put in the family grave a few days later, the nail is taken away and the body told it can move as much as it likes so as to return to the royal abode where the ancestors are waiting. When the grave is closed, the corpse moves a little, a long tail grows behind, the hands and feet change into small limbs with claws, and the skin becomes hard and scaly. Finally it becomes a crocodile, and goes off to the river. The family sacrifice a bull to it once a year.

A dancer's headdress worn in fishing rites by the middle Niger river. The wooden figure decorated with metal represents Faran, the master of the river. Musée de l'Homme, Paris.

Oracles and Divination

There are many kinds of oracles by which people try to discover the future or the unknown past, or the will of God and the ancestors. There was no writing in tropical Africa in the olden days, but there were complicated systems of divination which used notation that was a kind of writing or means of recording and communicating. Such systems are known from Senegal to Malagasy, but the most famous is the Ifa divination of the Yoruba of Nigeria, which has been borrowed by neighbouring countries. Ifa is a spirit often identified with a god called Orunmila, 'heaven knows salvation'. In some versions it was he who directed creation under the orders of God. When God had all the elements of creation ready, he sent the morning star to call the gods, but only Orunmila came. The morning star told him that the materials of existence were kept in a snail shell which was in the Bag of Existence, lying between the thighs of God. Orunmila took this, came down below, scattered soil and got a hen and a pigeon to spread it abroad, as in the other Yoruba creation myths (see page 21).

Another story says that after living on earth for some time Orunmila went back to heaven, stretching out a rope and climbing it. But since he had been interpreting the will of God to humans, they now found themselves helpless and without guidance. Then Olokun, the Owner of the Sea, came and destroyed most of the earth and it became unfit for habitation. So in pity Orunmila came down again and made it pleasant.

The Yoruba say that under the name of Ifa, a man-god, the oracle came from heaven and was born of superhuman parents who had never

Opposite left. Ivory divining rod from the Yoruba of Nigeria, used in worship and fortune-telling. The designs are usually in pairs, male and female, representing spirits, and some rods have little clappers at the end to invoke them. The diviner takes the heavy end in his hand and strikes the divining board with the pointed end, murmuring prayers and chants inviting the spirits to be present and hear the prayers. In the possession of the author.

Opposite above right. Divination board or planchette of the Yoruba, Nigeria, with figures of gods and animals round the edge. Powder or sand is sprinkled in the middle and the diviner marks patterns on it with his fingers. Museum of Mankind, London.

Opposite below right. The Yoruba made beautiful vessels to hold the seeds used in divination. This bowl is held in the hands of a characteristic Yoruba carving of a mother carrying a child. Museum of Mankind, London.

been to earth. He was sent by God to put the world right: give help in sickness and childbearing, teach the use of medicine, and give guidance on secret or unknown matters. Ifa came down, stopping at various towns on the way, setting up centres for consultation, but he was not satisfied till he got to the sacred city of Ilé-Ifé where he established his home, and this is still the centre of his worship. Ifa was a great linguist, knowing all the tongues of earth and heaven, and he can advise every nationality and bring messages from the gods. He was a great doctor, and songs and proverbs used in his worship speak of his powers. The Ifa divination is performed by casting nuts in combinations of four and sixteen, and marking a pattern on a divining board.

The Fon of Abomey, who have borrowed the Yoruba system of divination, have their own stories of the

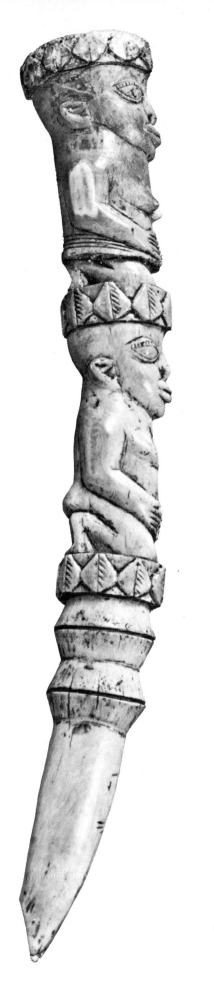

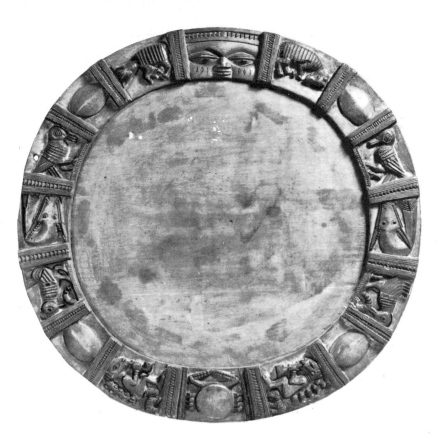

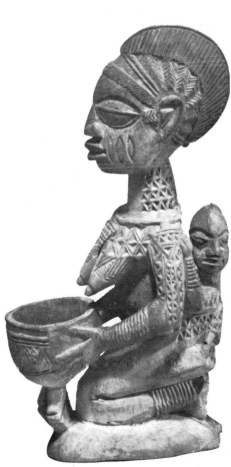

origins of the cult. They call it Fa, and say that after the creation of the world two men came down from heaven. In those days there were very few people on earth, no gods were worshipped and there was no medicine. So these divine messengers called men together and told them that God had said everyone must have his or her own Fa. When people asked what the Fa was, the men replied that it was the writing which God creates with each person, and by this they could find out what tutelary god to worship and how to do the will of God. The heavenly messengers selected a man, whom they taught how to work the oracle. They had brought from heaven some nuts of a special palm tree, which could be manipulated so as to reveal the messages of Fa. They showed the man how to throw the nuts from one hand to the other, trace patterns on a board according to the number of nuts left over from the throw, and so discover his destiny. They told him to gather up the sand which bore the resulting pattern, inscribe it on a piece of calabash, put it in a small cloth bag, and so keep the secret of his horoscope. Since that time divination has been performed on this pattern, both for ordinary occasions and to make a life horoscope.

This is the most complicated system of divination, though simpler methods of using strings with objects attached, and judging the oracle by the patterns made when they are thrown on the ground, are found in many places. In the Transvaal the Venda people use four pieces of flat ivory for divination, and other peoples use dice of wood carved with designs of beasts like crocodiles. The four dice represent members of the family: old man, young man, old woman, and young woman. They are thrown into sixteen possible combinations and diviners have interpretations for each combination.

Divining bowls, filled with water and an assembly of objects, are used for discovering secrets or detecting witches in parts of tropical Africa. But in southern Africa apparently only the Venda and the Karanga of Zimbabwe use such divining bowls, with patterns and pictures round the side of the bowl, and a cowrie shell in the middle which is called the umbilicus and represents the spirits of the mother. However in the ruined buildings of Zimbabwe similar soapstone bowls have been found, decorated with figures such as bulls.

A famous oracle was at Aro in eastern Nigeria, and during the time of the slave trade he was widely feared and called by Europeans the Long Juju. The oracles were given from a cave seven feet (2 metres) up the bank of a little river. Visitors stood in the river, while the priest was in or by the cave, and gave answers in a nasal voice, like the oracle at Delphi. People who were guilty of crimes, or declared to be so, were said to be 'eaten' by the oracle, and they passed through the cave or some other route to be sold into slavery. This trade was destroyed in 1900, though the oracle is still respected.

The greatest of the demi-gods of Buganda, Mukasa, was a great giver of oracles, a kindly deity who never asked for human sacrifice. Myths say that when Mukasa was a child he refused to eat all ordinary food and

disappeared from home, later being found on an island sitting under a large tree. A man who saw him there took him to a garden and lifted him on to a rock. People were afraid to take him into their houses, thinking he was a spirit, so they built a hut for him on the rock. They did not know what to give him to eat, for he refused all their food, but when they killed an ox he asked for its blood, liver and heart. Then people knew he was a god and consulted him in any trouble. Mukasa lived on the island for many years, married three wives, was cared for by priests, and at last disappeared as suddenly as he had come.

His temple was a conical reed hut, which was rebuilt at intervals on the express orders of the king. Originally it is said that Mukasa spoke his will directly to the priests, but later they used mediums who uttered his messages. The medium never entered the temple but had a special hut in front

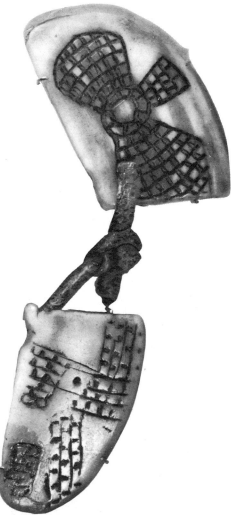

of it. When seeking to know the will of Mukasa she smoked some tobacco until the spirit came upon her, and then she announced in a shrill voice what was to be done. The medium was not allowed to marry, or walk about in the sight of men, or talk to any man but the priest, and once chosen held the office till death.

Connected with the oracles are often other messengers who act as intermediaries, between the gods and men. The Yoruba of Nigeria have many images of an intermediary spirit called Eshu, who is both a messenger and a guardian of human beings. His image is placed outside houses and villages. But he has an unpredictable character, and is often violent or crafty, and he may express the anger of the gods at human wrongdoing. Eshu is very powerful and only the Supreme Deity can curb his might. One day the Storm God was boasting that he could subdue every other spirit. Eshu asked if that statement included him. The Storm God at once apologised and said he did not count him in this category. Another god bought a slave without consulting Eshu, and when he found his slave strangled next morning he knew who was responsible.

A popular story tells how Eshu introduced discord into the house of a man with two wives with whom he lived at peace. Eshu did not like this, as he delights in confusion, and he laid a trap. Changing himself into a trader, he made a beautiful headdress and stood in the marketplace. One of the wives came down, saw the fine hat, and bought it. She showed it to

Left. Old ivory divining tablets of the Bushmen of the Kalahari desert, Botswana. The diviner beat the leather strips joining the tablets with his hand and invoked the oracle to tell the truth. Then the tablets were jerked from his hand and the direction and person at which they pointed gave the answer required. Museum of Mankind, London.

Opposite. Ivory statuette from Benin city, Nigeria, used in the cult of Oromila, whom the Yoruba call Orunmila. This is the spirit of divination and the female figure holds in her hands a box containing the nuts for casting in the Ifa system of divination. Museum of Mankind, London.

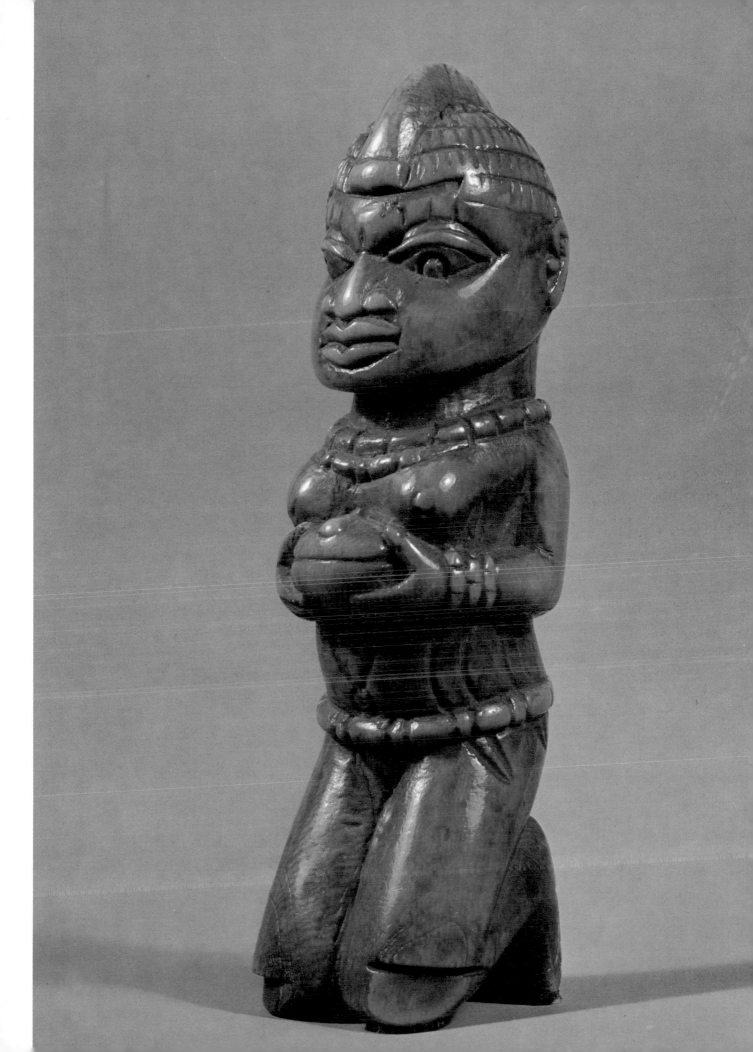

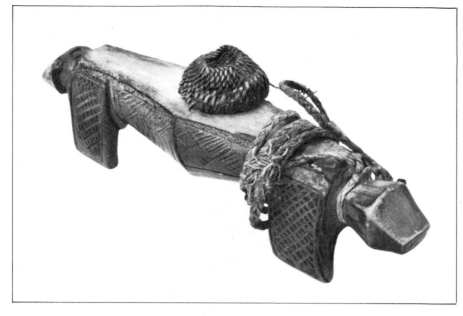

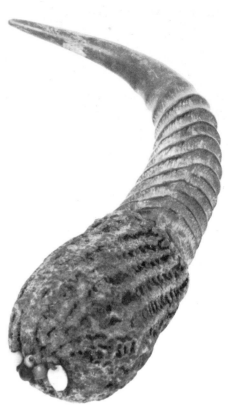

her husband and he favoured her in such a way that the other wife was jealous. She in turn went to the market, and found Eshu there with a hat far better than the first. She took it home and became her husband's favourite. Then the first wife went again, and the same thing happened; the second went later, and so on. The rivalry grew in intensity, with the husband's affections swaying first to one side and then to the other, till nobody knew where they were. Then Eshu left off going to market, the women were in despair, and the family was engulfed in strife.

The Fon of Abomey have similar beliefs about a kindred spirit called Legba. In the beginning Legba lived on earth with God and only acted on his orders. Sometimes God told Legba to do something harmful and then people blamed Legba for it and came to hate him. They never gave him credit for his good deeds but thanked God instead. Legba got tired of this and went to ask God why he should always be blamed, since he was only doing the divine will. God replied that the ruler of a kingdom ought to be thanked for good things and his servants blamed for evil.

Now God had a garden in which fine yams were growing, and Legba told him that thieves were planning to plunder it. Therefore God called everyone together and warned them that whoever stole his yams would be

killed. During the night Legba crept into God's house and stole his sandals, put them on and went into the garden. He took away all the yams. It had rained not long before and the footprints were clearly seen. In the morning Legba reported the theft, saying that it would be easy to find the thief from the prints. All the people were called but nobody's feet fitted the prints since they were too big. Then Legba suggested that perhaps God had taken the yams in his sleep. God denied this and accused Legba of his usual mischief, but when he consented to put his foot down it matched the prints exactly. The people cried out that God had stolen from himself, but God replied that his son had tricked him. So God left the world, and told Legba to come to the sky every night to give an account of what went on below.

A variant, giving another version of the stories of God retiring to heaven, says that when God and Legba lived near the earth Legba was always being reprimanded for his mischief. He did not like this and persuaded an old woman to throw her dirty water into the sky after washing. God was annoyed at the water being constantly thrown into his face and he gradually moved away to his present distance. But Legba was left behind and that is why he has a shrine in every house and village, to report on human doings to God.

Legba is closely associated in Fon story and ritual with the oracle Fa. One myth says that Fa had sixteen eyes, the nuts of divination. He lived on a palm tree in the sky. From this height Fa could see all that went on in the world. Every morning Legba climbed the palm tree to open Fa's eyes. Fa did not wish to convey his wishes by speaking out loud, so he put one palm nut in Legba's hand if he wanted two eyes open, and two palm nuts to have one eye open. Then he looked round to see what was happening. And so today one palm nut thrown by the diviner is a sign for two marks to be made on the divining board, and two nuts make one mark.

Later God gave Fa the keys to the doors of the future, for the future is a house of sixteen doors. If people used the palm nuts correctly they opened the eyes of Fa and showed the right door of the future. Legba worked with Fa, and when there was a great war on earth which threatened to destroy everything God sent Legba to teach the method of the Fa divination, so that people could consult the oracle and know the proper way of conduct.

Opposite left. Wooden figure used by Congolese diviners. The small circular piece is rubbed on the back of the figure and if it sticks at one place an answer is given according to the diviner's judgement. Horniman Museum, London.

Opposite right. Divining horn from Zambia, filled with leaves and adorned with beads, and used to find what sacrifice will avert sickness.

Right. A Yoruba carving of Eshu, the go-between. He is represented in the style of the Yoruba (Nigeria) king's messengers with the characteristic Yoruba dressed hair.

Below. Eshu, the messenger between man and the gods, wearing the cowrie shell strings by which he can read the future.

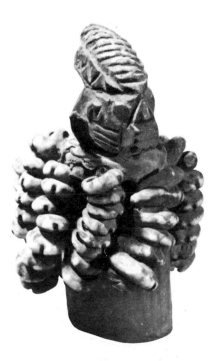

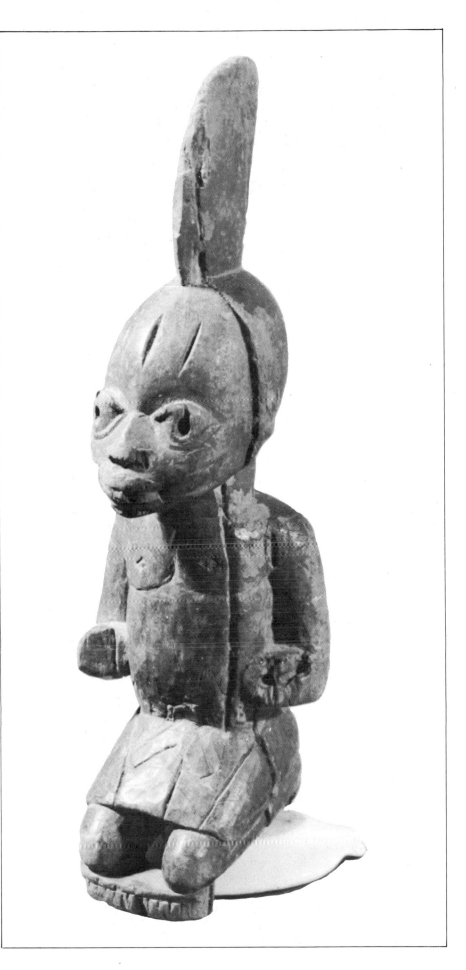

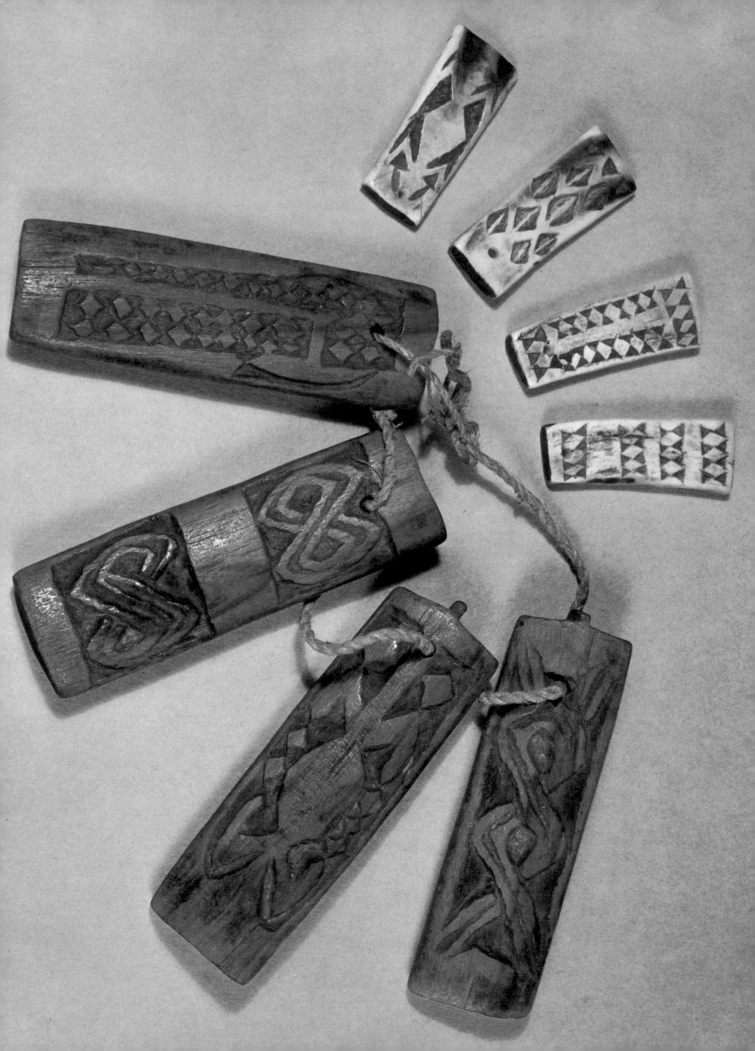

Witches and Monsters

Witchcraft is believed in throughout Africa. Basically it is the belief that certain people, chiefly women, have the power of changing themselves into other forms, when they prey on the bodies and souls of their enemies or even their relatives. It must be firmly said that it is a delusion. People do not leave their bodies or destroy the souls of others. So in fact there are no witches, though many people believe in them. Witch-doctors try to treat and cure those who are thought to be bewitched. Many African peoples distinguish witchcraft from magic and sorcery. Magic is the practice of making charms to help or

Opposite. Divining tablets from the Shona of Zimbabwe. Many kinds of tablets were used to discover secrets or predict the future, decorated with animal or human figures or combinations of numbers and patterns. These were interpreted by a skilled diviner according to the manner in which they fell to the ground. Museum of Mankind, London.

Below. A dance mask in carved and painted wood from Abomey. Such masks are worn during ceremonies performed to ward off the influence of sorcerers. Collection Bastide.

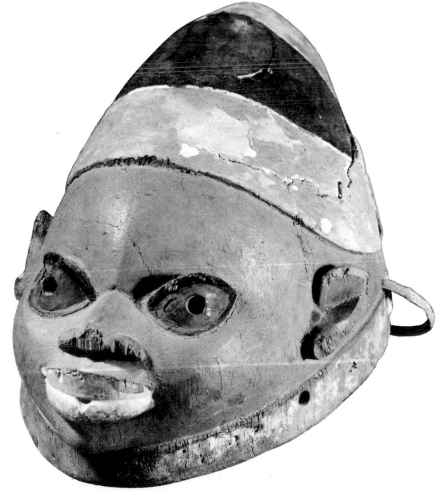

harm people, so the good magician, medicine-man or doctor is a respected figure. But the bad magician or sorcerer is hated by everyone and consequently works in great secret.

A Hausa story of Nigeria tells of a man who had three wives, all of whom had magical powers but only two were witches. They used to dance in the forest, and the two tried to persuade the third wife to do a witchcraft dance with them. She put them off by saying that the dance was too difficult and they must wait until she had given her husband a gift of cloth. Then she warned her husband of what was afoot and he pretended to go on a journey, but really he was rolled up in his mat and stayed quiet. When they thought he was gone the wives began to dance. The two witches chanted that they would offer up their husband to the witchcraft dance; one said she would have his liver and the other his heart. Then the husband jumped up, beating one wife and driving her out, and tying the other to the top of a tree. Then he lived in peace with the faithful one.

Another Hausa story tells of a witch who had nine mouths on her body, but of course they could not be seen. One day she went to get leaves from a forest tree and boiled them as broth for her husband and his father. When the husband opened the bowl of soup it cried out in warning, 'Cover me up, for if you do not you will die.' Then the husband's father uncovered his broth and it also cried out, 'Cover me up, for if you do not you will die.' So the husband got his own soup and his father's and threw both bowls over his wife's head. At once her nine mouths became visible, she was shown as a real witch, and she ran away.

Apparently circumstantial stories are told of people who have left their bodies at night and flown off on bats or owls to cannibalistic feasts in the tree tops. In the Ivory Coast a witch is said to have changed into an owl, though her body was still asleep on the bed. The owl flew out but was shot by a brave hunter, and at the same moment the witch died in bed. Another story says that a witch

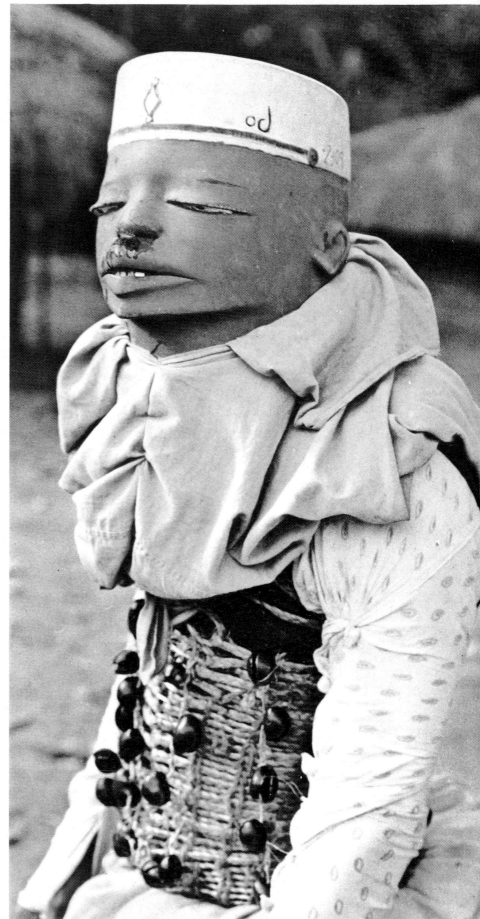

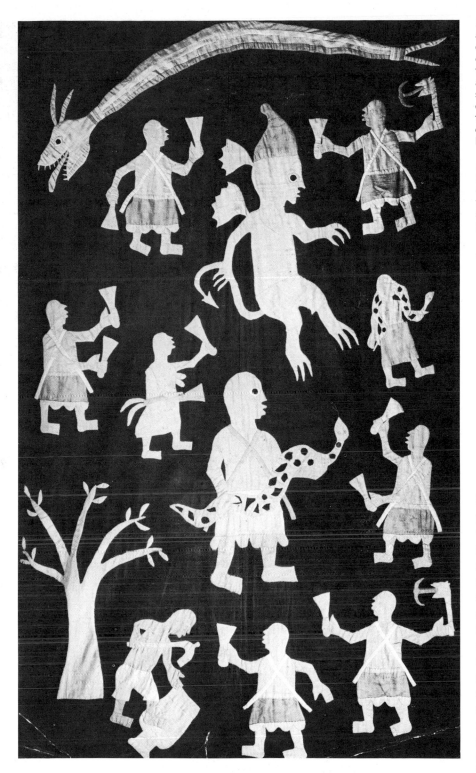

such a being is supposed to have haunted the forests, challenging any-one to wrestle with him, and offering medicines to a man strong enough to hold him down. Then there are 'little people', perhaps early Pygmies, though later regarded rather as fair-ies. Some lived on the highest moun-tains, like Kilimanjaro, which formerly were beyond the reach of human feet. Elsewhere there were mischievous imps, who could help or harm human beings.

In a Swahili story a girl found a beautiful shell on the seashore, and put it on a rock while she went on with her companions to look for more. Then she forgot it till they were nearly home, and asked her friends to go back with her. They refused and she had to go alone, in the dangerous dusk, so she sang to keep her courage up. On the rock she found a fairy, and when he heard her he asked her to come closer and sing the song again. Then he seized the girl and stuffed her into a barrel. He went along from village to village, offering to play wonderful music in exchange for a good meal. When the fairy beat the barrel like a drum the girl sang inside and people gave him plenty of food, but he gave none to the girl.

In time he reached the girl's own village. They had already heard of his fame and begged him to give them an entertainment. When the girl sang her parents recognised her voice, so they gave the fairy a great deal of wine afterwards to make him fall asleep. They rescued the girl, and put bees and soldier ants into the barrel, so

changed into a crocodile, and while a girl was bathing the crocodile seized her and dragged her into the water. But a man killed the reptile with an axe and at once the witch died in the house where her body had been lying. It was the witch's soul that went off in an animal body, and in many stor-ies it is not the victim's flesh that is thought to be eaten by witches but what is called 'the soul of the flesh'.

The forest, bush, plains or any lonely places are thought to be the lair of dangerous spirits. There are 'half-men' who have only one hand, leg, eye and ear. A Gikuyu story of Kenya tells of such a being whose body was half flesh and half stone. Elsewhere such men are said to be half human, half wax. In Malawi

that when the fairy next beat it he would be severely stung.

In southern Africa there are Xosa and Lesotho versions of this story, in which the parents put poisonous snakes into the barrel and the fairy dies. In another version he throws himself into a pool to get away from the snakes and a pumpkin tree grows on the spot. Later some boys take one of the large pumpkins home, but their elders are horrified, knowing what it is, and chop it to pieces.

Then there are dangerous animals that may take human form for a time, like the 'were-wolves' of Europe, though there are no wolves in tropical Africa but dangerous beasts like lions and hyenas. A story told with variants in Kenya, Zambia and Malawi, and no doubt elsewhere, tells of an obstinate girl who would never marry any of the suitors who came to her. Her parents were so angry that they offered to give her to anybody who presented himself. One day there was a great dance to which men came from other villages. A very tall and handsome youth arrived with a ring round his head like a halo. All eyes were drawn to him and the girl followed him all the time. The dancing continued for days, the girl danced with the beautiful young man a great deal, and fell in love with him.

But her brother happened to see that the fine youth had a second mouth at the back of his head, and warned his mother of danger. She ridiculed the idea that such a handsome man was evil, and when he demanded their daughter's hand both parents agreed with joy. The wedding was celebrated and some days later the girl and her husband set off for his home. But her brother followed at a distance, still feeling uneasy. As they got farther away the husband asked his wife if she could still see the smoke from her parents' house, and she said she could. Later he asked if she could see the hills behind her home, and she could just discern them. When they had at last disappeared the animal in human form told his wife to weep her last tears for he was going to eat her. But just then the brother shot at him with a poisoned arrow, saved his sis-

ter, and took her safely back home.

In similar stories the younger brother accompanies the sister and husband, and at night the husband goes out and changes into animal form, as a lion or a hyena. Having prowled around he tries to break into the house with other lions to devour the two humans. But the brother has strengthened the thorn-bush defences and they are safe for a time. When the animal in human form returns, the brother makes a drum, or a miniature boat, and by his magic forces it to rise in the air. He and his sister cling to it and thus escape.

There are many tales about monsters which swallow human beings and then are killed by a hero. In a Zulu tale there lived in a mythical river a female, bearded, humpbacked monster. One day the daughter of a chief went to bathe in the river with her companions, against the warnings of her parents. When the girls came out of the river they found that all their clothes had been taken, and each girl politely asked the monster to give them back. All succeeded, except the chief's daughter, who refused to plead with the monster and was seized and dragged into the river. When the chief heard the news he sent his young warriors to attack the beast and rescue his daughter, but they too were swallowed up. Then the monster went to the chief's village and devoured all the people, even eating the dogs and cattle.

The father of two beautiful twins escaped, however, and he swore revenge. He took his club and spear and went after the beast, who had disappeared. First he came across some buffaloes, who told him which way to go. Then he met some leopards, who directed him forward. Next he came to an elephant, who also sent him on. At last he met the monster, and she apparently hoped to deceive him, for she told him to stay on the same path and proceed. But the man was not fooled, he demanded his children, and stabbed the monster in her great hump. The wound was fatal and she died. Then all the people, the cattle and the dogs came out of her mouth, and last of all the chief's

daughter, who was restored to her father. In another version it is the girl herself who kills the monster and sets the people free, and in similar tales a herd-boy or young hero makes the beast so uncomfortable that she pleads to be cut open and all the victims are released.

Ghosts, particularly those of people who have not been properly buried, are believed to dwell in the bush and to trouble unwary travellers. Animals and trees have souls as well as humans and many have ghosts. A story told by the Dagomba of Togo says that a chief long ago wanted to show his people that he was greater than anybody else. So he called them all together and said that in future he would no longer ride a horse but a dappled antelope. His hunters were sent into the forest to catch such an animal, and after a long time they succeeded. But they did not know that their dappled antelope was a ghost. When the chief ordered his men to saddle the creature they encountered great difficulty, though they managed in the end. Then the chief leapt into the saddle, but the antelope at once dashed into the forest, with the chief clinging to its back.

The hunters pursued him as fast as they could, but both antelope and chief were lost from sight and have never been seen again. So it is said that whenever a chief from that town is about to die, people see a dappled antelope come in the night and stand outside the chief's house waiting to take him away.

Ebony figure of a doctor from Mozambique. The doctor may be a medicine-man who knows the secrets of nature and tends the sick, or a witch-doctor trying to cure those who are thought to be bewitched. Most gods of sky, earth and water have priests who perform sacrifices in their temples, and the doctor may be a priest as well. He is a wise man and much respected.

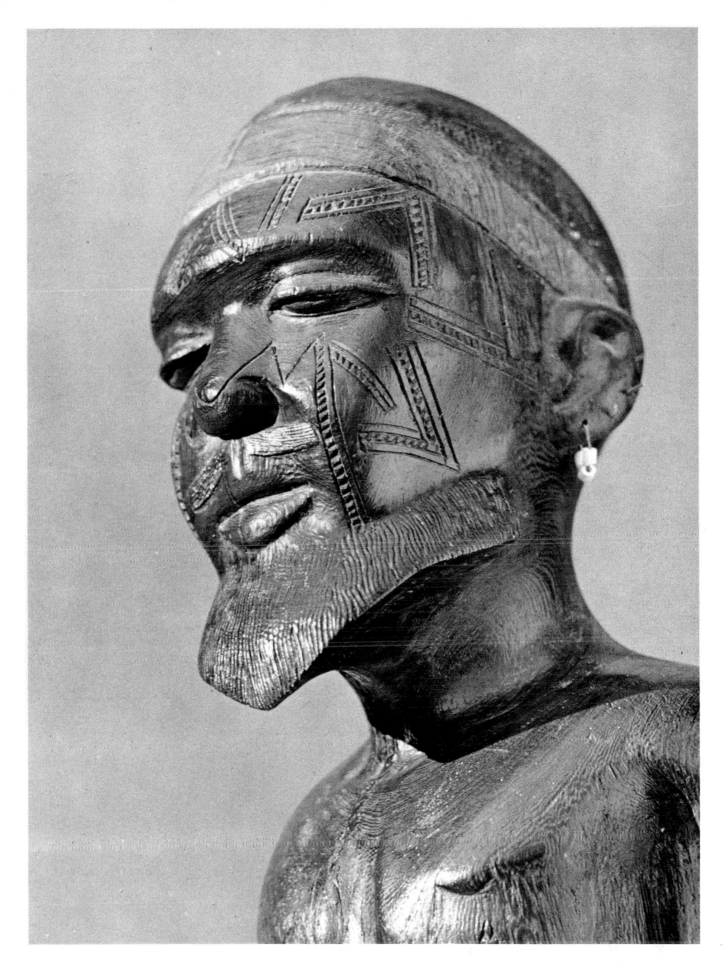

Secret
Societies
and
Ancestors

In many parts of Africa there are closed associations which are popularly called secret societies. They serve various purposes, of which the initiation of young people and the representation of dead ancestors are the most common. The masquerades of their officials, 'masked spirits', in fantastic dress, are some of the most striking and most photographed of all African religious ceremonials. The mythology of the secret societies is not easy to obtain since they are secret except to initiates. The great number of such societies would demand volumes to record even part of them. So as an example one of the best known is chosen here, the Poro, of the Mende people of Sierra Leone.

The Poro, meaning perhaps 'no end', can be traced back for several hundred years and is related to other West African societies. Various myths account for its origin. One says that long ago there was a rich old man who had a large family and so much land that he was looked upon as the chief of that place. But trouble came to him and he was struck with a disease of the nose, so that his voice became very harsh. The people had never seen such a disease before and they were afraid. They isolated the old man in the forest outside their village. Only his chief wife and youngest daughter were allowed to look after him, and when elders went to discuss business with the chief they went alone. Everyone else was forbidden to approach or to attempt to look on him. Eventually the men plotted to kill the chief and his wife and daughter, in order to seize his lands. He was already out of sight and all that could be heard was his harsh voice, so they planned to make an instrument that would imitate it. This

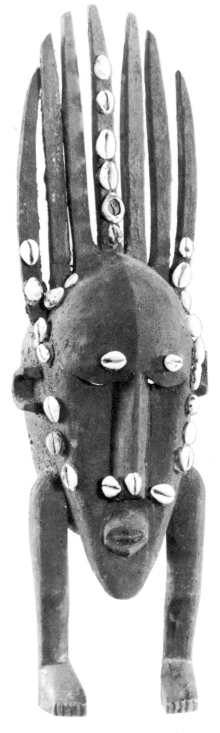

was done by making a hollow stick, with a piece of skin fitted over one end. Then the village people were told that the chief had become a spirit. Occasionally it was said that he was coming to the village to visit the rest of his family. A herald came announcing this and all the women and children were rushed out of sight into their houses. Then the herald called out that the chief needed rice, goats, and so on, and these were provided.

Another version says that the first chief of this people was very powerful, and when he died the elders were afraid that the whole community would break up if his death became known. So they kept it a secret and found a man who could imitate his voice. As the late chief had a strongly nasal tone it was easily copied. The first person to act as imitator was bound by oaths of secrecy, and when in due time others had to be told, they were bound to secrecy also.

More rational explanations, though not more likely, are given of the origin of the Poro society. One is that it came from groups of people hiding in the forest from slave-raiders and bound to mutual loyalty. Another suggests that it arose from chiefs holding meetings in the bush to avoid being overheard by women, or away from the spies of their enemies in wartime. Yet another suggests that very sick people were isolated in the bush, and even after their death their voices were heard, being copied by instruments made to frighten women and children into submission. The story says that the elders acquired all the man's property, but when his children grew up they were introduced to their father impersonated by a member of the society. The young men were taken one by one to a 'spirit', a masked robed figure, sitting on a tree trunk with the Poro horn, the pipe of office.

The Poro society is also found in neighbouring countries, and in Guinea this story is told of its origins. In the olden days there was a great famine and food was scarce and bad. There were some goods in the market but the women sellers demanded very high prices. The men got desperate, and at a secret meeting they decided to frighten the women away from the market and seize their provisions. So they carved human features on pieces of wood, put horns on some and horrid faces on others, and practised guttural sounds such as were never heard from human mouths. Then they went to the market, masked and screeching, while other masked figures interpreted their words. The frightened women gave them all they wanted and ran away. The masked figures beat all the men they met, and cut scars on their bodies, saying that this would assure their protection by the spirits. Since then men have made scars on their bodies and women always provide food for the masked Poro dancers.

These fanciful explanatory myths must not detract from the serious purpose of the Poro society. Its function is to fit every youth to play the role of an adult in society, and perpetuate the ancestral customs. The society is controlled by elders and arranged in a hierarchy, but differing in each village. It is said that the first Poro spirit before he died named his wife as leader of the women's section. Since then women have joined on the same terms as men, but are not usually officials. The Poro members meet in 'sacred bush' outside the village, where the founder of the particular group was buried. The chief masked spirit is the Gbeni, who may only be looked at by members of the society, and appears in public on special occasions, for example when a new group of boys is to be initiated, in a series of rituals lasting from November till May.

The initiation is a symbolical rebirth. The youth is swallowed by the Poro spirit when leaving his parents; this is like death, and marks are cut on his back to indicate the scars left by the spirit's teeth. The boys stay in a camp, with no modern comforts, sleeping on the ground, staying out in the rain, cooking their own food, and making wild cries if they see village people. They are instructed in family and social duties, and learn drumming and Poro songs. At the end of the training they return as reborn to

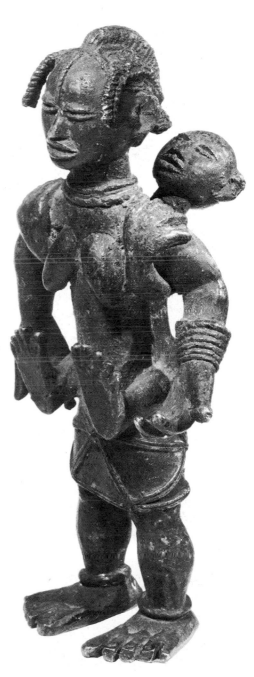

Opposite. A Bambara 'standing' mask from Mali. These strange constructions, of carved wood decorated with cowrie shells, were used in the initiation rites of the Ndomo society. Musée de l'Homme, Paris.

Below. A figure of a woman and child from an altar of the Poro society, Sierra Leone. The Poro is one of the most celebrated African 'secret societies'. It serves to initiate youths into the tasks of manhood, and continues ancestral customs. R. J. Hewett, Esq.

97

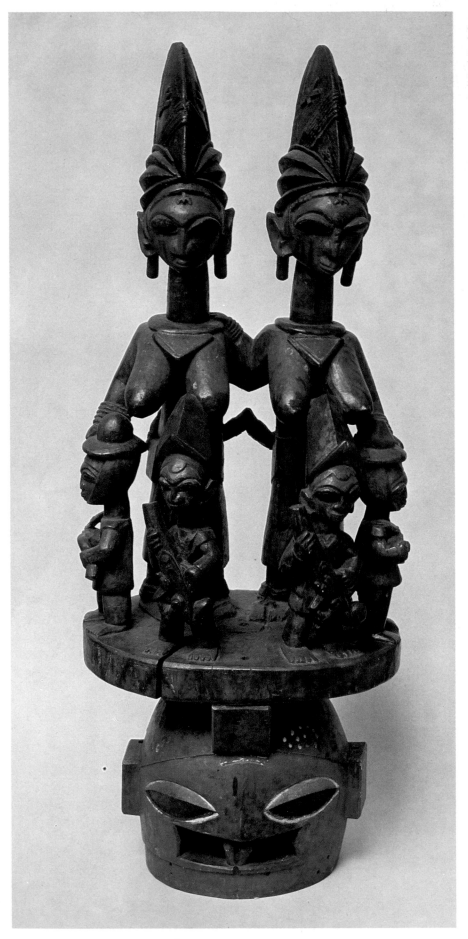

Left. Two sisters, or two wives, with their children, from the Yoruba, Nigeria. The figures stand on a mask of the Epa cult of ancestors. Carved of wood and carried on the head of a masquerader, it demanded skill from the wearer. As ritual objects they show links between family life in this world and the next. Museum of Mankind, London.

Opposite. Mask of the Poro society of Sierra Leone and Guinea. The members meet in 'sacred bush' to perform rituals for their ancestors and to initiate young men into adult secrets and duties. The masked spirits appear in public on great occasions when the whole body is covered with cloth or grass. Mrs Margaret Plass, Philadelphia, Pennsylvania.

their parents, having passed from childhood to manhood.

A parallel society, the Sandé, exists for the initiation of girls, with the same purpose of fitting them for adult life. The Sandé spirit appears masked in public on great occasions, with a wooden mask, and a robe of black cloth covered with strips of wood fibre and little bells fixed on the dress. These masked figures, though terrifying at first sight, are known to represent the spirits of the ancestors and of the societies, and are deliberately meant to show their supernatural character and power over men.

A story about the origin of masks is told by the Kono people of Guinea. An old woman used to make pots and went one day to get supplies of clay from the banks of a little stream far from her village in the forest. Her daughter was with her and as the woman dug she placed the clay beside her daughter. Suddenly she dug up a Thing, which surprised her, but she put it by her daughter and went on digging. A little later she came upon another Thing, female this time, the first having been male. The two Things said not a word, though the woman tried to make them talk by pinching them. The daughter ran off to the village to fetch other women and when all had arrived they decided to take the Things home with them. When they got there they shut all the men up in their houses, with the exception of a doctor whom they hoped would persuade the Things to speak. He told them to put the Things in a hut and burn pepper there.

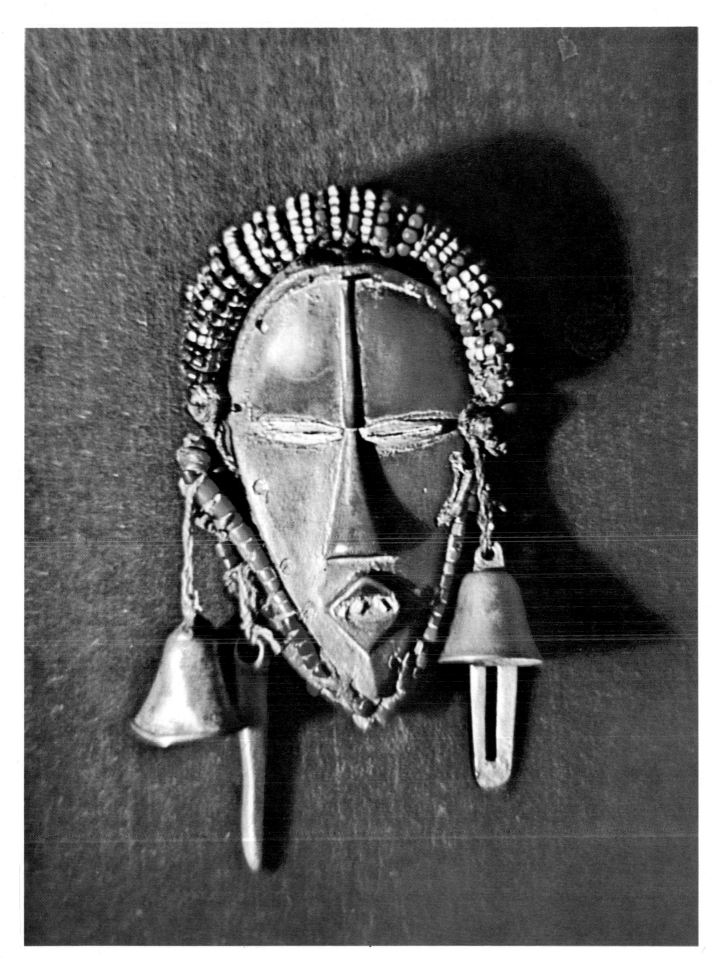

99

Before long the Things began to be stifled by the fumes of burning pepper, and the women heard a low growl from the male Thing, which said 'Shake your rattles!' At the sound of this voice the women fled, crying out to the men to save them. The men emerged from their houses and they heard the female Things singing sweetly. They took charge of the Things, and have held the secrets of their voices and masks ever since, while the women who discovered them lost control of the masks through lack of courage.

Another version says that the women found the spirits under the large leaves of a climbing plant. They brought them home and danced round them, but were terrified when the Things began to growl in menacing tones. Their men came with weapons, took the spirits to the forest, and ever since have known the secrets of the masks though women discovered them first. The stories suggest an earlier dominance of women, which men later overcame.

Many of the societies use a bull-roarer. This is a flat piece of wood or metal, which when twirled at the end of a cord gives off an irregular and frightening sound. A story told by the Dogon of Mali says that when the masked dancers performed the women came to watch, and even when men tried to chase them away the women peered from far off and imitated the dances. Then a man called Moyna found a flat piece of iron at the smithy. He tied a cord to it, and whirled it in the air and was struck by the sound it made.

On the night of the next dance there was a low growling sound, and the women looked round in fear, wondering what it was. Moyna whirled the iron faster and the women fled in panic. Next day Moyna got the blacksmith to make a better piece of iron, with a hole at the end. At night-time he went outside the village and whirled his bull-roarer faster than before. The women fled into the safety of their houses and Moyna went through the village, announcing that it was the Great Mask speaking, and any woman or child who came out would be eaten. Since that day women and children always hide indoors when the bull-roarer sounds. When Moyna died he passed the secret to his sons, and told them to sound the bull-roarer when any notable person died.

The rock paintings that are found in many parts of Africa often depict animals and people, and sometimes masked figures. A Dogon story says that a leopard was pursuing its prey, a gazelle. The chase became furious as the gazelle fled for its life and soon the two were far from their home in the bush. They came into rocky country and lost their way. But the chase continued fast and fierce, until the beasts found themselves confronted with a high and long wall of rock that even they could not leap over. So great was their speed that they both crashed into the wall and flattened themselves on it. Their pictures can still be seen, the smaller representing the gazelle, and the leopard with his neck and legs elongated by his speed. Another story says that a woman had

seen masked dancers and wanted to get hold of the pattern of their masks, so she drew it on the ground and her husband copied it on the rocks. More often it is said that the painting was made by an ancestor or a hero who wanted to teach his descendants the form of masks that he had learnt from spiritual beings. And more simply,

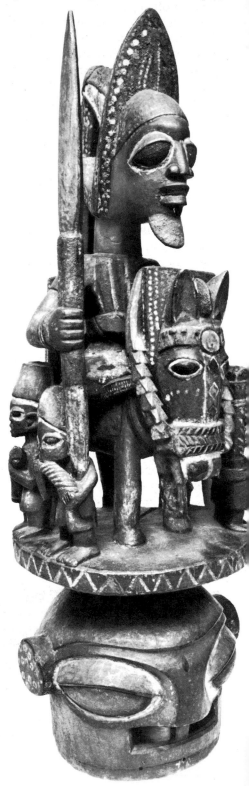

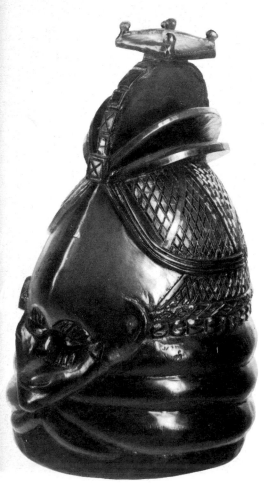

but perhaps no less truly, rock paintings are said to represent some outstanding event, or simply just some curious being.

Myths of the ancestors will be found under stories about the first men, and in the next section on legends from different parts of Africa. Stories of the gods have shown that they are often partially ancestors, and a further example may be given from the Songhay of the upper Niger. Zoa was a wise man and ancestor of the people and their protector. Once he heard some travellers say that if a pregnant woman is given sheep's liver to eat, it is the child in her belly who is eating it. He tried this on a slave, cut open her belly, and saw the child eating. Another day Zoa went hunting and came across a wounded lioness lying on an ant-hill. Zoa tended the wound and after that the lioness went hunting with him. When Zoa married and had a son he took the boy hunting with him. They saw a bird eating millet and Zoa said that the bird would fall dead at his word, and it did so. He said that the bird should be cooked on a fire, and a fire lit itself and cooked the bird.

But his son began to cry at the death of the bird and Zoa, in anger, told the earth to open. He called all the people of the village to the edge of the hole, and told them that his son would be chief in future. When the rains would not fall, or evil came, or war happened, they must bring a white sheep or a white bull and offer it to him, and he would do all they asked. But he forbade the deaf, the blind, bastards, and all people with hernias to visit his shrine. Then he disappeared into the earth and closed it up after him, and four trees grow in that place, in the directions of the compass. Every year people have gone to pay homage to Zoa, and when there is no harvest they have prayed and he has given them millet. If they have been spared from war it is because he had prevented it.

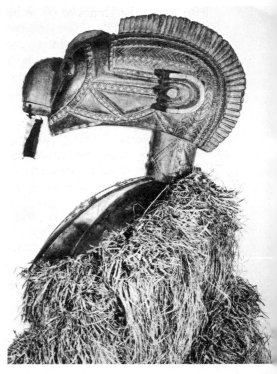

Right. A mask of the small Baga tribe of Guinea. It represents the goddess of maternity, protector of mothers, worshipped by the Simo society. The head is carried on the dancer's head, and he sees through holes in the chest, while his body is completely covered by a fibre dress. Musée de l'Homme, Paris.

Opposite right. A dance mask in carved wood. In spite of the weight – this one is over four feet (1.2 metres) high – they were carried on the head by dancers at Yoruba festivals. Museum of Mankind, London.

Opposite left. An elaborate wooden mask of the Sande female initiation society of the Mende of Sierra Leone. Called Bundu, it represents the ancestors which preside over the girl initiates. Glasgow Art Gallery and Museum.

Right. Mask of a white monkey called Ireli from the Dogon of Mali. The man who wears it leans on a stick and sits apart from the crowd in a melancholy attitude, but he is encouraged to dance by singers who chant: 'Monkey on a high tree full of fruit, all eyes are on you, the drum is beating for you, move your head, move your legs, all the people have their eyes on you.' Musée de l'Homme, Paris.

Below. A bull-roarer from the Nandi tribe of Kenya. Many African secret societies use this kind of instrument, which is also found in other parts of the world. When whirled rapidly in the air, it gives off a harsh and irregular sound, like a bull roaring or a dog barking, which is said to resemble the uncanny voices of spirits of the dead. Museum of Mankind, London.

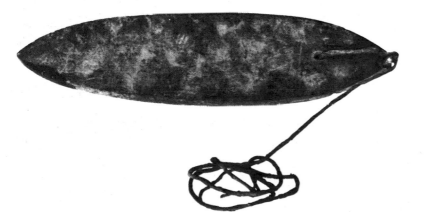

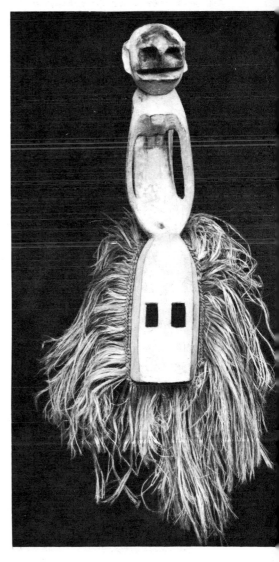

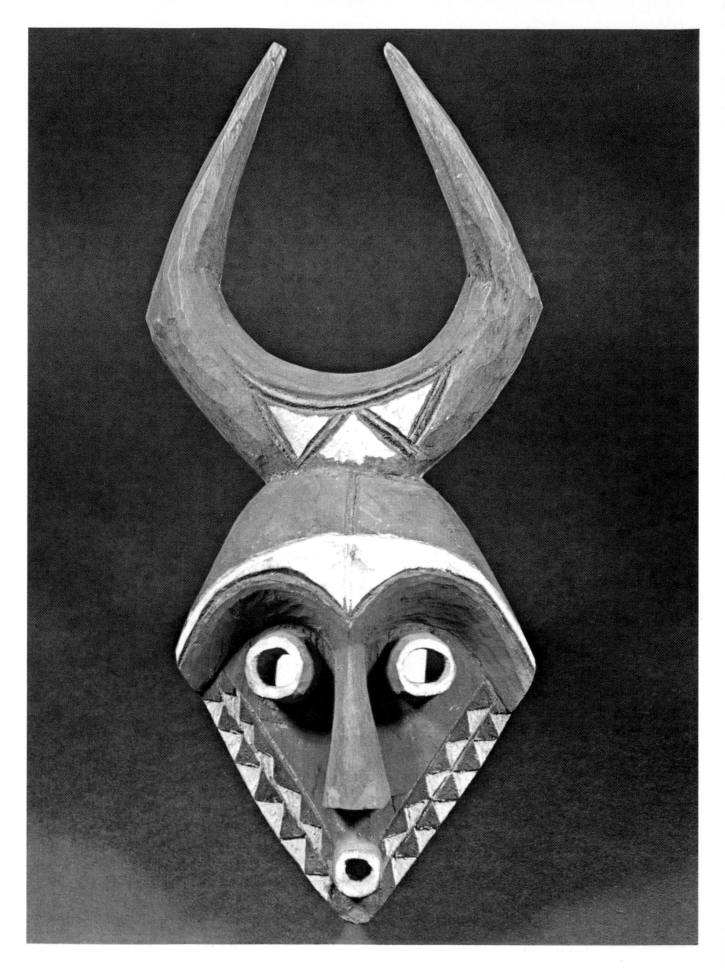

Right. Painted wooden mask of the Egungun society of the Yoruba, Nigeria, just one of the countless decorated masks with entwined figures, famous for their infinite variety of carved and coloured representations. The Egungun, 'bone' or 'skeleton', is a society of masqueraders whose members appear in public at special times of the year to demonstrate the continued existence of the ancestors, reveal their power and convey messages to survivors. Museum of Mankind, London.

Opposite. Many African masks represent in realistic and stylised form the heads of animals which are believed to have great power, concentrated in the head. The wearer is protected from evil by this power and dances like the animal. This painted animal mask comes from the Bapende of Zaïre. Museum of Mankind, London.

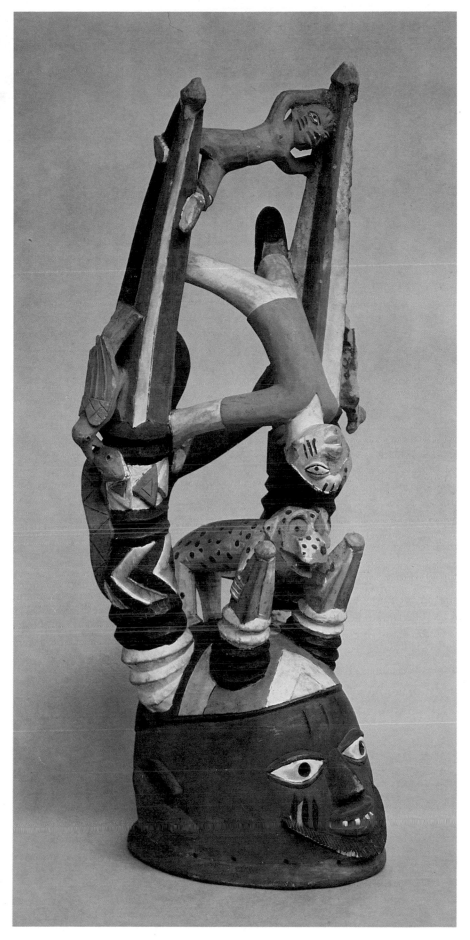

Legends of Old Africa

A myth is a story of supernatural or primeval beings which cannot be placed in recorded history. A legend is a traditional story, about historical or semi-historical people, even if the narratives are partly imaginary. Many stories include both myth and legend. No doubt every African people has legends of the founders of the group, or later heroes. Most of these are of great interest as illustrating thought and religion, as well as history and prehistory. Some well known stories are given here, selected from different parts of the continent.

The Golden Stool

Stools are traditional seats and symbols. In some places a man's personal stool is regarded as the shrine of his soul, and in funeral ceremonies it is carried into the family stool house, where regular offerings are made to the spirit of the ancestor. Stools are often highly carved, out of one block of wood, and there are many patterns, all of which have a name and meaning.

In the eighteenth century the fourth king of Ashanti, Osai Tutu, made his people into a great nation. They had been subject to a neighbouring kingdom, whose ruler had a clansman called Anotchi. Anotchi offended that king and fled the country. He took up the study of medicine and magic and became the greatest doctor in the land. He said that Nyame, the Supreme God, had given him the mission to make Ashanti a great people. He went to King Osai Tutu, and by means of his spiritual powers brought down from the sky, in a black cloud and amid thunder and dust, a wooden stool covered with gold. It slowly descended, to rest on the king's knees, and the monarch had four bells made to hang on each side of the stool. Anotchi told the king and the people that this Golden Stool contained the soul of the Ashanti people and that their health and welfare were in it. He made the king, queens and chiefs take a few hairs from their bodies and parings from their forefingernails. These were made into magical powder, some of which was drunk and some poured on the stool. Anotchi said that the stool must not be sat upon, though on great occasions the

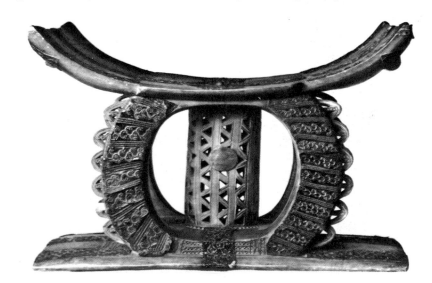

king might pretend to sit on it three times and rest his arm on it. When it went out in procession once a year it was carried under umbrellas and attended with royal state.

The Ashanti rebelled against their oppressors and totally routed them. It is said that the king of that country was sitting playing the game of wari (mankala, a popular African game) with one of his wives, wearing gold chains on his wrists, when the Ashanti soldiers burst in upon him. The royal couple were executed and the golden chains fastened to the Golden Stool. Another king had a copy of the Golden Stool made for himself, and the Ashanti were so angry that they made war on him, and had two golden masks made from his face and attached to the Golden Stool.

When the British fought Ashanti in 1896 it was feared that the Golden Stool would be damaged, so Ashanti submitted. But the new conquerors demanded to sit on the stool, thinking it to be the sign of government. A second war broke out in which many lives were lost and the Golden Stool disappeared. It was not heard of again until 1921. Then some workmen making a new road came upon two brass pans. Before they could dig them up the custodians of the stool came and frightened the men away,

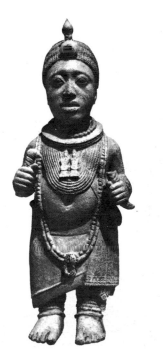

knowing that the hiding place of the stool had been discovered. They said the place was infected with smallpox, and the stool was taken to a new hiding place. But greedy people discovered it and stole gold ornaments from the stool and tried to sell them. They were recognised and there was a great uproar; the thieves were put in prison to save their lives. National mourning was declared and a revolution seemed imminent. Fortunately the authorities had learnt the significance of the Golden Stool, and it was restored to the royal palace at Kumasi, where it remains. When Princess Mary was married in 1922 the Queen Mothers of Ashanti sent her a silver stool, with a message saying that their love was 'bound to the stool with silver fetters, just as we are accustomed to bind our own spirits to the base of our stools'.

Ifé Art

The wealth of art found at Ifé in Nigeria has only become known to the wider world in this century. So much of the rest of African art seems stylised that the calm naturalism of the Ifé bronzes and terracottas makes a great contrast. The bronzes are usually dated from the thirteenth or fourteenth centuries and show the existence of schools of craftsmen whose works have very rarely been rivalled before or since. Other work has been done in ivory, clay and wood, and there are some fine royal stools in quartz.

The Yoruba regard Ilé-Ifé, the 'house of Ifé' as their place of origin, as told in the creation myths (see page 22). Another version of this story says that when Great God had been sent to earth he became very thirsty and drank palm wine, and lay down to sleep. As he was away a long time God sent his brother Oduduwa to continue the work of creation. This he did and supplanted Great God in ownership of the land. Oduduwa is regarded as the first king of Ifé and the founder of their race. He was a strong personality but little of any particular interest has survived about him except general stories.

The son of Oduduwa was Oranyan, who was a great warrior. In old

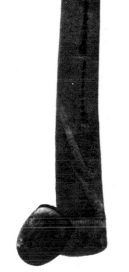

Above. The Staff of Oranyan, second king of the Yoruba of Nigeria, stands twenty feet (6 metres) high at Ifé. The white band and the pot at the base show that offerings have been made.

Left. A statue from Ifé, Nigeria, showing a royal figure. The face is probably carved from life but the shortened body is stylised and dressed in robes like those still used in coronation ceremonies. An axe in one hand and a horn in the other are symbols of power.

Opposite. The state stool of King Kofi of Ghana, taken from his palace in Kumasi in 1873. Made of wood, covered with silver, and shaped like a rainbow, it is the commonest pattern of royal stool. A proverb says that 'the circular rainbow encircles the neck of the nation'. William Rockhill Nelson Gallery of Art, Kansas City, Missouri.

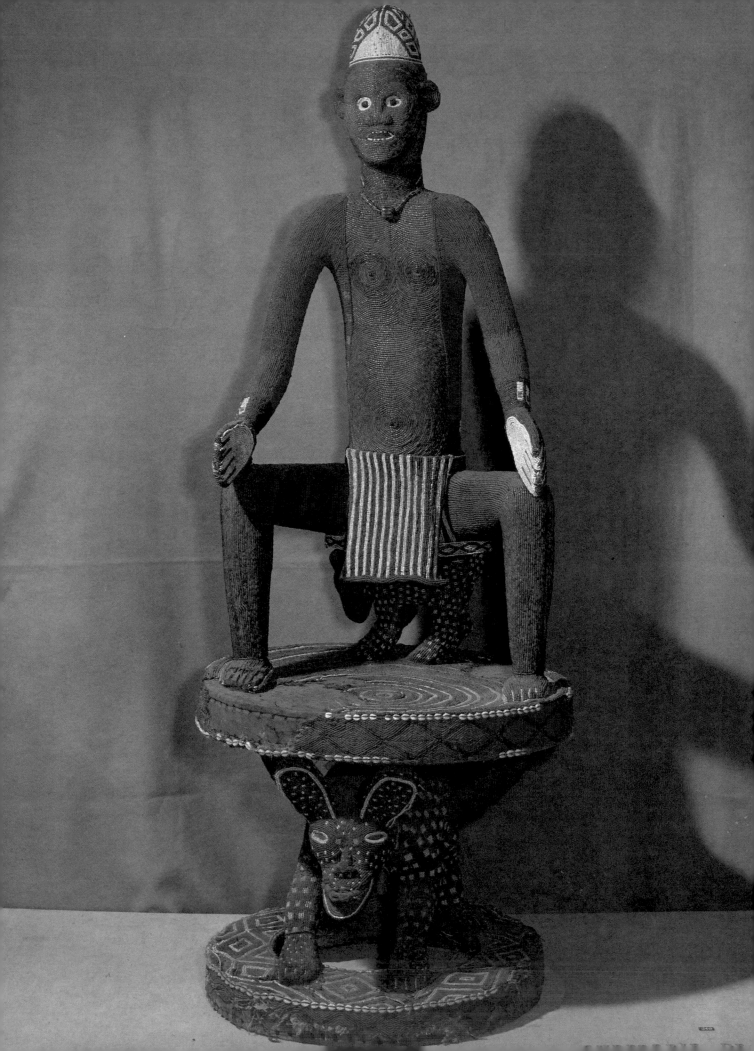

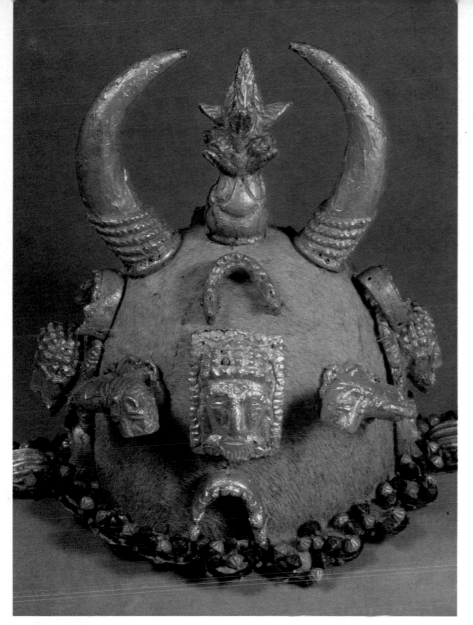

Above. The importance of gold in Ashanti, in the former Gold Coast, was to enhance the prestige of chiefs and powerful spirits. This gold cap could cover not only the head and upper face but by its horns and ornaments it suggested more than human powers and achievements. Museum of Mankind, London.

Opposite. Throne of state of the Bamileké of Cameroun, with a depiction of chief Néré in full size forming the back of a wooden stool decorated with abstract and shaped figures.

age he retired into a grove, but if his people were attacked he emerged and dispersed enemies single-handed. One day, however, during a festival when the city was full of people and some were drunk, a man called to Oranyan that they were being attacked. The old king came out on horseback and laid about the crowd, until the people begged him to stop destroying his own subjects. Then the shocked warrior drove his staff into the ground and said he would never fight again. It is said that it was turned to stone and so were he and his wife. Broken remains of stone have been dug up and fitted together to restore the pillar, 'the staff of Oranyan', which stands about twenty feet (6 metres) above ground, studded with iron nails whose pattern and meaning are disputed.

The later history of Ifé is not yet well documented, except for the fine bronze heads of kings which are still being unearthed. One of the best known is the Olokun head, discovered at Ifé in 1910, which represents a king, or the god of the sea whose clay images are still made in the region today.

Benin Bronzes

The craftsmanship of Ifé was passed on to Benin, now in Nigeria, which being nearer the sea was better known to early European travellers. Some of the early heads and royal masks are of modified naturalism. One of the best known is an ivory mask still worn by the king of Benin on ceremonial occasions. But from the sixteenth century Benin art developed in a baroque direction and became more elaborate and stylised.

Myths of Benin say that their kingdom was founded by the youngest son of the Supreme God. His elder brothers founded Ifé and other realms. When they left heaven each son was permitted to take some valuable object with him that would be useful on earth. The others chose tools, wealth and magic. But a bird told the youngest son to take a snail shell. When the sons arrived on the watery marsh here below, the bird told the youngest to turn up the snail shell, and sand fell out which covered the marsh. The debt of this story to the Yoruba creation myths is obvious. It justified the title of the king of Benin to the marshy land on which his realm was founded.

Myths say that the first people of Benin could not agree among themselves and for a time they were without rulers. At last they sent to the king of Ifé, Oduduwa, and asked him to send one of his sons to rule over them. Some say it was this son who brought the snail shell that gave him authority over the land, and the snail is modelled in brass and preserved in the royal palace. The son is said to have been Oranyan, whose stone staff is at Ifé. But after some years he renounced the rule of Benin in favour of his son and returned home. The date of the foundation of this kingdom is generally put in the twelfth or thirteenth century.

Brass-casting was brought to Benin from Ifé in the fourteenth century, and in 1472 the first Europeans arrived. They were merchant explor-

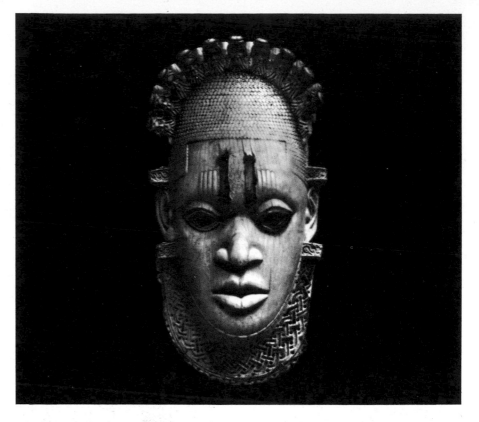

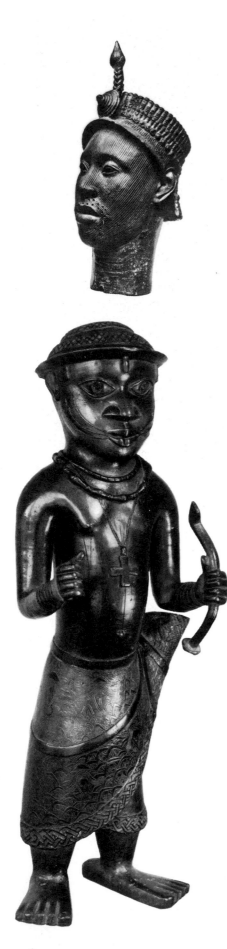

Above. An ivory mask representing a king of Benin, Nigeria, with a tiara of small heads depicting the Portuguese visitors who went to Benin from A.D. 1472. Museum of Mankind, London.

Above left. A famous bronze head from Ifé, Nigeria, where some of the finest African art flourished from the thirteenth century A.D. Sometimes called after Olokun, god of the sea, the head probably represents an early king. Museum of Mankind, London,

Left. A sixteenth-century Benin bronze figure of an archer. The cross is Portuguese and could have been acquired to be worn simply as a decoration, while the coral beads and skirt edged with a chain motif are characteristic of this part of Africa.

Opposite. The bronze panels from Benin, Nigeria, are notable for their characteristic style. Here a royal figure, with coral crown and necklet, bears a two-edged ceremonial sword, flanked by warriors and small attendants, carrying musical instruments. Musée de l'Homme, Paris.

ers from one of the Portuguese expeditions on their voyages of discovery round Africa. The fifteenth king of Benin was then on the throne.

In the sixteenth century, Benin art developed away from naturalism and became more elaborate, though still expressing meaning and not just stylised for its own sake as in some of the later art. Bronze panels were cast containing a number of figures. Some of them depict Olokun, the god of the sea and wealth (see page 82). Story connects him with a king who became paralysed in the legs and gave out that he had become the sea god. Thereafter on bronze panels two mudfishes are shown in place of the king's legs. Other bronzes showed the pointed headdress and the high collar imitating the red-coral bead crowns and necklets of the kings.

The Benin artists soon showed their adaptability by including figures who are clearly in Portuguese dress and carrying firearms. They show the impression made by Europeans and the skill of the artists in depicting new types. Bronze and wood work still continue, though much commercialised. Some of the most lively arts are those that cannot be exported: wooden posts carved for ancestral graves, and mud sculptures which are popular but fragile. There are mud reliefs on palaces and houses in Benin, comparable to those in old Dahomey though not so ancient. They give striking representations of kings and courtiers, soldiers and musicians, masked dancers and animals.

Spear Masters

Among the Dinka people of the upper Nile the Spear Masters are a hereditary priesthood, and their importance is shown by myths which unite political and religious ideas. One version says that long ago there were dances held by lions, and a man was dancing there when a lion demanded his bracelet. He refused, whereupon the lion bit off his thumb to get the bracelet and the man died. He left a wife who had a daughter but no son and she went weeping to a river. A river spirit asked why she was crying, and hearing that she had no son he told the woman to lift her skirt and brush the waves towards her so that they could enter her. He gave her a spear, the symbol of bearing a male child, and a fish for food, and told her to return home without delay. The woman bore a son called Aiwel, who had a full set of teeth at birth, a sign of spiritual power.

When he was still a baby his mother left him asleep on the floor, and on coming back she found that a full gourd of milk had been drunk. She accused her daughter of having stolen the milk and punished her. The same thing happened again and the mother became suspicious. She pretended to leave the baby alone with the milk and went out, but hid herself to watch him. She saw Aiwel get up from the floor and drink the milk. When she burst in and accused him, the child warned her not to tell anybody, else she would die. But the woman could not keep the secret to herself, and she died as Aiwel had predicted, for he already had the power of spear-masters in making his word come true, however terrible.

After his mother's death Aiwel would no longer live with his family and he went to stay with his spirit-father in the river until he grew up. Then he returned from the river as a man with an ox of many colours, representing great wealth and the colours of all the herds; but his chief colour was that of the rain clouds. The ox was called Longar, and from then on the man was called Aiwel Longar. He took up his abode in the village, tending the cattle that had belonged to his

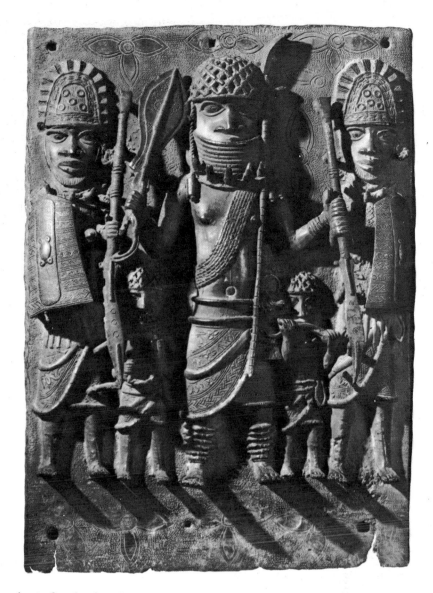

mother's first husband, who had died of the lion's bite. There came a drought on the land and people had to take their cattle far afield to find grass and water. Many of them became thin and died, but the cattle of Aiwel were fat and strong. The young men decided to spy on him to find out where he fed and watered them. They followed him to where some long-rooted grass was growing, and there he pulled up tufts of the grass to give his cattle the water that was underneath. Aiwel knew that the young men had spied on him and again his secrets were fatal, for when the youths revealed them to others they all died.

Aiwel Longar then told the village elders to leave their land where the cattle would die, and said he would take them to a promised land where

there was inexhaustible pasture and water and no death. But the elders did not believe him and set off on their own. So Aiwel went by himself, but it seems the people tried to follow him after all, for God put barriers of great mountains and rivers in their way. At one river where they tried to cross, Aiwel stood on the other side and killed the men with his fishing-spear as they passed over. The people were in danger of being destroyed altogether, until a man called Agothyathik thought of a ruse to save them. A friend took a large ox bone and held it out on a pole in front of him as he went through the reeds on the river bank. When Aiwel saw this he thought it was a human head and prepared to spear it. While he was occupied Agothyathik crept round to the back and grappled with him. For

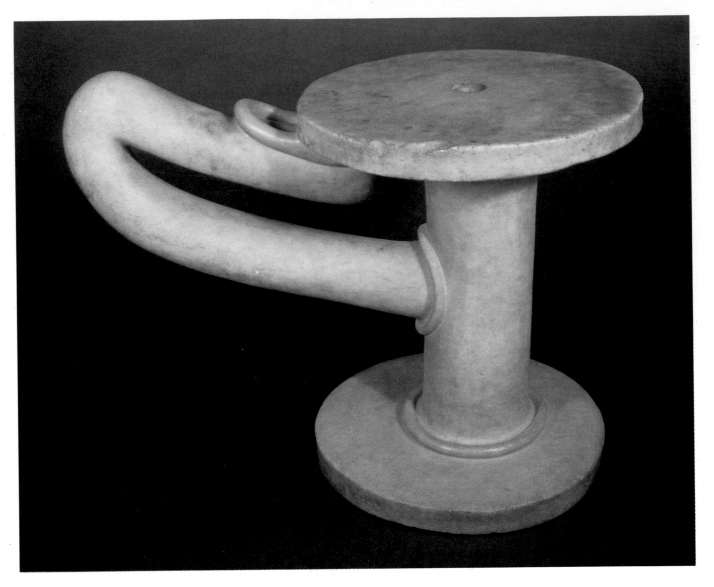

Quartz stool presented by Adelekan Olubushe, the Oni of Ifé, to the Governor of Lagos in 1896. This was probably the first time that any European became aware of the art of Ifé. Quartz stone is found at Ifé and is very brittle. This and similar stone stools were carved skilfully, with projecting loops whose function is unknown. The stool came from the shrine of a 'white god', Oluorogbo, who carried messages between heaven and earth. Museum of Mankind, London.

---

a long time they wrestled, till Aiwel was tired and gave up. He told Agothyathik to call the people over. Some were afraid, but to those who came Aiwel gave fishing-spears to carry when they prayed, and war-spears. He gave them other divinities to worship, and a sky-coloured bull whose thigh-bone would be sacred to them.

The men who received these gifts from Aiwel founded the clans which are now spear-masters, 'people of the fishing-spear'. Others who came later were 'people of the war-spear' and founded warriors clans. Aiwel Longar then left the spear-masters to rule the country, and said he would not intervene except in time of trouble.

There are other versions of this myth. One says that in the beginning all the people lived in the river, and the first to emerge was called Longar, the eldest son of God. He was like a spirit and like a man, the first to be created and the source of all life. Despite differences in the versions there are common themes, particularly the conflict with the divine figure who tries to kill the founder of the clan at a river-crossing, but who is outwitted and in the end gives his blessing. The fishing-spear is the symbol of priesthood, as explained by the myth. It shows that the original spear-master was a river man. Death and its avoidance also figure in the stories, as well as land and its ownership, still of primary importance for life.

Facing Mount Kenya

The Kikuyu, or more correctly, Gikuyu, people of Kenya say that in the beginning the Divider of the Universe, the creator God, made a great mountain as a sign of his wonders and a resting place for himself. This was Keré Nyaga, the 'mountain of Brightness' (or mystery), which Europeans call Mount Kenya. This was the earthly dwelling place of God, whose person cannot be seen and who is far away, though he is invoked at the crises of life. People turn towards the mountain in prayers, lift up their hands and offer sacrifices there.

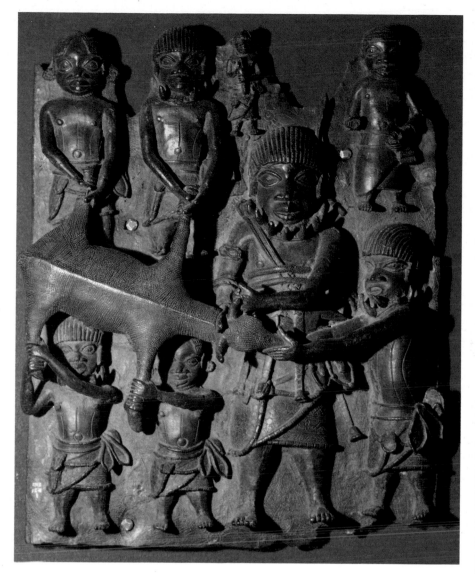

One myth says that God gave a choice to his three sons who were the fathers of the Kikuyu, Masai and Kamba peoples. He offered them a spear, a bow and a digging-stick. Masai chose the spear and was told to tend herds on the plains, Kamba chose the bow and was sent to the forest to hunt game, while Gikuyu selected the digging-stick and was taught the ways of agriculture. Another version says that God took Gikuyu to the top of the mountain and showed him the land with its valleys, rivers, forests, game, and all that God had made. Right in the middle of the country was a place where fig trees clustered and God told Gikuyu to make his home there.

When he got to the spot Gikuyu found that not only had God made a fine place, but he had also provided

Above. Bronze from Benin, Nigeria, depicting the sacrifice of a cow at the altar of the father of a family. Such offerings took place either where the father was buried or represented, often by a mask and ivory or wooden staffs. Museum of Mankind, London.

Right. Bronze head with carved elephant tusk from Benin city, Nigeria. Such bronze or brass heads were cast from about the fifteenth century and were made thicker and heavier when elephant tusks were inserted in them in honour of the dead chief or notable. An earthen altar was made over the grave, on which were placed wooden or bronze heads surmounted by elephant tusks carved with figures, especially of lizards and snakes. To this day such an altar may have several heads and tusks, with other carved figures. Museum of Mankind, London.

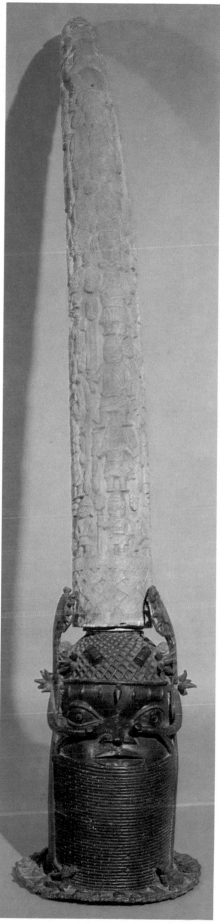

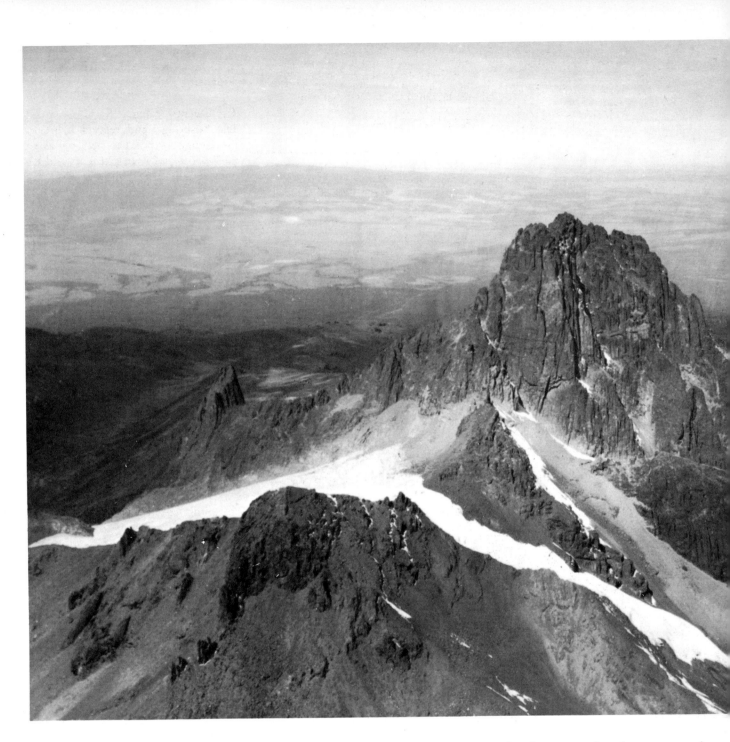

a wife for him. She was a beautiful woman, called Moombi, the Moulder or Creator, and she bore nine daughters to her husband.

Gikuyu was happy at this, but he could not help grieving that he had no sons. So he went to the mountain and called on God, asking his help. God told him not to worry but to follow his instructions. Gikuyu was to take a lamb and a kid, and sacrifice them under a large fig tree near his house. The fat and blood of the animals were to be poured on the

trunk of the tree, and the meat to be given to God by all the family as a burnt offering. Gikuyu did as God had directed and then took his wife and daughters home. When they got to the fig trees they found to their joy nine young men there. Gikuyu killed a ram and prepared millet for a great feast. They all ate, rejoiced, and then slept for the night. In the morning Gikuyu put the question of marriage to the young men. He offered them his daughters, but made the condition that if they accepted they must all live

in his home, under the system of matriarchal or female descent. The youths agreed willingly.

Then the Kikuyu all lived together in one group, which was named after the mother of them all, the family group of Moombi. When the parents died, the property was shared out equally among the daughters. Finally numbers became too great and the nine daughters each called her family together and made a clan bearing her own name. So were founded the chief Kikuyu clans, each still known by the

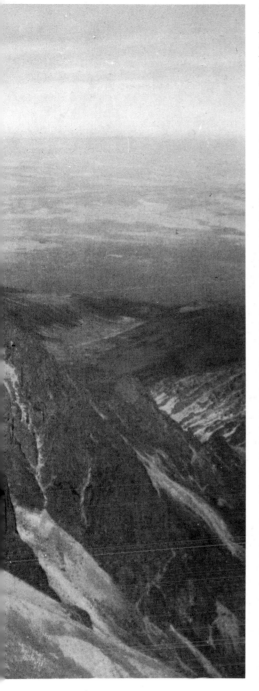

Mount Kenya, 17,000 feet (5200 metres) high, the Mountain of Brightness, which the Kikuyu say God chose as his earthly dwelling place. From here God showed the first man all the land that he had made, and told him to make his home in a cluster of fig trees in the centre.

name of one of the daughters, the whole being of the tribe of Moombi.

The women of Moombi's tribe practised polyandry, having several husbands each, a practice found in some other places, though it is more common for men to have several wives, a system called polygyny or generally polygamy. It seems that the men suffered under the women, they were afflicted with sexual jealousy and often guilty of infidelity, and they were punished and humiliated. So they planned to revolt, though it was

not easy, since the women were strong and good fighters. The men made a secret plot, which brought nature on their side, and was both ingenious and pleasurable. They all made love to the women and awaited results. After six months it was clear that nature had helped their plan and the women were in the family way. The men then broke out in open revolt and the women were too burdened to resist. So the men became heads of the community. They abolished polyandry, and instituted polygyny, taking several wives each. They also decided to change the names of the tribe and clan. The group of Moombi became the nation of Gikuyu, their first father. But when the men tried to alter the names of the female clans, the women in turn revolted. They threatened to kill all the male children that might be born to them, and to refuse to bear any more children after that. So the men had to yield, and the Kikuyu clans are still known by the names of the women who were the first founders of the clan system.

Time passed, families multiplied, and there was not enough room for everybody in the original Kikuyu settlement. Some of the people moved into the forest to get more land, but entry was barred for a time by Pygmies who lived there in caves under the ground. They were shy, and dug tunnels under the earth to avoid meeting people. The Kikuyu thought they were magicians who could open up the ground and disappear at will. In time they left the forest though stories are still told of little people underground. They were probably driven out by a race of hunters, Ndorobo, who traded animal skins and flesh and honey to the Kikuyu, in exchange for grain and fruit. When the Kikuyu wanted more land they bought it from the Ndorobo, so they not only

had the plains which God had given them but forest land which they had bought.

The Inventor King

The Bushongo and related tribes of the Congo tell of the beginnings of their people with an old man and his wife who had no children. One day the sky opened and a man of white colour came towards them. He asked where the other people were, and they replied that there were none and they were too old to have children. The visitor said he was the Lord, called Bomazi, and that a child would be born to them. The old folks laughed, but soon the woman gave birth to a girl, and when she was grown up the light-skinned Bomazi took her for wife. They had five sons, all of whom became chiefs of different peoples.

The first two children were twins, Woto and Moelo. When they grew up Woto had three wives, but coming back from the hunt one day he found his brother's son with his own wife and accused him of incest. The boy begged forgiveness but Woto found him sinning in turn with his other two wives. Woto was angry and went away into the forest, bewailing his loneliness. He was a magician and at his songs the forest trees opened and many little people came out of them. They exclaimed at the size of Woto; what big ears he had, what big eyes and nose. Nobody could subdue such a man, only women could enslave him. These were of course the Pygmies.

Woto wandered on and in time became father of all the Bushongo. But the stories are vague about his successors until the accession of the great King Shamba Bolongongo, said to be the ninety-third ruler, who lived about A.D. 1600. He is called Shamba of the Bonnet, and many inventions are credited to him. While still heir to the throne Shamba told his mother that he wanted to travel abroad to see other peoples. She warned him of the dangers, but Shamba replied that the king must be the wisest of men, and only by travelling could he learn about other people, admire what was good and learn to prevent what was

113

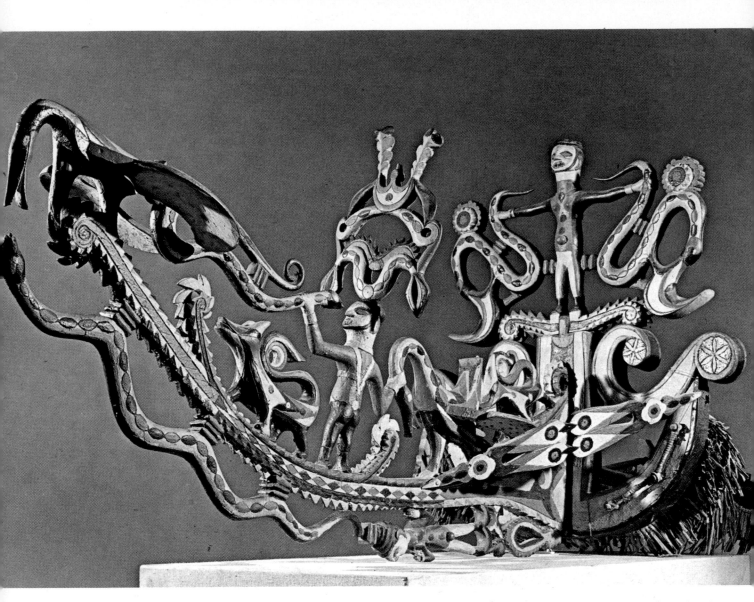

Above. The elaborate prow of a canoe from Douala, Cameroun. European figures and mythological motifs are combined in a design of remarkable vitality. Very striking is the encounter of the bird and the snake in the fore part. Staatliches Museum für Völkerkunde, Munich.

Opposite. Altar of the hand of an Oba, a ruler of Benin city, Nigeria. Different parts of the body – head, hands and feet – may be regarded as associated with spiritual powers. They need both physical and spiritual attention, being anointed with oil or blood. With the Oba are family and retainers, showing his complex social relations. Museum of Mankind, London.

evil. So he visited many countries, and came back after several years to introduce useful things that he had seen.

Shamba showed his people how to weave raffia fibre for clothing, in place of the rough bark cloth they had been using. He introduced the cassava plant, which the Portuguese had brought from America, and which needs long preparation to get rid of its poisons. He showed them embroidery and other crafts. Till then the Bushongo had been addicted to gambling, but Shamba showed them how to play the game of mankala, which came originally from the Arabs.

Shamba was a man of peace. He abolished bows and arrows for warfare, and particularly the terrible weapon called the *shongo*. This was

a throwing knife with four blades, which caused horrible wounds. Because of his peaceful ways Shamba and his people were respected and they were able to travel widely. If strange people attacked them, they had only to say that they were Bushongo and the thieves knelt to them as subjects of Shamba. But if it happened that a Bushongo was killed by brigands, then Shamba sounded the war-horn and his people swarmed out like locusts to find the criminals. Even then enemies were not killed unless they resisted, and women and children were spared. Shamba said that all people were children of God and had the right to live.

The Bushongo attribute almost all good things to Shamba. He introduced tobacco, and the oil palm tree bears the name Shamba. It is said that

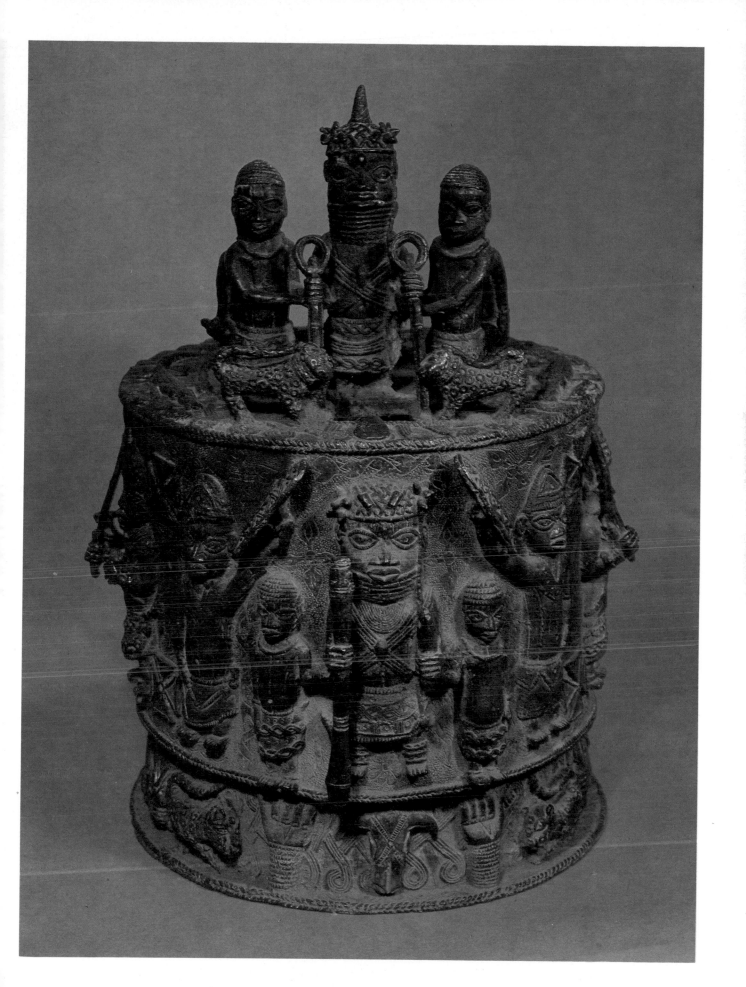

he compared palm wine to human nature, one of his many parables with a moral. When the first cut is made in a palm tree the wine is sweet but very weak, but as the flow increases it becomes stronger but harsh. That is like human life, youth is sweet but lacks wisdom, while old age is wise but lacks sweetness.

Many stories are told of Shamba's wisdom, and his judgements are remembered. If a guilty party did not appear in court he lost his case, because Shamba had said that a guilty man tries to avoid discussing matters. If a witness related hearsay and had not seen things himself, he was rebuked because Shamba had said that only he should speak who had seen with his own eyes. To bring peace to quarrelling wives Shamba told a story of a man who had two dogs, one black and the other red. Every day after his own meal he divided the rest into equal shares and gave them to the dogs. One day when a wild cow had been killed by the villagers the man was given a thigh bone for his share. He enjoyed the meat and gnawed away till only the bone was left. He tried to break it to get at the marrow, but it was too hard and he threw it to the dogs. Both dogs tried to grab the bone, and turned on each other in fury, fighting so hard that they died of wounds. Shamba said that each dog should have his own bone, and each woman her own husband, and then there would be peace at home.

A famous Bushongo wood carving shows King Shamba seated in front of a mankala board, his body decorated to show armlets and clothing, the hands roughly done, but all the attention is drawn to the face in its wisdom and peace.

Kintu and his Successors

The myth of Kintu has been told as the first man of Buganda, with a heavenly wife (page 44). When he was an old man Kintu went into the forest and disappeared. It was taboo for the chiefs to say that he had died, so they said he had vanished. They dug his grave secretly behind his house. The body was wrapped in cow hide and put in the grave without any earth on top, but thorns were placed over and around it as protection against wild beasts. The chief priest kept watch on the grave until he was able to remove Kintu's jawbone (a sacred bone, because it moved by itself), and this was put in a hill temple. The temple and its garden are sacred and animals may not be killed there; the ghosts of Kintu and his son act as guardians against wrong.

Kintu's son, who succeeded him, was also said to have been lost, this time on the plains. He was followed as king by his grandson, Kimera. Kimera's mother was the wife of a neighbouring king, who committed adultery with a visiting prince. Her lover died and she was saved from the king's anger by the help of a priest. This man said he had received a divine message to tell the king that if he heard of the misconduct of one of his wives he must not kill her, but banish her from the palace, and when her child was born throw it into a pit. This was done, but the child was saved from the clay pit by a potter, who could not bring up the child himself, but entrusted it to a nobleman whose wife cared for it. The child was Kimera, and when Buganda needed a new king they called for him and he was crowned. His mother came with him, but she stayed in a house outside the capital.

After some years Kimera sent an expedition, headed by his son, against a rich neighbour. The son died on the way, leaving a child called Tembo. When Tembo grew up his mother told him that his father had been killed by his grandfather, Kimera. She so worked on Tembo's feelings that he began to watch for an opportunity of killing his grandfather. One day the king was out hunting and got separated from his bodyguard. Tembo seized his chance, crept up behind the king and killed him with a club. He told the people that it was an accident, and that he had hit the king while aiming at an animal. The King's jawbone was enshrined on another hill, and Tembo succeeded him.

Some time later Tembo sent his son and daughter to be servants of one of the gods. But the young man became enamoured of his sister, they were united and she gave birth to twins. At the places where the children were conceived and born rivers sprang forth (see page 83). Later on Tembo became insane, but was cured by a

Opposite. In the ruins of the stone forts of Zimbabwe are numerous stone carvings, including a number of soapstone birds, similar to wooden figures found today among some Bantu people of South Africa. Lightning is thought to be like a giant bird. Museum of Mankind, London.

Below. A favourite African game, known by its Egyptian name of mankala. This fine board from Sierra Leone shows the twelve holes in each of which four nuts are placed. The two players sit on opposite sides and distribute the nuts all round the board in turn. If a turn ends at holes that already contain one or two nuts, the contents are taken by the player. He puts the nuts in the container at his end of the board, and the one who gains most nuts wins. Pitt Rivers Museum, Oxford.

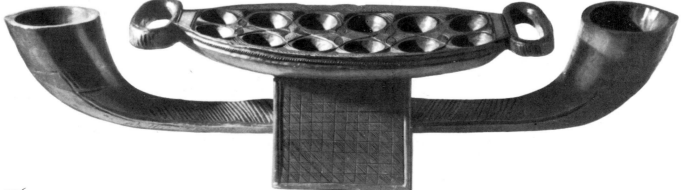

human sacrifice, and he wore anklets from the sinews of a man from the fish clan. His jawbone was preserved in another temple.

Some thirty kings of Buganda followed, but only a few legends can be mentioned here. The sixteenth king, Juko, so angered a priest that the latter commanded the sun to fall. Darkness covered the land, till one of the king's wives suggested that he should send for a god who lived on an island in Lake Victoria. The god came (or his priest and symbols), and restored the sun to its place. Then the king's brother took a wife against the advice of the priests, with the result that a child was born without arms or legs, which was said to be an incarnation of the god of plague. To appease the god a temple was built for him, but the king was told never to look at it. For years he obeyed, but then he forgot, and died after looking at the forbidden shrine.

The children of the eighteenth king died in infancy, and he was in despair. Then he was told by priests to restore a neglected temple, and after that his children survived. But the priests demanded enormous sums for their services, and the king was so angry that he ordered all the temples of the gods to be plundered and burnt down. Then he fled to the forest, but his people brought him back. It was found that he was possessed by the spirit of the greatest of the gods, Mukasa, and could give oracles. So the people built him a new palace where he lived and died.

It is said that the twenty-second king of Buganda was summoned with his queen by the ghost of the first king, Kintu. But just as they got to his temple another chief came up and Kintu's ghost fled. Later in his reign the king received a lying message that one of the old kings had risen from the dead and was coming to fight him. He sounded the war drums, and there was great confusion and slaughter among his people. A further revolt was encouraged by a priest who said that whoever stood on a magical charm would reach the throne, so the princes rebelled and killed the king.

The greatest monarch was Mutesa,

the thirtieth, both competent and ambitious. He built up a large army, with troops from every district, and introduced guns. His merchants brought back cottons, in exchange for ivory and slaves. Both Moslems and Christians entered the country during his reign, but modern times came and the slave trade was eventually destroyed.

The Zimbabwe Mystery

The mythology of the great stone buildings at Zimbabwe may appear more European than African, yet they are important both for that and for their place in the expression of African art. Seventeen miles south-east of Fort Victoria in Zimbabwe are three main groups of stone buildings that were made famous in Rider Haggard's *King Solomon's Mines*. Stone constructions are so rare in ancient tropical or southern Africa that writers have suggested they were built by Arabs, Jews, Indians, Chinese, in fact anybody but Africans. Similarly the naturalistic bronzes of Ifé used to be attributed to some castaway Portuguese, and it was not known then that comparable sculptures were made at Nok in Nigeria two thousand years ago. In fact over three hundred stone ruins have been found in Zimbabwe and neighbouring countries. All scholars are now agreed that the Zimbabwe ruins were the work of African builders, from the ninth century to the fifteenth. They were known to Portuguese travellers from 1513. That Indian and Chinese fragments have been found in the excavations simply shows that trade was going on through the Arabs whose boats plied between the coasts of Africa and Asia.

Zimbabwe lies in the country now occupied by the Shona people and they seem to have few stories linking them with the ruins. One of the Portuguese writers said that the people in his day ascribed these buildings to the Devil, but African mythology has no devil in the Christian sense. Later travellers were told that long ago white men put up the buildings but black men poisoned the water and they all died. These seem likely to

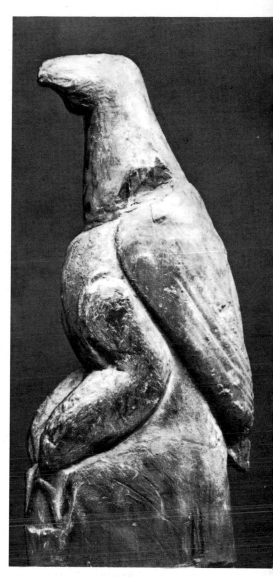

have been tales invented to please Europeans, and Africans are often reluctant to reveal their own traditional history. It may well be that the Zimbabwe buildings were made by other African tribes, or groups of tribes, who later moved further south, such as the Venda of Transvaal.

An empire led by Monomotapa in the sixteenth century included a number of tribes. According to Shona myths, fire was unknown to their ancestors until brought by the Rozwi, rulers of a large kingdom, perhaps the same domain as that of Monomotapa. They also brought grains and other seed. They lived in zimbas, or zimbabwe, a name which was applied to the residences or burial places of leading chiefs. There were many of these zimbabwes, which were occupied by Rozwi until recent times. But

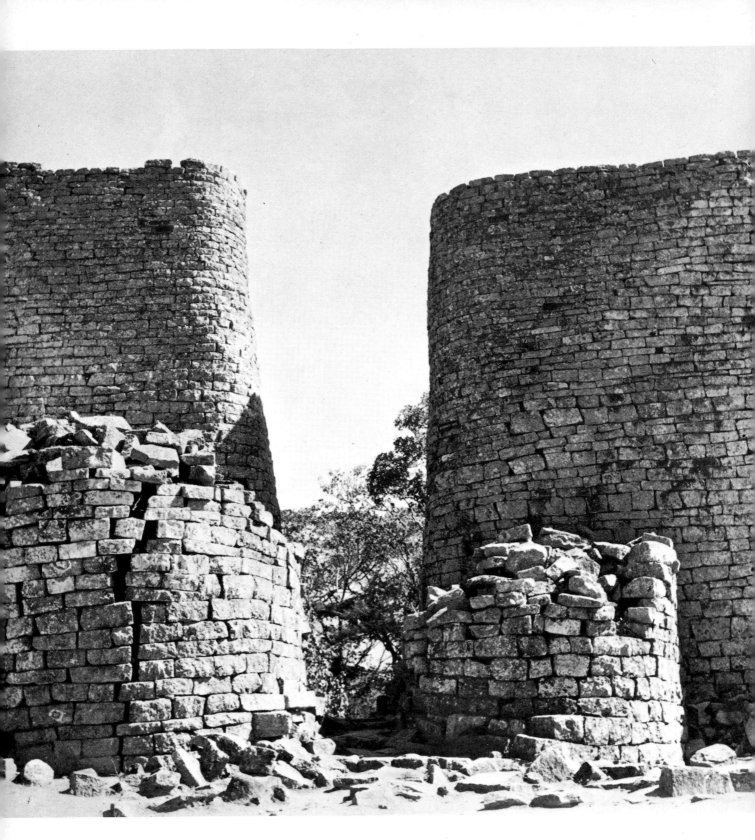

Above. Zimbabwe. Two of the massive conical towers flanking a gateway.

Opposite. King Shamba of the Bushongo people of the Congo, who lived about A.D. 1600. He is famed for the many inventions and new products that he brought to his people. He travelled widely, abolished cruel weapons, and was a man of peace. Shamba introduced tobacco, the oil palm and cassava, and taught weaving and embroidery. Here he sits calmly in front of the mankala board, a great African game with which he replaced gambling. Museum of Mankind, London.

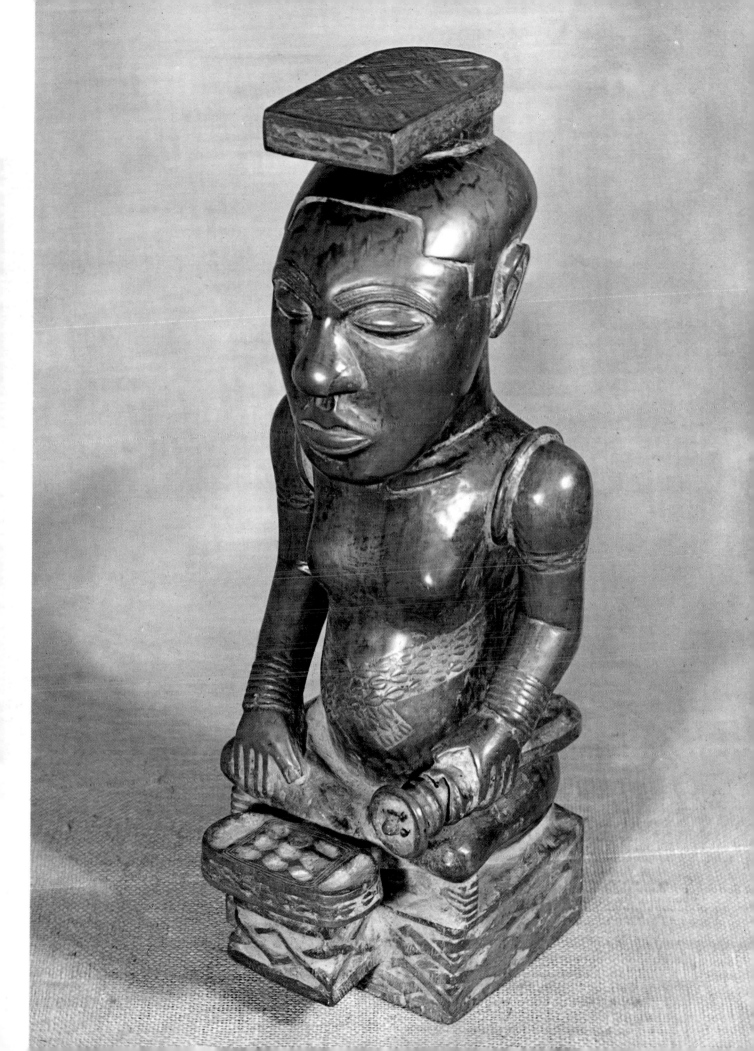

in the tribal and European wars of the nineteenth century the old kingdoms were broken up and many peoples left their ancient homes. Shaka the Zulu was extending his rule in South Africa, and the Matabele, though a powerful people, fled north and in turn went through the land of the Shona and the zimbabwes. The destruction of this culture was brought about by the twin effects of war and European occupation.

The nature of the ruins at Great Zimbabwe has been confused by romantic interpretations. There are three main groups: the largest is an elliptical 'temple' enclosing a conical tower, a fortified 'acropolis', and a mass of smaller stone enclosures called 'valley ruins'. There are stone carvings and a number of soapstone birds which are unusual, but wooden bird effigies on poles are to be found among a number of Bantu peoples today, the lightning being thought of as a giant bird. There are soapstone bowls, decorated with patterns of animals and geometrical designs, which resemble the wooden bowls used for divination by the Venda (see page 86). Perhaps some day a fuller African mythology will be recorded of Zimbabwe, or it may be lost for ever, leaving only the artistic works as evidence of the thought of vanished African peoples.

Rain Queen
The Lovedu are a Bantu tribe of the Transvaal, not numerous, but notable for their Rain Queen, Mujaji. The character of this queen, and the nature of the country where she ruled, suggested a theme and provided a location for Rider Haggard which he realised in the famous romance called *She*. Haggard suggested she must be of Arab stock but he knew little of the history.

The Lovedu have few cosmological myths. A rare story speaks of Khuzwane, who created the world and man, and left his footprints on rocks in the north while they were still soft. Another deity, sometimes identified with the first, is blamed for troubles such as sterility, and is a kind of destiny. But the chief object of rituals is the well-being of the family and the honouring of tribal ancestors.

About A.D. 1600, somewhere in the far north, the sons of a great king quarrelled and set up independent realms. One of them, Mambo, ruled in the area which is now called Zimbabwe. Mambo's daughter bore a son, though she was unmarried. She refused to disclose her lover's name, saying that the father of a prince should not be known. Tradition says he was her brother. When Mambo threatened his daughter she stole the rain charm and the sacred beads and fled south with her son, where they founded the Lovedu tribe. The son's child was named Muhale and he became a great king. He invited relatives from the north to join him and help in clearing the forests, and in teaching the original inhabitants the use of fire. Many of these inhabitants actually perished in a great conflagration, possibly because they did not know how to control the new element. But the Lovedu were safe; they had in the meantime discovered the 'place of the gods', and had prayed there, taking great care to appease the ancestors of the place.

The next king but one ruled in the mountains from a throne cut in the rock and surrounded by great walls, like those of Zimbabwe. He had a son, Mugodo, whom he treated like an outcast in public to deceive the people, but at night and in secret he taught him the secrets of the rain charms. However this disrespect brought division when Mugodo succeeded to the throne and his reign ended in confusion, terminating the rule of kings and inaugurating that of queens. Mugodo went to his favourite daughter and told her of a plan to save the kingdom, but she refused to believe that a sin could turn to good. Then he went to another daughter, Mujaji, and said that though unmarried she could give birth to the heir to the throne. She understood that Mugodo was to be the father and accepted his will. A daughter was born who became Mujaji II. Mujaji I had already gained ascendancy during her father's reign, but she lived in seclusion and hence men believed in her wisdom and immortality. She was called 'white-faced', 'radiant as the sun', 'one who gives water to wash the face'. Emissaries of other powers, the Sotho to the north and the Zulu to the south, came bringing gifts to the queen of the rainmakers.

Mujaji II was not so successful and her land was invaded by Zulus and Europeans. She tried to smite the Zulus with drought, and to deceive the Europeans by hiding herself and presenting a distant sister as 'She Who Must Be Obeyed'. But the sacred places were desecrated and in despair Mujaji II took poison and died. When Mujaji III came to the throne the Europeans discovered the previous deception and refused to recognise her till the other She had died. But conflict remained between the authority of the new conquerors and that of the Lovedu ancestors. However the Lovedu were one of the most peaceful in submission to the rule of the white people.

The Lovedu queen, now Mujaji IV, is more a rainmaker than a monarch, who gives rain to her own people and denies it to her enemies. She is 'Transformer of Clouds', who guarantees the cycle of the seasons, not only bringing rain in drought, but giving general care throughout the year. Her emotions, anger or satisfaction, are believed to affect her powers and help or hinder their working. People do not call on the queen every time rain fails, but in time of drought her advisers say that 'the people are crying'. They bring gifts and there are long dances. The queen does not work alone, but has a rain-doctor who tries to find the cause of drought by divination, and by his medicines tries to remove the forces which prevent the queen's powers from working. What objects and medicines she possesses are kept secret, for they are inherited and passed on to her successor just before the queen's death. There are also medicines which are burnt and produce black smoke to induce clouds to rise in the sky, just as in the Old Testament story Elijah caused fire and smoke to appear on Mount Carmel and shortly afterwards rain came.

The rain queen herself can only control rain by agreement with her ancestors, whose skins are said to be the most important ingredients of her rain-pots. If rains do not fall it is said to be because the ancestors are angry at neglect. People still believe in the power of the queen to bring rain and her health is vital to the maintenance of good seasons. God gives the queen her powers, which have been shown in the appearance of needed storms.

Swazi Kings

The Swazi people live to the northeast of South Africa. Names of their rulers go back thirty generations, though only the last eight can be clearly dated. There are many stories of early kings. One had two sons, Madlisa and Madlebe. The latter was son of a junior queen and was an unusual child; he was said to have been born wearing a magical bracelet, and, when he wept, tears of blood came and the bracelet cried in sympathy, 'Tsi, tsi!' One day the king called all his people and said that the son who could spit farthest he would make Little Chief. He hit them in turn with a hippo whip to make them spit far, but Madlisa's spittle only dribbled down his chest. Then the king hit Madlebe with his whip and his spittle went far away. There was a roar from the sky, Madlebe cried tears of blood, and the bracelet echoed 'Tsi, tsi!'

The king gave Madlebe a pot, a gourd and a spoon, and told him to place the pot on a high shelf for it must never be broken. One day Madlisa was hungry and tempted Madlebe to reach for the pot. At first he refused, but when he agreed and reached up the pot fell to the ground. The king was angry and sent his soldiers to execute Madlebe, who had fled to the forest. But when they lifted their hands to strike him the thunder roared and a lightning flash hit the earth. The warriors were afraid, and instead of killing him sent Madlebe away into another land. People thought he was dead and his mother mourned him.

When the king died Madlebe came back to his mother's house. There he saw a beautiful girl and they made love. In her ecstasy she wept blood, and Madlebe said 'Do you weep blood too?' Then the girl told her mother and the mother recognised Madlebe. The warriors recognised him too and were afraid, but the royal councillors made him king.

In more historical times the leader of one of the Bantu groups travelling down Africa was Dlamini, who founded the royal clan of the Swazi people and led them to the coast. They settled in what was later Mozambique, living peacefully with their neighbours and sometimes marrying with them. Their history is obscure until the reign of King Ngwane II, who is celebrated in the royal rituals of the Swazi, the first king to be so honoured. He decided to leave the coastlands and led his people into the forest-covered hills, chasing away the Lumombo tribes, as recalled in a praise song, 'O king, you scourged the Lumombo in your flight'. He brought his people south of what is now Swaziland and was buried in a hill covered with trees, where later kings also lie. The Swazi still call themselves 'The People of Ngwane'.

Ngwane's son and grandson were warlike rulers, and the latter came into conflict with the great Zulu king Shaka. Shaka's story belongs to history rather than mythology though it is one of the greatest of African endeavour. An unwanted child of an illegal union, he was born in 1787, and to overcome his shame he went through great ordeals. He built a huge army and in fifteen years conquered an area larger than Europe. He was notorious for his harsh and even cruel judgements, though these have been exaggerated, and he himself thought European punishments were inhuman. At the height of his career, when he was opening his empire to European ideas, Shaka was killed in 1828 by jealous brothers and in a few years his work was undone and his empire destroyed.

The Swazi tried to seal pacts with the Zulu by marriages. Shaka was received with lavish hospitality and took two Swazi women as wives, but when they were pregnant he had them

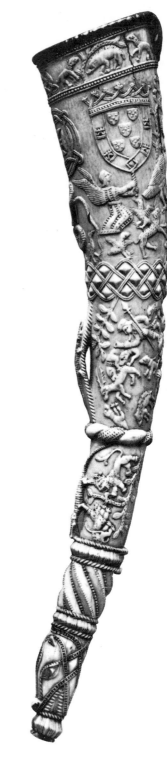

One of the beautiful ivory carvings which resulted from the meeting of African and European cultures in the sixteenth century. The African feeling is powerful and snakes and crocodiles can be seen. But the ivory also carries the arms of the Portuguese royal house, religious motifs, and a palpably European hunting scene. Museum of Mankind, London.

killed for fear of rivals. When the Zulu armies (*impis*) came raiding, the Swazi did not engage in pitched battles, and only fought them on the open plains after their power had been broken by the Boers in 1836. Finally the Swazi requested the protection of the Queen of England. The present king, Sobhuza II, rules over the most prosperous of the late protectorates.

Every year there is a great national ceremony, the Incwala, which celebrates the history and royalty of the Swazi people. The chief actor is the king, without whom there would be no Incwala; it is not held during a regency. The ritual is controlled by priests called 'people of the sea', because they fetch water from the sea and river to give the king strength. The time of the Incwala depends on the position of the sun and moon; old councillors study the sky and give the signal when the signs are right. It is in the December solstice, when the sun rests in its hut before leaping out on its northward journey; and this is correlated with the moon, thought of as a woman following her lord, the sun. A black ox is killed for the doctoring of the king, who spits to east and west to break the old year and prepare the new. There is a great deal of ritual, described in authoritative books on the Swazi. The Incwala aims at strengthening the king, and through him the people: a play of kingship which unites them against past foes and present decay.

As Others See Us

For nearly five hundred years Europeans have been trading with Africa, exploring it, and finally ruling over much of it for a time. These fair-skinned people with their strange ways have entered into African story. An amusing Yoruba tale says that when the Europeans arrived they were always the first at the market, and would sit there all day long till everybody else had gone home. The local people wondered why this was and planned to find out. They got up in the night and went to the market-place, and where the Europeans had been sitting were little holes. They

filled these with black warrior ants and hid behind trees to watch. At dawn the Europeans arrived, sat down, then jumped up and ran off with wild cries. The Africans laughed to see that the traders had tails.

More seriously, in Kenya, it is said that a great doctor used to predict future events. One night he had a dream from which he awoke trembling and bruised all over. His family called the elders to find out the trouble. They made a sacrifice and gradually the doctor recovered his voice and told his dream. God had taken him to a distant land where he had seen strangers coming out of great waters, in colour like yellow frogs and with wings like butterflies. They carried sticks sending out fire by magic. They brought a great iron snake, like a centipede, which spat fire, and stretched from the sea to the great lake. The doctor warned his people not to fight the strangers for that would bring disaster.

The elders and warriors were angry and said they would destroy the iron snake, but the doctor said they would not be able to do this, for it would repel their spears and arrows and destroy them in turn. The best thing to do would be to meet the strangers with courtesy but not to trust them, and especially not to bring them close to their homes and lands. But when Europeans did arrive, yellow and dressed in clothes like butterflies' wings, the Kikuyu did not know what to make of them. In time they forgot the advice of their prophet not to let the strangers come near their property. But they noticed that the yellow strangers were restless; they passed

through the country, came and went, and never seemed to stay long in one place. So the Kikuyu recited a proverb which said that no mortal thing lived for ever, and no doubt the foreigners would return to their own land.

King Mugodo of the Lovedu (see page 120), before his reign ended in confusion, had the war horns sounded and danced a great solitary dance before his prostrate people. He prophesied the coming of black ants who would bite the people but would be overcome, and red ants who would fight and conquer the Lovedu. The black ants were the neighbouring warlike tribes and the red ants the Europeans. These came in the reign of his successors, the Lovedu queens. The black ants, the Zulus, were put off by the power of the queen in sending drought, and deception was tried on the red ants by presenting them with the wrong queen. This imposter was called 'Chief of the Reds' by the Lovedu themselves, and the Europeans refused to recognise the rightful queen until the imposter died. The Lovedu helped her to her end.

King Sobhuza of the Swazi is also said to have had a dream which foretold the coming of the invaders from Europe. They were strange people, the colour of red porridge, with hair like the tails of cattle. They had houses built on platforms and pulled by oxen. They spoke barbarous languages and were utterly ignorant of human courtesies. They carried terrible weapons of destruction. The king's dream was interpreted as a warning sent by his ancestors that he must never fight these foreigners, because of their great strength in battle.

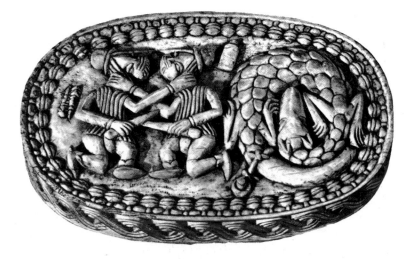

So it was that the Swazi looked upon Europeans as useful allies, and that eventually they requested the protection of England against other powers that threatened them.

The prudence of the African rulers appears in all these stories. Europeans were strange people, of abnormal colour, hair, dress, manners and needs. They were particularly to be treated with caution because of their superior weapons. There was a good deal of politic evasion, which was made easier by the real ignorance of the Europeans of the customs of the country.

Europeans tried to deal with the person they thought was king or queen. But it was remarked in Ghana that they took no notice of the old queen mother who crouched behind the king's throne and whispered to him not to have any dealings with the strangers. Even those who fought them, like Shaka, were willing to learn from European ways. Kindness and hospitality, too, are as much a part of the ordinary African people as the mythology suggests, and travellers like Livingstone journeyed practically unarmed across the whole continent. There is also the story of Mungo Park, who identified the Upper Niger. When he was alone and starving in the western Sudan, it was a simple old woman who had pity on the stranger, took him in, and fed him like a child.

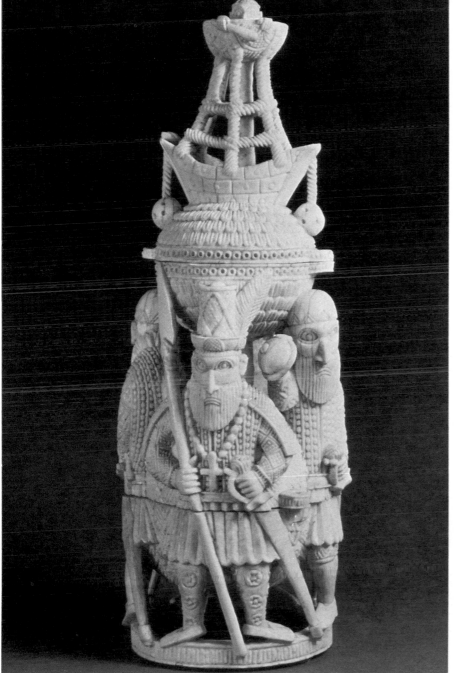

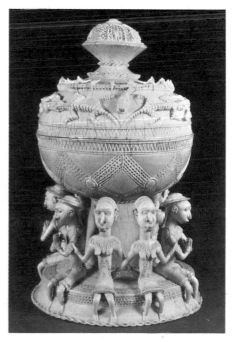

Left. Ivory salt-cellar from Benin, Nigeria. As one of the countries of western Africa earliest and most easily accessible to Europeans, the production of Afro-Portuguese objects here was understandable. This group shows a foreign soldier with a cross, sword and spear in the foreground, revealing the impression made by Europeans. The whole is surmounted by the kind of boat on which they sailed along the west African coast, but it was often thought that these strange creatures came out of the sea, being unlike other people. Museum of Mankind, London.

Opposite. Europeans went to Africa from the end of the fifteenth century onwards and did not always agree among themselves. This ivory box from Benin, Nigeria, shows two Portuguese fighting, possibly over possession of the crocodile seen on the ground beside them. The University Museum, Philadelphia, Pennsylvania.

Below. Ivory salt-cellar from Sherbro, Sierra Leone. The dominance of the African carving tradition is seen in the figures, and the bowl, while made for salt, could equally well have been used for divination nuts or ancestral relics. Museum of Mankind, London.

Animal Fables

Some of the most popular of all African stories are the animal fables, and these are innumerable. They show that humans are in close touch with nature, but the animals are pictured with human feelings. Some fables are pure fantasy, others are projections of human desire. There are many 'Just So' stories, of the kind that Kipling made popular with additions and a literary form of his own. African fables of this kind are explanatory: why the cock has fine feathers, why the ram paws the ground when it thunders, how the goat became a domestic animal, why bats hang downwards and only fly at night, why the crocodile does not die in water, why the mosquito lives in the forest, why frogs swell up and croak, why the lizard bobs its head up and down, why the chameleon's head is square, why the snake sheds its skin, why elephants live in the forest, why the sparrow flies into smoke, how the spider became bald, how the elephant's bottom became small and how the parrot's tail became red.

How the Leopard got its Spots
This is a characteristic story from Sierra Leone and says that at first the Leopard was friendly with the Fire. Every day the Leopard went to see the Fire, but the Fire never visited him in return. This went on so long that the Leopard's wife mocked her husband, saying it was a poor sort of friend who would never return a visit. When he went out next day she quarrelled with him and said it must be because his house was unworthy that his friend would never come to it. So the Leopard begged the Fire to come to his house on the next day.

At first the Fire tried to excuse himself, saying he never visited. But the

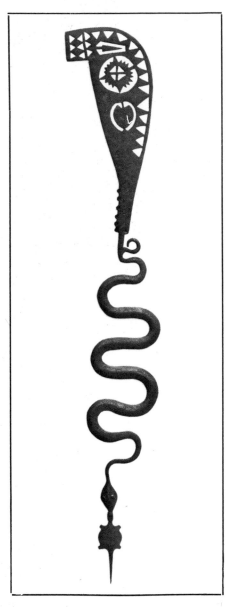

Above. Symbolical swords are used in state and religious rituals, and this finely decorated one from Ashanti, Ghana, has abstract patterns as well as a snake and tortoise. The sword is carried in front of a chief, and a man swearing loyalty is handed the sword, which he points to heaven and earth as his witnesses. Museum of Mankind, London.

Opposite. Bronze leopard from Benin, Nigeria. Staatliches Museum für Völkerkunde, Munich.

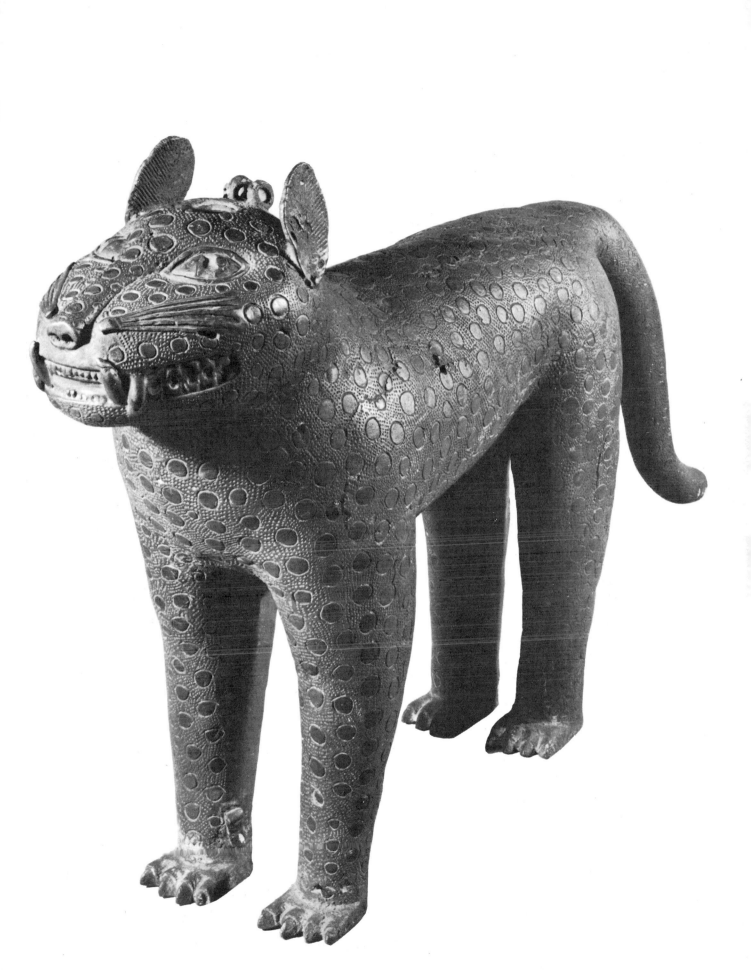

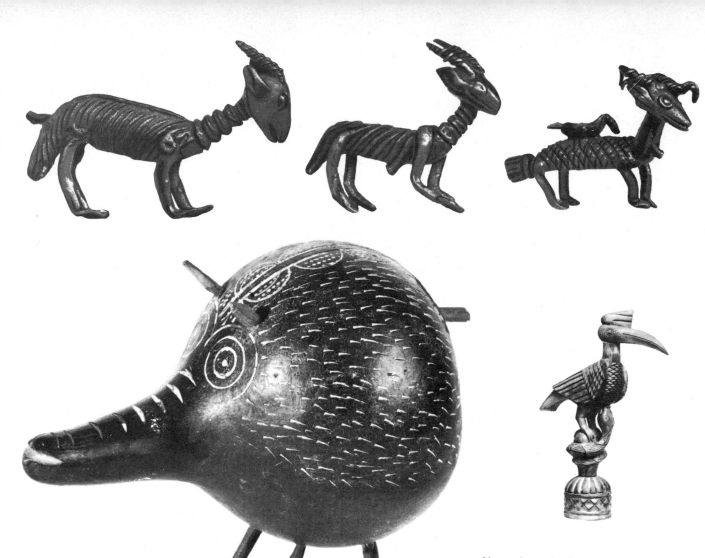

Leopard pressed him, and the Fire said he never walked but if there was a road of dry leaves from his house to the Leopard's then he would come. The Leopard went home and told his wife what to do. She gathered leaves and laid them in a long line from one house to the other. She and her husband prepared their house ready to do honour to the Fire. While they were waiting they heard a strong wind and loud cracks outside the door. The Leopard went to see what was the matter and it was the Fire at the door. His fingers of flame touched the Leopard, but he and his wife leapt backwards and jumped out of the window. Their house was destroyed, and ever since then the Leopard and his wife have been marked all over their bodies with black spots as a clear reminder of where the fingers of Fire touched them.

How the Goat was Domesticated

A Yoruba story from Nigeria says that the animals used to drink from a common pool, and once a year they all went to clean it out. Anyone who did not join in this work was to be killed. But one year the Goat did not go to the cleaning, for she had a baby kid and did not want to leave it. The other animals sent messengers to ask why the Goat was absent, and she prepared her excuses. When the Stag came to demand her reason the Goat said she had a kid. And the Stag then demanded if it was male or female. The Goat knew that the Stag's mother had died recently, so she said it was female. Then the Stag asked whose mother had been born again in the kid and the Goat replied that it was his own. The Stag could not harm the mother of his own reincarnated parent, so he went away.

Above. An umbrella top in carved wood from Ashanti, Ghana, which illustrates the proverb: 'The snake lies on the ground, but God has given him the hornbill bird.' Museum of Mankind, London.

Above left. Calabash toy from Madagascar, decorated to represent a porcupine. The calabash is a gourd which grows above the ground like a marrow and can be forced into different shapes. When ripe, the pulp inside is scooped out, and often dry seeds are put in to make a rattle used in music. Musée de l'Homme, Paris.

Top. Animal figures from Ashanti, Ghana, used in weighing gold, are in many different forms: human, animal, fish, bird, insect or abstract. Many are 'proverb' weights which illustrate situations in life. An animal with long horns may be called 'Had I known that, but it has passed behind me.' In other words, just as the animal's horns are behind it, so regrets are vain when a thing is past. Museum of Mankind, London.

Opposite. Ivory leopards with copper spots from Benin city, Nigeria. The apparently mild-looking leopards show their popularity in fable and as royal symbols, but their cunning and ferocity are dangerous to hunters. Museum of Mankind, London.

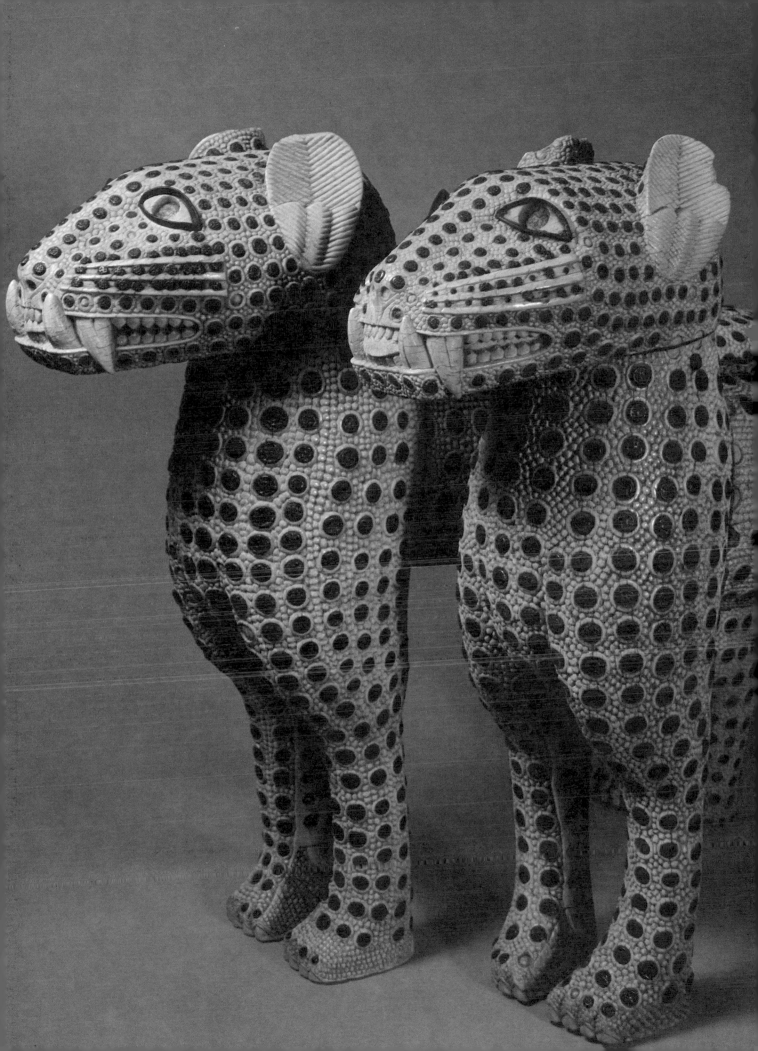

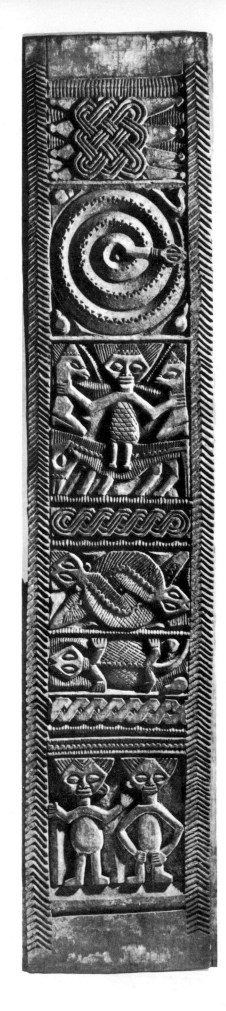

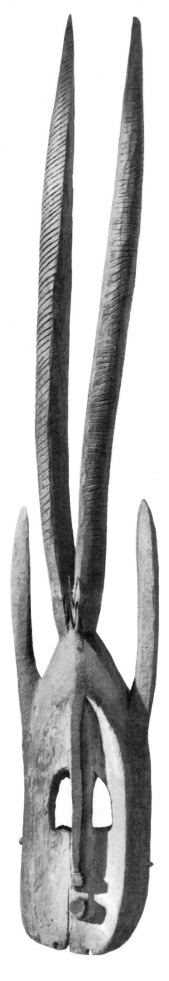

Then the Antelope came along and asked why the Goat had been absent and was told that she had a male kid. When he demanded whose father had been reborn, he was told that it was his own, so he too went away. All the animals came in turn, and the Goat told each one that it was some dead relative of theirs reborn. But the Leopard was suspicious, and he hid while the Goat answered two other animals. To one he said he had a male kid and to the other a female. So when he came to the Goat's house and asked whose parent had been re-born, the Goat said it was his mother, because she knew the mother had died not long before. But the Leopard said it could be his father, who was also dead, and he respected him more. When the Goat tried to change her story, the Leopard sprang at her with a roar. The Goat leapt sideways out of her house and ran with all speed to the village. Only there did the Leopard turn back, and the Goat has been quite content to live with human beings ever since, but the Leopard kills goats whenever it finds them straying outside a village.

Why the Tortoise is Taboo

A Malagasy fable says that one day a green Bird was hopping about in the bushes, looking for insects, when it saw a huge Sea Tortoise with a scaly shell come out of the water. The Tortoise told the Bird that it had always lived in the sea but would like to know the earth and its people. The Bird said that it was easily done and he would act as guide. So they set off for the interior. The Tortoise found it hard to walk, because of its flat feet, and began to complain. But the Bird had no trouble, jumping from tree to tree and resting in the shade. It laughed at the Tortoise at first, but then took pity on it. The Bird said it was a magician and would make better feet for the Tortoise. This was done and they went on with their journey. A little later the Bird dropped some dirt on the Tortoise, by accident, and the Tortoise called it filthy. The Bird got angry and flew off leaving the Tortoise to find its way back by itself. That is how the Sea Tortoise became a Land Tortoise. Ever since then the Land Tortoise and its children have wandered about, without finding the sea. So its flesh is taboo, for God made it for salt water, and humans can only eat animals that live on land.

Tales of Spider and Hare

All across Africa fables are told of the cleverness, deceit and triumph of the Spider or the Hare, called by various names according to the language. These yarns were taken to America by the slaves and became the Brer Rabbit tales related by Uncle Remus. There are no rabbits in tropical Africa, and the clever animal is really a hare, which depends on its speed and cunning to protect itself against the dangers of the open Sudan and savannah country. Its chief enemy is the Hyena, the Brer Fox of the American versions.

In the forest regions it is the Spider, the Annancy of America, which plays the role of the clever animal. In these stories the weak but guileful creature overcomes the powerful but stupid larger beasts. Perhaps he is the ordinary man, oppressed by harsh rulers or foreign conquerors, who projects himself into the parts of the agile Hare or Spider, taking revenge on the great ones of the earth. To score off the police or the government is a great delight, and always arouses laughter from the listeners to these village tales as they sit around in the moonlight. But they have their sad side too, and the Hare who is caught in deception, or going beyond his powers, is severely punished by authority. Since he is often a thief or a practical joker, laughing at the morality of sober people, he suffers for his folly when caught.

Rubber Girl

This is a well-known Hare or Spider tale, the Tar baby of the Brer Rabbit stories. The Hausa of Nigeria tell it about the Spider. One day the Spider told his wife to measure out some ground-nuts and he would plant them in his field. When they were ready he took his hoe, but arriving at the field he sat down by a shady stream, for it was hot and he was a lazy animal who preferred somebody else to work. He had a drink, began nibbling the nuts, finally ate them all, and fell asleep. When he awoke evening had come. He got some mud from the stream, plastered it all over his body, went home, and told his wife that he had come in dirty from work and wanted some water for a bath. The same thing happened on the following days, till the time for gathering the ground-nuts was at hand. Then the Spider's wife said that the neighbours were digging up their nuts and she would go and get their own. But her husband answered that as he had planted the nuts it was his right to dig them up. He went off and stole nuts from his neighbour's field; he took so many that the neighbour kept watch and saw him.

Then he laid a trap for the Spider, in the form of a Rubber Girl made out of the sticky resin from the rubber tree. When the Spider came along he saw the Rubber Girl, with a beautiful long neck and large breasts. He came up to her, put out a hand and touched her breast, and his hand was held fast by the sticky rubber. 'Oh, you must want me badly,' he said, and put his other hand on her other breast. That hand stuck tight, and he exclaimed, 'You girls hold a man too tight. I will kick you.' He did this and the rubber caught his foot. Then he was angry and called the Rubber Girl an illegitimate child of low parents, and kicked her with the other foot. That stuck too and he was clasped tight to her body. He tried butting with his head and that stuck also to the Rubber Girl. Then the neighbour, who was watching from a hiding place, saw the Spider securely held and gave thanks to God. He cut a pliable switch from a tree, warmed it in a fire, rubbed it with grease, and beat and beat the Spider till his back was raw. Then he released the Spider and told him that if he came stealing again he would kill him. So the Spider suffered for his laziness and thieving.

In a Sierra Leone version the Spider wanted to eat rice but also to save himself the toil of working, so he pretended to die, having first made his wife promise to bury him on his farm. Then the rice from his neighbour's field started disappearing, for the Spider came out of his grave at night after the others had gone home, and

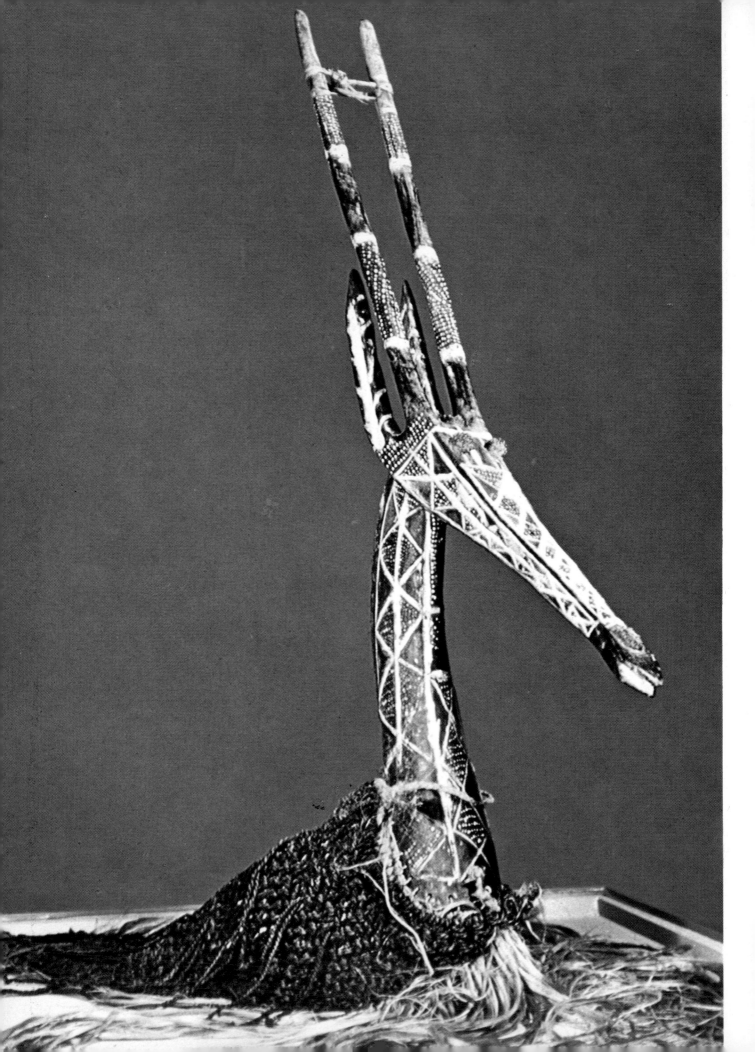

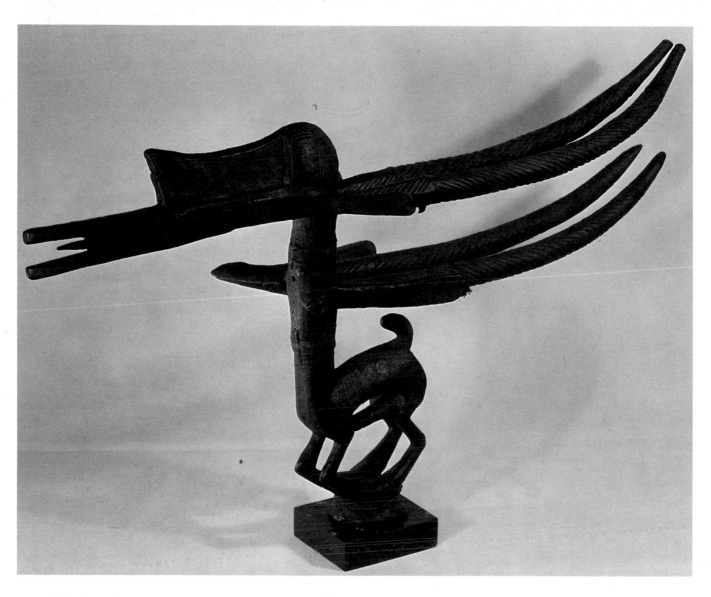

ate all he found. His wife asked the advice of a diviner, who told her to make a girl of wax from a tree that had sticky gum. The Spider was caught as before. Then all the people came up and beat him till the Spider's body became flat as it is today; formerly it was round and sleek.

In a Yoruba version of Nigeria the Hare figures in a tale of a great drought. All the animals decided that they would cut off the tips of their ears, and the fat from them would be used to buy hoes so that they could dig a well. Everyone did this except the Hare, who hid away. The other animals dug their well, and when it was finished the Hare came along beating a calabash, and making such a noise that the animals ran away without waiting to see who it was. Then the Hare drank his fill of water

from the well, and not content with that he washed himself in the water and made it dirty. When he had gone the animals saw that they had been tricked, and they made an image of a girl and covered it with bird lime. The Hare was caught in the usual way and well beaten. Then he was driven away and has lived in the grasslands ever since, and that is the reason why he has ears so much longer than those of any other animal.

In a version from Angola the owner of the farm was a Leopard, who made a wooden image of a girl and smeared it with gum from a wild fig tree. He caught both the Hare and the Monkey, and gave them a thorough beating. Since then they have always slept in secret places to keep away from the Leopard: the Hare sleeping in a hole and the Monkey in a tree.

Above. Complex antelope head on a mask from the Ivory Coast. As creatures of grace and speed, much sought after by hunters, antelopes are one of the most popular symbols in African art and mythology. They suggest the power and elusiveness of the spirits. Musée National des Arts Africains et Océaniens, Paris.

Opposite. Graceful antelope-like headdress, with seeds inlaid against the blue paint, made by the Kurumba of Upper Volta. It is used in a ceremony of dispersing ancestral spirits after a time of mourning. Museum für Völkerkunde, Vienna.

In southern African stories the Hare is caught by the Tortoise, who hid in the bottom of a well and smeared his shell with bird-lime. The Hare came to bathe his feet and was caught fast, and then his hands and face were caught too. All the other animals came up and beat him for deceiving them and stealing their goods.

Tug of War

One of the most popular of the Hare stories tells how by his cunning he deceived larger but more stupid animals. It is sometimes told about the Tortoise, and in America it is Brer Tarrypin who challenges the Bear, and since he can find no animal of equal size, he ties the other end of the rope to a tree.

In a West African version the Hare was improvident and always borrowed from his neighbours. He had taken so much from the Elephant and the Hippopotamus (the Crocodile in some versions) that both got very angry. But the Hare managed to calm them down by promising to give them all and more than he owed, with interest. He went away and made himself a rope of liana from the forest trees, then taking one end to the Elephant the Hare told him that he had only to pull it and he would find a great treasure chest on the end. Quickly he took the other end to the Hippo in the river and told him the same. The two animals took the strain, the Hare running backwards and forwards to cheer them on. As the Hippo was in the river and the Elephant in the trees, and both are short-sighted, this went on for a long time. But finally the Elephant got thirsty and went to the river for a drink, and the Hippo came out of the water, and they recognised each other, while the Hare ran off in safety.

In other versions it is a plain trial of strength, to which the Hare challenged the Rhinoceros and the Hippopotamus in turn. They ridiculed the idea that he was stronger than they were, but they pulled against each other from opposite sides of a bush-covered island until the rope broke,

or the Hare cut it in the middle, and both competitors fell over and Hare claimed his forfeit. In an Ila version in Zambia the Rhino and the Hippo had been enemies before, but now they became reconciled, and so the Rhino goes to the river to drink and the Hippo comes out to eat the grass where the Rhino feeds.

An additional narrative from Togo says that the Elephant and the Hippo were so angry at their deception that they vowed to prevent the Hare from eating any grass on land or drinking water from the river. The Hare was in a fix, and while he was thinking over his problem he met a Deer and asked for the loan of the horns from his head. Putting the horns on his own head the Hare went to see the Elephant. The Elephant asked if the Hare was ill, since horns had grown out of his head. The Hare started spitting all over the place and said the sickness came from his mouth. The elephant was frightened and ran away, and the Hare ate as much grass as he liked. Then he went to the Hippo and told him the same story, with the same result, and had plenty of water to drink.

Strength and Cunning

One day the Hare went hunting with the Hyena (Brer Fox), and they agreed to share all their catch. But whenever the Hare killed a beast the Hyena took it and put it in his own bag. As the Hare was so much smaller and weaker he was in no position to complain. He was particularly annoyed when the Hyena caught a fine red deer and kept it to himself. So the Hyena had a great bag of fine game and the Hare had nothing. They set off home, but having no bundle the Hare went on ahead.

Just outside their village he found some red earth and plastered his body with it, and got some white earth and put spots all over himself. Then he climbed on top of an ant-hill and waited for the Hyena to pass by. When the Hyena came along he saw this strange thing and was afraid to pass. He called out, 'O Something-on-the-hill, shall I give you some meat that I have caught?' The Hare just

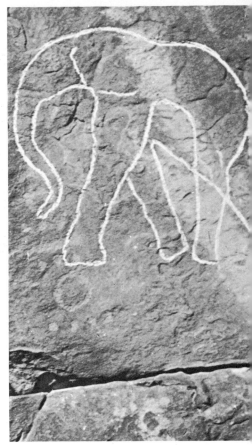

growled, 'Mm, Mm,' and the Hyena drew out a large piece of meat and laid it in front of him. But the Hare did not move away, and the Hyena called out again, and gave him another piece of meat. He kept on doing this till nearly all the meat was gone. Then the Hyena called out, 'O Something-on-the-hill, I have given you all my meat. Can I pass on?' But the Hare growled, 'You still have some meat left.' So the Hyena drew out the red deer, laid it down, and ran off. The Hare had all the good meat, and it had been carried to his door as well.

King of Beasts

In a Hausa story of Nigeria, similar to others told in many parts of the world, the small animal defeated the King of Beasts, the Lion. In the American Uncle Remus Stories the Hare defeated the Wolf. The Hausa say that the animals were all being eaten by the Lion and they took counsel to see what could be done to save themselves from extinction. They went to the Lion and asked if he would be

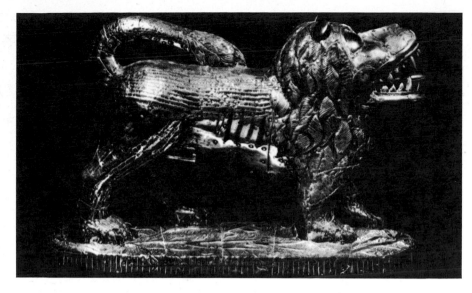

content to eat one of them every day and leave the rest alive. As the Lion is proud but lazy he accepted the offer, and the animals drew lots each day to decide who should be the victim. First the Gazelle was chosen, and they seized her and took her to the Lion, who ate her with pleasure but did not touch the other animals. Then the Roan Antelope was drawn and taken to execution, and the same went on every day among all the animals.

Finally the lot fell on the Hare, and when the others were going to carry him off he persuaded them that he was going calmly to his fate and did not need to be dragged there. So he marched off but went to his hole and fell asleep till midday. Then the Lion felt hungry and got up in anger and went roaring through the forest looking for the chosen animal. The Hare had meanwhile climbed up a tree overlooking a well, and as the Lion drew near he shouted to him to stop.

'Why are you making all that noise?' he asked. The Lion replied that he had waited all morning and his servants had not brought the promised food. Then the Hare from the top of the tree said, 'Well, I was chosen for you by lot, and I was coming along with a present of honey as well, when another Lion met me and took the honey out of my hand.' 'Where is this other Lion?' roared the Lion angrily. The Hare said, 'He is in the well, but he is not afraid of you, for he says he is much stronger than

you.' The Lion became even more furious, and looking into the well he saw another Lion looking up at him, and angry as well. The Lion insulted him, but there was silence. He abused him, slandering the honour of his parents, but still there was no answer. The Lion became mad, and sprang on the other Lion in the well – and was drowned. Then the Hare went back to the other animals and told them that he had killed the Lion, and that he had now assumed the title of King of Beasts.

In a story from Zambia the Hare was out with the Lion one day. He laid himself down on an ant-hill, and asked the Lion to set light to all the grass around it. While the Lion was doing this the Hare slipped down a burrow underneath the ant-hill and was saved from the flames. When they had died down he came out, rolled in the black ash, and went to find the Lion. 'See, I am not hurt; look at this ash,' he said. The Lion was astonished and asked if he could have some of the Hare's magical medicine. So the Hare gave him some leaves, looked round for another ant-hill with plenty of grass on it, and told the Lion to lie down there. Then he set fire to the grass all round. When the fire got near him the Lion cried out in alarm, but the Hare told him not to cry – that would spoil the power of the medicine. Then the fire reached the Lion, it singed his hair, burnt his body, set fire to him all over, and he died. So the Hare ran off and

told the other animals that he was now their king.

Other fables tell more of Hare's victories over lions, how he broke all the lion's teeth, ate his children, wore a lion's skin, killed many lions, and caused the chief Lion to be stung to death by bees. Another tale from Zambia says that one day the Hare found the Lions eating meat, and he asked if he could stay with them and simply pick the fleas out of their tails. Of course he was deceiving them as usual, and instead of picking out fleas he was digging holes underneath them. As the lazy animals lay stretched out, gorged with their meal, the Hare buried their tails in the holes and rammed them down with soil. Then he went home, fetched out a big drum, and began to beat it. The Lions thought that men were coming and jumped up suddenly to run away, breaking off their tails which were fixed in the holes. Then the Hare enjoyed the rest of the meat which they had left.

Hare and Tortoise

This story of the famous race is known in many versions in Africa; sometimes it is the Hare who races the Tortoise, sometimes the Elephant or some other animal. One day the Hare was boasting as usual, and the Tortoise said that he could jump farther than the Hare. The Hare laughed at the very idea, so the Tortoise challenged him to a trial and it was agreed for the next day. The Tortoise hurried off, found his wife, put her in the bushes near the spot that had been decided. When the Hare arrived early

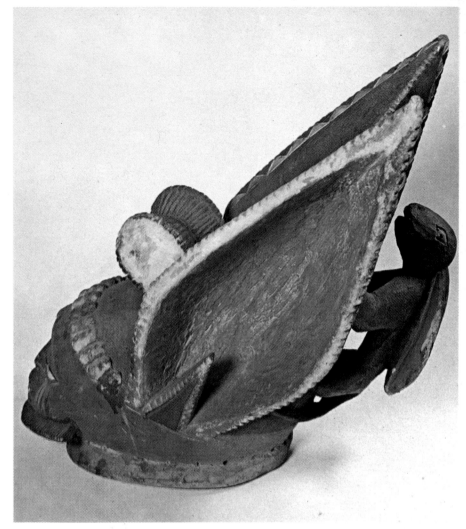

next day he found that the Tortoise was waiting for him. He asked the Hare to jump in a certain direction, and the lively beast took a great leap. Then the Tortoise called out that he was coming, slipped into the grass, and his wife appeared in the distance, far ahead of the Hare. The Hare was amazed and said he had not seen the jump, but the Tortoise said that was because his eyes had not been quick enough.

So the Hare acknowledged defeat, but challenged the Tortoise to a foot race which he knew he could win. The Tortoise agreed, but said he was too tired that day and it would have to be the next morning. Then he went home and collected all his family, and spent the night placing them along the road and telling them what to do. Next morning the Hare and the Tortoise started off together and the Hare was soon far ahead. He called back, 'Tortoise', and to his surprise heard a voice ahead saying, 'I am here.' The same happened all along the road, and, since it was circular, when the Hare arrived panting he found the original Tortoise calmly sitting waiting for him.

Other versions of a race between a slow and fast animal appear in the stories of the messengers of life and death (see pages 56–59), where the slow Chameleon, or another animal, arrives before the fast Dog, but with a less happy message. There are stories of the Tortoise and Baboon, Lizard and Leopard, with the slower always scoring off the faster. Other animals, birds, snakes and other reptiles figure in countless stories. But the cycles of fables about the Hare and the Spider are the most popular.

Anansi and the Corn Cob

In West Africa, where the Spider is called Anansi, the Annancy of America, he is the cleverest of animals and often appears in a mythology where he is the chief official of God though at first he has no name. One day Anansi asked God for one corn cob, a stick of maize grains, promising to bring him a hundred slaves in exchange for it. God laughed but gave him the cob. Anansi set off from heaven to earth and stopped at the first village, requesting a night's lodging from the chief. Before he went to bed he asked the chief where he could put the corn cob safely, explaining that it belonged to God and must not be lost. The chief showed him a hiding place in the roof, and they all went to sleep. But in the night Anansi got up and gave all the corn from the cob to the fowls. When he demanded his cob next morning it had gone, and

he made such a fuss that the chief gave him a whole basket of corn to pacify him.

Anansi continued his journey and after a time sat down by the roadside, since the basket was too heavy to carry far. Along came a man with a chicken in his hand and Anansi easily persuaded him to exchange it for all the corn. When he reached the next village the chief put him up, and Anansi asked where the fowl could be hidden, since it belonged to God and must be kept safe. The bird was put in a quiet fowl-house and everybody went to sleep. But Anansi got up, killed the fowl, and daubed its blood and feathers on the chief's door. At dawn he made a great cry, shouting that the bird was gone and he would lose his place as God's captain. Everybody started looking and Anansi suddenly pointed to the blood and feathers on the chief's door. The chief

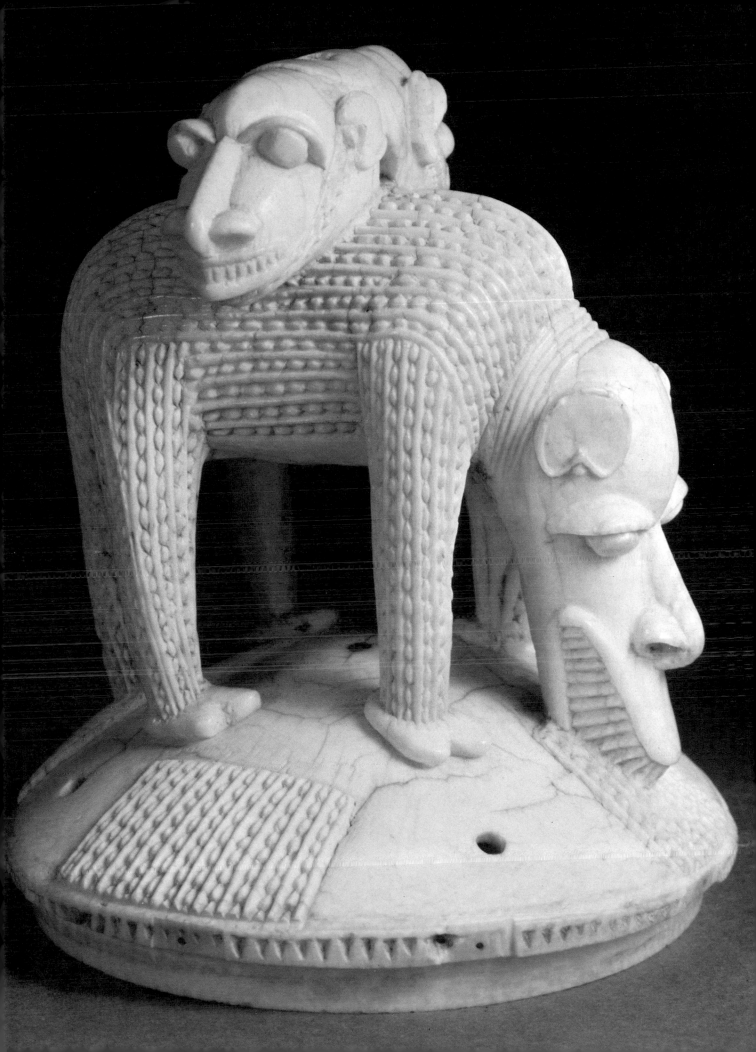

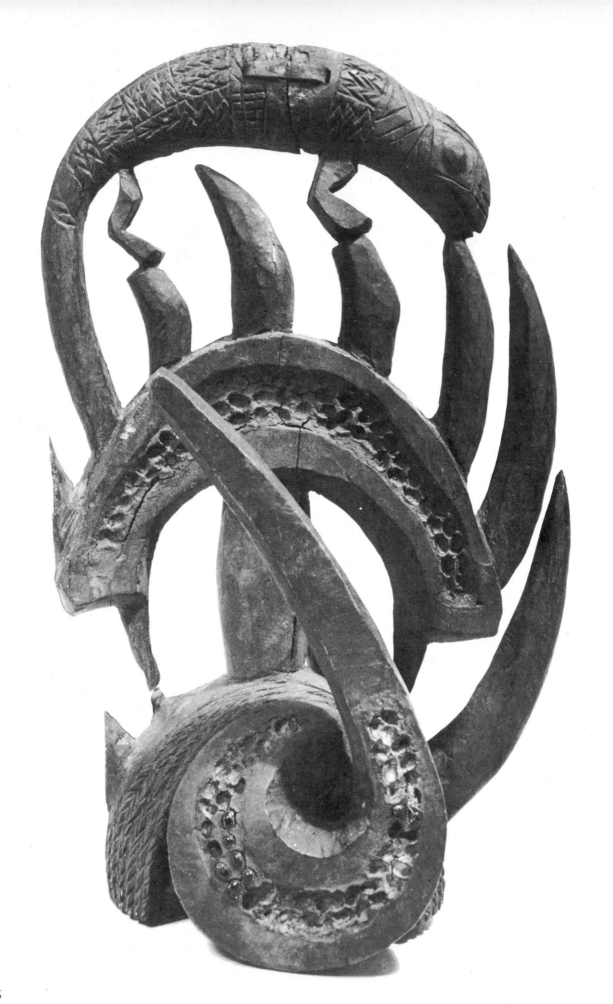

136

and all his people begged Anansi to forgive them, and gave him ten sheep to calm his anger.

Anansi went off and rested on the way to graze the sheep. Along came some people carrying a corpse, and when Anansi asked whose it was they replied that it was the body of a young man who had died far from home and they were taking him back to the family. Anansi said he was going that way, and offered to take the body if they would take his sheep. They were glad to agree and Anansi went on with the body to the next village. There he asked the chief for rest and explained that he had with him the favourite son of God, who was asleep and needed a hut to rest in. The chief prepared his best room for God's son, and after feasting and dancing they all went to bed.

In the morning Anansi asked some of the chief's children to wake God's son, saying that they might have to shake and even beat him, for he slept heavily. When they came and said they could not wake him, Anansi told them to flog him harder. Still the boy did not wake up, and at last Anansi uncovered the body and cried out that he was dead. He said that the sons of the chief had killed the favourite child of God with their rough beating. There was great wailing among the people, and they were terrified to think of the anger of God. The boy was buried that day, on Anansi's advice, and he said he would try to think of a plan to appease the divine anger. At night he called the chief and said he would have to report the matter back to God. But the chief must give him a hundred young men, to witness that they and not Anansi were responsible for the boy's death. The chief and people gladly agreed, and Anansi set off and finally arrived back in heaven with the youths. He told

God how from one corn cob he had gained a hundred fine young slaves, as he had promised.

God was so pleased that he confirmed him as chief of all his host, and gave him the special name of Anansi which he still bears.

How Anansi tricked God

Anansi, the spider, was very conceited and this was often his undoing. When he had been made captain of the divine hosts he began to boast that he was even more clever than God himself. God heard this and was angry. He sent for Anansi and asked him to bring him 'something'. He would not say what it was and Anansi puzzled all day without success to find out the mysterious object that was needed. In the evening God laughed at him, saying that he had boasted that he was as clever as himself, so he must prove it and find the 'something' without any further help.

Anansi left the sky to look for this 'something' on earth, and after a time he had an idea. He called all the birds to him and borrowed a feather from each of them. He made the feathers into a splendid cloak, flew back to heaven, and perched in a tree against God's house. When God came out he saw the brilliant bird and called all the people together to find out the name of the bird. Nobody could tell him, not even the Elephant who knows all the beasts of the forest. Somebody said that Anansi might know, but God explained that he had sent him away on an errand. All the people asked what the errand was and God said that Anansi had boasted that he was as wise as God so he had been sent to get 'something'. The people asked what the 'something' was and God told them that it was the Sun, Moon, and Darkness.

Anansi in the tree heard this, and when God and the people had gone he came down from the tree, threw away his fine feathers, and went off to look for the Sun, Moon and Darkness. It is said that the Python was the only one who knew where they were and he gave them to him. Anansi put them in a bag and went back to

God. God asked if he had brought 'something', and Anansi said, 'Yes', and brought Darkness out of his bag. Then he drew out the Moon, and people could see a little. Finally he took out the Sun, which was so brilliant that some of the people were blinded, and others could see only a little. So it was that blindness came into the world. But others had their eyes shut and the Sun did them no harm.

Anansi and the Chameleon

Anansi and the Chameleon lived in the same village. Anansi was rich, with plenty of children and a large farm, while the Chameleon was poor and alone, and had only a small field to cultivate. But one year the rain fell on the Chameleon's field and not at all on Anansi's farm. Anansi was envious and asked the Chameleon to sell him his field, and when he refused he threatened revenge. Chameleons walk with curious steps over grass and bushes and do not make roads like other people, so there was no path to the Chameleon's field. Anansi therefore got his children to make a wide roadway from his house to the Chameleon's field during the night. In the morning he went there and started pulling up the crops. The Chameleon came and protested and was told to go away – the field belonged to Anansi. The Chameleon made a complaint at the chief's court and Anansi was called to account for his action. When both animals claimed the field, the chief asked for proofs. Anansi demanded that they agree it was true that he always made a path while the Chameleon made none, and the latter agreed. The chief sent his servants to see if there was a path, and when they reported back he awarded the field to Anansi.

The Chameleon had to go home without field or food, and shut himself up in his house plotting revenge. He decided to dig a great hole, deeper than anyone had seen before, covering it with a roof and leaving just a small hole. Then he set to work to catch hundreds of large buzz flies, which he tied to dried vines and made into a large cloak. When the chief

137

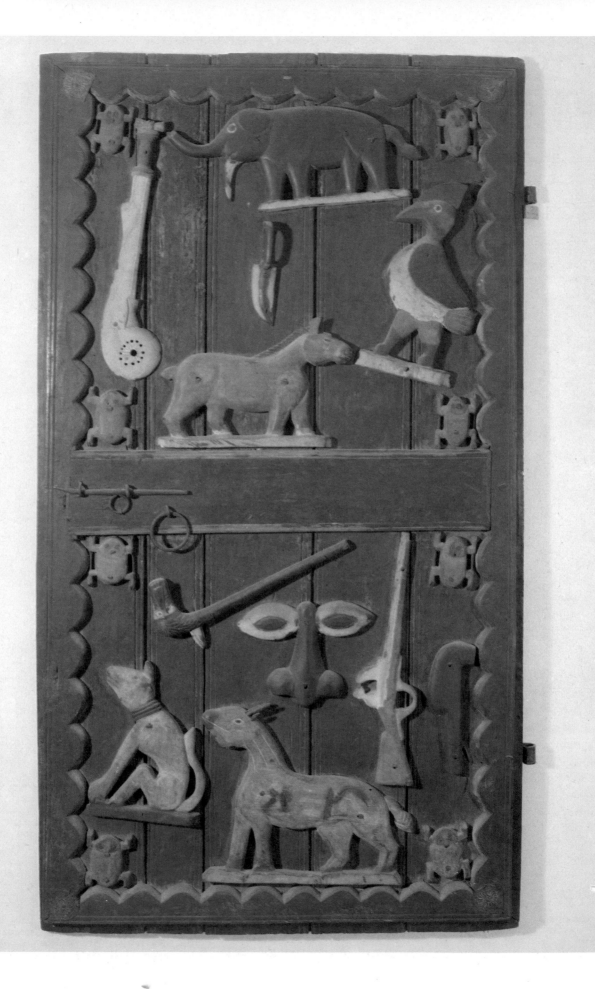

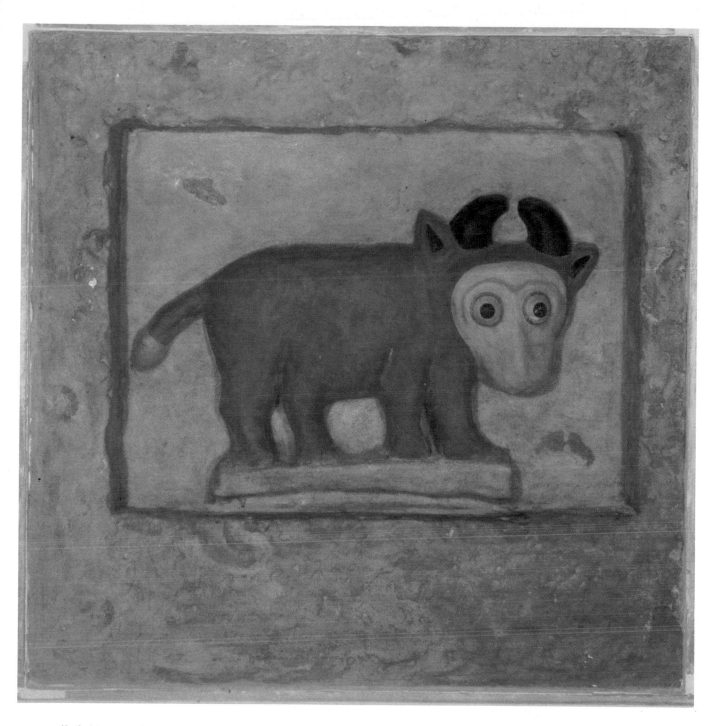

next called his people together the Chameleon went along, walking slowly and proudly in his strange brilliant costume, with the flies buzzing and shining in the sun. The chief himself wanted to buy the cloak but the Chameleon refused. But when Anansi heard of it he promised the chief he would buy it for him, since he was rich. He went to the Chameleon and asked the price. At first the Chameleon refused, but later he relented, saying he was so hungry that if Anansi would give him the food he

needed he could have the cloak. He did not want much food, just enough to fill the little hole of his store.

Anansi looked at the tiny opening and promised to send his children with enough food to fill it twice over. So Anansi's children came with loads of food next day and poured the grain into the hole, but the more they brought the less the hole was filled. For days and weeks they brought food, while the Chameleon stood by and reminded Anansi that he had promised to fill the hole twice over.

Above. There are two interpretations of this colourful clay relief from a wall of the old palace at Abomey. The first is that it is an allegory of King Ghezo as a buffalo, recalling his victorious war against the Mahi people at Dassa to the north. The other view is that the figure is a ram representing the thunder god, So, who 'roars his anger in the clouds'. Musée de l'Homme, Paris.

Opposite. Door from the former royal palace at Abomey, now a museum. The figures nailed to the wooden frame show different animals and weapons used in hunting. The frogs in the corners serve as decoration, like the snails on the door on page 71. Musée de l'Homme, Paris.

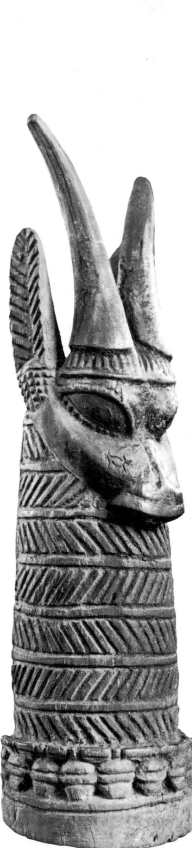

Anansi was vexed, and kept his children at work till his granaries were empty. Still the hole was not filled, and to keep his word Anansi sold his sheep and cows, and all he had to buy grain to fill the hole. At last the Chameleon declared he was not a hard man, and though the hole was still not full, he would let Anansi off the rest of the debt. He took the cloak out of a box and gave it to him. But during the long time that the cloak had been put away the vines had rotted, and when Anansi took the cloak outside the wind blew it about and all the flies flew away, leaving Anansi with a few withered vines and no crops or money. All the people laughed at him, and since that time Anansi hides in the corners of houses and no longer goes out proudly in the streets as before.

How Anansi became a Spider

Another fable explains why Anansi became so small. He was once a man, and there was a king who had a magnificent ram, larger than any other, and he forbade anybody to touch it, no matter what it did or ate, under pain of death. Anansi had a large farm and a fine crop of corn was growing there. But one day when Anansi went to look at his corn he was horrified to find that part of the field had been trampled down and the young corn shoots eaten. In the middle of the field, and still munching, was the king's ram. Anansi was so angry that he threw a stone at the ram and killed it. Then he was afraid, for he knew the king's orders.

As he stood under a tree wondering what to do a nut fell on his head, and he picked it up and ate it. Then another nut fell, and he had an idea, like Newton with the apple. He picked up the ram and climbed up with it into the tree, hanging it on one of the branches. Then he went to call on a friend, who was a large Spider. He showed him a nut and promised to show him where he could find others. They went back to the tree and Anansi told the Spider to shake it, and the dead ram fell down with the nuts. Anansi exclaimed that the Spider had killed the king's ram, and the Spider

asked what he should do. Anansi said the best thing was to confess his crime and hope that the king would be in a good mood.

The Spider picked up the dead ram and set off. But on the way he stopped to tell his wife what had happened, in case he did not see her again. Anansi stayed outside while the Spider went in to speak to his wife. She said her husband was stupid. Had he ever seen a ram climb trees? There must be some trick, and so the Spider must go on alone to the king, return without seeing him, but report to Anansi that all was well. The Spider did this, and when he came back he told Anansi that not only was the king not angry, but he had actually given him some of the meat of the ram to eat. Anansi cried that this was not fair. He himself had killed the ram and ought to have a share of its flesh. Then the Spider and his wife seized Anansi and took him to the king. Anansi fell to the ground and begged for mercy, but the king was furious and kicked him so hard that he broke into a thousand pieces. That is why Anansi is much smaller now, and is found in every corner of the house, like a creature broken into many pieces.

African Story

These animal fables are genuine African story, though many of them have travelled far away, to America and Europe. African mythology has not only exported but also imported tales from other parts of the world. Some of the very old stories, though they cannot be dated, may have entered the tropical regions of Africa with Negro migrants from the north thousands of years ago. Others came later, with the traders. Some clearly arrived from the Moslem world and there are versions of stories from the Arabian Nights, particularly down the coast of East Africa. A few stories can be traced across to India, to such great collections as the Hindu *Pancha-tantra* or the Buddhist *Jataka* tales. Other yarns came from Europe. Portuguese narratives are found particularly in Angola and Mozambique, and English and French influences are clear elsewhere. Grimm's fairy tales are told in many African schools today, so the ancient mythology of Europe enters the African world. In modern times fresh details appear in many stories, such as taking letters up to heaven where the older versions would simply say that messages were sent.

But there is still a great mass of African mythology untouched by any foreign influence, and it is to be hoped that as many myths as possible will be recorded, before they change too much. For they reveal African views of the world, of God and of human behaviour and hopes, that are still of great power in the lives of African people in the modern world.

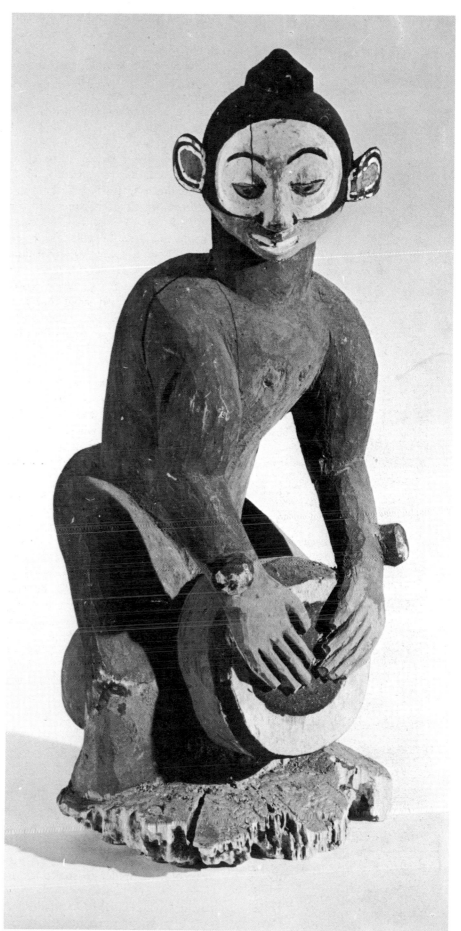

Right. Monkey carved in wood. The figure represents the drummer who traditionally beats the drum to announce the opening of the circumcision and initiation ceremony among the Nkanu of the Kwango area (Zaïre). It decorated, with other carved figures and painted wooden panels, the shelter where initiation took place. Koninklijk Museum voor Midden Afrika, Tervuren.

Opposite. Wooden ram's head from Benin, Nigeria. It is pierced at the back and fitted on a staff when in ritual use. The University Museum, Philadelphia, Pennsylvania.

Further Reading List

Arinze, F. A. *Sacrifice in Ibo Religion*. Ibadan University Press, 1970.

Arnott, K. *African Myths and Legends Retold*. Oxford University Press, 1962.

Cardinall, A. W. *Tales Told in Togoland*. Oxford University Press, 1931.

Davidson, B. *The African Past*. Penguin, London, 1954.

Evans-Pritchard, E. E. *Nuer Religion*. Oxford University Press, 1956.

Forde, D. (Ed.) *African Worlds*. Oxford University Press, 1964.

Griaule, M. *Conversations with Ogotemmêli*. Oxford University Press, 1956.

Herskovits, M. J. *Dahomey*. Augustin Company, New York, 1938.

Idowu, E. B. *Olodumare, God in Yoruba Belief*. Longmans, London, 1962.

Itayemi, P. & Gurrey, P. *Folk Tales and Fables*. Penguin African Series, London, 1953.

Kenyatta, Jomo. *Facing Mount Kenya*. Secker & Warburg, London, 1953.

Krige, E. J. & D. D. *The Realm of a Rain-Queen*. Oxford University Press, 1943.

Kuper, H. *An African Aristocracy: Rank among the Swazi*. Oxford University Press, 1947.

Lienhardt, G. *Divinity and Experience: The Religion of the Dinka*. Oxford University Press, 1961.

Little, L. L. *The Mende of Sierra Leone*. Routledge & Kegan Paul, London, 1951.

Parrinder, E. G. *West African Religion*. Epworth Press, London, 1949. *African Traditional Religions* S.P.C.K., London, 1974. *Witchcraft, European and African* Faber & Faber, London, 1963.

Rattray, R. S. *Ashanti*. Oxford University Press, 1923. *Religion and Art in Ashanti*. Oxford University Press, 1927.

Rouch, J. *La Religion et la Magie Songhay*. Presses Universitaires, Paris, 1960.

Schapera, I. *The Khoisan Peoples of South Africa*. Routledge & Kegan Paul, London, 1930.

Schebesta, P. *Les Pygmées du Congo Belge*. Duculot, Brussels, 1952.

Smith, E. W. and Dale, A. M. *The Ila-speaking Peoples of Northern Rhodesia* Macmillan & Company, London, 1920.

Smith, E. W. and Parrinder, E. G. (Eds). *African Ideas of God* (3rd edition). Edinburgh House Press, London, 1967.

Tempels, P. *Bantu Philosophy*. Présence Africaine, Paris, 1959.

Turner, V. W. *The Drums of Affliction*. Oxford University Press, 1968.

Verger, P. *Dieux d'Afrique*. Institut Français, Dakar, 1954.

Werner, A. *Myths and Legends of the Bantu*. Harrap, London, 1933.

Acknowledgments

Photographs. P. Almasy, Neuilly-sur-Seine 46, 75 right; Art Centrum, Prague 12 right; Art Institute of Chicago, Illinois 53 left, 61 bottom; Arts Council of Great Britain, London 18 left, 70 left, 79 left, 136; British Museum, London 8, 13 right, 14 top, 15, 25 bottom, 28 right, 45, 48, 55, 66, 85 bottom right, 86, 108 top left, 108 top right, 117, 119, 121, 123 left, 123 right, 124, 126 top, 126 bottom right; Brooklyn Museum, New York 21 bottom; Photographie Giraudon, Paris 30 right, 36, 43, 47 left, 51, 68, 91, 106, 131, 138, 139; Glasgow Museum and Art Gallery 100 left, 128 left; Hamlyn Group Picture Library 6, 9 centre, 10, 11, 14 bottom, 18 right, 20, 21 top, 22 left, 23, 24, 26 right, 27, 30 left, 34 right, 38, 42, 54 top, 61 top left, 62 bottom, 70 right, 72, 75 left, 85 left, 85 top right, 87, 88 left, 88 right, 89 left, 89 right, 101 bottom left, 102, 114, 125, 128 right, 134; André Held, Ecublens 64 centre, 93, 133; Michael Holford, Loughton 39, 90, 98, 103, 107, 110, 111 left, 111 right, 115, 127, 135; Holle Verlag, Baden-Baden 22 right, 31, 58, 63, 78; Koninklijk Museum Voor Midden-Afrika, Tervuren 69, 141; M. Lancaster 74; Mansell Collection, London 62 top; Musée de l'Homme, Paris 9 left, 12 left, 25 top left, 25 top right, 28 left, 32, 34 left, 35, 41, 47 left, 50, 57, 64 left, 65, 71, 83, 96, 100 right, 101 top, 101 bottom right, 109, 126 bottom left, 128 centre, 132; Museum für Volkerkunde, Berlin 70 centre; Museum für Volkerkunde, Vienna 130; Museum of Primitive Art, New York 16, 26 left, 53 right, 60, 64 right, 76; Nigerian Government 108 bottom; Geoffrey Parrinder 54 bottom; Pitt-Rivers Museum, Oxford 9 right, 116; Mrs Margaret Plass 99; Paul Popper, London 105 left, 105 right, 112, 118; Rijksmuseum voor Volkenkunde, Leiden 81; Sotheby Parke Bernet, London 13 centre, 61 top right, 97; United Africa Company, London 79 right, 80; University Museum, Philadelphia, Pennsylvania 13 left, 29, 44, 56, 122, 140; William Rockhill Nelson Gallery of Art, Kansas City, Missouri 104; ZEFA, Dusseldorf 92, 95.

Line drawings. International African Institute, London 27, 48, 49, 51.

Index